HOMŒOPATHIC

DOMESTIC MEDICINE.

BY

J. LAURIE, M.D.,

MEMBER OF THE ROYAL COLLEGE OF SURGEONS, EDINBURGH.
SENIOR PHYSICIAN TO THE WESTMINSTER AND LAMBETH HOMŒOPATHIC
MEDICAL INSTITUTION AND DISPENSARY.

ARRANGED AS A PRACTICAL WORK FOR STUDENTS.

CONTAINING
A GLOSSARY OF MEDICAL TERMS.

FIFTH AMERICAN EDITION, ENLARGED AND IMPROVED,

BY
A. GERALD HULL, M. D.

NEW-YORK:
WILLIAM RADDE, 322 BROADWAY.
PHILADELPHIA:—RADEMACHER & SHEEK, 239 ARCH-ST.
BOSTON:—OTIS CLAPP, 12 SCHOOL-ST.
ST. LOUIS:—FRANKSEN & WESSELHOEFT.
1850.

H. LUDWIG AND CO., PRINTERS, N.Y.

PREFACE TO THE AMERICAN EDITION.

The editor recommends laymen who make use of this book, to resort to lower dilutions in the treatment of acute attacks of disease in preference to those set down in the text.

For example: where *Aconite*, *Belladonna*, or *Chamomilla* of the 24th or 30th attenuation, are prescribed by Dr. Laurie, the editor would put one drop of the tincture of either of these remedies in a tumbler full of water and give a tablespoonful at a time; but in chronic maladies the editor earnestly recommends the doses set forth in the text.

The editor considers the tinctures, and the first, second and third, dilutions, when used in water, as nearly of the same medical power; perhaps, however, it is best to put two or three drops of these dilutions to the tumbler of water when they are applied in the place of the tinctures. When the triturations are contained in a medicine chest,—instead of the higher dilutions, which are preferred to them,—one grain of any of them can be dissolved in a tumbler of water, and used as above indicated.

In general, it may be best to repeat the doses of these solutions at the same intervals of time as are prescribed in the work; but the editor respectfully suggests, that in very severe cases of acute diseases, as in convulsions, or rapidly exhausting diarrhœa, or hemorrhage, it is proper to make the intervals much shorter than the author prescribes. It is quite probable that the water solutions can be repeated at shorter intervals, *cæteris paribus*, than the pellets or powders; and for this reason physicians often dissolve the pellets themselves in water, and repeat the spoonful doses twice or thrice as frequently as they would give them dry.

The editor's mode of using this work in acute diseases, then, is to put one drop of the tincture, or two drops of a first, second, or third dilution, into a tumbler of water, and to administer of this solution a tablespoonful to an adult, and a teaspoonful to a child as a dose. Or, again, when a trituration (a dry powder) is preferred, to stir one-third of an ordinary penknife blade full (about equal to one grain in weight) of it in a tumbler of water, and use the same doses.

And finally, when the pellets are good, and are preferred by the prescriber, the editor recommends that five or six of them be dissolved in a tumbler of water, and that they be repeated twice as frequently, as a general rule, as the dry pellets are ordered in the text.

The water should be very pure, and the glasses and spoons should be scrupulously cleansed before using them for medicines.

In all instances of additions made to this volume by the American editor (as, indeed, with all the foreign works edited by him), where he has not specified his own experience or given the authorities, he wishes to be understood to have compiled the same from the best practical results of the school at large, without formal signs of quotation.

A. G. H.

PREFACE TO THE THIRD EDITION.

From the favourable reception, and the rapidity of sale, of the last edition, the Author at first contemplated making little or no alteration in the contents of the present one, concluding that the aforenamed circumstances might be held as satisfactory indications that the work had been found sufficiently copious for domestic purposes. As, however, on the preceding occasion, he entered upon the experiment of bringing out the work in such a form, that it might prove of some slight service to the medical man commencing to make a practical inquiry into the *homœopathic* system, and having since had reason to determine that his hopes have not been disappointed, he has on that account been induced to change his original intention, and will feel amply rewarded for the additional labour which he has bestowed, should he thereby be the means of leading an increased number of his professional brethren to become converts to the all-important reformation in medicine effected by Hahnemann.

In compiling this, and the past editions, the Author has derived considerable aid from Jahr's 'Manual' (Nouveau Manuel de Médicine Homœopathique), and Hartmann's Acute and Chronic Diseases, as also from Constantine Hering's 'Hausarzt,' or Domestic Physician.

It being impossible to give minute and infallible directions for the treatment of all the various forms that diseases, even of daily occurrence, are so liable to assume, the author has added, at the termination of most of the chapters, a few of the medicines which the medical reader may, in many cases, either complicated or otherwise, find useful to refer to in the Materia Medica and Chronic Diseases of Hahnemann,—which every student who wishes to acquire a proper knowledge of Homœopathy ought to possess, and make a constant habit of carefully studying and consulting, if he wish to avoid falling into an indolent and unsafe method of practice.

J. L.

12 *Lower Berkeley Street*, *Portman Square*.

PREFACE TO THE SECOND EDITION.

In offering to the public a Second Edition of this work, of which an impression of upwards of one thousand copies has been sold in less than eighteen months, the Author feels that a few words of explanation are required.

On a comparison with the first edition, the reader will find a great number of serious and acute affections added, some others more deeply entered into, several alterations in the potencies prescribed, and more explicit directions given for the administration and repetition of the different remedies.

When the Author first committed this work to the press, it was simply intended to be, what its name implied, a Treatise on Domestic Medicine, by which individuals might be enabled to treat themselves or their families in slight affections, or even, in case of necessity, in more serious diseases, subject to the restriction mentioned in the preface to that edition. Since that time, however, the Homœopathic system has been daily attracting more attention from the medical world, and the want of a work which might serve for a practice of Physic for beginners, has been repeatedly a subject of complaint. In order *partially* to supply this want, the Author has materially added to the number of diseases treated, and prescribed the potencies found most useful in practice in the more severe forms of disease; he has also given the book a more medical character by the addition of the diagnosis of disease, causes, &c., and the employment of medical terms; but in order not to interfere with the utility of the work, a *glossary* has been added for the non-professional reader.

The non-medical public who confine themselves to their proper sphere, viz., the treatment of slight and ordinary ailments, will still find this Treatise useful as a Domestic Medicine; in such cases the globules at medium and high potencies are amply sufficient. It may be remarked, moreover, that the globules are much better adapted for *keeping* than the tinctures, and, with proper precautions, will retain their medicinal virtues for *many years*.

At the request of several friends, directions have been given for the administration and repetition of the medicines in each disease; some remarks, also, are made upon this important point, in the *Introduction*, to which, and the article upon the *Potencies of the medicine*, the attention of the reader is *particularly* requested.

PREFACE TO THE FIRST EDITION.

In presenting this little work to the public, the Author may be allowed to state, as briefly as possible, the motives that have led him to the undertaking.

Of these, the principal are, the present paucity* of homœopathic practitioners; the refutation, by a plain statement of the treatment of *acute disease*, of the too prevalent idea, that Homœopathy is available only in *Chronic* affections; and the hope that this work may, under proper restrictions, prove of service in cases of ordinary derangement, or where the advice of a homœopathic physician is unattainable; and by assisting in the selection of the proper remedy, save many from having recourse to allopathic modes of relief, such as aperients, &c., which are so calculated to undermine the strongest constitution, and convert trifling affections into permanent maladies.

From the first-mentioned motive, (the present want of homœopathic practitioners,) the Author has found himself compelled to include many acute diseases, which fall more particularly within the province of the physician; in so doing, he has given a range of treatment that will meet a great variety of cases, and in almost all so far obviate immediate danger, and place the malady in such a position, as to give time, when imperatively necessary, for seeking suitable advice.

In cases that require prompt and decided measures, such as "Convulsions," "Croup," &c., the treatment has been pretty fully

* I have sincere gratification in remarking, that even since the first publication of this work, this want has been, to some extent, diminished, by the great number of medical converts who are daily joining our ranks, and whose extensive practice, wherever they have settled, holds out most cheering prospects for the future. Still, in many of the great towns and densely-populated districts of this empire, as well as in our possessions abroad, a homœopathic practitioner would be eagerly welcomed. Much has been, but more remains to be done.—Author.

gone into. In others, such as "Inflammation of the Brain and Lungs," the course to be pursued to ward off all *immediate* danger, has been briefly, but it is to be hoped, clearly pointed out. Other acute or dangerous maladies, such as "Puerperal Fever," "Phlegmasia Alba Dolens," (puerperal tumid leg,) "Epilepsy," "Cancer," &c., have been slightly glanced at, or wholly omitted; convinced, that to do justice to their several treatments, would carry the work far beyond its intended limits and purpose, and that an imperfect sketch would be rather productive of injury than benefit.

In many instances Domestic Medicines do considerably more harm than good, by inducing individuals to rely too fully upon their own resources, and to omit having recourse to those who have made the diseases of mankind their peculiar study; but still greater injury results *from an ill-regulated perusal of elaborately written medical works, which require the previous education of the physician fully to comprehend, and his practical experience properly to apply.*

To the Student, still at the threshold of our science—to the Allopathist, willing by *fair experiment* to put the system to the test—it is hoped that this little work may prove peculiarly valuable.

It may be here remarked, that the beautiful simplicity and harmonious uniformity of the homœopathic system, conjoined with its invariable rule of administering only one medicinal substance at a time, have misled many into the idea, that it is so much easier of practice than the old system, as scarcely to require the qualification of a medical education; acting upon these false premises, many amateurs, after having studied a few of the leading medicines, although wholly destitute of other physiological or pathological knowledge, imagine themselves qualified to prescribe for every variety of ailments, and their presumption is generally in exact ratio with their ignorance. No doubt, from the inherent excellence of the system, some of these zealous individuals have cured diseases that have defied allopathic mode: but generally, from the absence of a medical education, and of a perfect knowledge of the *Materia Medica*, by a circuitous route; whereas the practised mind of the physician, frequently detecting the exact *nature of the disease*, and at all times carefully discriminating the primary from the purely sympathetic, or secondary symptoms, is thereby enabled to make a more ready selection of a *specific* remedy, and save the patient from a course of needless suffering.

If such be the case in Chronic, how much more so in severe

and complicated Acute diseases ; such, it is evident, no individual, not fully competent, should take upon himself the serious responsibility of treating, unless coerced by an imperious necessity, and then with the *closest attention to, and most minute observance of, the symptoms.*

Under such conditions, the Author hopes that this work may prove useful ; and when the symptoms are *perfectly* in accordance with those given under the different medicines, the administration of the latter will be always marked with decided benefit.

In conclusion, it may be observed, that from the unfair impressions of the science, that have been so industriously propagated, Homœopathy has been too frequently treated as a species of charlatanism, to which people resort only when every other mode of promised relief has utterly failed. After enduring with patience a long and ineffectual treatment under the old system, they feel disappointed if Homœopathy does not work an *immediate* cure ; nay, in acute diseases, when danger appears to threaten, some individuals fall back upon allopathic measures, and undo all that the Homœopathist has effected : perhaps again seeking his assistance when the mischief has been rendered irremediable by their own fatuity. Others, who have seen members of their families (whose diseases were beyond the power of medicine) die during homœopathic treatment, reproach the science with failure ; whereas their minds would have felt perfectly satisfied, had such a misfortune occurred under the old system ; forgetting that, in many instances, the patient only sought Homœopathy as a last resource, in cases where the affection was of its own nature incurable, or had been rendered so by a long course of improper treatment.

What Homœopathy stands upon, is the simple fact of success in thousands of cases, in which every other mode has signally failed—upon the firm and irrefragable basis of a multitude of unimpeachable and incontrovertible proofs.

CONTENTS.

PART I.

INTRODUCTION.

PAGE

Regimen 1
Clothing and Habits 4
Potencies of the Medicaments 5
Administration and repetition of the Medicines . . . 9
Pharmaceutical Signs 12
Synopsis of the Rules for Diet 14, 20

PART II.

ON THE SYMPTOMS, CHARACTER, DISTINCTION, AND TREATMENT, OF DISEASES.

FEVERS.

General consideration of Fever, &c. 17
Causes 19
General Treatment and Diet 20
Simple or Ephemeral Fever, *Febris simplex* 20
Inflammatory Fever. *Synocha* 22
Nervous Fever. *Febris nervosa*. Typhus 24
Congestive Fever 26
Putrid Fever, or Typhus. *Typhus putridis* 36
Contagious Fever, or Typhus. *Typhus contagiosus* . . . 37
Accessory Treatment (*during typhus*). Prophylaxes, &c. . . 38
Intermittent Fevers. Ague. *Febres intermittentes* . . . 39

ERUPTIVE FEVERS.

Scarlet Fever. *Scarlatina* 48
Purpura rubra 55
Scarlatina Miliaris . . . . . . ib.
Scarlet Rash . . . . ib.
Measles. *Rubeola* 59
Smallpox. *Variola* 63
Chicken-pox. *Variola spuria, Varicella* 71
Miliary Fever. *Miliaria* 72
Nettlerash. *Urticaria* 75

DISEASES OF ORGANS CONNECTED WITH THE DIGESTIVE SYSTEM.

Toothache 77
Sore Throat, or Quinsy. *Angina* 81

Ulcerated Sore Throat. *Angina maligna* 89
Mumps. *Parotitis. Angina parotidea* 93
Bilious Complaints 95
Indigestion. *Dyspepsia* . . . . . . ib.
Want of Appetite. *Apepsia. Anorexia* 101
Derangement of the Stomach, Eructations, &c. . . . 107
Flatulence 110
Spasms of the stomach. *Gastrodynia, Cardialgia* . . . 112
Heartburn. *Pyrosis* 119
Vomiting of Blood. *Hematemesis* 119
Constipation. *Obstructio Alvi* 123
Piles. *Hemorrhoids* 128
Protrusion of the intestine. *Prolapsus Ani* 132
Colic. *Enteralgia* 133
Looseness of the Bowels. *Diarrhœa* 137
Dysentery. *Dysenteria* 141
Suppressed Dysentery 148
Cholera 149
——— Asiatic 152
Cholerine 155
Liver Complaint . . . . ib.
Acute Inflammation of the Liver. *Hepatitis* 156
Liver Complaint. *Hepatitis chronica* 160
Jaundice. *Icterus* 161
Inflammation of the Spleen. *Splenitis* 162
Inflammation of the Stomach. *Gastritis* 165
Chronic ditto. *Gastritis Chronica* 168
Inflammation of the Bowels. *Enteritis* 168
Inflammation of the Peritoneum. *Peritonitis* 175
Inflammation of the Kidneys. *Nephritis* 177
Inflammation of the Bladder. *Cystitis* 180
Worms. *Helminthiasis* 181

DISEASES OF ORGANS CONNECTED WITH THE RESPIRATORY SYSTEM.

Catarrh, or Common Cold 187
Hoarseness. *Raucitas* 191
Chronic Laryngitis. *Laryngitis chronica* 193
Cold in the Head . . . . ib.
Cough 196
Hooping-cough. *Tussis convulsiva* 204
Croup. *Angina membranacea* 210
Influenza 219
Determination of Blood to the Chest. *Congestio ad Pectus* . . 221
Inflammation of the Mucous Membrane of the Bronchial Tubes.
——— *Bronchitis* 225
——— *Bronchitis Chronica* 232
Inflammation of the Lungs. *Pneumonia, Peripneumonia, Pneumonitis* 234

Pneumonia Notha Occulta 239
Typhoid, or Congestive Pneumonia 240
Consumption, or Incipient Phthisis 241
Inflammation of the Pleura. *Pleurisy, Pleuritis* . . . 242
Pleurodynia. *Pseudo-Pleuritis* 251
Spitting of blood. *Hæmoptysis* 252

DERANGEMENTS OF THE CEREBRAL SYSTEM.

Determination of the Blood to the Head. *Congestio ad Caput* . 260
Apoplexy. *Apoplexia* 266
Inflammation of the Brain and its Tissues. Brain Fever. *Phrenitis Encephalitis* 271
Tetanus 276

CUTANEOUS DISEASES.

St. Anthony's Fire. Rose. *Erysipelas* . . . 280
Boil. *Furunculus* 283
Carbuncle. *Anthrax. Furunculus malignans. Pustula nigra* . 285
Chilblains. *Perniones* . . . . . . ib.
Corns. *Clavi pedis* 287
Abscess. 288
Itch. *Scabies* 291
Whitlow. *Panaris. Paronychia* 293
Irritation of the Skin 294
Ringworm. *Herpes circinnatus* 296
Ringworm of the Scalp 297
Ulcers 301

GENERAL DERANGEMENT OF THE SYSTEM.

Gout. *Arthritis* 307
Rheumatism. *Rheumatismus* 310
Lumbago 314
Inflammation of the Psoas Muscle. *Psoitis* . . . 315
Sciatica 316
Pain in the Hip. *Coxalgia, coxagra* 318
Hip-disease. *Morbus coxarius* 320
Determination of Blood to the Abdomen. *Congestio viscerum abdominis, congestio ad abdomen* 323
Acute Inflammation of the Eyes. *Ophthalmitis* . . 324
Short Sight. *Myopia.* 331
Swelling of the Lip . . . . . . ib.
Scirrhus . . . . ib.
Warts on the Face 332
Hordeolum, Stye . . . . ib.
Inflammation of the Ears, and Ear-ache. *Otitis, otalgia* . . 333
Bleeding of the Nose. *Epistaxes* 337
Swelling of the Nose 340
Canker of the Mouth. *Cancrum oris* 343
Scurvy. *Scorbutus* 345

Inflammation of the Tongue. *Glossitis* . . . 346
Offensive Breath 348
Face-ache. *Neuralgia facialis* 349
Palpitation of the Heart 351
Cramp in the Legs 352
Goitre . . . . ib.
Sweating Feet 353
Sleeplessness. *Agrypnia* 354
Nightmare. *Incubus* 357
Acute Inflammation of the Spinal Cord and its Membranes. *Myelitis*. 358
Palsy. *Paralysis* 361
Rupture. *Hernia* . . . . ib.
Fainting. Swooning. *Syncope* 367
Headache. *Cephalalgia* 370
Pains in the Loins. *Notalgia* 391
Delirium Tremens Potatorum . . . . ib.
Epilepsy. *Epilepsia* 394
Asthma 395

CASUALTIES.

Concussion, Bruises, Sprains, and Wounds, &c., . . . 403
Burns and Scalds 417
Fatigue 419
Stings of Insects 420
Sea-sickness 420
Apparent Death. *Asphyxia* 422
Hydrophobia 426
Poisons 434
Mental Emotions 438

PART III.

TREATMENT OF INFANTS AND CHILDREN, AND OF THEIR PECULIAR AFFECTIONS.

Introductory remarks 441
Treatment after Birth 442
Asphyxia 443
Swelling of the Head 444
Navel Rupture in Infants . . . . . ib.
Meconium, Expulsion of 445
Suckling of the Infant 446
Choice of a Nurse 448
Diet during Nursing . . . . . ib.
Supplementary Diet of Infants 449
Duration of Suckling and Weaning 451
Sleep. Sleeplessness 452
Exercise 455

DISEASES OF INFANCY.

Inflammation of the Eyes in New-born Infants . . . 458
Hiccough 458
Cold in the Head 459
Crying and Wakefulness 460
Regurgitation of Milk 462
Spasmodic Asthma 463
Milk Crust 464
Thrush, or Aphthæ 466
Constipation. *Obstructio alvi neonatorum* . . . 467
Bowel Complaints *Diarrhœa neonatorum* . . . 468
Excoriation *Excoriationes neonatorum* . . . 474
Jaundice. *Icterus neonatorum* . . . 474
Induration of the Cellular Tissue. *Erysipelas neonatorum* . . 475
Lockjaw of Infants *Trismus nascentium* . . . 476
Derangement during Teething 478
Convulsions in Children 480
Water in the Head. *Hydrocephalus* . . . 484
Asthma of Millar 486
The Rickets *Rachitis* 488
Infantile Remittent Fever . . . . . ib.
Atrophy. *Atrophia.* 493
VACCINATION 494

PART IV.

TREATMENT OF FEMALES AND THEIR PECULIAR AFFECTIONS.

Chlorosis. *Emansio mensium* 495
Amenorrhœa. *Suppressio mensium* 498
Menorrhagia 499
Dysmenorrhœa 501
Hysterics. *Hysteria* 501

OBSERVATIONS ON PREGNANCY.

Introductory remarks 503
Air and Exercise 505
Clothing 506
Diet 508
Employment of the Mind and Habits . . . . ib.
Influence of External Objects upon the unborn Infant . . 509
Mental Emotions . . . . . . ib.

DERANGEMENTS DURING PREGNANCY.

Menstruation 511
Morning Sickness 512
Constipation 513
Diarrhœa . . . . . . ib.
Fainting and Hysteric Fits 514

Toothache 515
Swelled Face 516
Swelled Veins. *Varices* 517
Pains in the Back 518
Miscarriage. *Abortus* . . . . . ib.

TREATMENT BEFORE PARTURITION.

Preparation of the Breasts 524
Remedies before Labour 525
False Pains 526
Parturition 528
Tedious or complicated Labours 528
Spasmodic Pains, Cramps, and Convulsions 531

TREATMENT AFTER DELIVERY.

Introductory remarks 532
After-pains 534
Duration of Confinement 535

DISEASES FOLLOWING PARTURITION.

Suppressed Secretion of Milk 536
Excessive Secretion of Milk 537
Perspiration after Delivery 537
Milk Fever 538
Irregularities of the Lochial Discharge 540
Diarrhœa in Lying-in Women 541
Abdominal Deformity 542
Falling off of the Hair 543
Leucorrhœa after Parturition . . . . . ib.
Internal Uterine Swelling and Prolapsus 543
Weakness after Delivery 544

OBSTACLES TO SUCKLING.

Disinclination of the Infant 545
Excoriation of the Nipples 546
Inflammation of the Breast 547
Mental Emotions affecting the Milk 548
Deficiency in the Secretion of Milk 548
Deterioration and Discoloration of Milk . . ; . 549
MOTHERS NOT SUCKLING THEIR CHILDREN . . . ib.
GLOSSARY 550
Index . . : 562

N. B.—$\frac{000}{3}$ or $\frac{00}{30}$, indicates : *three* globules of the *third*, or *two* globules of the thirtieth dilution.

TABULAR INDEX

OF THE

MEDICINES, THEIR ABBREVIATIONS, SYNONYMES, AND ANTIDOTES.

AC-HYDR.—ACIDUM HYDROCYANICUM. Prussic acid. (*Ammon. carb. Camph. Ipecac. Coff Opium.*)

AC-M.—Acidum Muriaticum. Muriatis Acidum, s. Hydrochloricum. Muriatic acid. (*Camph. Bryonia.*)

ACON.—ACONITUM NAPELLUS. Aconite. Monk's Hood. (*Camph. Nux vom. Wine, Vinegar, Paris*)

AC-SULPH.—ACITUM SULPHURICUM, s Sulphuris Acidum vitrioli. Sulphuric acid Vitriolic acid Oil of Vitriol (*Pulsatilla.*)

ALUM—ALUMINA. Argilla Pura. Aluminum oxydatum. Alumine (*Bryonia. Camph. Chamom Ipecac*)

AM-C.—AMMONIUM CARBONICUM. Carbonas (sub) ammonii. Sal volatile Carbonate of Ammonia. (*Arnica Camph. Hepar sulph.*)

AM-CAUST.—Ammonium Causticum. Caustic Ammonia. (*Dilute Vinegar.*)

AM-M—AMMONIUM MURIATICUM. Murias, s Hydrochloras Ammonii, Sal Ammoniacum. Muriate of Ammonia. Hydrochlorate of Ammonia, Sal Ammoniac. (*Camph Hepar sulph.*)

ANT-C.—ANTIMONIUM CRUDUM. Stibium Sulfuretum Nigrum. Antimonii Sulfuretum. Crude Antimony. Sulphuret of Antimony. (*Hepar sulph. Mercur.*)

ARN.—ARNICA MONTANA. Arnica. Leopard's Bane. (*Camph. Ignatia. Ipecac.*)

ARS.—ARSENICUM ALBUM. Acidum Arseniosum. Sesquioxide Arsenic— White Arsenic. (*China. Ferrum met. Graph. Hepar. Ipecac. Kali carb. Nux vom. Samb. Verat.*)

AUR.—AURUM FOLIATUM. Leaf Gold. (*Bellad. China. Cuprum met. Mercur.*)

BAR-C.—BARYTA CARBONICA. Carbonas (sub) Barytæ. Carbonate of Baryta. (*Camph*)

BELL.—BELLADONNA. Atropa Belladonna. Deadly Nightshade. (*Coffea. Hyosc. Hepar. Pulsat.*)

BOV.—BOVISTA. Lycoperdon Bovista. Puff-ball. (*Camph.*)

BROM.—BROMINIUM. Bromine. (*Coffea. Opium. Camph.*)

BRY.—BRYONIA ALBA. White Bryony. (*Acon. Chamom. Ignat. Nux-vom.*)

CALC-C—CALCAREA CARBONICA. Calcis Carbonas, Carbonate of Lime. (*Camph. Nitr. ac. Nitr. spir. Sulph.*)

CAN.—CANNABIS SATIVA. Hemp. (*Camph.*)

CANTH.—CANTHARIS. Cantharis Vesicatoria, Meloe Vesicatorius. Cantharides. Lytta Vesicatoria, Spanish Blistering Fly. (*Camph.*)

CAP.—CAPSICUM ANNUUM. Cayenne, Capsicum, or Guinea Pepper. (*Camph.*

CARB-A.—CARBO ANIMALIS. Animal Charcoal. (*Camph.*)

CARB-V.—CARBO VEGETABILIS. Carbo Ligni. Wood Charcoal. (*Arsen. Camph. Coffea. Lach.*)

CAUST.—CAUSTICUM. (Tinctura acris sine kali.) Caustic. (*Coffea. Colocyn. Nitr spir. Nux vom.*)

CHAM.—CHAMOMILLA. Matricaria Chamomilla. Wild Chamomile. (*Acon. Coccul. Coffea. Ignat. Nux vom. Pulsat.*)

CHINA. Cinchona Officinalis. Chinæ Cortex. Quinquina. Yellow Bark. (*Arnica. Arsen. Bellad. Calcar. Carb. veg. Ipecac. Sulph.*)

CIC.—CICUTA VIROSA. Water Hemlock. (*Arnica. Tabacum.*)

CINA. Artemisia Santonica. Worm Seed. (*Ipecac.*)

COCC.—COCCULUS. Menispermum Cocculus. Cocculus Indicus, Cocculus Tuberosus. Indian Berries. (*Camph. Nux vom.*)

COFF.—COFFEA CRUDA. Coffea Arabica. Mocha Coffee Berries. (*Acon. Cham. Nux vom.*)

COLCH.—COLCHICUM. Colchicum Autumnale. Meadow Saffron. (*Nux vom. Coccul. Pulsat.*)

COLOC.—COLOCYNTHIS. Cucumis Colocynthis. Bitter Cucumber, Colocynth. (*Camph. Caust. Coffea. Chamom.*)

CON.—CONIUM. Conium Maculatum. Hemlock. (*Coffea. Nitr. spir.*)

CROC.—CROCUS. Crocus Sativus. Saffron. (*Opium.*)

CUPR.—CUPRUM METALLICUM. Copper. (*Bellad. China. Ipecac. Mercur. Nux vom.*)

CUPR-A.—CUPRUM ACETICUM. Acetas Cupri. Acetate of Copper. (*Bellad. Calc. carb. China. Coccul. Ipecac. Mercur. Nux vom.*)

DIG.—DIGITALIS. Digitalis Purpurea. Common Foxglove. (*Nux vom. Opium.*)

DROS.—DROSERA. Drosera Rotundifolia. Round-leaved Sun Dew. (*Camph.*)

DULC.—DULCAMARA. Solanum Dulcamara. Bitter Sweet, Woody Nightshade. (*Camph. Ipecac. Mercur.*)

EUPHR.—EUPHRASIA. Euphrasia Officinalis. Eye-bright. (*Pulsatilla.*)

FERR.—FERRUM. Ferrum Metallicum. Pure Iron. (*Arnica. Arsen. Bellad. Ipecac. Mercur. Pulsat.*)

FER-AC.—FERRUM ACETICUM. Ferri Acetas. Acetate of Iron. (*Arsen. Bellad. Mercur. Nux vom.*)

GRAPH.—GRAPHITES. Plumbago. Pure Black Lead. (*Arsen. Nux vom. Vinum.*)

HELL.—HELLEBORUS NIGER. Black Hellebore, Christmas Rose. (*Camph. China.*)

HEP-S.—HEPAR SULPHURIS. Hepar Sulphuretum. Sulfuretum Calcis. Liver of Sulphur, Sulfuret of Lime. (*Acetum. Bellad.*)

HYOS.—HYOSCYAMUS. Hyosciamus Niger. Henbane. (*Bellad. Camph. China.*)

HYPER.—HYPERICUM PERFOLIATUM. (*Mesmerism.*)

IGN.—IGNATIA AMARA. Strychnos Ignatia. Faba Ignatia. St. Ignatius' Bean. (*Pulsat. Chamom. Coccul. Arnica. Camph. Vinegar.*)

IOD.—IODIUM. Iodine. (*Arsen. Camph. Coffea. Phosphor. Sulph.*)

IPEC.—IPECACUANHA. Cephaelis Ipecacuanha, Ipecacuanha Root. (*Arnica. Arsen. China.*)

JAL.—JALAPPA. Convolvulus s. Ipomœa Jalappa, Ipomœa Macrorrhiza. Jalap. (*Camph.*)

KALI-B.—KALI BICHROMATUM. Bichromate of Potash.

LACH.—LACHESIS. Trigoncephalus Lachesis. Lance-Headed Serpent, (poison of the). (*Alum. Arsen. Bellad. Nux vom. Rhus tox.*)

LED.—LEDUM PALUSTRE. Rosmarinus Sylvestris. Wild Rosemary, Marsh Tea. (*Camph.*)

LYC.—LYCOPODIUM. Lycopodium Clavatum. Lycopodii Pollen. Club Moss. Wolf's Claw. (*Camph. Pulsat.*)

MAGN.—MAGNESIA CARBONICA. Carbonas (sub) Magnesiæ. Carbonate of Magnesia. (*Camph.*)

MERC.—MERCURIUS SOLUBILIS. Mercurius Hahnemanni. Black Oxide of Mercury. (*Arnica. Bellad. Camph. Hep. sulph. Iod. Laches. Sulph.*)

MERC-V.—MERCURIUS VIVUS. Hydrargyrum. Quicksilver. (Vide *Mercurius Solubilis.*)

MEZ.—MEZEREUM. Daphne Mezereum. Mezereon. (*Camph. Mercur.*)

MOSCH.—MOSCHUS. Moschus Moschiferus. Musk. (*Camph. Nux mosch.*)

NATR-C.—NATRUM CARBONICUM. Carbonas (sub) Sodae. Carbonate of Soda. (*Arsen. Camph.*)

NATR-M.—NATRUM MURIATICUM. Murias Sodæ. Hydrochlorate of Soda. (*Arsen. Camph. Nitr. spir.*)

NIT-AC.—NITRI ACIDUM. Acidum Nitricum. Nitric acid. (*Calc. Carb. Conium. Camph. Hep. sulph. Sulph.*)

NUX-V.—NUX VOMICA. Strychnos Nux Vomica. Nux Vomica. (*Acon. Camph. Coffea. Pulsat.*)

OP.—OPIUM. Papaver Somniferum. Opium. White Poppy. (*Camph. Calc. carb. Hep. sulph. Mezer. Sulph.*)

PETR.—PETROLEUM. Rock Oil. (*Acon. Nux vom.*)

PLUMB.—PLUMBUM METALLICUM. Lead. (*Alum. Bellad. Hyosc. Opium.*)

PHOSPH.—PHOSPHORUS. Phosphorus. (*Camph. Coffea. Nux vom.*)

PHOSPH-A.—PHOSPHORI ACIDUM. Acidum Phosphoricum. Phosphoric Acid. (*Camph. Coffea.*)

PLAT.—PLATINA. Platinum. (*Pulsat.*)

PULS.—PULSATILLA. Anemone Pratensis. Meadow Anemone. Pasque Flower. (*Cham. Coffea. Ignat. Nux vom.*)

RHAB.—RHABARBARUM. Rheum. Rhubarb. (*Camph. Cham. Nux vom.*)

RHUS-T.—RHUS TOXICODENDRON. Sumach. Poison Oak. (*Bellad. Bryon. Camph. Coffea. Sulph.*)

SABAD.—SABADILLA. Veratrum Sabadilla. Caustic Barley. (*Camph. Pulsat.*)

SABIN.—SABINA. Juniperus Sabina. Savine. (*Camph.*)

SAMB.—SAMBUCUS. Sambucus Niger. Elder. (*Arsen. Camph.*)

SQUIL.—SQUILLA. Scilla Maritima. Squill. (*Camph.*)

SEC.—SECALE. Secale Cornutum. Ergot of Rye. (*Camph. Opium.*)

SENEG.—SENEGA. Seneka. Snake Root. (*Arnica. Bellad. Bryon. Camph.*)

SENN.—SENNA. Cassia Senna. Senna. (*Chamom.*)

SEP.—SEPIA. Sepia Succus. Inky juice of the Scuttle Fish. (*Acon. Nitr. spir. Vinegar.*)

SIL.—SILICEA. Silex. Siliceous Earth. (*Camph. Hepar. sulph.*)

SPIG.—SPIGELIA. Spigelia Anthelmintica. Indian Pink. (*Camph. Aurum.*)

SPONG.—SPONGIA. Spongia Usti. Spongia Marina Tosta. Burnt Sponge. (*Camph.*)

STANN.—STANNUM. Pure Tin. (*Coffea Pulsat.*)

STAPH.—STAPHYSAGRIA. Delphinium Staphysagria. Stavesacre. (*Ambra. Camph.*)

STRAM.—STRAMONIUM. Datura Stramonium. Thorn Apple. (*Bellad. Nux vom.*)

SULPH.—SULPHUR. (*Acon. Camph. Mercur. Nux vom. Pulsat.*)

SULPH-T.—SULPHURIS TINCTURA. Spiritus vini Sulphuratus. Tincture of Sulphur. (*Vide Sulphur.*)

THER.—THERIDION CURASSAVICUM. Black Spider of Curacoa. (*Camph.*)

TART-E.—TARTARUS EMETICUS s. Stibiatus, Antimonium Tartaricum. Tartras Potassii et Antimonii. Tartrate of Antimony and Potassa. Tartarized Antimony. Tartar Emetic. (*Coccul. Ipecac. Pulsat.*)

THUJ.—THUJA OCCIDENTALIS. Thuj., Arbor vitæ. Tree of Life. (*Camph. Pulsat.*)

VAL.—VALERIENE OFFICINALIS. Valerian. (*Bellad. Camph. Coffea. Mercur.*)

VER.—VERATRUM ALBUM. Helleborus Albus. White Hellebore. (*Acon. Arsen. ac. Camph. Coffea. China. Mercur.*)

VIO-T.—VIOLA TRICOLOR. Jacea. Pansea. Hearts'-ease. (*Camph.*)

VERB.—VERBASCUM THAPSUS. Mullein. (*Camph.*)

ZINC.—ZINCUM. Zincum Metallicum. Zinc. (*Camph. Hep. sulph. Ignat.*)

NOTE. In the SELECTION OF THE REMEDY, it is not necessary that *all* the symptoms noted should be present; at the same time, care must be taken, that there are no symptoms of any consequence not covered by the medicine, or more strongly indicative of another.

When symptoms are met with, *not* covered by a remedy, which nevertheless appears indicated, the TABULAR INDEX may, with advantage, be availed of, in order that it may be ascertained if the symptom required to complete the group, is given under the medicament in any other part of the work. In other cases, where different medicines are pointed out as useful in an affection, the table may be made use of, for, by carefully noting the symptoms given under them elsewhere, the reader may thereby be enabled to select the remedy most clearly indicated.

HOMŒOPATHIC

DOMESTIC MEDICINE.

PART I.

INTRODUCTION.

THE principal points we have to notice in this part are, the Regimen to be observed under treatment—Clothing, and Habits—the Administration and Repetition of the medicines—and the Potencies in general use.

REGIMEN.

The excellence of the homœopathic rules on regimen has wrested approbation even from our own opponents, although at the same time they disingenuously make use of it as a handle against the science itself, and ascribe the cures effected to its observance, rather than to the efficacy of the medicines employed.

To individuals unacquainted with Homœopathy, the regimen is represented as extremely rigid: to that assertion a plain statement of the course to be pursued in general cases will prove the best refutation; and it may also be observed, that at the first sight the self-denial imposed seems more stringent than it would prove on being carried into effect, and that many individuals in the Author's own experience have pursued the same system of diet, after they have had no furthur occasion for medical assistance, thus continuing from choice what they had begun from necessity.

The homœopathic regimen consists merely of the avoidance of medicinal and indigestible substances during treatment, both as calculated to interfere with the actions of the medicines and the proper functions of the alimentary system. Consequently, among liquids the articles generally proscribed are green tea or strong black tea, coffee, malt liquors, wine, spirits, and stimulants of every description; lemonade, or other acid or alkaline drinks, and natural or artificial mineral waters; cocoa, unspiced chocolate, toast, rice, or barley water, oatmeal gruel sweetened with a little sugar, or raspberry or strawberry syrup, if desired, whey, milk and water, or pure milk not too recent from the cow, boiled milk, and in some instances buttermilk, or in fact any non-medicinal beverage, is allowable.*

In animal food, pork, young meats—such as veal, lamb, &c.; and among poultry, ducks and geese—had better be avoided, particularly when derangement of the digestive function exists. Beef, mutton, venison, and most descriptions of game, if not too long kept (high), pigeons, larks, rabbits, are allowable at discretion. (Vide Synopsis.) Ham, and neats' tongues, under certain restrictions.

Fish is a wholesome article of diet, and may in most cases be partaken of without scruple, with the exception of the oleaginous species, such as eels, salmon, &c., or shell fish, as oysters, lobsters, &c.

Eggs, raw, or soft boiled; butter, if free from rancid or unusual taste; cream, plain unseasoned custards, and curds.

Stimulating soups and made dishes are so evidently opposed to homœopathic regimen, as scarcely to require further notice. Beef-tea, veal, or chicken broth, &c., thickened with rice, maccaroni, or sago, and seasoned merely with a little salt, are of course allowable.

* The idiosyncrasies in some individuals in respect of diet are very remarkable; as for example, some cannot take the smallest quantity of milk without serious inconvenience; others throw out a rash after partaking of fish; and, again, others loathe the very sight of animal food. These peculiarities should not only be attended to in prescribing a suitable course of regimen, but should also be taken into account in the selection of the remedies.

Among vegetables, all of a pungent, aromatic, medicinal, or indigestible description, or greened with copper, are prohibited; such as onions, garlic, eschalots, asparagus, radishes, horse-radish, celery, parsley, mint, sage, mushrooms, tomatoes, beets, artichokes, parsnips, etc.; but others free from such qualities, such as potatoes, French beans, green peas or beans, cauliflower, spinach, seakale, etc., may be used with the needful precaution of avoiding any particular article of diet, whether of the animal or vegetable kingdom, that may seem to disagree with the individual. Lemon or orange-peel, laurel leaves, bitter almonds, peach leaves or kernels, fennel, aniseed, marjoram, are objectionable; acids, and the ordinary condiments, such as pepper, mustard, pickles, etc., and salads, ought either to be sparingly partaken of, or entirely abstained from, particularly by the dyspeptic. Salt and sugar in moderation are admissible.

Acid or unripe fruits are clearly objectionable, and even ripe fruits possessing little or no acidity, if fresh, or prepared by cooking, such as peaches, raspberries, sweet cherries, grapes, and dried or preserved fruits, as figs, prunes, apples, pears. should be used in moderation, particularly by dyspeptic individuals; and by those subject to colic or diarrhœa, not at all. Cold fruits, such as melons, and raw vegetables, such as cucumbers, etc., are inhibited; nuts of every description are forbidden.

All kinds of light bread and biscuit, free from soda or potash and such like, not new-baked; also simple cakes composed of flour or meal, eggs, sugar, and a little good butter; or light puddings, such as bread, rice, sago, semalino, without wines, spices, or rich sauces, are admissible: but coloured confectionary, pastry, and also honey, are not so. Regularity in the hours of meals should be observed, and too long fasting, as well as too great a quantity of food at one time, should be avoided.

During fevers and inflammatory affections, the patient must of course be kept upon a low regimen: gruel, barley-water, etc.; and at the commencement of convalescence a light pudding, with a little weak beef-tea or mutton or chicken broth, should form the whole of the nourishment given. Nature, however, is our best guide; and when she takes away appetite, thereby intimates the necessity of not taxing the digestive functions.

CLOTHING AND HABITS.

Upon the first point it were scarcely worth while entering into any observations, were it not simply to remark upon the impropriety of wearing garments impervious to air, and fitting closely to the shape, and the custum of exposing the extremities and chests of young children to the chilling atmosphere of our peculiarly variable and humid climate, under the absurd idea of making them hardy. The evil consequences arising from the check given to perspiration, by the first mentioned practice, are too well known to require any particular comment; but as the other is an error widely prevalent, I consider it my duty to mention it; and feel assured, that if mothers will only reform their system, and clothe their children in a more rational manner, they will make no slight advance towards the prevention of serious affections, not only during childhood, but in after life. Linen, cotton, or even leather, worn next to the skin, is generally preferable to flannel.

As regards habits, it may be briefly observed, that a systematic course of life, avoiding ill-ventilated apartments, late hours, dissipation, over-study, anxiety, and other mental emotion, and taking sufficient air and exercise, are the best preservatives of health.

The frequent use of hot-baths is injurious, and liable to retard the cure uuder homœopathic treatment. The idea that sea-bathing is almost universally beneficial is exceedingly erroneous; there are many constitutions on whom it produces far other than a salutary effect. Medicated baths, either natural or artificial, are, it is scarcely necessary to observe, strictly forbidden. Bathing the whole frame daily with a sponge or wet towel, with cold or scarcely tepid water, and the use of the flesh-brush, are by no means objectionable, and frequently indeed strongly to be recommended.

The use of any medicinal or aromatic substances in the arrangement of the toilet, such as camphorated or otherwise medicated dentrifices, lip-salves, smelling salts, or cosmetics, is detrimental to the action of the medicines, and had therefore better be avoided.

The deleterious gas that flowers emit during night, renders their presence in bed-chambers highly reprehensible.

POTENCIES OF THE MEDICAMENTS.

In homœopathic practice there are three points which merit the most particular attention: the first and principal is the CHOICE of the PROPER REMEDY; the second the *potency* at which it should be exhibited, and the third its *administration* and *repetition*. I shall now proceed to the consideration of the second; the selection of the potency, attenuation, or dilution, and give such directions as may serve for a guide in general cases, premising at the same time that much depends upon the discrimination of the administrator, and that it is impossible in this case to give any rule to which there are not exceptions.

The principal points to be attended to are, the susceptibility of the patient to medicinal influence, how far modified by circumstances, the age, sex, temperament, and habits—the disease itself, and further, the nature of the medicament employed.

As regards the first, the susceptibility of the patient, we find four classes:

First class. Those who are comparatively insensible to medicinal influence, particularly at high potencies, upon whom the medicines show neither marked action nor re-action. Such individuals are generally of what is denominated the leuco-phlegmatic temperament; they require generally low potencies and frequent repetition—such cases are not without their parallel in allopathic practice. Also, in disease, we find some persons who appear to enjoy a peculiar exemption from infections and even contagious influence. To this rule, however, of giving the low potencies in such cases, there are exceptions : I have found in practice, after a careful study of the individual, and a selection of a remedy suitable to temperament, a marked action and re-action produced by a very high potency, where a lower of the same medicament had failed to elicit any apparent effect, and *vice versâ*.

Second class. A marked susceptibility to medicinal action without a corresponding reflex action : such patients are generally of a highly nervous temperament, exceedingly difficult to treat, and require particular study; here the higher potencies are generally called for, although we frequently find benefit in resorting to the lower.

Third class. Those in whom no marked or a scarcely perceptible medicinal action declares itself, but a well-marked re-action; in such cases we must be guided by other indications in the selection of the potency; watch the effect carefully, and avoid too frequent a repetition.

Fourth class. Those in whom the medicines show a well-marked action and re-action; here, also, we must be guided by other circumstances in the selection of the potency, so as to obtain the greatest possible benefit without materially increasing the sufferings of the patient.

We generally find a particular susceptibility to medicinal influence, at any potency, in persons dwelling in the country, of robust frame, simple habits, and regular lives, who are not subject to any peculiar dyscrasia. In towns, particularly in large, densely-populated cities, this susceptibility is greatly developed, but the re-action less evident; however much depending upon the individual's employment, habits, and pursuits, it is difficult to give any fixed rule.

AGE. In infancy and early childhood, we find a marked receptivity to medicinal influence, a decided action and speedy re-action, consequently the higher potencies are the most applicable in their diseases, and they rarely require so frequent a repetition; however, in acute diseases of any of the more noble organs, we may exhibit lower potencies, particularly of some of the less energetic medicines : for example, *Sambucus, Ferrum, Ipecacuanha, Chamomilla,* etc., a globule constituting the maximum dose. Some further remarks upon this subject have been made in Diseases of Infancy.

SEX. Females, for the most part, possess a higher degree of susceptibility than males, in which they approach nearer to children; for them the higher and medium potencies are generally most suitable; to this rule, however, there are many exceptions, particularly in those who are engaged in laborious employments.

TEMPERAMENTS. In the *Sanguine* temperament, there is considerable susceptibility to all the potencies, and a speedy re-action. In the *Nervous*, we find great susceptibility, sometimes without an equivalent re-action: here we should be cautious in administering, and generally use the higher potencies. In the *Bilious*, there is generally but little susceptibility, but the re-action, when roused, is powerful and prolonged; hence a necessity for low potencies, generally given at long intervals. The *Lymphatic* being the least susceptible of all temperaments, the medicines may be given at low potencies, and frequently repeated till some effect is produced.

Since these temperaments often occur in a mixed form, the rules above given must be modified accordingly.

I may observe that the remarks above made refer principally to chronic and subacute diseases.

THE DISEASE. In severe acute diseases I am generally in the habit of resorting to the low potencies, and in tinctures, from the circumstance that I have usually found them more certain in their effect in such affections. In the cases of children, an exception may be made, as already observed. In ordinary cases the best range is from the third to the twelfth potency; this rule should, of course, be modified according to the remedy itself, the disease, and the individuality of the patient.

THE NATURE OF THE REMEDY. Medicaments which in their crude state possess little or no appreciable medicinal property, but whose virtues have been developed by trituration and segregation of particles, such as *Lycopodium*, *Natrum muriaticum*, *Calcarea carbonica*, *Sepia*, *Carbo vegetabilis*, *Silicea*, etc., should generally be used at the higher potencies. Others also which have been found from experience to display considerable efficacy, even when greatly attenuated, such as *Phosphorus*, *Sulphur*, *Lachesis*, *Acidum nitricum*, *Arsenicum*, etc. On the contrary, some which have a short-lived, but well-marked action, may be used in some cases in the original substance; for example, *Moschus*, *Valerian*, and *Camphor*, but in exceedingly small doses. Others again have been found most useful at the first, second, or third potency, such as *Tartarus emeticus*, *Ferrum*, *Ipecacuanha*, *Hepar sulphuris*, *Stannum*, *Rhus toxicodendron*, *Opium*, and in many cases *Cinchona*. Still, all these remedies in peculiar cases act well at the higher.

Throughout this work I have given a variety of potencies, specifying those which the nature of the affection treated of seemed to require; but I beg it to be understood that I by no means insist upon a strict observance of what I have laid down, for it is undeniable that when a remedy is *correctly chosen*, whatever may be the potency, it will in most instances be followed by the desired results. From the tenor of the foregoing remarks, however, as well as from what will be found stated under the succeeding paragraph, the importance to practitioners and others who make an extensive use of the homœopathic remedies, of being in possession of several potencies of nearly every medicine, will be rendered sufficiently obvious. In highly perilous acute affections, and, indeed, in all cases, our great point is to obtain as speedy an effect with as little suffering as possible; and when the physician succeeds in effecting this, he may rest satisfied with himself, even although it was by the assistance of a low potency, of a powerful drug, and given in drops. But I must warn the *tyro in our system* not to imagine that because with a *minute* dose he has done much, that by *increasing* it he may do more; the faults of most beginners is to fly too hastily to very low dilutions, and repeat too frequently —patience, coolness, firmness, and attentive observation, are necessary to make a good homœopathist. For my own part, I consider the whole range, from the *first attenuation to the thirtieth, and even upwards*,* useful, according to the nature of the case, and the properties of the remedy, and moreover, that a rigid adherence to any particular dilution in all instances, savours rather of the empiric than of the professor of a liberal art.

ADMINISTRATION AND REPETITION OF THE MEDICINES.

Upon this subject I will offer a few remarks, premising at the same time that it is almost impossible to give any general rule that will serve in all cases, much more depending upon the

* Hahnemann, in his latter years, was much in favour of an extension of the scale of potencies ; and Grosse and other continental homœopathists of repute have recently spoken strongly of the striking results obtained from *Arsenicum* and other medicines at the 200th and even the 1800th attenuation! Their opinions and recommendations, being derived from experience, are at all events well worthy of considerate attention and careful investigation, whatever the *material-headed reasoners* may say to the contrary.

If tinctures are used, put one drop, or three or four drops of the first dilution, into a tumbler full of pure rain water, (or spring water, if very pure,) and give of this solution a teaspoonful for a dose, which is to be repeated according to the rules. The dose may be increased to a dessert or tablespoon, or even more, if the patient be of a strong bodily constitution, and especially if he be of an insusceptible temperament.—The dose is one or two grains of the powdered remedies, according to the strength and susceptibility of the patient ; and this quantity is to be mixed with twice or three times as much powdered sugar of milk. A grain is about as much as will lie on the point of an ordinary penknife blade. In cases of doubt, as to which of two or three remedies, named in this book in any given case. ought to be applied, we recommend a resort to *Jahr's New Manual of Homœopathic Practice.* Turn to the Clinical Chapter, (always in Vol. II,) which precedes the tabular exposition of the effects of medicines upon the part affected in the case, and find the disease under which the patient is labouring ; this chapter alone will often contain the desired information. But if it do not, the table following the Clinical Chapter must be studied, and if this do not suffice to determine the choice satisfactorily, the notices of the remedies in question contained in first volume may be read.

discrimination of the administrator, and a careful observance of the symptoms, than routine.

However, throughout this work I have given directions for the exhibition and repetition of each medicine; these are intended, of course, to be modified according to circumstances, not blindly adhered to; the following observations may, therefore, prove useful:

In *acute* diseases, we must carefully watch the symptoms, and when we feel assured we have chosen the proper remedy, if no perceptible medicinal aggravation or amelioration declare itself, but the disease seems to gain ground, *repeat* the medicine. In cases of high inflammatory action, *Aconite* has sometimes to be repeated every two hours, hour, or even less.

If a *medicinal aggravation* take place, followed by *amelioration, we must let the medicine continue its action, until the amelioration appears to cease,* and the disease again make head; if new symptoms set in, we must then have recourse to the medicine thereby indicated. Should, however, no perceptible *medicinal aggravation* take place, but an *amelioration* follow, we may safely await its approach to its termination, ere we again administer. If any symptoms remain, from the remedy first selected having afforded only partial relief, we must have recourse to some other medicine which seems best fitted to meet them; *but refrain from changing the remedy as long as benefit results from its employment.*

In chronic, sub-acute, and indeed almost all cases, when a very striking improvement takes place, it will generally be found advantageous to cease to administer the medicine as long as the improvement continues, and only to repeat as soon as the slightest symptoms of activity in the morbid phenomena reappear. But when a sudden or marked improvement of comparatively short duration follows the first dose of a remedy, and, on repeating the dose, the symptoms of the complaint increase instead of subsiding, as they did in the first instance, it may be concluded that the medicine does not answer, and that another must accordingly be had recourse to, in the selection of which it will be necessary to choose one *related to* the remedy first prescribed.

The distinguishing of the medicinal aggravation, from that of the disease, being a point of material consequence, we will here give the usual characteristics of each. The *medicinal aggravation* comes on *suddenly and without* previous amelioration; the aggravation of the disease more *gradually*, and frequently *following* an amelioration. Moreover, in the former, several of the *medicinal* symptoms, some of which we may meet under the *indications* for the remedy, and not *before* remarked, declare themselves.

I feel I cannot lay too much stress upon the necessity of carefully watching the effects of each dose, as in addition to the temporary aggravation of the symptoms which sometimes sets in, a development of collateral or pathogenetic signs occasionally takes place, particularly after frequent repetition of different remedies in susceptible patients: by a want of attention to this important point, we may incur confusion, and may be unconsciously treating a medicinal disease of our own creation. Such, unhappily, but too frequently occurs in allopathic practice, from ignorance of the real properties of the drugs employed. We must also guard against falling into the opposite extreme, and allowing the disease to gain head unchecked.

Slight diseases are often removed by a single dose of well-chosen medicine, but more severe and deeply-seated disorders require a frequent repetition.

In severe acute affections, we may often repeat the *same medicine at the same dose, at regular intervals, as long as it does good;* but this rule has many exceptions, and the directions already given at the commencement of this article should be borne in mind.

In chronic cases, by a long-continued administration of the same medicine, the patient often becomes less susceptible; in such instances, if the improvement remain stationary, or progress slowly, we may gradually increase the dose, or, still better, give at suitable intervals some other remedy or remedies of as nearly analagous medicinal properties to that first administered as possible, and then return to the original remedy, if needful; if, on the other hand, decided amelioration follows each administration, we should allow a longer interval to elapse before repeating, by which means the system gradually recovers itself, and the susceptibility to the medicinal influence remains unimpaired until the cure is completed.

In rare cases, this susceptibility increases; in such instances a higher potency should be selected,—provided the remedy still appears to be appropriate,—and the *intervals* between the exhibitions *lengthened.* This occasionally occurs when the medicine has been frequently repeated, and given in solution. When the beneficial effect of a medicine is interrupted by an attack of cold, diarrhœa, &c., some other medicine must be given for the new affection, on the removal of which, the medicine which was previously acting favourably must be recurred to.

In the Selection of the Remedy, it is not necessary that *all* the symptoms noted should be present; at the same time taking care, that there are no symptoms not covered by the medicine, or more strongly indicating another.

Remarks. When it is requisite to keep a medicine in solution for some days, a few drops of proof spirit may be added to the water, which should be as pure as possible, in order to preserve it from decomposition.

It may be scarcely necessary to explain the PHARMACEUTICAL SIGNS used in this work, to signify the potency and quantum of the dose; but as the book may fall into hands otherwise wholly unacquainted with the science, we do so as a measure of precaution; it will therefore be sufficient to remark, that Belladonna $\frac{0\,0}{3}$, means two globules of the third potency, $\frac{6}{6}$, six of the sixth, and the same with any other medicine.

In conclusion, it is necessary to state that the medicines should be taken fasting, and food or drink, as also excessive bodily or mental exertion, abstained from for half an hour to an hour afterwards. The homœopathic remedies should be kept in a clean, dry, dark place, free from odours. Every description of allopathic medicine, patent or domestic, is prohibited; likewise bleedings, blisters, medicated fomentations, perfumery and everything containing camphor. In cases of obstinate constipation, recourse may be had to an enema or lavement of cold, or of tepid water when the former disagrees, to which may be added, if necessary, a tablespoonful of olive oil.

It has repeatedly been found that some remedies act very beneficially when administered after the previous employment of certain others.

The subjoined list affords a few such examples, and may prove useful in the treatment of particular cases: the remedy to be selected must be in accordance with the symptoms.

ACIDUM NITRI. *Calc.*, *Petr.*, *Puls.*, *Sulp.*, are often used with success after *Acidum nitri.*

ACIDUM PHOS. *China*, *Lach.*, *Rhus*, *Verat.*, are sometimes suitable after *Acidum phos.*

ACIDUM SULP. *Puls.* is sometimes useful after *Acid. sulph.*

ACONITE. *Arn.*, *Ars.*, *Bella.*, *Bryon.*, *Cann.*, *Ipec.*, *Spong.*, *Sulp.*, &c., will frequently be found of use after *Aconite*, whether given from the commencement or in the course of treatment.

ALUMINA. *Bryon.* is often of great use after *Alumina*, when it is indicated.

ANT. CRUDUM. *Puls.* and *Merc.* sometimes answer well after *Antimony.*

ARNICA. *Acon.*, *Ipec.*, *Rhus.*, *Sulp. ac.*, are sometimes suitable after *Arnica.*

ARSENICUM. *China*, *Ipec.*, *Nux vom.*, *Sulp.*, *Veratr.*, will sometimes be found beneficial after *Arsenic.*

BELLADONNA. *China*, *Con. Dulc.*, *Hepar.*, *Lach.*, *Rhus.*, *Seneg.*, *Stram.*, *Valer.*, are sometimes the most appropriate medicines after *Belladonna.*

BRYONIA. *Alum.* and *Rhus* will sometimes be found suitable after *Bryonia.*

CALCAREA CARBONICA. *Lycopodium*, *Nitr. ac.*, *Phos.*, and *Silicea*, will be found most useful after *Calcarea.*

CARBO VEGETABILIS. *Arsen.*, *Kali.*, *Merc.*, will often be found suitable after *Carbo vegetabilis.*

CAUSTICUM. *Sepia*, and *Stann.*, will sometimes be found of service after *Causticum.*

CINCHONA. *Arsen., Bella., Puls., Veratr.*, are sometimes suitable after *Cinchona.*

CUPRUM. *Calc.* and *Veratr.* are sometimes of service after *Cuprum.*

HEPAR SULP. *Bella., Merc., Nitr. ac., Spong., Silicea,* are sometimes suitable after *Hepar sulp.*

IPECACUANHA. *Arn., Ars., Chin., Cocc., Ign., Nux,* are sometimes suitable after *Ipecacuanha.*

LACHESIS. *Alum., Ars., Bell., Carb. v., Caust., Con., Dulc., Merc., Nux vom., Phos. acid.*, are sometimes useful after *Lachesis.*

LYCOPODIUM. *Graph., Ledum, Phos., Puls., Silic.*, are sometimes serviceable after *Lycopodium.*

MERCURIUS. After *Mercurius, Bell., China., Dulc., Hepar, Lach., Nitr. acid., Led., Sulph.*, are sometimes suitable.

NUX VOMICA. *Bryon., Puls.*, and *Sulp.*, will frequently be found efficacious after *Nux vomica.*

OPIUM. After *Opium, Calc., Petr., Puls.*, will sometimes be found of use.

PHOSPHORUS. *Petr.* and *Rhus* will be found suitable after *Phosphorus.*

PULSATILLA. *Asa., Bryon., Nitr. ac., Sepia,* are sometimes suitable after *Pulsatilla.*

RHUS TOXICODENDRON. *Am. c., Ars., Bryon., Calc., Con., Phos., Phos. ac., Puls.*, and *Sulph.*, are sometimes useful after *Rhus tox.*

SEPIA. After *Sepia., Carbo v., Caust., Puls.*, are sometimes suitable.

SILICEA. After *Silicea, Hepar, Lach., Lyco., Sepia,* are sometimes of service.

SPONGIA. *Hepar sulph.* is sometimes suitable after *Spongia,* (in the croup.)

SULPHUR. *Acon., Bell., Calc., Cupr., Merc., Nitr. ac*, *Puls., Rhus., Sepia, Sil.*, are sometimes suitable after *Sulphur.*

TARTARUS EMETICUS. After *Tartar emetic, Bar-c., Ipec., Puls., Sep.*, are sometimes useful.

VERATRUM. After *Veratrum, Ars., Arn., Chin., Cupr., Ipec.*, are sometimes suitable.

SYNOPSIS

OF THE

RULES FOR DIET, UNDER HOMŒOPATHIC TREATMENT.

ALIMENTS ALLOWED.

Soup or broth made from the lean of beef, veal, and mutton; to which may be added, well boiled, sago, tapioca, vermicelli, rice, semolina, or macaroni, seasoned merely with a little salt.

Meats. Beef, mutton, (poultry, rarely,) pigeons, larks, rabbits, (venison, and game in general, may in most cases be partaken of in moderation, but never when high,) plainly cooked and roasted, broiled, or stewed, in preference to boiled. Ham or neat's tongue rarely.)

*Fish.** Soles, whiting, smelts, trout and flounders, broiled in preference to fried; when cooked in the latter manner, the white must alone be partaken of, and the outer or fried portions rejected.

Vegetables. Potatoes, brocoli, green peas, cauliflower, spinach, turnips, French beans, seakale, vegetable marrow, stewed lettuce, well cooked, and prepared with the gravy of meat, where required, instead of butter.

Eggs lightly dressed; all kinds of light bread not new-baked, and biscuit free from soda or potash and the like.

Light puddings, such as those made from vermicelli, semolina, fecula of potato, sago, arrow root, rice; simple cakes composed of flour or meal, eggs, sugar, and a little *good* butter.

Fruit. Baked, stewed, or preserved apples or pears: also gooseberries, raspberries, grapes, or any other fruit not of an acid quality, fully ripe, preserved, or in the form of jelly, may occasionally be partaken of.

* From the extensive varieties of American fish may be most safely selected—shad, king-fish, striped bass or rock-fish, Otsego bass (shad salmon,) lake trout (salmon trout,) halibut, haddock, sea bass or black-fish, sheep's head, pike, pickerel and perch.—Ed.

Beverage. Water, milk, cocoa, chocolate, (unspiced), arrowroot, or gruel, made thin, toast-water, barley-water, milk and water, sugar and water, rice-water.

Salt should be used in moderation.

ALIMENTS PROHIBITED.

Soups. Turtle, mock-turtle, ox-tail, giblet, mulligatawny, and all rich and seasoned soups.

Meats. Pork, bacon, calf's head, veal, turkey, duck, goose, sausages, kidney, liver, tripe, and every kind of fat and salted meats.

Fish. Crab, lobster, oysters,* and shell-fish in general; and almost all other fish not specified in *Aliments allowed.*

Vegetables. Cucumber, celery, onions, artichokes, radishes, parsley, horse-radish, leeks, thyme, garlic, asparagus; and every description of pickles, salads, and raw vegetables, or vegetables greened with copper.

Pastry of all kinds, whether boiled, baked or fried.

Spices, Aromatics, and *Artificial Sauces,* of all kinds; as also the ordinary condiments, mustard and vinegar.

Cheese.

Chestnuts, filberts, walnuts, almonds, raisins, and indeed almost the entire complement of a dessert, except what has been mentioned in *Aliments allowed,* under *Fruit.* (See also REGIMEN, p. 1.)

The above regulations are subject to considerable modifications in particular cases; but only under the direction of the medical attendant. Regularity in the hours of meals should be observed; and too long fasting, as well as too great a quantity of food at one time, should be avoided.

* The inhibition of the *European* OYSTER is justly demanded on account of its flavour and effects; but the American oyster, according to our experience, is one of the most valuable esculents that, at times, can be furnished either to the invalid or convalescent.—*Ed.*

PART II.

ON THE SYMPTOMS, CHARACTER, DISTINCTION, AND TREATMENT OF DISEASES.

FEVERS. *Febres.*

GENERAL CONSIDERATION OF FEVER.

CAUSES, TREATMENT, AND DIET TO BE OBSERVED.

PERHAPS no form of disease has more occupied the attention of pathologists, or given rise to a greater number of theories, than fever. Many authors consider fever and inflammation as synonymous terms, others as mere modifications of the same pathological state of the system. The investigation is certainly one possessing peculiar interest, but, fortunately, in the homœopathic system, no theory can in the slightest degree affect the practice, since in the treatment of this class of disease, the external phenomena present sufficient indications for the selection of the proper remedies.

Acute diseases have always been considered as the true touchstone of every system of therapeutics. Homœopathy has been submitted to this test, and the results have at once proved the bold assertion of its founder, that its principle was a law of nature,—the minute doses in these cases act with a promptness and certainty scarcely to be credited, except by those who have either witnessed or experienced their power; under this system the disease is brought to a salutary crisis before any great expenditure of vital energy has taken place; from this, and the absence of debilitating measures, the period of convalescence is greatly shortened, and in many instances scarcely perceptible, the patient being, as it were, at once restored from a state of disease to one of perfect health.

Although I shall avoid entering into any of the theories respecting fever and inflammation, I cannot but render the tribute of my admiration to the gifted men who have devoted so much of their time and energies to the elucidation of this difficult point, since every new pathological discovery serves to throw light upon the specific action of medicinal substances. Practically speaking, when we find a medicine produce a change of health resembling that present in fevers, we know that in such fevers it is curative: still it would be a satisfaction to be enabled to trace the connexion more closely, and to show the perfect affinity between medicinal and morbid action. There is no doubt that, if a perfect theory of fever be ever given to the world, it will be found in perfect accordance with the homœopathic law.

In all forms of acute diseases fever is present; in fever, properly so called, there is generally functional disturbance, accelerated action of the vascular, with the participation of the nervous system, and a tendency to increased development of heat. The symptoms common to most fevers are—at first, a feeling of coldness or shivering, then heat, accelerated pulse, thirst, restlessness and languor. Fever also possesses the property of passing from one species into another. Thus inflammatory fever may, by severe antiphlogistic measures, be altered into a low typhus; or, on the other hand, a simple fever, by injudicious treatment, into an inflammatory one, and that again assume the intermittent form; also, one attack may present all these different phases.

Fevers terminating fortunately and running a regular course, may be divided into five stages; the accession, increase, crisis, decrease, and convalescence. When the result is fatal, it may arise from a metastasis, the exhaustation of a vital energy of the patient, or the disorganization of some important function.

The belief in critical days is of very ancient origin, though there is some difference in the calculations of physicians upon that point; some counting from the day the shiverings declared the onset, others from the first hot fit; except in cases where a marked periodicity exists, as in quotidian and other forms of ague, such distinctions are of little value, inasmuch as the homœopathic treatment is directed to forwarding the crisis, and thereby materially shortens the duration of the disease. Statistics prove that the average continuation of acute affections is much shorter under the homœopathic system than it is where they are treated allopathically, or left to nature; consequently, any calculations based upon other modes of treatment are not to be depended upon, and the best plan for the physician to follow is to watch attentively the disease before him, and apply the remedies his knowledge and experience point out as best calculated to conduct it to a satisfactory issue.

A crisis may declare itself by diarrhœa, profuse perspiration or increase or alteration of other secretions, or by the appearance of an eruption, after which, if salutary, the skin becomes moist and resumes its functions, and the pulse returns to its usual standard.

Fevers have been differently classified by various medical writers. The arrangement we shall adopt is as follows: simple irritative fever, inflammatory fever, typhus, putrid, and gastric or bilious fevers, intermittent fevers, and then eruptive fevers, such as scarlatina, measles, etc.

Although this mode of classification is adopted for the sake of convenience, the author has no intention of generalizing disease: every febrile attack presents peculiar features, and is to be treated as an individual affection, and according to the nature of the symptoms presenting themselves, not by a blind adherence to the mere nomenclature of disease.

Causes of Fever. It cannot be denied but that there exists in certain individuals, a particular predisposition to acute diseases, and, as before remarked, in introduction, the sanguine, nervous, and bilious temperaments possess this susceptibility in a far more marked degree than the phlegmatic.

The exciting causes are numerous. Miasms, epidemic influences, contagion, powerful mental emotions, derangement of some important organ, external lesions, excess or errors in diet, heat or cold, or alterations of temperature, exposure to cold or damp, repercussed exanthemata—in fact, anything that causes derangement of the equilibrium of the system may produce fever.

GENERAL TREATMENT IN FEVER, AND DIET.

The great essentials in the treatment of fever are:

Perfect rest, mental and bodily.

Pure air and a cool apartment; the temperature of the patient's room should never exceed 55 degrees.

Feather-beds should be discarded, and mattresses substituted, when practicable, and the bed-clothes be light but sufficient.

Nature herself generally prescribes the regimen to be observed by taking away appetite, while the thirst present, as an eminent medical writer has well observed, may be considered as her voice calling for fluid. Water is the best diluent; no solid food, broth, or even gruel and the like, should be permitted in cases where the inflammation runs excessively high; and the utmost caution is to be observed, in allowing gruel or weak broths during the decrease: an error in this respect often causes irreparable mischief, and it is always safer to err a little on the side of abstinence than on that of indulgence.

A little toast-water, or weak barley or rice-water, sweetened with a little sugar, raspberry or strawberry syrup, may be allowed when the fever is somewhat abated, though then we must still carefully avoid incurring the risk of a relapse, by giving any aliment likely to tax, in however slight a degree, the digestive powers.

SIMPLE OR EPHEMERAL FEVER.

Febris Simplex.

The disease seldom presents any distinct character, and generally runs its course in twenty-four hours; as, however, it frequently forms the initiative of other more serious disorders, it deserves attention. Before attacks of scarlatina, measles, small-pox, etc., it is generally present, although occasionally showing itself as a distinct affection.

Diagnosis. Shivering, followed by heat, restlessness, thirst, accelerated pulse, general uneasiness and lassitude, terminated by profuse perspiration.

In allopathic practice, unless they could trace the immediate cause of the affection, for instance indigestion, the treatment is occasionally hazardous; for, if the simple fever was merely the commencement of an attack of severe inflammation, they incur the risk of increasing it by using stimulants, under the idea of its being a precursor of typhus; or acting upon the opinion of its being a forerunner of inflammation, of weakening the constitution by antiphlogistic methods, if it should unfortunately run on to the former. In this case the safer plan was to await quietly the development of the affection, to see if it would terminate in a crisis, or take upon it a more virulent form, and so deal with it accordingly.

Therapeutics. Throughout this work the disease will be found treated of, when arising from indigestion or cold, and found as the precursor of other affections; but when it is encountered along with the symptoms already detailed, and cannot be traced to any particular exciting cause, and particularly when *hot, dry skin* is present, Aconite $\frac{0}{6}{}^{0}$ may be administered* in a teaspoonful of water, which, if it be simple fever properly so called, will speedily dissipate all the symptoms; and if it be the forerunner of any more severe disorder, either at once check its further progress or materially modify its malignancy. The former is more peculiarly the case with purely inflammatory attacks: the latter holds good as far as relates to typhus, exanthematic diseases, and some other affections which run a regular course.

* In all cases where directions for the *administration* of a medicine are given, the attention of the reader is directed to the article on that subject in the introduction.

INFLAMMATORY FEVER. *Synocha.*

Diagnosis. Shivering or chill (generally considerable) followed by burning heat; pulse strong, hard, and greatly accelerated; dryness of the skin, mouth, lips, and tongue; the latter generally of a bright red, in some cases slightly coated with white; thirst; urine red and scanty; constipation; respiration hurried, in accordance with the pulse; amelioration of symptoms as the pulse assumes a more normal state. It runs its course with rapidity, rarely exceeding fourteen days, and progressing with regularity to a crisis, which shows itself in profuse perspirations, critical urine, diarrhœa, or hæmorrhages, principally epistaxis. The period mentioned is its ordinary average of duration, but under homœopathic treatment, the perfect crisis is considerably hastened, without the long convalescence entailed by the usual antiphlogistic means.

It is peculiarly apt, if not carefully treated, to change into typhus, or by metastasis to fix upon some important organ.

Causes. Sudden chill or check of perspiration, exposure to damp or wet, dry easterly winds, violent mental emotion, high living, external injury or lesion, local inflammation, and slight febrile attacks mismanaged.

Individuals of what is denominated a plethoric habit are particularly subject to this disease; it generally attacks between the ages of 15 and 30 years.

Under the *diagnosis* we have given the pathogonomic symptoms of synocha; we, however, find it complicated, in the majority of cases, with more or less cerebral disturbance, which we shall consider more in detail under Inflammation of the Brain and its tissues.

Therapeutics. Although throughout this work the author purposes to confine himself to pointing out the remedies most valuable in disease, without entering into any disquisition upon their efficacy, or the principle of their employment, yet he cannot refrain in this instance, from briefly noticing a medicament which has so successfully superseded all the antiphlogistic measures of the old school, subduing inflammation without lowering the vital energy. No one who compares the pathogenetic symptoms of ACONITE given in the *Materia Medica Pura* of Hahnemann, and carries in mind the principle of its application, can forbear being struck with the close resemblance which they present to those of pure inflammatory disease; and by this powerful auxiliary the author has no hesitation in declaring, that disease of the said description is brought so fully under the control of the physician, as to be in a great measure divested of its malignancy, and in *no case* is the superiority of Homœopathy more strongly evidenced.

ADMINISTRATION.* When, therefore, the symptoms above mentioned are present, we should at once administer **ACONITE**, six globules of the third potency, in an ounce of pure water, a dessert-spoonful to be given every quarter of an hour, every half or every two or three hours, according to the intensity of the fever, and the *pulse carefully* watched, lengthening the intervals according to the effect produced, till marked benefit results.

A slight degree of delirium is frequently present in this affection, chiefly at night, which, unless it threatens to run on to inflammation of the brain, in which case Belladonna must be had recourse to, *Aconite* is of itself sufficient to subdue. When, however, during the course of the affection other symptoms besides those mentioned develop themselves, we may find it necessary to have recourse to different remedies, such as *Belladonna, Bryonia,* &c.

BELLADONNA. When there is *great heat in the head*, with violent cephalalgia, particularly in the *forehead, and redness of the face; distention of the arteries of the neck and temples;* nocturnal sleeplessness, with furious *delirium;* eyes red, shining and fiery; general internal and external heat; burning thirst, and agonizing restlessness.

ADMINISTRATION. Six globules of the third potency in an ounce of water; a dessert-spoonful exhibited every four hours until amelioration takes place, or we observe unequivocal symptoms, of *medicinal aggravation;* in which latter case we

* Vide note, page 21.

must cease to prescribe altogether until the reaction has taken place; and in the former, lengthen the intervals of repetition as the improvement advances.

Bryonia. This medicament is indicated when, in addition to the usual symptoms of inflammatory fever already given, we find a heavy stupifying headache, with a sensation as if the head would burst at the temples, much aggravated by movement, *vertigo and giddiness on rising up or moving; burning heat, redness* of the head and face, with redness and swelling of the latter; delirium; *oppression at the pit of the stomach;* excessive thirst, sometimes followed by vomiting; *constipation;* aching or shooting pains in the limbs. dry cough, or cough with adhesive phlegm tinged with blood, stitches in the chest or side, and laborious breathing; when these latter symptoms are present, we may infer that the pleura or lungs are affected. In the latter case the practitioner should test the diagnosis by auscultation.

Administration. Six globules of the third potency may be added to an ounce of water, and a dessert-spoonful given every four or six hours; few cases are so particularly urgent as to require more frequent administration of the remedy; indeed, when the virulence of the disease has been subdued, a single dose is generally found sufficient, and no further exhibition should take place as long as the patient manifestly continues improving.

When inflammatory fever seems to arise from a primary inflammation of some important organ, such as the Head, Lungs, Liver, or Stomach and Bowels, the treatment will be found under the head of Inflammation of the function most evidently the seat of the disorder.

It is sometimes the result of severe lesion, in which case the patient is to be treated as prescribed under External Injuries.

NERVOUS FEVER. *Febris Nervosa.* TYPHUS.

It is sometimes extremely difficult, particularly when it arises from some local affection of the more important viscera, to discriminate at the commencement between a nervous or inflammatory attack, so as to give a decided prognosis. However, in such cases, the marked advantages of the homœopathic system is again shown: by exhibiting medicines in accordance with the symptoms that declare themselves, we run no risk of weakening the vital energies, should we err in diagnosis, and treat it on its first appearance as an inflammatory attack —or of stimulating the inflammation by what is commonly denominated an anti-nervous treatment, should the precursory symptoms lead us to consider it typhus, and it afterwards assume the inflammatory form.

Diagnosis. Typhus rarely sets in with such marked symptoms as announce the approach of inflammatory fever—instead of severe chill or shiverings, we first find a complaint of general uneasiness, a sensation of chilliness, occasionally followed by a greater or less degree of heat. The patient either complains but little, or of pains in his head, chest, and abdomen, and frequently an unusual degree of drowsiness is present, arising from a comatose state of the brain—there is also occasionally a slight dyspnœa; after various alternations of cold and heat, the former sensation predominates in the feelings of the patient, while to those around him he appears hot; the extremities, however, on examination, are found cold. Different characters of pulse present themselves; sometimes it is full and soft, at others accelerated, frequently about the natural standard or below it, or quick and weak, but not strong and hard as in inflammatory fever. The difference between the action of the pulse and heart is worthy of notice: the former may be so weak as scarcely to be perceptible, and the action of the latter strong; the pulse also may be hurried and the respiration natural. As the disease progresses, the tongue, at first moist, becomes thickly coated, dry, glazed, and tremulous; there is faintness, cephalalgia, giddiness, and vertigo: the delirium, at first slight, and manifesting itself only at night, becomes unintermitted, and is characterized rather by wandering and low muttering, than fury and violence: we may also meet with spasms and convulsions. All these symptoms, if the disease is allowed to gain ground, increase in malignancy, the evacuations become involuntary, the weakness and lassitude excessive, and the patient sinks down to the bottom of the bed—an evidence of complete prostration of strength, while all endeavours to rouse him are fruitless, and he is perfectly blind to all around. Tenderness of the abdomen or pain in the region of the cœcum is also frequently met with.

Some only of the above symptoms may be present, or the fever may be complicated with others: when only a few of the less virulent symptoms declare themselves, it is called mild typhus; when complicated with considerable disturbance of the vascular system, great heat and quick hard pulse, inflammatory typhus: a distinction is also found in the type, as in continuous and intermittent typhus; in the accidental circumstances or exciting causes present, as in the gastric and catarrhal complications, which, although generally treated as gastric or catarrhal fevers with typhoid symptoms, may be considered as modifications of this affection,—this difference in arrangement can, however, make none in practice, as we must be guided by the symptoms that present themselves in selecting our remedies.

The CONGESTIVE FEVER of some authors may be considered as a variety of typhus, in which, from the balance of the circulation being destroyed, the blood is determined to some particular organ—the external heat of the body diminished, and the pulse becomes slow and oppressed. The symptoms vary according to the organs attacked. It may be remarked, that in most forms of this malady, the course is extremely irregular,—the precursory symptoms may precede the disease only a few days or several weeks, and its duration is also uncertain.

Death may take place from exhaustion of the vital energies, paralysis of the whole system, or of the brain, apoplexy, disorganization of some of the nobler viscera, or a change to the putrid form.

CAUSES. Densely populated neighbourhoods, where a number of individuals are crowded into small apartments, and the air rendered impure by exhalations from decomposed animal and vegetable matter, stagnant water, and a want of circulation, are the very hotbeds of typhus; deficiency and improper quality of food are often added to the above, and are of themselves sufficient to produce it; other causes are, over-exertion, either of body or mind, or excesses of any kind, the prevalence of cold or damp weather, mental emotions, and contagion.

In fact, anything tending to depress the vital energies may be productive of typhus; it may consequently arise after inflammatory fever treated by bloodletting or other severe antiphlogistic measures, or even by the reaction of the organism, or an imperfect crisis after the same affection. We shall now proceed to consider the treatment of this malady, and under the indications for the different medicaments used, will be found the symptoms that declare themselves under the various phases which the disease presents.

THERAPEUTICS. At the commencement, where gastric symptoms set in, such as headache, giddiness, nausea, vomiting, watery, yellow, or *greenish*, slimy evacuations; particularly when attended with slight chills, alternately with heat or considerable shivering with slight heat, or marked heat with but little shivering, we may administer—

ADMINISTRATION. IPECACUANHA $\frac{\Omega\Omega\Omega}{3}$ in a teaspoonful of water, and repeat it every three or four hours.* Or *Pulsatilla* may be selected at this stage of the disorder, when there is frequent shivering, bitter taste, whitish tongue, loss of appetite, nausea, vomiting of mucus, slimy evacuations, and particularly when the above symptoms occur in phlegmatic subjects, with extreme depression of spirits, and tearfulness. Two globules of the sixth potency in a little water every three to six hours.

NUX VOMICA. Gastric or bilious symptoms, constipation with frequent inclination and ineffectual efforts to evacuate. *Nux vomica* is further indicated when the spasms, which not unfrequently accompany this disease, are confined to the

* Vide note, p. 21.

stomach and intestines, particularly the rectum, a frequent cause of the above-mentioned constipation; painful pressure, and tension in the epigastrium and hypochondria; sensation as if the limbs were bruised; general nervous excitability, with great nocturnal restlessness and slight delirium; weakness, and exacerbation of the symptoms in the morning. Temperament, sanguine or bilious; disposition, irritable and impatient.

ADMINISTRATION. Two globules of the sixth potency every twelve hours.

When the disorder assumes the asthenic form of *abdominal* typhus, or when the inflammatory diathesis is more lymphatic than arterial. from the occurrence of the disease in venous-lymphatic subjects. with pale or yellowish appearance of the face, severe headache, or sensation as if a tight band were across the forehead; thickly-coated tongue; bitter or foul taste; little thirst; sensibility of the scrobiculus or umbilical region to the touch. and distention of the abdomen; evacuations *copious*, *watery*, flocculent, and even bloody, sometimes attended with *tenesmus;* at first dry burning skin, followed by profuse debilitating *sweats;* depressed pulse, and great prostration; extreme restlessness and anxiety, with constant tossing about in bed; disturbed unrefreshing sleep, with anxious dreams, — MERCURIUS will be found a most efficient medicine.

ADMINISTRATION. Three globules of the sixth in a little water every two hours, until the evacuations become diminished in number, and improved in appearance, and the tenderness and pain in abdomen, etc., relieved.

CINCHONA. This remedy is frequently of service in the first stage, or when there is paleness of the face, lancinating, rending, aching, or pressive headache, cloudiness of vision, buzzing or roaring in the ears, dulness of hearing; yellow or white coating on the tongue, dryness of the mouth, insipid, clammy, or bitter taste; inclination to vomit; sensibility and distention of the abdomen; thin, yellow, watery motions, occasionally intermixed with undigested substances; urine scanty, pale, or dark coloured, and cloudy; oppression at the chest; dragging shooting pains in the limbs; anxiety, sleeplessness, and general coldness and shivering. In an *advanced stage* of the disease, china is moreover occasionally of considerable value, especially when the attack has become lengthened and tedious, and the following symptoms have set in: nocturnal sweats, obstinate diarrhœa, but with clean tongue, and absence of abdominal pain; followed by *Sulphur*, should the sweats not yield.

ADMINISTRATION. Three globules of the third potency every six hours, until benefit result.

When inflammatory symptoms declare themselves from the commencement, *Aconite* and *Belladonna* are the best remedies; when the disease becomes more developed, and still retains the inflammatory character, *Bryonia* and *Rhus* will generally be found more useful. For the employment of *Aconite*, we have given the fullest indication under Inflammatory Fever; and in all cases where these decided symptoms are present, it is imperatively called for, and should be administered as there prescribed. The following symptoms indicate BELLADONNA:

Alternate heat and chills, or general heat externally and internally, with redness, burning heat or bloated appearance of the face; violent throbbing of the carotids, redness, sparkling, and protrusion of the eyes, with dilatation of the pupils, extreme sensibility to light, and strabismus; singing or noises in the ears to a greater or less degree; wild expression of the countenance, with uneasy glancing around, as if from fear, sometimes attended with a marked inclination to run away; violent shooting pains in the forehead, or dull heavy pain, causing the patient to put his hand frequently to his head; furious delirium or loss of consciousness; silent delirium and carphologia, or spasmodic or convulsive attacks; parched lips, sorenesss of the corners of the mouth, redness and dryness of the tongue, which is sometimes also foul and covered with a yellow coating; skin hot and dry; bitter taste in the mouth, intense thirst, difficulty of deglutition, especially of liquids, nausea, pressure at the pit of the stomach; meteorismus; and constipation, or watery motions; scanty and red or amber-coloured urine, rapid respiration, pulse full and accelerated, or quick, hard, and wiry; parotid glands inflamed and tumid.

STRAMONIUM may be given when, in addition to the above symptoms, we find twitching of the muscles of the face, subsultus, strabismus, trembling of the extremities, tremulous motion of the tongue on protrusion, burning heat of the body, suppression of the urine, fantastic gesticulations, and risus sardonicus.

HYOSCYAMUS, with similar symptoms, and moreover, twitching of the tendons, strong full pulse, fulness of the veins, burning heat of the skin, sensation of pricking all over the body, and constant delirium; frequent *but ineffectual urging to urinate.*

ADMINISTRATION. Of the three last mentioned remedies, six globules of the third potency may be added to an ounce of pure water, and a dessert-spoonful given every three or twelve hours, according to the violence of the malady or the improvement that ensues. When the skin continues *hot and dry,* and the bowels relaxed, or the motions even passed involuntary; or when there is phlegmonous inflammation of the tonsils; the alternate administration of *Belladonna* and *Aconite* every two or three hours until the skin becomes moist, etc., will be attended with a desirable result.

We will now proceed to the consideration of the two medicines, ***Rhus*** and ***Bryonia,*** whose value in typhus, in the form in which it appeared in Germany in 1813, was proved by Hahnemann's treatment of 183 patients, not one of whom died, while thousands perished under the means employed by the professors of the old system of medicine. The two medicines above mentioned possess many striking points of similarity, but also many of difference; they may on some occasion be administered alternately with great advantage in the manner below described; for the several employments the indications are as follows:

BRYONIA. More particularly when the disorder assumes the character of a ***Febris nervosa versatilis,*** or ***Typhus cerebralis,*** with *violent stupifying* headache, as from a blow, and pain across the temples, as if the head would burst. *Aggravation* of these sensations by *movement—continued* delirium, violent, with excessive febrile heats, foul thickly-coated yellow tongue, with dryness of the mouth and great thirst, and vesicles on the mouth or tongue, furred lips, nausea, inclination to vomit, or vomiting of mucous and bilious matter; tenderness of the scrobiculus when touched; general heat of the whole body, dryness of the skin, redness of the face, and *profuse perspiration* during the fever; sensibility of the epigastric region, distended abdomen.—*Constipation,* or relaxed stools; urine of a deep orange colour or bright yellow, with yellow sediment; sensation as of a plug in the throat, with difficulty of hearing; stitches in the side; drowsiness or disposition to sleep during the day; sleeplessness, fugitive heat and excessive restlessness, or continued drowsiness or coma, with startings and unpleasant dreams; painful shootings and soreness of the limbs, *aggravated by movement,* trembling of the hands; pulse *quick,* soft, *frequent;* or irregular, *small* and *intermitting.* Petechiæ, IRRITABILITY, IRASCIBILITY, *despair of recovery.*

RHUS TOXICODENDRON. This medicine is more peculiarly suitable to the *debile* form or stage, the *Febris nervosa stupida,* as is Bryonia to the *inflammatory;* but will frequently be found serviceable in all the stages of the disease, particularly when there is *diarrhœa,* and congestion to the head and great weakness. The headache is generally of a stupifying nature, with a feeling as if from a bruise, but not so *severe* as that of Bryonia; the tongue presents nearly the same character, *less* nausea and inclination to vomit exists; *violent pain* is present at the epigastrium, especially when *touched.* Constipation as in *Bryonia,* but more particularly, *copious yellowish or loose* sanguineous evacuations; the symptoms of general heat, and those of the face, resemble those given under *Bryonia,* but *without* the perspiration, or at most, a clammy feeling of the skin. The urine is hot, *dark coloured,* or at first clear, and afterwards turbid, the symptoms of the ears the same; sleep also the same; *difficult deglutition of solids,* as if from *contraction* of the throat and œsophagus; *general trembling, debi-*

lity and prostration, almost amounting to paralytic weakness of the different limbs, shooting pains in various parts of the body, *aggravated* when at *rest* or at night, and *momentarily relieved* by *moving* the part affected; pulse quick and small, or weak and slow. In the *morale* we may notice, excessive anguish, anxiety, extreme lowness of spirits, and inclination to weep. Petechiæ, as in Bryonia, are frequently present.

Administration. As before remarked, *Rhus* is particularly suitable in the debile form or low typhus; we may add six globules of the third potency to an ounce of water. In some extreme cases, however, the practitioner will find it necessary to prescribe a more frequent administration of the dose, and at a still lower potency, (such as the second dilution, or even the mother tincture,) and administer one dessert-spoonful every three to four hours in ordinary cases, lengthening the intervals as improvement ensues, and then quietly awaiting its action. The *Bryonia* may be given in the same manner when it appears indicated, and in many cases it will be found useful to give these medicines alternately at six hours' interval, a dessert-spoonful of the mixture above mentioned as a dose.

Arsenicum. This is decidedly one of the most important remedies in *abdominal typhus*, sometimes restoring the patient when almost beyond the reach of hope, and renovating the vital spark. The chief indications for its employment are EXTREME PROSTRATION OF STRENGTH, falling of the lower jaw, open mouth, dull and glassy eyes, burning thirst, and colliquative diarrhœa, pulse scarcely perceptible and intermittent.

Administration. Six globules of the third, sixth, or twelfth potency may be added to an ounce of water, and a dessert-spoonful given every quarter, or half hour, until improvement is perceptible, when the intervals between the doses may be extended.

Carbo vegetabilis is another remedy of great utility in these desperate cases; it is indicated where we find drowsiness with rattling respiration, face pinched, sunken, and deathlike, pupils insensible to light, pulse scarcely perceptible, and rapidly sinking, cold perspiration on the face and extremities, involuntary and offensive evacuations, deep red urine, with a cloud floating in it or rising towards the surface.

ADMINISTRATION. Six globules of the sixth potency in the same quantity of water as the preceding, administered in the same manner. An alternate administration of these two medicines, at intervals of from four to eight hours, has been attended with the most fortunate results.

ACIDUM PHOSPHORICUM. When at the very commencement of the disease, we find great exhaustion and prostration, with wandering even when awake; or in almost hopeless cases, either alone, or still better in alternation with *Rhus*, when the patient is always found lying on the back in a comatose state, and either gives no reply when talked to, or if he does it is in an incoherent manner; constant loquacious delirium, or low muttering; carpologia, fixed look; seeming efforts to escape from some alarming object; black incrustations on the lips; dry, hot skin, continued *copious watery diarrhœa;* the motions are generally passed involuntarily; sanguineous evacuations; frequent, weak, and occasionally an intermitting pulse. Should the debilitating sanguineous evacuations continue, *Acid. nitricum* should be administered, or *Cantharides*, should strangury also be present.

ADMINISTRATION. Same as the above.

SULPHUR may often be had recourse to with advantage when *Bryonia*, *Rhus* and *Acidum phosphoricum* have been fruitlessly administered; the following, however, are its characteristic indications in this disease: pale and collapsed countenance, burning itching eruptions on the lips, dryness of the mouth; foul, dry tongue; bitter taste; slimy or bilious vomiting; tenderness of the epigastrium, and pain in the umbilical region increased on pressure; borborygmus; frequent watery, flocculent or yellow evacuations; cloudy urine, depositing a reddish sediment; stitches in the chest, oppressed breathing; dry cough, worse towards evening and at night; sleeplessness, or whining during sleep, dry heat during the day, with moderately quick pulse, profuse sweating at night.

ADMINISTRATION. Six globules of the sixth in an ounce of water, a dessert-spoonful every six hours.

OPIUM. Great drowsiness, or coma with stertorous breathing, open mouth, half closed eyes, or fixed look, slight delirium or muttering; CARPOLOGIA; the patient is in a continual state of sopor from which it is extremely difficult to rouse him, and is scarcely aroused ere he relapses into his former state; dry offensive stools, which together with the urine are passed involuntarily.

ADMINISTRATION. Six globules of the third potency in half an ounce of water, a teaspoonful every three hours.

CALCAREA C. may sometimes be administered advantageously, alternately with *Belladonna, Arsenic* or *Rhus*, according to symptoms; it is further sometimes a most efficient remedy in cases in which debilitating diarrhœa or epistaxis will not yield to such remedies as, *Ac. phos., Rhus, Cinchona*, etc.: when the nasal hemorrhage does not yield to *Calcarea, Hepar sulphuris* is generally the most appropriate remedy to follow up with, provided the entire feature of the disease is not better embraced by *Pulsatilla, Belladonna, Rhus*, or *Sulphur*.

PHOSPHORUS. When the disease becomes as it were concentrated in the lungs, and there is consequently congestion with extremely laborious breathing and excessive anxiety, dulness on percussion, mucous rale, stitches during respiration; cough with copious expectoration of mucus mixed with blood, or even offensive pus; more benefit may be looked for from this than from any other remedy.

ADMINISTRATION. Six globules of the third in an ounce of water, a dessert-spoonful every four hours.

ACIDUM MURIATICUM. Weakness, with *a constant tendency to sink down in the bed*, with groaning during sleep, almost paralytic state of the tongue, rendering it almost impossible for the patient to speak, even when in a collected state, and great dryness of the mouth.

ADMINISTRATION. The same potency and in the same manner as *Arsenicum*.

After severe cases of Typhus, a period of debility generally supervenes of greater or less duration, according to the violence of the attack. In such instances CINCHONA $\frac{000}{6}$, in a little water, repeated in five days, followed by VALERIAN in about four days to a week, according to the result produced. Of this latter medicine, three or four globules of the third potency may be given in a glass of water, and repeated every two days, if necessary, until the desired result is attained.*

An alteration of these two medicaments, at intervals of twenty-four hours, has also been found very useful in these cases. When debilitating sweats supervene, Cinchona should be administered, followed by Sulphur if required.

Should symptoms of deranged digestion remain after the fever has been subdued, *Nux vomica* and *Pulsatilla* will be found most serviceable according to the temperament of the individual, and the symptoms present. (See article INDIGESTION.) The other medicaments mentioned under the head referred to, may also be advantageously consulted. Where a peculiar morbid state of the constitution exists, denominated by some Homœopathists, a psoric tendency, a drop of the third potency of the TINCTURE OF SULPHUR in three dessert-spoonfuls of water, one daily, and the medicine then allowed to act from one to three weeks, according to circumstances, may be administered.

DIET. In a disease that presents so many varieties, it is difficult to give any rules upon this head applicable to all cases. When a marked inflammatory character is present, the same abstinence should be enjoined as already noted under Fevers; and in all cases, either during the progress of the disease or the period of convalescence, the greatest possible care should be taken to avoid taxing the digestive functions; the diet should be light and simple, and the patient never allowed to indulge the appetite to its full extent.

PUTRID FEVER, OR TYPHUS.

Typhus Putridus.

We have already alluded to this form of the disease under *Typhus*, particularly in the indications given for the employ-

* Vide note, p. 21.

ment of Arsenicum and Carbo vegetabilis; but consider it of sufficient importance to be remarked on separately, although of course, except in cases of decided emergency, no individual not properly qualified would think of treating so serious an affection.

Diagnosis. The symptoms of Typhus already given, running on to the colliquative state; extreme debility, pulse exceedingly small and weak, so as to be scarcely perceptible; a peculiar sensation of burning pungent heat, communicating itself to the hand when placed upon the body of the patient, heavy cadaverous smell of the whole body, putrid odour of the breath, perspiration, and secretions in general; profuse oily and clammy sweats; involuntary evacuations; colliquative or sanguineous diarrhœa; dark and bloody urine; epistaxis, petechiæ, and other marked tendencies to organic dissolution. The patient is always found lying on his back, and continually shrinks down to the foot of the bed, a sign of utter helplessness and prostration.

Therapeutics. Arsenicum corresponds closely to the foregoing symptoms, and is, therefore, our principal remedy when the disease assumes this form, particularly when we find involuntary and sanguineous evacuations and tenesmus. *Carbo vegetabilis* may also be with advantage alternated with it, when the symptoms already given under Typhus for the exhibition of that medicine are present; *Mercurius* is called for in case of *great tenesmus*, and when the discharge of blood is principally alvine, followed by *Acid. phosph.*, *Acid. nitr.*, or *Cantharides*, should sanguineous diarrhœa continue. (See nervous fever, p. 29.)

Administration. When *Arsenicum* itself is found called for, we may add one drop of the third potency to an ounce of water, and administer a dessert-spoonful every six hours, or even every hour if the patient seems sinking, until an improvement takes place. If, however, from the symptoms given under that medicine, an alternation with *Carbo vegetabilis* seem desirable, they may be thus exhibited at intervals of from six to twelve hours, according to the urgency of the case; in some instances, where *Arsenicum* does not produce all we could desire, this mode has been adopted with success.*

CINCHONA will be found useful when the more dangerous symptoms have been in a great measure subjugated, but at the same time great weakness remains from the loss of humours; it is also useful when the little nutriment the patient may have partaken of passes off undigested.

ADMINISTRATION. Six globules of the third potency in an ounce of water, a dessert-spoonful every four hours. In those cases where *Arsenicum* and *Carbo vegetabilis* seem to fail, the employment of the Mother Tincture of Rhus, one drop in a tea-spoonful of water every three hours, has, in a number of instances, been found most efficacious.†

CONTAGIOUS FEVER, OR TYPHUS.

Typhus Contagiosus.

DIAGNOSIS. The symptoms of typhus caused by infection or contagion.

THERAPEUTICS. The same as already given under Typhus. We may, however, here remark upon one remedy of especial value in this form of the disease, namely, OPIUM, indicated by drowsiness or coma.—Coma somnolentum, especially,—stertorous breathing, mouth partly open, eyes open or partially closed, loss of speech, rigidity of the limbs, smallness or in-

* It may here be remarked that Gross and others have recently recommended, and are in the habit of administering, *Arsenicum* at extremely high potencies (the 200th and even the 1600th) in typhus and other diseases, when the vital energies seem rapidly sinking. See also "*Potencies of the medicaments*" in the Introduction.

† Many of the remedies, along with the indications for their employment, which have been given in the preceding chapter, will also be found equally appropriate in particular cases or in certain stages of so-called *putrid fever*—the attention of the practitioner is therefore particularly called to them in such circumstances.

termission of the pulse, meteorismus, involuntary evacuations, or constipations.

Administration. We may add six globules of the third potency to an ounce of water: give a dessert-spoonful every three or four hours until a favourable change is observed.

When in addition to the above-named paralytic affection, we find jerkings in individual limbs, we should have recourse to ***Hyoscyamus*** or ***Stramonium***. administered in the same manner, choosing the remedy which most closely approximates to the symptoms we have given for their individual use, under Typhus (p. 30.)

It may be remarked, that whenever the symptoms given under *Opium*, and the other medicines, present themselves in Typhus, *from whatever cause arising*, the remedies are of course indicated.

Accessory Treatment—Prophylaxes, &c.

We need hardly insist upon what every practitioner knows to be essentially adjuvant in the treatment of this affection, a constant supply of fresh and continually renewed air.

Prophylaxes, during the prevalence of Typhus. Cool pure air, thorough ventilation, the avoidance of dark or dismal-looking apartments into which the genial daylight does not freely penetrate; and the removal of all causes generating the disease, such as stopped sewers, or collection of decaying vegetable and animal matter; a plain wholesome diet, with a moderation in the use of fermented liquors or wine, and total abstinence from spirits; refraining from late hours, intense study, and excessive mental or corporeal exertion; exercise in open situations, with proper precautions against exposure to cold or damp; and finally, the preserving a healthy tone of mind and cheerful temper.

The absurd practice of keeping the bowels constantly open by means of aperient medicines, and the use of sudorifics, cannot be too strongly reprobated; both these practices weaken the system, and predispose to the disease.

Standing between a fire or open window and the bed of the patient is to be avoided, as unnecessarily increasing the risk of taking the infection.

The safest plan for the physician to pursue in epidemic or endemic typhus, is to form an aggregate of the symptoms by carefully collating those of individual sufferers, so as to present a perfect image of the existent malady, and to choose his remedies accordingly, which should be administered directly on the premonitory symptoms declaring themselves, without waiting for the further development of the disease.

It may be remarked, that *Bryonia* and *Rhus* cover a great number of the symptoms of typhus, as met with in this country; when, therefore, this point has been ascertained, they may be given alternately, BRYONIA $\frac{00}{6}$ and RHUS $\frac{00}{3}$ each in one dose, at intervals of twenty-four hours, which will often either check the malady at its outset, or materially modify its virulence—in some cases one of these remedies is of itself sufficient, according to the leading symptoms of the reigning epidemic; in a great variety of instances, ARSENICUM may prove a valuable *prophylaxis*; but at the same time, the indications we have already given of the several medicaments should be carefully consulted, as the same rule holds good for them all.

INTERMITTENT FEVERS—AGUE.

Febres Intermittentes.

We have now to enter upon a class of fevers differing essentially from those already considered, in possessing a marked character of their own, in the simplicity of their form, the periodicity of the different stages, and the uncertainty of their duration.

DIAGNOSIS. A chill or cold fit, followed by heat, and terminating by perspiration, more or less profuse; these three stages constitute a paroxysm; after which for a certain period, called the *Apyrexia*, the patient is generally free from suffering.

These periods are generally of definite duration;—if the paroxysms return at regular intervals of *twenty-four* hours, the fever is termed a Quotidian; of *forty-eight*, a Tertian; of *seventy-two*, a Quartan; even longer intervals have been observed between the attacks; hence the Octanæ of some writers,—if two paroxysms take place within each period, the ague is said to be doubled, as a double Quotidian or Tertian.

These fevers are sometimes found existing in the simple form above noted, and at others complicated with other forms of disease, as in intermittent catarrhal or gastric fevers.

They are exceedingly indefinite in duration, and frequently assume a chronic form. An individual once attacked with ague is frequently liable to a return in after-life, if the disease has not been radically cured at the commencement; nay more, any attacks of disease he may be hereafter subjected to, are peculiarly apt to assume the intermittent form.

Nervous or inflammatory fever may change into an intermittent, or the latter take upon itself, if it continue, the character of either of the two former, or become remittent; this frequently happens in hot climates.

Ague is rarely dangerous in this country, except when of long continuance, by the weakness it occasions and the injury it inflicts upon the constitution; it may, however, lead to obstructions and indurations of the more important viscera, particularly of the liver and spleen, or induce dropsical affections.

But in hot climates or in low marshy countries, this disease is exceedingly fatal; and on dissection, the brain and its tissues, the mucous coat of the stomach and bowels, the lungs and peritoneum, have been found affected; in such instances, when the disease gains ground, the patient loses strength and becomes emaciated, every fresh paroxysm entails an increase of suffering, and the perspiration fails to relieve; he complains of a sense of weight in the hypochondria, particularly the right, with griping pain in the bowels, flatulent distention of the abdomen, diarrhæa, or constipation, and constant thirst; or of headache, cough, and dyspnœa: the tongue is furred, and dry at the tip; the skin hot, harsh, and dry; the urine scanty, the abdomen tumid, the extremities become dropsical, and sleep is restless or broken.

Death may ensue from collapse in the cold stage, the absence of perspiration, and the disease passing into continued or remittent fever, or from disorganization of some important function, such as the brain, lungs, spleen, or liver.

We shall now proceed to a general consideration of the three stages of the disease, premising that the various modifications of the symptoms will be found more in detail under the medicaments when we enter into the therapeutic treatment.

Premonitory symptoms. Sense of languor, or general uneasiness; yawning, headache, stupor, pains in the limbs or dorsal region, the toes and fingers becoming numb, and the nails blue.

Cold Stage. Coldness of the extremities, with a feeling as of a stream of cold water running down the back, and extending itself to the chest and abdomen; general prostration of strength, insupportable coldness, external and internal tremors, chattering of the teeth, respiration laboured and hurried, with inability to draw a full inspiration, and oppression at the chest. The head is variously affected, sometimes with headache, at others with coma, stupor, or delirium; the pain noticed in the premonitory symptoms are generally present, and in some instances the patient complains of pain all over; the tongue is moist, the eyes are heavy and sunken, the features pinched, and the lips and cheeks livid; the rigors sometimes run on to convulsions.

The pulse is weak and oppressed, sometimes slow, at others quick, and frequently intermitting, and often, from the severity of the rigors, scarcely perceptible.

The heat of the body, except at the extremities, is generally above the natural standard, while the patient complains of cold.

Sometimes the patient feels only a slight degree of cold, without tremors, but accompanied with symptoms of functional derangement, and in a few hours the hot fit declares itself. The duration of the cold stage is from an hour to four hours; and it runs into the hot without any marked interval.

The *Hot Stage* presents all the characteristics of a modified inflammatory attack, with hot, dry skin, and thirst, oppression at the chest, hurried and anxious breathing, and acute pain in the head, region of the spleen, liver, &c.; there is also occasionally a degree of cerebral disturbance, or even delirium.

The general duration of the hot fit is from four to twelve hours, when it terminates in the sweating stage; when this does not take place, it is apt to run on to continuous fever, or take the form of a remittent,—a not uncommon issue of this disease in warm climates.

Sweating Stage. After the hot fit has continued a longer or shorter period, profuse perspiration sets in, commencing in the forehead and extremities, and quickly diffusing itself over the whole body; as soon as it makes its appearance, the uneasiness and other symptoms begin to disappear, and the patient, in simple ague, continues free from suffering until the next paroxysm.

Causes. Marshy districts are noted as being the hot-beds of this malady; a continuance of fish or farinaceous diet is also apt to produce it; it may, moreover, arise from taking cold, indigestion, internal obstructions, peculiar constitutional tendency, or local irritation.

The medicines should generally be administered in the apyrexia or interval between the paroxysms.

Therapeutics. The following remedies have been found most appropriate in ordinary cases of this affection:

Cinchona, Arsenicum, Ipecacuanha, Nux vomica, Pulsatilla, Antimonium crudum, Bryonia, Veratrum album, Cocculus, Sabadilla, Ignatia, and Carbo vegetabilis.

Cinchona. This well-known but too frequently abused remedy, is undoubtedly of the greatest efficacy in those fevers which owe their origin to the influence of marsh miasm, and are peculiarly prevalent at particular seasons of the year. It may be given as soon as the *precursory symptoms* manifest themselves, when we find a degree of fever, with anxiety, palpitation of the heart, headache, sneezing, great thirst, bulimy, or nausea, and pain in the bowels. It is also indicated when the fever has set in by adypsia *during* the cold stage—but thirst AFTER the heat and *during* the sweating. It is *contra-indicated* when thirst exists *during* the hot stage.

ADMINISTRATION. When properly selected, a single dose of this medicine (three or four globules of the third potency) will generally remove the fever; but in other cases frequent repetitions and still lower potencies will sometimes be found necessary.*

ARSENICUM is indicated when the different stages are not definitely marked, but the fever, and heat, and shivering, appear simultaneously—or we find cold shuddering alternately with heat, or a sensation of cold internally, with heat, or an *imperfect development* of the paroxysms ; or burning heat, as if molten lead were coursing through the veins, communicating an unpleasant sensation of heat (*calor mordax*) to the hand when placed upon the body of the patient—great restlessness ; and excessive, almost *insatiable thirst*, obliging the sufferer to drink constantly, although but little at a time; depression, *marked prostration of strength* and anxiety; nausea, desire to vomit, retching, and even vomiting; severe and burning pains in the stomach, and insupportable pains all over the body, especially in the limbs.

A marked characteristic of *Arsenicum* is, that all the sufferings of the patient, pains in the limbs, &c., increase in intensity *during* the paroxysm, and others develop themselves ; another is, its marked *periodicity*, generally either Tertian or Quartan, and the rigors generally setting in towards evening.

It is therefore called for in these cases where we meet with *a well-marked periodicity of imperfectly developed paroxysms*, with some or any of the symptoms above mentioned.

ADMINISTRATION. Of this medicament $\frac{000}{6}$ given during the apyrexia, will be generally found a sufficient dose ; however, in some cases, when the vital energies of the patient

* Vide note, p. 21.

seem insufficient to rally, and the cold fit continues, *two drops* of the tincture of the third potency may be added to an ounce of water, and a dessert-spoonful given every four or two hours, or every twenty minutes, according to the exigency of the case. Such cases are happily rare in this country, but I have thought it advisable to touch upon the means to be employed when they do occur; in such instances also *Veratrum* (which see) is occasionally useful.*

IPECACUANHA. This remedy will be found useful in most cases of this affection, for although it may not always prove competent to the entire removal of the complaint, yet when administered at the commencement it rarely fails to prove of considerable benefit, and in many instances, when judiciously selected, it of itself performs a cure,—the most marked results have been derived from its ADMINISTRATION with *Nux vomica* in the following mode: exhibit IPECACUANHA $\frac{0\,0\,0}{3}$ in a little water, and repeat the dose in three hours; NUX VOMICA $\frac{0\,0\,0}{6}$ twelve hours after, and if possible, in the evening. Should, however, the apyrexia take place towards evening, lengthen the intervals, giving the *Ipecacuanha* every five hours, allowing twelve hours to intervene, and administering the *Nux vomica* in the evening, and if the attack be quotidian, repeating the latter medicine in the apyrexia preceding it.

Either of these remedies is of itself sometimes found sufficient to shorten the duration of the disease; the indications for IPECACUANHA are as follows: much shivering, with but little heat, or vice versâ; *increase of the shivering by external warmth*; oppression at the precordial region; *adypsia*, or at least, little thirst; dryness of the mouth, nausea, vomiting, and other symptoms of deranged digestion.

For NUX VOMICA. Giddiness, with feeling in the head as if from intoxication, desire to lie down, with trembling of the limbs, or a feeling of a paralytic weakness and prostration, with cramps in the different extremities, particularly the calves of the legs and feet, difficulty of breathing, anxiety, irascibility, fear of death, and even slight delirium; gastric derangements, such as anorexia; dislike to bread; bitter and

* Vide note, p. 37.

sour eructations, tension of the abdomen, or spasms of the abdominal muscles, and constipation. *During the fever:* Coldness and blueness of the skin, desire to be constantly covered, even during the access of heat and perspiration; occasionally stitches in the side, shooting pains in the abdomen, aching in back and limbs, and *dragging* pain in abdomen during the rigors. During the *hot fit* particularly, headache, buzzing in the ears, heat in head, face, with redness of the cheeks, and thirst.

Administration. In most cases the dose before mentioned will be found sufficient; but when the disease is violent, a few globules or a drop at the third potency may be added to an ounce of water, and a dessert-spoonful taken every night to the day a return is expected.

Pulsatilla, like the two remedies last mentioned and *Antimonium crudum, Bryonia* and *Ignatia*, is an excellent remedy in Agues complicated with gastric or bilious symptoms, whenever the slightest dyspeptic attack brings on a relapse; its more peculiar indications are: adypsia all through the fever, or thirst *only* during the hot fit; simultaneous heat and shivering—aggravated *in the afternoon or towards evening;* shivering when uncovered; anxiety and oppression of the chest during the shivering. *During the hot stage,* redness and swelling of the face, or redness of the cheeks only, and perspiration on the face. The presence of diarrhœa, and the patient being of a mild disposition, are corroborative indications for its employment.

Administration. In ordinary cases $\frac{000}{6}$ may be given in a dessert-spoonful of water during the apyrexia; in very severe attacks, a few globules, or a drop or so of the third potency, may be added to an ounce of water, and a dessert-spoonful given every six or twelve hours during the same period; in some instances, it will be sufficient to give a dose about three hours before the expected attack.

Antimonium crudum. The indications for this remedy closely resemble those of Pulsatilla, but it is particularly called for when *the perspiration breaks out simultaneously with the accesses of heat, and then suddenly disappears, leaving the skin dry and hot.* It may be exhibited at the same potency and the same manner as *Pulsatilla.*

Bryonia is indicated by headache and vertigo, with dry heat preceding the attacks of shivering; by the predominance of cold or shivering, with redness of the cheeks, heat in the head, and headache; or marked heat followed by shivering; by stitches in the side, excessive thirst, thickly coated tongue, bitter taste in the mouth, disgust at the sight of food, nausea or vomiting, and constipation.

Administration. Bryonia may be exhibited at the same potency and in the same manner as Nux vomica, (which see,) with the distinction of administering it when practicable in the morning, instead of at night.

Veratrum album is indicated by the predominance of *external coldness, with heat internally, cold clammy* perspiration, especially on the forehead, or general coldness of the whole body; or by shivering followed by heat and perspiration, and then relapsing into shivering; coldness, great thirst, deep-coloured urine, diarrhœa with griping, or constipation; sometimes nausea or vomiting and vertigo, and pains in the dorsal and lumbar regions.

Administration. This medicament may be exhibited in the same manner as *Arsenicum,* if the cold fit continues beyond the usual time; or may be had recourse to either singly or in alternation with that medicine, as circumstances may point out.

Cocculus $\frac{000}{6}$ in a little water, at the customary period, when, in addition to the usual symptoms of Ague, we find during the apyrexia, symptoms of spasmodic affections, particularly of the stomach and abdomen, such as cramp-like pains at the epigastrium, or constrictive pinching, or tearing, burning, colic-like pains in the hypogastrium.

Sabadilla has been found useful in cases where the attacks return always at the same hour, with chills of short duration, then thirst followed by heat; also where thirst is present just at the close of the cold stage, and in such affections as consist entirely of chills.

Administration $\frac{000}{3}$ as given under *Arsenicum.*

IGNATIA is indicated when with heat of some parts of the body there is coldness, chill, and shuddering of others, also where the heat is only external. Its best characteristic is, when the chills are *easily relieved by external warmth, and attended with thirst.*

ADMINISTRATION, $\frac{000}{6}$ at the same potency and in the same manner as *Pulsatilla.*

CARBO VEGETABILIS, in constitutions with a peculiar morbid tendency, will be found a most useful remedy. It is particularly indicated when thirst is present *only* during the shivering; and there are rheumatic pains in the teeth or limbs before or during the attack, nausea, giddiness, redness of the face during the hot fit.

ADMINISTRATION. $\frac{000}{12}$ may be dissolved in a little water, and given morning and evening during the apyrexia.

When the hot-fit continues long without perspiration supervening, and the intermittent threatens to change into a remittent or inflammatory fever, we must have immediate recourse to ACONITE, of which we may give $\frac{00}{6}$, and if no relief follows in three or four hours, add six globules of the third potency to an ounce of water, and administer a dessert-spoonful every hour until perspiration sets in, or the pulse is reduced.

Arsenicum, Carbo vegetabilis, and *Lachesis*, are three of the most important remedies against intermittent fevers which return every year.

The preceding are the medicines that have been found useful in ordinary cases of this affection; but as the disease is frequently found complicated with other complaints, it has only been found practicable to give a general statement of the course to be pursued when met with in its more simple forms, and merely to allude to the others—there being scarcely a disease known that may not assume the intermittent type, as there *is scarcely a proved medicine that does not also partake of the same character.* All the author has endeavoured to do, in the preceding pages, is to give a clear idea of the treatment of ague, commonly so called, as frequently met with; as he feels it would be vain to attempt to enter upon the many various forms and appearances which this malady presents.

ERUPTIVE FEVERS.

UNDER this head, I intend to treat of those diseases possessing the common property of febrile symptoms, preceding an eruption which is present during a part of their course, that eruption varying in character according to the nature of the affection.

In this class are comprised scarlet fever, purples, measles, small-pox, chicken-pox, miliary fever, and nettle-rash.

SCARLET FEVER.

This disease, in its simple generic character, consists of a contagious fever, with swelling of the face and a scarlet appearance of the skin—(hence its name)—which is of a bright raspberry colour, or of a hue resembling a boiled lobster, *smooth and glossy*, upon which the finger being pressed leaves a white imprint, which almost immediately disappears. However, in the present day, we seldom meet with it in this simple form, but more frequently complicated with severe or ulcerated sore throat, delirium, congestive or violent inflammatory symptoms, and often with more or less deviation from the characteristic efflorescence above described.

DIAGNOSIS. Fever with extreme quickness of pulse; a feeling of soreness or pain in the throat; and in one or more days, the appearance of an eruption of the colour above mentioned, in large indefinitely marked patches, gradually growing paler towards their margins, and often extending over entire limbs with an uniform scarlet colour; the efflorescence disappears in five or six days, when the skin desquamates, and comes off in large pieces.

We sometimes find scarlet fever with scarce any, or even no external redness, but at the same time marked angina and bright redness of the tongue; in such cases the disease, instead of showing itself on the skin, has fixed upon the mucous membrane; end even the angina and redness of the tongue present in most cases of this disease may be considered as an internal scarlatina.

Scarlatina was formerly confounded with measles, from the resemblance which the two eruptions bear to each other at their commencement; but they are easily distinguishable, even without taking into consideration the peculiar appearance of the skin above mentioned—characteristic of the disease,—by the eruption in scarlet fever generally developing itself in from twenty-four to forty-eight hours from the commencement of the fever, whereas that of measles rarely sets in before the third or fifth day; and moreover by the absence of catarrhal symptoms, such as cough, sneezing, lachrymation, the usual precursors of measles. The greatly accelerated pulse, which denotes the approach of scarlatina, is also never met with to the same extent in any other disease.

THERAPEUTICS. In those cases in which it appears in its simple form, BELLADONNA is a specific remedy. We may dissolve four globules of the sixth potency in four teaspoonfuls of water, and administer one every six or even three hours, if the fever run high, lengthening the intervals as it decreases in intensity, only repeating when a cessation of the amelioration takes place. We ought to watch carefully after each administration, for if the fever increases soon after, we may conclude it is a medicinal action, and avoid aggravating it by a repetition of the dose.*

The next form which we shall treat of is, when the scarlatina becomes a severe and dangerous disease, when the throat is considerably affected (*Scarlatina anginosa*), and high fever or congestive symptoms set in, which, if not properly treated, may assume the malignant type (*Scarlatina maligna*), attended with ulcerated sore throat, extension of the inflammation to the air-passages, delirium, spasm, &c. (Vide ULCERATED SORE THROAT.)

The fever and sore throat increase with the eruption in mild cases, and cease with its decline; but in the more severe, con-

* Vide note, page 21.

tinue; it is when the disease appears principally to attack the head, throat, thoracic or abdominal viscera, that it becomes dangerous.* The eruption frequently does not appear before the third day, and then only in isolated patches:

BELLADONNA should therefore be administered as soon as the throat and tongue become affected with dryness and burning; and there is desire, but complete inability, to swallow even drinks or saliva, with sense of suffocation; further, when the throat presents a *bright-red* appearance, sometimes excoriated, with white specks, *or* stringy mucus, *or* appearance like thrush; tonsils swollen, and the tongue of a *bright fiery red*, sometimes interspersed with dark red patches, but generally appearing later in the disease, if at all; also when delirium is present.

ADMINISTRATION. We should dissolve six globules of the third in six teaspoonfuls of water, and exhibit a teaspoonful every four hours; to a child under twelve years of age, $\frac{0}{6}$ in a teaspoonful of water repeated as above, which will generally be sufficient to bring about a speedy amelioration.

If the disease have taken a favourable turn, we may allow the *Belladonna to continue its action*;† but if we *clearly* perceive an appearance of *ulceration commencing*, with increase of mucus, and swelling of the throat and tongue, we must have immediate recourse to MERCURIUS.

ADMINISTRATION. One grain of the third trituration in six dessert-spoonfuls of water, one dessert-spoonful every four hours; but when the ulcers present a livid appearance about the edges, and emit an offensive odour; or when there is excessive thirst, with great dryness of the mouth, and *extreme prostration of strength*, we must exhibit ARSENICUM $\frac{000}{6}$ in a little water, every four or six hours, according to the effect produced, and follow it with NUX VOMICA $\frac{000}{6}$, in the same manner, if the former prove inadequate to complete the cure. (Vide ULCERATED SORE THROAT.)

* When scarlatina anginosa occurs in complication with pneumonia, phrenitis, or enteritis, the remedies mentioned under these different heads must be had recourse to.

† See the article on the "*Administration of the remedy*" in the Introduction.

When the fever assumes a clearly inflammatory type, and the pulse runs high, we may administer ACONITE,* at the same potency and in the same manner as already given under *Inflammatory Fever*, which see.

When the quickness of pulse and other inflammatory febrile symptoms are subdued, and the affection of the throat again appears prominent, we may return to *Belladonna*, especially if the skin retain the peculiar scarlatina hue.

OPIUM may follow the administration of *Belladonna* when there is burning heat of the skin, drowsiness, stupor, stertorous breathing, open mouth, eyes half closed, restlessness with vomiting, or convulsions.

ADMINISTRATION. Six globules of the tincture of the third potency, added to an ounce of water, a dessert-spoonful every four hours; if, however, a marked improvement follow the first dose, we may allow the remedy to continue its action.

We may here notice a remedy which has been found particularly efficacious in a peculiar affection of the brain, that frequently declares itself in cases of repercussed exanthemata, and which if not speedily checked, may terminate in paralysis of that organ. We shall therefore treat of this remedy here, and refer to this place, when we may hereafter have occasion to allude to it. The discovery of its value in such cases is

* ANTIMONIUM TARTARICUM. The indications for Tartar emetic, according to Dr. Gray, are: a soporose condition from which the patient does not of itself fully arouse, and when awakened by the attendant, answers correctly without confusion or delirium; intense heat with nausea or spasmodic jerks or general convulsions, and varying colour of the skin from pallor to deep redness, with imperfect patchy development of the eruption. The occurrence of sweat around the mouth, with pallor of the perspiring parts, increases the balance in favour of the Antimony. The Doctor gives it when Aconite proves unavailing, the indications for the latter being present.

Our own views and results fully corroborate those of Dr. Gray.

Dr. George W. Cook strongly commends the Antimony in his essay on Scarlet fever (Homœopathic Examiner, new Series, p. 133, vol. I.). He presents the following indications for its use: convulsions which often precede the cutaneous efflorescence, colliquative diarrhœa, cold clammy skin, hurried respiration, hippocratic countenance, hoarse voice, retchings and vomiting of glairy mucus.—ED.

due to Dr. Schmid of Vienna, whose formula for its exhibition we shall give herewith.

Cuprum aceticum. When the eruption during efflorescence is suddenly repercussed, the result of which is frequently fatal, this medicament may be almost considered *specific;* or at least the substance with which the greatest degree of certainty can savė the patient; if in this condition death should happen, it is in consequence of paralysis of the brain.

Symptoms indicating its employment: Quick, small, weak irregular pulse; temperature of the skin considerably reduced, in more severe cases chilly, and covered with perspiration. *Affections of the nervous system are never absent;* to this belong convulsive movements of various parts of the body, distortion of the eyes, face, mouth, head, &c., spasmodic affection of the chest, sometimes even eclampsia; as well as great restlessness, frequent change of position, sopor, delirium, &c.

It displays its efficacy in reproducing the eruption, when the cerebral affection disappears, and the disease runs its usual course.

Formula. One grain of the Cuprum aceticum triturated with one hundred, one hundred and fifty, or two hundred grains of sugar of milk previously triturated so as to feel as fine as flour; the process should occupy from twenty to thirty minutes. Of this preparation take from three to four grains, dissolve in a tumbler of pure water, and administer in table-spoonfuls, every quarter, half, one, or two hours, according to the violence of the disease.*

Pulsatilla, when derangement of the stomach and digestive organs is a prominent symptom, the face pale, red, or bloated; also constipation—or looseness, especially at night,—occasionally with pains in the bowels, and shivering; disposition fretful and sensitive, or melancholy.

Administration. We may exhibit to an adult $\frac{000}{6}$, and

* The remarks made on this medicine are taken from the translation of Dr. Schmid's paper on the subject, in that excellent and useful medical periodical, the British Journal of Homœopathy, No. III., page 233, to which the reader desirous of further information is referred.

repeat in six hours if no improvement takes place; to a child, one globule of the same potency.

We frequently find this affection in a complicated form, distinguishable from pure scarlet fever by the absence of the peculiar hue of the skin, of which we have spoken at the commencement, and by the pressure of the finger leaving no white imprint. This so widely different type of the disorder will be found treated of in the succeeding chapter, under the denomination of *Purpura miliaris* or *Scarlatina miliaris.*

In strumous habits, or in instances when the disease has been allopathically treated from the commencement, many troublesome sequelæ are frequently left. And we may remark, that even after the desquamatory process is completed, the whole of the danger is not altogether passed, any exposure to cold or infringement of dietetic rules being likely to entail unpleasant and even dangerous consequences.

CHAMOMILLA may be employed with advantage, either alone or alternately with Belladonna against rawness of the face, &c.

ADMINISTRATION. Six globules of the sixth or third potency in six dessert-spoonfuls of water, one twice a day.

AURUM. Against the offensive and purulent discharge from the nose with soreness and swelling of the interior.

ADMINISTRATION. $\frac{oooo}{6}$ in half an ounce of water, a teaspoonful taken morning and evening.

MERCURIUS VIVUS against soreness of the nose and face with swelling of the submaxillary glands; followed by Hepar sulphuris, Silicea, Sulphur, and Calcarea if necessary.

ADMINISTRATION. Half a grain of the third trituration in six dessert-spoonfuls of water, one three times a day.

Against the following, *Belladonna* is extremely efficacious: Puffiness of the face, swelling of the hands and feet, lingering fever in the evening, glandular enlargements, chaps about the mouth, severe headaches, stammering, &c.; and may frequently be advantageously alternated with the medicines just mentioned.

Dropsical swellings of the whole body is not an unfrequent

sequela, sometimes requiring a most careful and discriminating treatment. The following remedies will generally be found the best adapted to the successful treatment of the same: *Helleborus*, *Arsenicum*, *Belladonna*, and, in obstinate cases: *Arnica*, *Bryonia*, *Phosphoric acid*, *Digitalis Baryta m.*, *Sulph.*, *Lycopod.* Against Otitis, or Otorrhœa: *Belladonna*, *Hepar sulphuris* or *Pulsatilla* :—and in the case of Boils, *Arnica* followed by *Bryonia* and *Sulphur* when necessary :—Deafness, *Belladonna*, *Pulsatilla*, *Dulcamara*, *Sulphur*, chiefly.

Scarlet fever is chiefly dangerous when a latent constitutional virus is called into activity, and associates itself with the disease; in such cases, the allopathist finds himself baffled by an evil against which he possesses no specific remedy, and the utmost skill of the homœopathic practitioner is called into play. Such, it is evident, are far beyond the sphere of a work of this nature:

We may, however, remark, that *Ammonium carbonicum*, *Arsenicum*, *Secale cornutum*, and *Acidum phosphoricum*, have been found very useful in scarlatina when it assumes the typhoid form; and *Arsenicum* in frequently repeated doses,—or *Acidum nitricum*, *Aconitum*, *Lycopodium* and *Belladonna* alternately, a dose of each remedy being given every hour, or oftener if necessary, to rouse the vital force to new efforts, for several successive hours,—in the severe and dangerous *sore-throat* which accompanies malignant scarlatina; the amygdalæ being swollen into hard tumours, often as large as apples, with difficult, snorting, breathing, enlargement of the neighbouring glands, remitting pulse, and sopor.

Belladonna is valuable as a preservative against *pure* scarlatina when epidemic, and moreover greatly assists in modifying the character of the disease, in such individuals as do not wholly escape its attacks; with children $\frac{00}{12}$, in a teaspoonful of water, and with adults, or robust children above ten years of age, $\frac{00}{6}$ every three or four days, for from two to three weeks at farthest, which will generally be found sufficient to obviate any risk; should the disease continue to rage, the treatment may in some instances be renewed: if the ruling epidemic be scarlatina in a complicated form, that is, not possessing the clear scarlatina hue, we should alternate this medicine with Aconite, one or two globules of the 6th potency, according to the age, allowing the *Aconite* an action of about twelve hours, and afterwards proceeding with the *Belladonna* as before. While taking these medicaments, the patient must adhere strictly to the homœopathic diet, particularly avoiding *wine* and *acids*. *We must, in administering prophylaxes, carefully watch their effects, and if a medicinal action set in, discontinue immediately.*

Diet. During the course of this malady, the greatest possible attention must be paid to this point. In the more severe accesses of fever, no other nourishment must be given than toast-water or weak barley-water; and after the fever has abated, every care must be taken, and a return be gradually made to a more nourishing diet, as negligence in this respect may be productive of the most serious consequences. In mild attacks the patient may be allowed gruel or weak broths.

PURPURA RUBRA *s.* MILIARIS HAHNEMANNI.

Scarlatina miliaris. Miliaria purpurea.

SCARLET-RASH.

This affection is sometimes met with in complication with smallpox, measles, and scarlet fever, more particularly the latter, of which disease, indeed, it is regarded by many as a mere modification.

It is easily distinguishable from pure scarlet fever, by the dark redness of the efflorescence, by the slight pressure of the finger leaving no white imprint, and by the small granular elevations, the cause of the dark red hue, which are felt on passing the hand over the affected cutaneous surface.

This eruptive fever does not run a defined and regular course, like other exanthematic fevers. The efflorescence often disappears suddenly, and is then productive of extreme danger, frequently terminating in a fatal result. The extent of the efflorescence does necessarily add to the danger, as the latter is often greatest when the efflorescence is scarcely perceptible.

Sweat is only met with on the surfaces affected with the eruption, and it is consequently only when the eruption covers the whole body that the sweat is general.

Those who have been affected with the disorder are by no means exempt from future attacks. Soreness of the throat is chiefly encountered when the eruption is altogether wanting, but it is also frequently met with before the outbreak of the rash, becomes trivial during the full bloom, and again very severe on the disappearance of the same.

This disease, dissimilar though it be to the true scarlatina, has yet been frequently confounded with it by careless observers. It requires a totally different treatment, and Belladonna, the specific in scarlatina simplex, will in this case neither be found to be a preventive nor an indispensable curative remedy, but simply an auxiliary in some complicated cases.

Aconitum. When the disorder occurs in an idiopathic form, there are few exceptions in which any other remedy but Aconite is required for the entire removal of the disorder. In administering it, we may dissolve three globules of the sixth potency in as many teaspoonfuls of water, and give a teaspoonful every three or four hours. Sometimes it is found necessary to administer a dose of *Coffea* ($\frac{000}{3}$) a few hours after the first or second dose of *Aconite*, when the patient complains of severe pain in the head, trunk, or extremities, and is extremely restless, fretful, agitated, and disposed to shed tears; and then again to return to *Aconite*, after a similar interval; and so on, alternately, until the cure is completed; which, under favourable circumstances, is speedily accomplished by means of these remedies.

When, however, this eruptive fever occurs in complication with scarlatina, smallpox, or measles; or when it breaks out in unfavourable seasons, during the prevalence of one or more of the said exanthemata, it generally becomes a much more serious disorder, and requires the aid of other remedies in addition to the above mentioned Amongst these: *Ipecacuanha, Pulsatilla, Bryonia, Dulcamara, Belladonna, Arsenicum, Phosphorus*, and *Rhus*, are the most important, preceded by *Aconite*, when symptoms of inflammatory fever, or the following, present themselves: Slight, general fever chills, with rapidly alternating redness and paleness of the face; quick, full pulse; slight confusion of ideas, increasing to a mild degree of delirium at night, combined with dryness of the mouth and lips, and thirst; eyes somewhat inflamed; oppression at the chest, short cough, sometimes attended with reddish sputa, and followed by a shooting pain under the ribs; occasional vomiting; *angina pharyngea*. In such cases, then, a dose or two of Aconite, at intervals of four hours, will be found of considerable service, if not sufficient to put a check to the further progress of the affection.

Ipecacuanha $\frac{000000}{3}$. In many instances, either at the commencement of the attack, *before* the appearance of the eruption, or during its full development, but particularly the former, this is a most efficient remedy. It is indicated when there is a sensation of *distressing tightness of the chest*, with laborious breathing, and heightening of the febrile action towards evening; with symptoms of nausea, or even vomiting; extreme restlessness and agitation; deep sighing, or moaning; disposition to tearfulness or whining in children; diarrhœa, colic.

When the oppression at the chest and excessive restlessness have been removed by *Ipecacuanha*, but considerable nausea or frequent fits of vomiting remain, *Pulsatilla* will generally put an early termination to the latter.

Bryonia $\frac{000000}{6}$, is frequently more efficacious than either *Coffea* or *Ipecacuanha* in relieving the extreme anxiety, restlessness, deep sighing and moaning, which so generally attend this affection; it should therefore be had recourse to in all cases in which these remedies fail to afford speedy relief. In some rare cases even *Bryonia* is not sufficient, and it is then found necessary to administer *Cinchona*, followed by *Phosphorus*. *Bryonia* is further indicated when the accompanying fever partakes of a nervous character, attended with delirium and other symptoms mentioned under *Bryonia* in the article on

Nervous fever—which see. The excessive and continual urging to urinate, which sometimes sets in, in the course of the disease, is often very readily subdued by *Bryonia* or by *Conium*.

BELLADONNA $\frac{000000}{6}$. When the disorder is met with during the prevalence of Scarlatina, (as also when symptoms more or less characteristic of the latter affection make their appearance in the course of purpura miliaris,) this remedy is a most efficient auxiliary; it is, moreover, a most important remedy when symptoms of cerebral disturbance exhibit themselves; or when the patient complains of the throat, which, on being examined, is found to be in a state of phlegmonous inflammation. *Mercurius* may follow *Belladonna* when the tonsils become much inflamed and tumefied, or ulceration supervenes; in this latter instance, however, *Arsenicum* or *Acid. nitricum* may become necessary under particular circumstances. (Vide SCARLATINA, p. 47; SORE THROAT, p. 84; and SCARLATINA MALIGNA, p. 50.)

PHOSPHORUS $\frac{000000}{6}$. This remedy is very useful in cases in which there are symptoms of congestion in the chest, with extreme anxiety and oppression, and also when there is considerable cerebral irritability, characterized by over-excitability of the senses; further, when the patient appears extremely listless and apathetic, and complains of burning sensations in isolated parts, causing a frequent change of posture necessary. Phosphorus is often of great utility after Bryonia or Belladonna.

DULCAMARA $\frac{000000}{6}$. When severe aching or gnawing (rheumatic) pains are complained of in the back or extremities, either in the course of the disease or at its termination, and when, in addition, there is an apparent complication of Scarlatina with this affection, *Dulcamara* should be administered.

ARSENICUM $\frac{000000}{6}$, may be had recourse to in any advanced stage of the complaint if the vital power seems rapidly sinking, and the organs which perform the act of deglutition are as it were paralyzed, so that the patient is incapacitated from swallowing; or when, from a metastasis to the throat, the latter has become so rapidly and seriously affected, as to have assumed a gangrenous aspect. (See ULCERATED SORE THROAT.)

When the disease, in cases of a bad type, takes on a nervous or even a putrid character, with extreme offensiveness of all the excretions, and hemorrhage from the nose, mouth, &c. The medicines mentioned under fevers of the said description, (which see, p. 32,) must here also be employed. *Cuprum aceticum* and *Kreosote* have been found useful in some of these almost hopeless but fortunately somewhat rare cases; the former particularly, when the efflorescence appears and disappears suddenly in the course of the disease.*

ADMINISTRATION. Six globules of the remedy indicated, at the potency mentioned, may be dissolved in about an ounce of water, and one dessert-spoonful administered every three, four, or six hours, according to the urgency of the case.

The remedies required for the occasional sequelæ, are the same as those enumerated at the conclusion of the chapter on Scarlatina.

MEASLES. *Rubeola.*

This disease generally reigns as an infectious epidemic, and for the most part confines its attack to children, in which cases it is seldom, when properly treated, either severe or dangerous; when it occurs in adults it generally assumes a more critical character. It rarely attacks an individual a second time.

Measles is not to be so much dreaded for itself, as for the deleterious consequences it, under an improper mode of treatment, frequently entails, or to use the technical term, the *dregs* it leaves after it, in many constitutions developing an inherent disposition to consumption.

* *Rhus* and *Sulphur* may also be mentioned as having been found useful in this disorder; the former when the exanthema degenerated into a species of vesicular erysipelas, attended with lethargy, great thirst, and strangury; and the latter in cases where *Belladonna* had failed to effect all that could be expected. In the event of repercussion of the eruption, *Bryonia, Phosphorus, Sulphur,* and *Cuprum aceticum,* have been recommended as the most useful.

Diagnosis. *Catarrhal symptoms,* such as short dry cough, lachrymation, with redness of the eyes, and a degree of fever, more or less marked, preceding the eruption from three to five days, and generally continuing as long after, or all through the disease.

Eruption of a number of small red spots (frequently papular), the skin in the intervals between them generally preserving its natural colour, and sometimes exhibiting a faint reddish hue. We often find them in the shape of small irregular arcs. They for the most part make their first appearance on the face and neck, become confluent, and extend themselves gradually downwards over the rest of the frame. About the sixth or seventh day from the time of sickening, the eruption begins to turn pale on the face, and afterwards on the rest of the body, and generally entirely disappears about the ninth day, with a *bran-like* desquamation of the epidermis, a distinguishing sign of this disease.

Aconite has been regarded, in some instances, as almost specific against measles, and in its mild form will frequently be found sufficient, in a few doses, to conquer the disease, or at least materially to shorten its duration; it is particularly indicated when the fever assumes an inflammatory form, attended with dry heat of the skin, heat in the head, with confusion and giddiness, redness of the eyes, intolerance of light, general weakness or prostration; and is more or less useful throughout the course of the disease, either alone or in alternation with *Pulsatilla,* or any of the other remedies which may be better indicated, whenever marked febrile or inflammatory action becomes prominent. (*Coffea* or *Hepar* are frequently useful after *Aconite,* when there is a distressing, dry cough.)

Administration. $\frac{00}{6}$, or to very young children $\frac{0}{6}$, in a teaspoonful of water, every twelve hours; or in severe cases, exhibit it as under Inflammatory Fever, (which see,) and continue the treatment till we find an amelioration, should none of the symptoms hereafter mentioned, indicate the necessity of having recourse to another remedy.

Pulsatilla is also very efficacious, and even specific, in this disease, and is frequently indicated in the commencement, from the strong resemblance which some of its pathogenetic * properties bear to the *catarrh* attendant upon measles, together with the characteristic exacerbation of the symptoms towards evening, &c. † This remedy is moreover of great utility in bringing out the eruption when it is longer than usual in making its appearance; but whilst the fever is high, *Aconitum* must be administered; and if the febrile irritation does not diminish after a dose or two of *Aconitum*, *Sulphur* may be given; after which, if the fever return with increased force, *Aconitum* will rarely fail to answer our expectations.

When there is great oppression at the chest, before the eruption is evolved, a dose or two of *Ipecacuanha* is very useful.

ADMINISTRATION. Of *Pulsatilla* $\frac{000}{3}$ in an ounce of water, giving a dessert-spoonful every four hours while the same indications continue, until amelioration sets in. *Pulsatilla* is also valuable when any gastric derangement is present, or when the cough which so generally accompanies the disease, is worse *towards evening* or in the *night*, and is attended with considerable mucous ronchus, or copious, thick, yellowish or whitish expectoration, sometimes followed by vomiting, or symptoms of threatening suffocation; further when there is coryza with a thick yellowish or greenish nasal discharge. (*Sulphur* is frequently of considerable service after Pulsatilla, particularly in strumous subjects.)

BELLADONNA. When the inflammation attacks the throat, presenting many of the throat symptoms, we have given for this medicine under Scarlet Fever, attended with great thirst, which the patient is often prevented from indulging by the acute *shooting or pricking pain in the throat* produced by swallowing; and further, when there is a hoarse, *dry*, barking, and somewhat spasmodic cough, *worse at night*, with mucous ronchus, great restlessness and high nervous excite-

* *Pathogenetic* symptoms. Those caused by the action of a medicine upon a healthy individual.

† *Pulsatilla* and *Bryonia* are two of the most important remedies when there is prominent bronchitic complication. (See also BRONCHITIS.)

ment; also in those cases of measles where no eruption declares itself, but simply headache and catarrh, with *inflammation of the eyes*, which present a glassy appearance, are bloodshot, or streaked, and watery; finally, when evident signs of *cerebral irritation*, &c. set in.

Administration as under Scarlet Fever, (which see.)

Bryonia is an excellent remedy when the eruption is faint, or imperfectly developed, and the respiration much oppressed and laborious; achings in the limbs, also when there is dry cough, and the patient complains of shooting pains in the chest, increased by a full inspiration. (Vide Pleuritis.)

Administration. In mild cases $^{0}\frac{0}{6}{}^{0}$ in a teaspoonful of water, given when practicable in the morning, and repeated in twenty-four hours; but in severe attacks, we may find it requisite to add six globules, or in some cases a drop or so of the third potency, to an ounce of water, and administer a dessert-spoonful every six hours until improvement set in.

This disease has frequently terminated fatally, from the eruption being driven in by sudden exposure to cold or change of temperature; in such cases, Bryonia, administered as above, is generally found efficacious in re-evolving the eruption, and preventing this disaster; if diarrhœa, with mucous discharge, follow the suppression, Pulsatilla is indicated; if the *vomiting* with great oppression at the chest be the more prominent symptom, Ipecacuanha should be substituted, and followed in turn by *Arsenicum* if symptoms of improvement do not speedily show themselves.—In the case of children, *Chamomilla* is to be preferred to *Ipecacuanha* when there is dyspnœa and diarrhœa with colic and vomiting: When symptoms of cerebral disturbance supervene, *Cuprum aceticum*,* *Belladonna*, and *Stramonium*, or *Helleborus niger*, *Arsenicum*, and *Sulphur*, have proved of the greatest utility:—And in the case of pulmonic inflammation, *Phosphorus*, *Bryonia*, or *Sulphur*. In those comparatively rare cases in which *typhoid* symptoms manifest themselves, either during the course of the disease, or at its termination, *Bryonia*, *Arsenicum*, and *Phos-*

* Vide Scarlatina, p. 52.

phorus will be found useful, where any chance of recovery remains. (Vide TYPHUS.)

For the treatment of coughs which measles sometimes leave after them, *Sulphur, Sepia, Carbo v., Conium, Chamomilla, Drosera, Dulcamara, Hyoscyamus, Ignatia, Nux-v., Belladonna,* &c., are very serviceable. (See COUGHS.)

For the diarrhœa remaining under similar circumstances, *Cinchona, Pulsatilla, Mercurius,* and *Sulphur,* are in general the most appropriate: For their indications, see DIARRHŒA. Otitis or Otorrhœa: *Pulsatilla, Carbo v., Sulph., Merc.,* and *Hepar sulphuris,* chiefly. Parotitis: *Arnica,* and *Phos.* Tenderness of the skin: *Mercurius.* Miliaria alba: chiefly *Nux v.* Burning, itching, rash, which bleeds after scratching: *Arsenicum* and *Sulphur.*

As a precautionary measure against the attacks of this disease, when epidemic, we may administer PULSATILLA $\frac{00}{6}$, in a little water, followed by ACONITE $\frac{00}{6}$, three days after; allow the latter medicine to act for twenty-four hours, and continue the alternation for a fortnight, renewing it when necessary at the termination of a week or ten days. This treatment will frequently be found sufficient in warding off this disease, or, if taken, it will generally be in an extremely mild form.

DIET. In this respect we may follow the rules given under SCARLET FEVER.

SMALLPOX. *Variola.*

This disease is, by pathologists of the present day, divided into two varieties—the *distinct,* when the pustules on the face are clearly defined, and do not run into one another; the *confluent,* when they coalesce and form one continuous whole.

When the symptoms are less severe than those properly characteristic of the disease, and the eruption on the face slight, it is called the modified smallpox. We generally find this description in such persons as have been properly vaccinated, which precaution, although not always a preservative from the attacks of variola, greatly lessens its virulence, and gives a milder character to the complaint when taken.

Diagnosis. This disease is frequently very sudden in its attacks, commencing with chilliness and shivering, followed by febrile symptoms, with headache, severe pains in the small of the back and loins, languor, weariness and faintness; the patient also complains of headache, oppression of the chest, and acute pain in the pit of the stomach, *increased by pressure*. The eruption makes its appearance at the close of the third day, first on the face and hairy scalp, then on the neck, and afterwards spreads over the whole body. Catarrhal symptoms, as sneezing, coughing, wheezing, and frequently difficulty of breathing, often accompany this disease.

The eruption first appears in the shape of small hard-pointed red elevations, which become depressed in the centre as they enlarge, and contain a semi-transparent fluid, with inflamed circular margin; about the sixth or eighth day, the lymph in the pustule becomes converted into pus, and the depression in the centre disappears.

When the pustules are very numerous on the face, it generally becomes much swollen, and the eyelids are frequently closed up. On the first day, a small lump like a millet-seed may be felt in each of the elevations above noticed, distinguishing this eruption from all other exanthemata. The pocks continue coming on the first three eruptive days, and each pock runs its regular course; thus, those which first appeared are dying off, while the others are suppurating; and as the first dry and form into scab on the eleventh day from the commencement of the disease, the seventh from the appearance of the eruption, the general desiccation happens on the fourteenth day.

When the pustules have attained their full development, they generally burst, in mild cases emitting an opaque lymph, which dries into a crust and falls off; in severe ones, we find a discharge of puriform matter, forming scabs and sores, which leave, on their healing, permanent marks or pits. Red stains, caused by increased vascular action, always remain for a while after the eruption; but if no ulceration has taken place, they disappear in process of time.

In Confluent Smallpox, all the precursory symptoms are more severe, the fever runs high, and frequently continues so throughout the course; the pain in the pit of the stomach, and difficulty of breathing, are more complained of, and in children the eruption is frequently preceded by convulsions and delirium; the latter symptom is frequently present with adults during the suppurative or secondary fever, which frequently assumes a typhoid character, and sometimes carries off the patient on the eleventh day; and all cases in which we have a deeply-rooted morbid constitutional taint to contend against, require the utmost skill of the experienced practitioner to ward off a fatal result.

Salivation, with soreness of the throat and aphthæ, or pustules on the tongue and pharynx, frequently declares itself in both forms of this disease, but more particularly the confluent.

Before we come to the medicines to be administered in the different stages of the disease, we may say a few words upon the treatment of the patient.

Cool and fresh air are our best auxiliaries, the variolous virus is one which rests upon the organism, and warmth is calculated to increase its activity. So beneficial is cool air found in this malady, that taking a child to an open window when attacked with the convulsions, frequently present, will generally be found to afford immediate relief. Great cleanliness must also be observed, and the linen frequently changed.

When the vesicles declare themselves, and begin to form into pustules, the room ought to be kept as dark as possible, to aid in preventing the risk of disfigurement, a precaution deducible from common experience, since we find that the parts of the frame exposed to the action of light are always those most strongly marked by the ravages of the disease.

To avoid the cicatrices and consequent disfigurement left by this disease, many physicians have adopted a mask or plaster for the face, of different substances, such as gum, mucilage, calamine, &c. We have, however, in general course of practice, found the specific action of the medicines, and the precaution above mentioned, sufficient materially to obviate all evil consequences of this nature.

THERAPEUTICS. In the first or febrile stage of the disorder, COFFEA is valuable in allaying the nervous excitability generally present.

ADMINISTRATION. $\frac{0\,0}{3}$ in a dessert-spoonful of water, repeated in four hours, if necessary.*

ACONITE may either follow or precede this medicine when the fever runs high, and visceral congestion threatens. Administration as in INFLAMMATORY FEVER, page 23, (which see.)

CHAMOMILLA is often of great service at this period, or during the course of the disease, in children, when there is dyspnœa and diarrhœa, with colic and vomiting; or when *startings* or *convulsions* set in prior to the appearance of the eruption; and again during the maturative stage, when the nights of the little patient are much disturbed by a troublesome cough. Should *Chamomilla* afford but slight relief, *Belladonna* may be administered.

When considerable tightness and oppression at the chest, sometimes attended with *nausea* and *vomiting*, are experienced before the appearance of the eruption, the alternate use of *Ipecacuanha* and *Antimonium tartaricum* affords speedy relief; the latter remedy is, moreover, well indicated in this disease from the close analogy which the eruption it is capable of producing, bears to that of smallpox, and may therefore be also administered with advantage during the eruptive and maturative stages, unless some other remedies should be more urgently called for by the nature of the symptoms; the existence of a hollow-sounding cough, with *loud mucous ronchus*, is an additional index for the employment of *Antimonium tartaricum*.

ADMINISTRATION. Three globules of the sixth potency of each remedy, in a dessert-spoonful of water, alternately every one, two, or three hours, according to the severity of the

* Vide note, p. 21.

symptoms, until symptoms of improvement set in. When *Antimonium tartaricum* is given alone, it will be sufficient to repeat the dose every three to six or even twelve hours, according to circumstances.

Bryonia is sometimes useful in assisting the natural course of the eruption; it is also indicated when considerable symptoms of gastric derangement are present, such as bitter taste in the mouth, foulness of the tongue, headache, *rheumatic pain in the limbs, increased by motion,* constipation and irritability of disposition; also when there are occasional shooting pains in the chest, especially during inspiration.

Rhus is equally serviceable at this stage of the disease, and particularly when the acute pains in the head, back, and loins, are aggravated when in a state of rest, and temporarily relieved by movement.

Administration. In slight cases, $\frac{0\,0}{6}$ in a teaspoonful of water, given every twelve hours, as the eruption continues developing itself; in severe cases, six globules at the third potency to an ounce of water, a dessert-spoonful every six hours; it may be preceded or followed by Aconite, should there be considerable fever, with dry heat of the skin, the medicine being administered as above ordered until these symptoms are abated.

Belladonna. This remedy may follow *Aconite, when the latter has been indicated,* should symptoms of cerebral disturbance have set in, characterized by flushed countenance, intolerance of the eyes to light, headache and delirium; great thirst, nausea and vomiting; or when there is redness of the tongue at the tip and margins; abdomen tumid and painful, particularly at the epigastrium, with sensibility on pressure; prostration of strength, stupor, &c.

For further indication for the employment of this remedy, and the mode of exhibition, see Inflammation of the Brain and its Tissues.

Opium is useful when there are symptoms of stupor or strong *inclination to somnolence.* $\frac{0\,0\,0}{3}$.

Should vomiting set in attended with diarrhœa, we may administer Ipecacuanha $\frac{0\,0}{3}$, followed by *Pulsatilla* $\frac{0\,0}{6}$, if the symptoms become aggravated towards evening and the patient be of a mild and phlegmatic temperament.

If *Antimonium tartaricum* and *Ipecacuanha* do not succeed in allaying the nausea and vomiting, and the patient complains of *excessive thirst and dryness of the mouth, the tongue being at the same time very foul and dark, and the prostration of strength excessive,* we may administer ARSENICUM $\frac{00}{6}$ in a teaspoonful of water, and repeat the dose every two or three hours, if required; but the remedy must be discontinued as soon as decided benefit has resulted from its action. The last symptom generally occurs after the maturation of the eruption and secondary fever.*

PULSATILLA is occasionally of considerable utility in confluent smallpox, when an efflorescence similar to that of measles precedes or accompanies the eruption, with nausea or vomiting, and aggravation of all the symptoms towards evening.

An occasional dose of *Stramonium* $\frac{0}{1}\frac{0}{2}$ is *sometimes* useful, when some pustules are already formed, in forwarding the eruption and shortening its duration.

During the filling up of the pocks, a secondary or suppurative fever frequently sets in, particularly when the pustules are thick, and evince a disposition to run into the *confluent* form; when, moreover, there is swelling of the head, inflammation of the eyes, throat, and nose, with salivation, hoarseness, and impeded deglutition; tenderness of the stomach; diarrhœa, with tenesmus, and sometimes sanguineous stools; having, if called for, first attacked the more prominent febrile symptoms with ACONITE, exhibited as above prescribed, we should administer on the same day, MERCURIUS, a grain of the third trituration in half an ounce of water, a dessert-spoonful every six hours, until amelioration declares itself. When the fever runs high in confluent smallpox and threatens to continue so,

* In some cases, and especially those of a bad type, livid spots or diffused ecchymoses are observed on the skin prior to the evolution of the eruption (*variolæ nigræ.*) *Arsenicum* is here also of considerable service, the more so when great weakness and languor, thirst, nausea, or vomiting, with pain in the epigastrium, are present.

as it often does throughout this form of the disease, *Aconite* must repeatedly be had recourse to, and given in alternation with *Sulphur*, when not sufficient of itself to mitigate the excessive febrile action.

While the disease is running its course, particularly during the distention of the pustules, should no other remedies be imperatively called for, and also towards the period of their bursting, we may safely administer an occasional dose of *Mercurius* as above, in the latter case, followed by a dose or two of SULPHUR to assist in the desiccation.

When rheumatic pains in the back and extremities, which become worse at night, and are somewhat relieved by movement, are complained of at this period, *Rhus* may be advantageously alternated with *Sulphur*. *Rhus* is moreover extremely serviceable in confluent smallpox when the fever assumes a typhoid type, attended with the signs denominated putrescent; *Mercurius* and *Arsenicum* are equally useful, however, in the latter case, when indicated by the character of the symptoms. (Vide TYPHUS).*

During the period of desiccation, continual laving with tepid water and bran, and gently drying it afterwards, will be sufficient; cleanliness being then the great requisite, with a careful attention to diet.

REPERCUSSION OF THE ERUPTION. When this has taken place, and the symptoms of cerebral disturbance, given under the head of the medicine about to be mentioned, (see SCARLET FEVER, page 42,) set in, we must have immediate recourse to *Cuprum aceticum*, and employ it as there directed. Some physicians in their treatment of the affection divide it into two distinct stages; we have, however, contented ourselves, when necessary, with slightly referring to them. To the practitioner they are sufficiently well known: and the

* When *Pleuritis* or *Pneumonia* intervene during the progress of the disorder, the remedies mentioned under these different heads must be called to our aid. The invasion and progress of the latter disorder is sometimes so insidious, that, unless the aggregate signs of pneumonia be narrowly looked for, disorganization of the lung may take place before the existence of such a complication is detected.

non-medical administrator must be guided by the *symptoms* that present themselves from time to time, in the selection of the remedy, by which mode he is less likely to fall into error than he might be were he to act by mere routine. Against the cough which sometimes results from an attack of smallpox, *Belladonna, Mercurius,* and *Arsenicum,* are three of the most appropriate remedies in most cases, (the particular indications for which will be found in the article on COUGHS, which see;) and against asthmatic symptoms attended with mucous rattling in the chest, *Tartarus emeticus,* followed by *Senega,* should the former not effect a cure.

Cinchona and *Phosphorus* have repeatedly been found specific against the diarrhœa which occasionally results. And against the Ophthalmia, *Conium, Belladonna, Hepar sulphuris, Euphrasia, Sulphur, Calcarea, Arsenicum, Pulsatilla, Mercurius, Nux vomica,* and *Rhus toxicodendrum,* have been found the most useful.

MODIFIED SMALLPOX is merely a mild description of the above, and as we have before said, is the form the disease generally assumes when it attacks those who have been properly vaccinated. We must regulate our treatment according to the symptoms, being guided in the selection of the remedies by the indications before given.*

DIET should be regulated by the virulence of the attack; but in all instances the beverages should be cold, as a warm regimen and neglect of the precautions before mentioned, may convert the mild into the malignant form; and after recovery it is necessary that the patient abstain for a considerable time from animal food.

It may be remarked, that after recovery from an attack of malignant smallpox, the patient's constitution frequently re-

* I have given in detail the treatment which has been generally adopted by Homœopathists, and with great success. But it may here be added, that Vaccinine, given internally, has obtained much repute as an important and eminently successful remedy, in the treatment of variola; the most virulent cases having been reported to have yielded to it with a promptness and certainty that afford another great proof, if such were needed, of the truth of the homœopathic law.

quires a thorough renovation, and that he should be put under a course of medicine best calculated to attain that result.

CHICKEN-POX. *Variola spuria, Varicella.*

Diagnosis. A disease bearing a considerable resemblance in its external character to smallpox, but differing in its duration, and symptomatically, being considerably milder, generally requiring no medical assistance, but merely attention to diet, and but rarely becoming dangerous, except when it extends itself to the lungs or brain. The fever, however, occasionally runs high.

When this affection attacks an individual, and smallpox is epidemic, which is not unfrequently the case, it is often mistaken for that disorder, but it soon discovers its real character by the rapidity with which the eruption declares itself; the pustules (in many instances closely resembling those of the smallpox) being generally fully matured by the third day, and the whole eruption disappearing at the end of the fourth or fifth, without leaving any mark.

Therapeutics. When much fever is present, we should check it by the administration of Aconite $\frac{0}{6}{}^{0}$, repeated from time to time as required, or Coffea, $\frac{0}{3}{}^{0}$, also occasionally repeated if there be simply extreme restlessness and anxiety. When cerebral symptoms threaten, Belladonna; for the employment of this medicine, see Inflammation of the Brain. When attended with convulsions in children, particularly during dentition, see Convulsions. *Antimonium tartaricum* may be given to accelerate the eruption.

Mercurius $\frac{0}{6}{}^{0}$ may be given when the lymph of the pustules becomes converted into pus, as in the smallpox, and is also beneficial if strangury be present. When the eruption has been driven in, see Repercussion of the eruption in Smallpox. In anomalous cases, where other symptoms supervene, more closely resembling Smallpox, we may consult the remedies mentioned under that disease.

MILIARY FEVER. *Miliaria, miliaria alba. Miliaris sudatoria. Sudor miliaris.*

Diagnosis. A great number of exceedingly small round, transparent vesicles, afterwards becoming opaque, and ending in scurf, irregularly scattered, of the size of millet-seeds, (hence its name,) which, when the hand is passed over the surface, feel as if they were small grains of sand beneath the cuticle.

This affection is sometimes idiopathic, but more frequently associated with fever, and even occasionally present in various chronic diseases, in which latter instance it may generally be considered as an evidence of some internal constitutional taint; it is also not uncommon with women at the period of confinement, arising from the room being kept at too high a temperature—a frequent cause of this malady. This, like other cutaneous affections of the same nature, is generally preceded by febrile symptoms; the eruption appearson the fifth or sixth day; from the commencement of the fever we frequently find profuse perspiration, with a putrid sour odour; previous to the vesicles evolving themselves, there is a tingling or itching of the skin, occasionally attended with a sensation of burning, together with a numbness of the extremities; the patient complains of a sense of oppression at the chest, sometimes with short dry cough, and stitches in the side, and not unfrequently of severe or fugitive rheumatic pains in the limbs and teeth. Low spirits are a frequent accompaniment of this affection.

Therapeutics. In consequence of the numerous diseases with which it is complicated, it requires a variety of medicaments. When it appears in a simple and apparently idiopathic form, and is attended with anxiety and restlessness, which seem to depend upon an accelerated circulation of the blood, with great internal and external heat, Aconite is a specific remedy; and when the above seems more particularly to arise from high nervous excitability, Coffea is indicated.

Belladonna $\frac{0}{6}^{0}$, when the accelerated circulation is attended with considerable determination of blood to the head, and delirium. Arsenicum $\frac{0}{6}^{0}$, when the eruption is accompanied with *excessive anxiety.*

When the disease is found conjoined with puerperal or other fevers, and is preceded by oppression, lassitude, anxiety and a sense of weight about the chest, restlessness, sighing, &c., it is generally speedily subdued by IPECACUANHA $\frac{00}{3}$, or should the symptoms which precede the eruption be accompanied by *constipation*, or shooting pains in the chest, BRYONIA $\frac{00}{6}$ should be selected.

When this disease comes on in children, brought about by the same cause, viz., excessive warmth, or even errors in diet, attended with a greenish or watery yellowish diarrhœa, we may administer CHAMOMILLA $\frac{00}{6}$, followed, if no alteration takes place, by TINCTURE OF SULPHUR $\frac{00}{6}$.

ADMINISTRATION OF THE MEDICINES. When this disease appears in an idiopathic form, it is rarely so severe as to require a very frequent repetition of the medicines, if the accessory treatment about to be pointed out be carefully attended to—in most cases a globule or two at the potency above given, repeated in from four to twelve hours, according to the intensity of the disease, will be found sufficient. And in many instances, a single dose will dissipate all the symptoms, or at least so modify them that we may safely trust to nature to perfect the cure.

REMARKS. When it exhibits itself in complication with other affections, Miliaria may be either symptomatic or critical, and the physician should always bear in mind that an improper treatment of other affections may develop it. When *symptomatic*, it may be recognised by appearing either very early or late in the original affection, which so far from being relieved by the eruption, is frequently exacerbated by the excitement of the nervous system consequent on its appearance. Even when *critical*, in which case, after the eruption has been fully developed, amelioration takes place, it is still dangerous from its liability to retrocede. When a proper attention is paid to keeping the patient cool by light covering and the *removal of feather beds*, and allowing a free supply of pure air, this troublesome concomitant will rarely show itself. When, however, it appears critical, we must be most careful not to check it, and a moderately warm temperature must be kept up.

REPERCUSSION OF THE ERUPTION. When this has taken

place, we must carefully watch the result: sometimes Nature herself provides for it by an increase of some other secretion; but when symptoms of cerebral disturbance, &c., present themselves, (see *Cupr. acet.*, article SCARLET FEVER, p. 48.)

DIET. Same as already given for FEVER, modifying it according to the violence of the symptoms; when repercussion threatens to take place, the patient's beverages should be given moderately warm.

NETTLE-RASH. *Urticaria.*

DIAGNOSIS. Spots or wheals, flat or prominent, and of a dull white colour like the sting of a nettle, or redder than the surrounding skin, generally encircled with a rosy areola, disappearing in warmth, and reappearing when exposed to cold, evolved suddenly and continually changing their situation.

This eruption is brought to the surface by various causes, not unfrequently arising from indigestion, caused by the use of improper articles of food. Before the eruption discloses itself, the patient is affected with restlessness, languor, oppression, and want of appetite, derangement of the digestive functions, and fever. When the eruption breaks out, the above symptoms become relieved, but considerable suffering arises from heat and itching; sometimes swelling of the parts affected; this disease, in almost all cases arising from a constitutional cause, requires for its total eradication a regular course of treatment.

THERAPEUTICS. In acute cases, the remedies found most useful are *Dulcamara, Aconite, Nux vomica, Pulsatilla, Antimon. crud.*, *Belladonna, Hepar sulph., Rhus tox.*, and *Bryonia.*

DULCAMARA when the exciting cause has been cold or damp, when the affection occurs in wet weather, or when we find considerable fever with bitter taste in the mouth, foul tongue, diarrhœa, pains in the limbs, and extreme itching, with a burning sensation after scratching.

ACONITE when the febrile symptoms are more intense, the pulse high, the skin hot and dry, restlessness and anxiety present.

NUX VOMICA when there is considerable gastric derangement, with constipation, more especially when arising from wine, stimulants, or indigestible substances; it may, if necessary, follow

Aconite in eight or twelve hours after the febrile symptoms are somewhat modified.

PULSATILLA deserves a preference under similar circumstances, when the bowels are relaxed, and the patient of a quiet disposition and lymphatic temperament, and the attack has apparently been excited by indigestible food.

ANTIMONIUM CRUDUM may follow *Pulsatilla*, should the latter have failed to relieve the affection.

BELLADONNA is indicated when the affection is attended with a severe throbbing headache, with redness of the face.

HEPAR SULPHURIS, when cold in the head, and particularly if affecting only one nostril.

RHUS TOXICODENDRON is one of the most useful remedies in a great majority of cases of this eruption, and especially when the affection has apparently arisen from some idiosyncrasy of constitution, in which the eruption has been thrown out by the use of some particular article of food. See article on DIET in Introduction.

ADMINISTRATION OF THE MEDICINES. In ordinary cases we may dissolve four globules of the sixth potencies in six dessert-spoonfuls of water, and administer one morning and evening, except in the case of *Aconite*, which may be more frequently repeated when the febrile symptoms seem to demand it. (Vide note, p. 21.)

In this, as in every other cutaneous eruption, great care ought to be taken against driving in the eruption, by external applications or lotions; their sudden suppression, as before noted under SCARLATINA and SMALLPOX, being frequently attended with fatal consequences. When, however, from improper treatment we have reason to dread this having taken place, we should administer BRYONIA$\frac{00}{6}$, repeated every four hours until the eruption reappears, which will generally be found sufficient to bring back the rash, and prevent further dangerous consequences. Should, however, marked cerebral symptoms declare themselves, see SCARLET FEVER, *Repercussion of the eruption.*

URTICA URENS has been found useful in some cases. In those of a chronic or extremely obstinate character, *Calc.*, *Lycopod.*, *Sulph.*, *Carb. v.*, *Caustic.*, *Acid. nitric.*, *Conium*, *Natr. m.*, &c.; the latter two, particularly when the eruption is liable to reappear after violent exercise or exertion of any kind; *Calc.*, when exposed to cold fresh air; and *Acid. nitric.* on going into the open air, after having kept within doors for a day or two.

GASTRIC FEVER.—Symptoms: sensation of fulness and weight in the epigastrium; flatulent distention of the epigastric region, with inclination to vomit; eructations of offensive flatus, and sometimes vomiting of ingesta and tenacious mucus mixed with bile; thickly furred, dirty yellow tongue; abdomen soft; bowels costive; but in the advanced stage of the disease the evacuations are often very offensive, and contain a portion of undigested food; frontal headache; languor; sickly and distressed expression of countenance, with yellow discoloration of the albuginea; more or less chilliness, succeeded by heat and dryness of skin; urine thick, cloudy, and dark coloured.

BILIOUS FEVER.—Symptoms: more heat of the skin; restlessness and thirst excessive; constant desire for acid drinks; the epigastrium is distended with flatus; the tongue is coloured at first with a pale yellow fur, which assumes a deeper or brownish colour; the taste and eructations are bitter, and the substance vomited consists of a greenish, bilious matter; the bowels are either confined or relaxed, in the latter case a yellow, green, or brown colour; the face exhibits an earthy, somewhat jaundiced aspect; sometimes there is also a greater or less degree of sensibility, hardness, tension, burning in the hepatic region; the urine is dark brown, bilious.

THERAPEUTICS. In Gastric Fever: *Puls.*, *Nux-v.*, *Ipec.*, *Antim. c.*, *Bryon.*, *Cham.*, *China*, *Cocc.*, *Tart-c.*, *Rhus-t.*, *Sulph.*, *Arsen.*, *Verat.*, *Coloc.*, *Acid. phos.* (See Dyspepsia, p. 95.) When mental emotions have given rise to the disorder: *Cham.*, *Bryon.*, *Coloc.*, *Acid. phos.*—*Cham.* and *Bryon.* in consequence of a fit of passion; *Coloc.* from indignation or mortification. *Staphys.* when vexation is combined with indignation. *Acid. phos.* if grief, care, anxiety, have been the causes. (See Mental emotions.)

In Bilious Fever: Acon., *Cham.*, Puls., Nux-v., China, Cocc., Digit., Bell., Arsen., Coloc., Merc., Staph., Colch., Tarax., Ignat., Asar. (See dyspepsia hepatitis, mental emotions, nervous and putrid fevers.)

DISEASES OF ORGANS

CONNECTED WITH

THE DIGESTIVE SYSTEM.

TOOTHACHE. *Odontalgia.*

WHEN we find a *constant disposition* to this distressing malady, on the slightest exposure to cold, without any presumable cause, or what is generally called *rheumatic toothache*, we are warranted in concluding that some taint lurks in the constitution; and until means are taken for its eradication, even the remedies most clearly indicated under other circumstances fail for its relief, or at most but temporarily alleviate its pangs. Another obstacle to the selection of the proper remedy is the difficulty we find in obtaining from the patient a perfectly clear description of his sensations. We shall, nevertheless, mention a few of the remedies which have proved most efficacious in the relief of toothache, and when the symptoms of the sufferer approximate closely to the indications given for the medicine, they will, in very many cases, afford a prompt relief.

THERAPEUTICS. Among these, *Belladonna*, *Chamomilla*, *Mercurius*, *Nux vomica*, *Pulsatilla*, *Sulphur*, *Carbo vegetabilis*, *Hepar sulphuris*, and *Arsenicum*, hold a high rank.

ADMINISTRATION. The medicine selected may be taken dry, or dissolved in a teaspoonful of water; and if an *aggravation* of pain is experienced soon after taking the medicine, it must not be repeated, as this is generally succeeded by considerable relief; but when the pain threatens to get worse again, the same remedy may be repeated, provided the symptoms are of a similar description to what they were before taking the remedy; if they have altered, select another medicine.

Belladonna $\frac{000}{30}$, is particularly indicated when the pains are very severe, of a *drawing, tearing,* or *shooting* nature, extending to the face and ears; *becoming aggravated in the evening,* and *especially at night,* with gnawing or boring pain in the carious teeth, swelling of the gums and cheeks, *dryness of the mouth with excessive thirst,* with or without salivation; renewal of the pains from intellectual labour, or after eating; aggravation of suffering *when masticating; also in the open air; congestion to the head, with heat and redness of the face,* also pulsation in the head and cheeks.

Chamomilla $\frac{000}{12}$, when there are severe drawing, jerking, pulsative or shooting pains; *heat and redness, especially of one of the cheeks:* the pain becomes *almost insufferable, especially at night in the warmth of the bed:* shooting and pulsative pains in the ear and side affected, *the pains are aggravated by eating or drinking anything hot or cold, but especially the former;* great agitation and loss of self-control from pain, or *excessive weakness,* sometimes amounting to fainting; great irascibility, and disposition to shed tears during the paroxysms. *Chamomilla* is useful in cases of toothache which have arisen from abuse of Coffee,* in which affection *Nux vomica* and *Pulsatilla* are also valuable when indicated by the symptoms. *Rhus* and *Dulcamara* frequently answer best after *Chamomilla* in toothache from cold, where the former remedy has not removed the attack. And when the toothache returns after every exposure to cold, *Sulphur* is generally the best remedy; in some cases *Cinchona.*

* Those who are subject to toothache, ought to abstain from coffee altogether; as also from very hot or cold drinks, stimulants of every description, sweetmeats and acids; they ought farther to refrain from using medicated tooth-powders, particularly if they wish to derive any benefit from homœopathic treatment; the toothpick ought to be catiously used if required, and the mouth well rinsed with tepid water (or about the same temperature as that of the mouth) night and morning, and after each meal.

Mercurius $\frac{000}{12}$ is particularly indicated when the *pains affect carious teeth*, or exist in the *roots of the teeth*, and consist of *tearing*, *shooting* pains, occupying the *whole side of the head and face* of the part affected, and extending to the ears; loosening of the teeth, and a feeling as if they were too long; the pain becomes almost insupportable towards evening, and especially at *night* in the *warmth of the bed;* aggravated when eating or drinking, particularly *after anything cold*, also by exposure to cold or damp air; *swelling and inflammation of the gums;* nocturnal perspiration, peevishness and inclination to tears; it is especially useful in persons who are subject to glandular swellings.

Nux vomica $\frac{000}{30}$ is useful for persons who are habituated *to wine, coffee, or other stimulants*, or addicted to *sedentary life or study ;* of *lively or irritable temperament, dark* or *florid complexion;* sufferings increased by intellectual labour. The pains generally occur in *carious teeth*, and are of *a drawing* and *jerking or gnawing* description, occasionally diffusing themselves to the head and ears, sometimes attended with painful enlargement of the submaxillary glands; gums *swollen and painful*, accompanied with *throbbing and pulsation*. The toothache is more liable to come at *night* or on *awaking in the morning*, sometimes *also after dinner* or in the *open air*.

Pulsatilla $\frac{000}{12}$ is peculiarly adapted to persons of a *mild or phlegmatic* disposition. The pains are digging and gnawing, attended with *pricking* in the gums, extending to the *face, head, eye* and *ear* of the side affected; this remedy is particularly efficacious in toothache, attended with *earache*, with *paleness of the face*, and when the toothache has been excited by taking cold, or *where* we find *shortness and difficulty of breathing ;* the pains are sometimes of a *drawing, tearing, shooting*, or *jerking* description, and occasionally produce a sensation as if the nerve were drawn tight, and then suddenly relaxed; the pain is much aggravated in the *evening or after midnight*, generally *increased by warmth* and when *at rest*, and mitigated by *cold air* or *cold applications* to the mouth.

Tincture of Sulphur $\frac{00}{3}$. This remedy is particularly valuable in strumous habits, with a tendency to constipation;

pain, sometimes attended with *swelling of the cheek* and *shooting pains in the ears, congestion of blood to the head,* and *pulsative headache;* the pain is of a *tearing, jerking, pulsative* description, affecting both *carious* and sound teeth; aggravated in the *evening* and at *night,* or by exposure to the *open air,* also by the application of *cold water,* or by mastication; loosening, sensation of elongation, and setting on edge of the teeth; the gums are *swollen,* affected with *pulsative pains,* and bleed easily.

Bryonia $\frac{000}{18}$ is also a useful remedy in this affection, particularly with persons of lively, choleric, and obstinate disposition. Its indications are *loosening* and *sensation of elongation* of the teeth, especially during or after eating; shooting in the ears, with *inclination to lie down,* pains aggravated by taking anything hot in the mouth, mitigated by lying on the affected side or exacerbated by the contrary position.

Carbo vegetabilis $\frac{000}{30}$ is indicated by toothache, with dragging-tearing, or constrictive and throbbing pains excited by anything *hot, cold,* or *salt;* chronic looseness of the teeth; receding, ulcerated and suppurating gums, (particularly after the abuse of mercurial preparations, such as calomel, etc.,) bleeding from the teeth and gums, with tendency of the teeth to decay *rapidly.*

Hepar sulphuris ½ gr. of the third trituration, is indicated by dragging jerking toothache, increased by approximating the teeth (clenching), by masticating, or from sitting in a warm room; swelling of the gums, with tenderness on pressure, abscess in the gums; (especially useful in cases where hurtful doses of *Mercury* have previously been taken under allopathic treatment.)

Arsenicum $\frac{000}{30}$ by nocturnal pain, which extends into the ear, cheek, bones of the face, and temple; *aggravation of the pain by lying on the affected side;* amelioration from the warmth of the fire; aching in the teeth so excessive as *almost to drive to madness or distraction;* sensation of elongation and looseness of the teeth; grinding of teeth; and bleeding of the gums.

Aconite, Belladonna, Chamomilla, Coffea, and *Ignatia,* are the most useful in affections of this nature with children.

ACONITE $\frac{000}{24}$. When the pains are difficult of description, attended with great agitation, feverish sensation, blood to the head, heat and redness of the face, and when the pains are described as of a pulsative, throbbing nature.

COFFEA $\frac{000}{30}$. Against violent pains with great excitability and almost distraction in adults; also when the patient is conscious that the excitement is disproportionate to the pain suffered.

For *Chamomilla* we have already given indications; if it prove insufficient, has been caused by a chill, and is attended with diarrhœa, we may substitute DULCAMARA $\frac{00}{24}$.

IGNATIA $\frac{000}{30}$ is suitable to those cases presenting similar indications to those of *Nux vomica* or *Pulsatilla*, but more particularly applicable to mild or sensitive dispositions with alternation of high and low spirits.

TARTARUS EMETICUS. 1 gr. of the third trituration in about an ounce of water, a dessert-spoonful three times a day;—in toothache occurring *during cold, wet weather*,—particularly in women, with nocturnal exacerbations, or aggravation of the pain when drinking any cold liquid.*

SORE THROAT, or QUINSEY. APHTHOUS SORE THROAT.

Angina faucium, Tonsillitis phlegmonoides, Cynanche tonsillaris,—Angina aphthosa,—etc.

QUINSEY.—DIAGNOSIS. Inflammation of the throat, denoted by swelling and red colour of the back part of the throat, accompanied with difficulty of swallowing, impeded respiration, alteration of the voice, and fever.

In the incipient stage of this affection, there is a sense of

* In rheumatic or arthritic toothache with *nocturnal* aggravations, or increase of pain on partaking of *cold* or warm drinks, but temporary relief on the *external* application of heat; also in toothache which returns every spring or autumn, during the prevalence of easterly winds, (and then continues sometimes for several weeks,) the pain being occasionally confined to one tooth, which is extremely sensitive to the slightest touch, and often accompanied with acute shootings into the ear, *Rhododendron chrysanthum* is a useful remedy, in repeated doses.

constriction about the throat, with a feeling of soreness, and sometimes of obstruction in the act of swallowing the saliva; if it runs its course, the difficulty of swallowing and breathing increases, the tongue swells and becomes foul, the tonsils assume a redder hue, occasionally a number of small yellow eminences appear at the back of the throat, and particularly on the tonsils; the patient complains of thirst, and the pulse is high, strong, and frequent; sometimes the cheeks swell and become florid, and the eyes inflamed, and in severe cases delirium is not an unfrequent occurrence. As the local affection progresses, the majority of the foregoing symptoms become aggravated, the tonsils tumefied, and suppuration ensues if resolution be not speedily effected.

When suppuration takes place, the pain is instantly relieved on the bursting of the abscess; it sometimes happens, however, that scarcely has the patient been relieved from suffering by the latter event, before the state of the other tonsil gives indications that a similar train of symptoms are about to be encountered there. This affection, occasionally, if not properly treated, dangerous in its simple form, becomes particularly critical when it puts on the putrid type. In such instances, the attendant fever generally assumes a typhoid character; when this takes place, we may always infer a peculiar constitutional tendency.

THERAPEUTICS. The following are the principal remedies used in the treatment of this affection:—*Aconitum, Belladonna, Mercurius, Carbo v., Acidum nitricum, Lachesis—Pulsatilla, Nux v., Arsenicum, Chamomilla, Ignatia, Dulcamara, Hepar sulphuris, Silicea, Sulphur.* When this affection is at the commencement attended with considerable fever, thirst, and dry heat, deep redness of the parts affected, painful and difficult deglutition, pricking sensation in the throat, with aggravation of the symptoms when speaking, we should have recourse to ACONITE.

ADMINISTRATION. This must be regulated by the intensity of the inflammation; in many cases a dose of $\frac{0\,0}{6}$, repeated in six hours, if necessary, will be found sufficient; but if the inflammatory symptoms are very violent, we may add six globules of the third potency to six dessert-spoonfuls of water, and administer one every hour or half hour, according to the urgency of the case. Should, however, deglutition of liquids prove extremely distressing, or almost impracticable, we may give $\frac{000}{3}$ dry upon the patient's tongue, at similar intervals. This rule will hold good for the other remedies about to be mentioned in this complaint.*

The next medicament we shall mention, *Belladonna*, as may have been observed in the treatment of Scarlatina, Measles, &c., is one of the best remedies we possess against phlegmonous inflammation of the throat. When the above symptoms have been subdued by *Aconite*, or should the following symptoms have existed from the commencement, we should have immediate recourse to its administration.

Pain in the throat as if from *excoriation*, attended with scraping, and a sensation of enlargement, and burning or *shooting* pains, principally experienced during the *act of swallowing;* these pains sometimes extend to the ears. Other characteristic indications for this remedy are—sense of *spasmodic constriction* or *contraction* of the throat, with *constant desire to swallow saliva;* occasionally there is violent thirst, with dryness of the throat, but *a dread of drink* from the suffering it occasions. Sometimes a complete inability to drink exists, and the liquid *returns by the nostrils.* On examination, the throat presents a *bright red colour*, with swelling of the palate, uvula and *tonsils;* also accumulation of *slimy whitish mucus* in the *throat* and on the *tongue*, obliging the patient to spit frequently; *swelling of the muscles and glands of the neck*, severe headache, chiefly confined to the forehead, sometimes determination of blood to the head, and delirium. (After *Belladonna*, *Mercurius*, *Lachesis*, or *Pulsatilla*, are often suitable.)

Administration. The same as *Aconite*, but allowing a longer interval between the doses, say from four to twelve hours, according to the violence of the affection.

This remedy frequently succeeds in speedily removing the

* Vide note, p. 21.

whole of the above group of symptoms, or, at least, so far subdues them as to enable *Mercurius* to complete the cure.

Mercurius, frequently valuable at the commencement of the disease when so indicated, or in alternation with *Belladonna* in troublesome cases, is one of the most valuable remedial agents; following that medicine, when necessary, to complete the cure. Its indications are *violent shooting in the throat and tonsils*, especially when *swallowing;* these pains extend to the *ears*, and *glands before the ears*, and under the jaw; inflammatory redness and swelling of the affected parts of the throat, burning in the throat, desire to swallow, attended with a sensation of an obstruction existing in the passage; accumulation of thick and tenacious mucus in the throat, difficult deglutition, especially of liquids, which sometimes escape through the nostrils; *swelling of the glands*, and muscles of the neck, and of the posterior part of the tongue; occasional swelling of the gums; unpleasant taste in the mouth, which is filled with *saliva* more or less *inspissated;* throbbing of, and matter forming in the tonsils; (confluent, or small, isolated, round, white specks or vesicles on the tonsils; indolent *ulcers in the throat;*) (*Angina aphthosa;*) offensive odour from the mouth, aggravation of symptoms at *night*, when speaking, and in the *evening; chills*, and *shivering*, sometimes alternated with heat. (*Lachesis, Hepar sulphuris, Carb. v.* or *Ac. nit.* are often suitable after *Merc.*)

Administration. Six globules of the sixth potency, or in severe cases with small ulcerations,—a grain of the third trituration dissolved in an ounce of water, and a dessert-spoonful given every six to twelve hours, according to the results; if an alternation with Belladonna seem advisable, we may allow a similar interval to elapse between the exhibition of the two medicines.

Lachesis. One of the characteristic indications for this remedy is, *aggravation* of the *pain in the throat from the slightest external pressure;*—it is moreover an excellent remedy in all cases of tonsillitis in which *Belladonna* or *Mercurius* have afforded relief, but seem incapable of effecting resolution; and also in aphthous sore throat with considerable ulceration, when *Mercurius* has afforded only partial relief.

Administration. Six globules of the sixth potency to an ounce of water, a dose every twelve hours in ordinary cases; in the more virulent, at intervals of three to six hours, according to the effect produced.

Carbo vegetabilis. This remedy may either follow, or be selected in preference to *Mercurius*, after a previous dose or two of *Aconite* when necessary, in *Aphthous* sore throat characterized by the appearance of small white specks or pimples, on the enlarged and protuberant tonsils, (which if not checked become confluent and spread beyond the throat,) *when* the *patient complains* of severe *burning* and *pricking pain*, with great thirst.

Administration. Six globules of the sixth to be dissolved in about an ounce of water, a dessert-spoonful to be administered twice a day. A dose or two of *Sulphur* is sometimes required after *Carbo v.* or *Mercurius* in very obstinate cases.

Acidum nitricum. After *Aconite* and *Mercurius* in *Aphthous* sore throat, characterized by superficial ulcerations in the throat, should the small white or *gray* ulcers not put on a healing appearance a few hours after the use of *Mercurius*.

Administration. Six globules of the third potency in an ounce of water, a dessert-spoonful every six, then every twelve or twenty-four hours until the cure is complete.

Nux vomica. This remedy is especially useful when the sore throat appears to arise from or to be accompanied by symptoms of deranged digestion, and when a sense of *scraping* or *excoriation* exists in the throat; also when a feeling of contraction is experienced in the upper part of the throat *during empty deglutition; swelling* and *elongation* of the *uvula*, producing a constant desire to swallow; at times only a *sensation of swelling*, with pressure and pains; or when cold has been the exciting cause, and the affection is attended with dry cough and headache, chiefly in the morning, and pains under the lower ribs during the cough. This remedy is also indicated likewise when there are small offensive ulcers of the throat, or considerable debility is present. (Vide Ulcerated Sore Throat, page 89.) *Sulphur* is frequently useful after *Nux vomica*.

Administration. $\frac{00}{6}$ in a little water exhibited in the evening when practicable; in *severe* cases repeated every six hours, until improvement results.

Pulsatilla is frequently serviceable after *Belladonna*, when there is an increased secretion of viscid mucus in the fauces: but it is more particularly when the following symptoms are met with that this remedy is called for: gastric derangement, with *dark livid redness* of the throat and tonsils; a *sensation as if the parts affected were much swollen*, or a feeling of an enlargement of the upper part of the throat, as also, of excoriation and scraping, with dryness of the throat *without thirst*, *shooting* pains in the throat when not swallowing, aggravation of the symptoms *towards evening*, attended with *shivering;* also *accumulation of adhesive mucus* in the throat. This remedy is more particularly suitable for females, or for individuals of a mild and phlegmatic temperament.

Administration. $\frac{00}{6}$ in a little water, repeated in twelve hours, if no amelioration takes place within that interval.*

Chamomilla is a remedy particularly useful in the sore throat occurring in children, and especially when the disease has been brought about by *checked perspiration*, when there are shooting or burning pains, with sensation of a *swelling of the throat*, deep redness of the parts affected, inability to swallow solid food, especially when lying down; thirst, with dryness of the mouth and throat, swelling of the tonsils and glands before the ear and under the jaw; cough excited by constant *tickling of the throat*, attended with *hoarseness;* fever towards evening, with alternate heat and shivering, *redness of one cheek*, great excitability and tossing about.

Administration. $\frac{00}{6}$ administered every twelve hours, until amelioration takes place.

Ignatia is indicated when there is a sensation as *of a plug in the throat*, with red and inflammatory swelling of the tonsils, or palate; burning pains in deglutition, as if a substance were passing over an excoriated surface, or partially obstructed by some foreign body in the throat. Liquids are

* Vide note, p. 21.

more difficult to swallow than solids; there are also *shooting pains in the cheeks, thence extending to the ears, when* NOT *performing the act of deglutition;* induration of the tonsils, or evolution of small pustules upon them.

Administration. The same as Pulsatilla.

Dulcamara. An almost specific remedy when sore throat, particularly in the form of tonsillitis, has arisen from EXPOSURE TO WET. It may be followed by *Belladonna* or *Mercurius,* should it not wholly remove the affection, and should any of the symptoms given under these medicines present themselves.

Administration. $\frac{0\,0}{6}$ repeated in twelve hours, and if no symptoms of increased pain or swelling present themselves, allowed an action of thirty-six hours from the last exhibition, during which period a marked amelioration, if not a perfect cure, sometimes preceded by a temporary aggravation, frequently develops itself. This medicine, if taken *immediately* after a severe wetting, often succeeds in preventing any unpleasant consequences.

Coffea cruda. Sometimes useful as an intermediate remedy; when many of the symptoms enumerated under *Belladonna,* with the exception of the external swelling of the throat, are present; and also by a sensation as if the uvula were elongated or loaded with mucus, causing a constant inclination to swallow. One of the best indications for its employment in this, as *in other diseases,* is an extreme over-excitability of the nervous system, characterized by sleeplessness, great restlessness, sensitiveness, disposition to weep, and peculiar impressibility to external agents.

Administration. A few globules of the sixth or thirtieth potency.

Arsenicum. The indications for the employment of this remedy in sore throat have been already given under Scarlet Fever, p. 48, and under Malignant Sore Throat, p. 89.

Hepar sulphuris is valuable in *bringing the matter to a head,* when resolution cannot be effected, and the quinsey has attained to such a height that its bursting is desirable from the painful sensation of suffocation which arises in consequence of the tumefied condition of the tonsils.

ADMINISTRATION. One grain of the trituration, third potency, added to an ounce of water. One dessert-spoonful every two hours until the quinsey bursts.

SILICEA. This remedy is in some instances more efficacious than *Hepar in rapidly forwarding the suppurative process, and causing the ripened abscess to burst.*

ADMINISTRATION. Six globules of the sixth in an ounce of water, a dessert-spoonful every two hours.

MERCURIUS may follow the above medicine after an interval of a few hours, to facilitate the healing. In obstinate cases, such as are occasionally met with in bad constitutions, the healing of the cavity after the matter has been discharged goes on very unfavourably, and even fresh abscesses form in succession: *Sulphur*, *Hepar s.* and *Psoricum*, repeated every eight or twelve hours, have chiefly been recommended in these fortunately rare cases. *Sulphur* in ordinary cases; *Hepar s.* when the patient has been previously subjected to an abuse of *Mercury* under allopathic treatment, and *Psoricum* when *Sulphur* has been taken in excess.* Half a grain of the trituration to an ounce of water, a tablespoonful every twelve hours.

THE DIET of the patient must be regulated according to the degree of inflammation present.

If required, the throat may be gargled with a little warm water, and when much pain is present, inhalation of the vapour from boiling water will often afford considerable relief; but at the same time, it may be observed, that all medicinal gargles, blisters, leeches, or other topical applications, are rendered unnecessary by proper homœopathic treatment. While we thus free the patient from a considerable degree of annoyance and needless suffering, we, at the same time, by a careful attention to the symptoms, and the exhibition of the proper remedy, effect a speedy cure.

* *Brit. Journ. of Homœopathy*, No. vii.

ULCERATED SORE THROAT.

Malignant Quinsey, Malignant, putrid or gangrenous Sore Throat.—Angina Maligna, Tonsilitis Maligna, Cynanche Maligna.

Diagnosis. This serious disease is also known by the name of *Scarlatina Maligna*, from the eruption with which it is frequently attended. It is usually epidemic, of a highly contagious nature, and generally occurs in damp and sultry autumnal seasons.

It sets in with cold and shivering, succeeded by heat, and accompanied with great languor and oppression at the chest; nausea or vomiting and sometimes purging; eyes inflamed and watery; deep red colour of the cheeks; the nostrils are also more or less inflamed and secrete a thin acrid discharge, frequently causing soreness or excoriation of the nose and lips; pulse indistinct, or very weak, small, and irregular; tongue white and moist.

The deglutition is painful and difficult, and on examining the throat early in the disease, it is observed to be of a bright red, and much tumefied; but this state is very soon altered, and numerous ulcers of various sizes will then be observed to be interspersed over the parts, which become covered with a white, grayish brown, or livid coat. In some cases these ulcerations spread so as to extend over the whole fauces into the nostrils, or downwards even to the glottis and gullet, &c., and assume a sloughing appearance as they increase in size: The prostration of strength, considerable from the first, is now excessive; the tongue, lips and teeth are covered with brown or blackish incrustations, and there is more or less delirium; the breath is extremely fetid, and the patient himself complains of a disagreeable odour. The neck appears swollen and of a livid colour, and an efflorescence of a faint scarlet hue, or blotches of a dark or livid red sometimes intermixed with petechiæ, break out on various parts of the body, and usually, though not necessarily, add to the danger,—as many are carried off, particularly children or persons of an advanced age, without any eruption,—when the local symptoms are severe and the fever high: But the appearance of livid spots or petechiæ, and other indications of so called putrescency, with frequent shivering, weak fluttering or intermittent pulse, *sunken countenance, severe purging*, extreme prostration, and bleedings from the nose, mouth, &c., must decidedly be regarded as symptoms of imminent danger.

When the local symptoms are mild, the danger is rarely great; and even in the severe forms of the disease, when a gentle sweat breaks out about the third or fifth day, when the sloughs throw off in a favourable manner, leaving a clean florid healthy-looking bottom, and the respiration becomes more gentle and free, the expression of the face more lively, and the pulse stronger and more equal, a salutary result may be held in expectation.

Therapeutics. The remedies to be employed are nearly the same as those which are commonly used in scarlet fever of a bad type, or in typhus. The following will generally be found adequate to subdue the various forms which the malady assumes, where any prospect of a cure may reasonably be entertained from the commencement: *Aconitum, Belladonna, Mercurius, Acidum nitricum, Pulsatilla, Arsenicum, Lachesis, Nux v., Carbo vegetabilis, Sulphur, &c.*

The accompanying fever being generally of a low typhoid character, *Aconite* is rarely necessary in this complaint; however, there are cases, and particularly when the fever runs high from the commencement, in which advantage is found to result from a dose or two of this remedy, followed by *Belladonna* as soon as the patient complains of dryness, with impeded deglutition and a sense of constriction or choking in the throat, which latter, on examination, is observed to be swollen and to present a florid red appearance.

Belladonna is also indicated when the fever continues to run high; when the face is bloated and the eyes much inflamed; when the patient is affected with considerable delirium, and is occasionally only with difficulty to be restrained from leaving the bed or commiting acts of violence; or farther, when the rash, which sometimes breaks out in this disorder about the third day, presents a scarlet hue.

In cases in which the symptoms are mild, or in which the above-mentioned symptoms have been reduced by means of the remedies quoted, and an increased secretion of mucus supplies the place of the previous dryness, while the patient is at the same time afflicted with nausea and bilious vomiting, a dose or two of *Pulsatilla* may be administered with effect; the progress of matters in the throat must however be carefully watched, and as soon as the presence of small ulcers, or still better, their incipient formation, can be detected, a dose of *Mercurius* should be prescribed, followed by *Acidum nitricum*, when from the increasing size and painfulness of the ulcers, *Mercurius* does not promise to arrest their progress or cause them to take on a healthy aspect.

In the milder forms of this disease, the two last-named remedies will frequently be found sufficient to conduct it to a speedy and successful termination.

But in those much more dangerous forms which the complaint so readily assumes when it rages as an epidemic, and where the patient at the commencement is seized with vomiting and purging, attended with such prostration of strength as to render it impossible for him to leave the recumbent posture without feeling faint, and compelled to fall back exhausted by his efforts:—Where, moreover, the ulcerations spread with alarming rapidity, and early take on a sloughing character:—in such cases, the conducting of the disease to a happy issue becomes obviously a much more serious and difficult task. Here the symptoms must generally at once be attacked by administering *Arsenicum*:—

Sometimes, however, a little benefit will be found to result from a dose of *Pulsatilla* at the commencement, when there is an excessive degree of bilious vomiting; but *Arsenicum* must unhesitatingly be had recourse to when there is that marked "*prostration of strength*" so characteristic of this disease, accompanied with nausea or vomiting; or when the ulcers present a *livid hue.* This important remedy is also indicated in a more advanced stage of the disease, when the ulcerations are covered with dark sloughs, surrounded by a livid margin; the teeth and lips encrusted with sordes; the pulse small and irregular; and there is delirium or constant muttering, with frequent hanging of the lower jaw; laborious respiration; acrid discharge from the nostrils, causing excoriations; the eyes dull and glassy; the skin hot and dry, and the thirst excessive; yet the patient drinks but little at a time, and appears to perform the act of deglutition with great pain and difficulty; finally, when the *prostration of strength is so extreme* that the patient seems rapidly sinking, and a rash of a livid colour breaks out in blotches, here and there intermingled with petechia.

Lachesis will frequently be found very useful after, and in some cases alternately with *Arsenicum,* should the patient complain of great pain in the throat, which is aggravated by the slightest external pressure; or should the sloughs not seem disposed to cast off in a kindly manner; and the neck become much swollen and discoloured. When the tendency to gangrene continues, and the patient is still affected with considerable prostration accompanied with debilitating sweats, *Cinchona* will often be found of service. *Nux vomica* is frequently serviceable after *Arsenicum* when the diarrhœa has been checked, but numerous small, foul, offensive ulcers are seen in the mouth and throat,—succeeded by *Carb. v.,* should a copious fetid ichor be discharged from the ulcers; with extreme exhaustion, and small, indistinct, or scarcely perceptible pulse. *Secale cornutum* may sometimes be administered with advantage in alternation with *Carb.* when the latter appears to afford but temporary benefit. *Rhus* is also occasionally useful in extreme cases, particularly if there be great muscular weakness, with trembling of the extremities, especially on movement; sopor and other symptoms described under this remedy in the Chapter on Typhus.

When from the beneficial effects of *Arsenicum,* or any of the other remedies above mentioned, the strength of the patient becomes invigorated, the countenance more animated, and the sloughs are thrown off in a kindly manner, yet the ulcers threaten to become indolent ; they will generally very speedily acquire a clean and florid bottom, and begin to cicatrize, on the administration of *Acid. nitricum*.

For further particulars in the treatment of malignant sore-throat, the reader is referred to page 54 of this work.* It remains but to be added, that in conducting the cure, the utmost cleanliness, combined with free ventilation, ought to be strictly observed,—for the double purpose of removing all malignant excretions and effluvia, and thereby putting a check to the ready extension of the contagion, as well as for the comfort and well-being of the patient.

The diet should consist of semolina, sago, gruel, and such like.

MUMPS. *Parotitis, Angina, Parotidea.*

Diagnosis. Inflammation with swelling of the parotid and submaxillary glands, sometimes running high, and extending to the throat and tonsils, with danger of suffocation.

This affection generally affects individuals under the age of puberty, and frequently declares itself as an epidemic during the prevalence of cold damp weather. When properly treated it is rarely dangerous, but particularly apt, if not carefully attended to, to attack some more important organs by metastasis; for example, suddenly disappearing in the glands mentioned, and painfully affecting those of the breast, etc.: these metastases may occur either from fresh exposure to cold, or by the application of saturnine, camphorated, or other repellent lotions.

This affection is generally ushered in by the ordinary symptoms of mild catarrhal fever, after which the swelling declares itself, sometimes interfering with the motion of the jaw; and by the extension of inflammation to the tonsils, affecting the hearing and impeding inspiration.

* See also Sore Throat, page 81.

THERAPEUTICS. MERCURIUS may almost be termed the specific remedy in the idiopathic form of this disease.

ADMINISTRATION. In many cases a single dose $\frac{000}{6}$ will be found sufficient to effect the cure; in other cases it will be found necessary to repeat the dose every twenty-four hours, for three or four successive times. When *Mercurius* does not promise to produce much benefit, after a dose or two, which is frequently the case in those who have been formerly salivated by *Mercury* under allopathic treatment, *Carbo vegetabilis* should be administered, particularly if the affection be accompanied by a considerable degree of hoarseness.

When through any neglect in taking proper precautions against cold, a metastasis to the brain has taken place, characterized by a sudden disappearance of the swelling of the glands, followed by a loss of consciousness, delirium, or other symptoms of *Inflammation of the Brain*, (which see,) we should have immediate recourse to *Belladonna*, *Hyoscyamus*, or *Cuprum aceticum*, as *there* prescribed.

Belladonna is moreover indicated when the swelling is red and presents an erysipelatous appearance; and should the inflammatory symptoms not readily yield to *Belladonna*, *Hyoscyamus* may be given; and after the latter, *Rhus*, *Bryonia*, *Sulph.*, *Arsenicum*, *Lachesis*, or *Silicea*, according to circumstances.

Should, however, the disease in the same manner be transferred to the stomach, CARBO VEGETABILIS is usually a most useful remedy; when it fails to afford all the desired relief, *Cocculus* may be had recourse to.

ADMINISTRATION. Six globules of the sixth potency, added to an ounce of water; a dessert-spoonful every two hours, until improvement declares itself. Should this glandular enlargement occur as a sequelæ of the following disorders, the practitioner will generally find the remedies thereafter mentioned the best adapted to effect resolution when practicable: of TYPHUS, *Bella.*, *Sulph.*, *Calc. c.*; of MEASLES, *Arnica*, *Bryonia*, *Rhus*; of SCARLATINA, *Hepar s.*, *Dulc.*, *Baryta*, *Bella.*, *Rhus*, and *Arsenicum*, *Carb. v.*, *Silicea*, *Lycopodium*, *Hepar*, *Conium*, *Aurum*, *Sulp.*, *Calc.*; in general cases, according to circumstances.

During the treatment of this affection, every care should be taken that the patient be kept *moderately* warm, exposed neither to damp, cold draughts, nor vicissitudes of temperature, and the jaws and neck should be protected by a worsted or flannel bandage.

BILIOUS COMPLAINTS.

Bilious complaints have of late years become the popular term for almost all derangements of the digestive functions; and by common consent, all these disorders have been at once unhesitatingly ascribed to a superabundance or deficiency of the important secretion of the liver. This opinion, although sufficiently plausible on its first appearance, will, on a careful examination, be found erroneous; for although in the disease which is commonly denominated, in severe cases, liver complaint, this organ is powerfully affected, yet it is generally only by sympathy; and the real seat of the disorder is in the stomach and bowels. When we succeed in restoring them to a normal state, the liver will, in most instances, again resume its natural functions.

Having premised thus much, we shall proceed to the consideration of Dyspepsia or Indigestion; under which will be found all the symptoms ascribed to the two imaginary and opposite causes of derangement, inactivity of the liver and too great a secretion of bile.

INDIGESTION OR DYSPEPSIA.

This disease appears in so many different phases, that we shall simply content ourselves with an enumeration of some of the principal exciting causes, and refer to the symptoms given under the different medicaments for its Diagnosis. The following are among the principal exciting causes:

Irregularities in diet—such as an over-indulgence in the pleasures of the table, partaking of rich and indigestible food and stimulating soups, excessive use of wine, malt and spirituous liquors, tea, coffee, and other stimulants; imperfect mastication of food, irregularity of, or too long fasting between meals, indolent or sedentary habits, exhaustion from intense study, keeping late hours, mental emotions, &c.

The foundation of this disorder is frequently laid in early life, by the baleful practice of the administration of large doses of calomel, and other deleterious drugs; and the evil is perpetuated in more mature age, by a continuance of the same absurd and dangerous system.

THERAPEUTICS. The principal homœopathic remedies for the treatment of this affection are, *Nux vomica*, *Sulphur*, *Pulsatilla*, *Bryonia*, *Chamomilla*, *Ipecacuanha*, *Ignatia*, *Carbo vegetabilis*, *Cinchona*, and *Hepar sulphuris*. Of these, *Nux vomica* and *Pulsatilla* are the chief.*

ADMINISTRATION. In dyspeptic cases we may dissolve seven globules of the third or sixth potency of each medicine, with the exception of *Nux vomica*, in fourteen teaspoonfuls of water, taking one morning and evening for a week, and cease its administration as long as we find manifest improvement; or if a medicinal aggravation come on, await the result. Of *Nux vomica*, we may dissolve three globules in seven teaspoonfuls of water, and take one each evening on going to bed; or when people are in the habit of taking supper, from half an hour to an hour before that meal. It will be found useful in many cases to vary the potency of the medicines chosen, the high acting better upon some constitutions, and the low upon others; but the principal point is the correct selection of the remedy.†

An abuse of coffee and tea is a frequent cause of many descriptions of sick and nervous headache, attended with excitement and dyspeptic symptoms, which will frequently disap-

* *Calcarea carbonica* is, in our estimation, one of the most valuable medicaments for Dyspepsia. It is indicated for the principal phenomena contained under *Nux vomica*, although, in regard to temperament, sex, &c., it accords more generally with *Pulsatilla*. It is peculiarly available as a transient or long-working remedy, after the use of either of these two medicines, especially when their impressions become by repetition evanescent.—ED.

† Vide note, p. 21.

pear of themselves on the disuse of these beverages; however, should not this speedily be the case, for the effects of coffee we may have recourse to *Nux vomica*, *Pulsatilla*, *Chamomilla*, or *Ignatia*, under which the sufferer will find his symptoms indicated. Against the effects of tea, *Cinchona* will generally be found an antidote, followed by *Ferrum* if necessary; in other cases, *Ipecacuanha*, *Thuja* or *Selenium* will be found useful.

NUX VOMICA covers the following symptoms, either when they have arisen in consequence of sedentary habits, excessive mental exertion, long watching, or the abuse of wine or ardent spirits: the *head confused*, with occasionally a *feeling* as if from *intoxication*, and *giddiness*, with sensation of turning and wavering of the brain; headache, unfitting for, and increased by, mental exertion; tearing, drawing, or jerking pains in the head or cheeks, and pulsative pains, and a sensation as if a *nail were driven into the brain*; congestion of blood to the head, with humming in the ears. The headaches are often deeply seated in the brain, or in the back part of the head, frequently confined to one side, or over the eyes, and at the root of the nose, coming on chiefly in the morning, after a meal, or in the open air. EYES, yellowness of the lower part of the whites, with a mist before them; a sensation as if one were about to fall; sparks, or small gray or black spots before the eyes; short-sightedness. FACE *pale* or *yellowish*, especially about the mouth and nose, frequent headache, and redness of the face, impaired powers of digestion, with insipidity of food. TONGUE foul, *dry*, *white*, or yellowish; *thirst* with water-brash, particularly after acids or rich food, accumulation of slimy mucus, or of water in the mouth; metallic, salt, sulphurous, herbaceous, mucous, *bitter*, *putrid*, *sour*, *sweetish*, or *putrid* taste, chiefly in the morning, or after meals; *bitter eructations*, or continued *nausea*, especially after *meals*, or even after drinking cold water or milk,—or on going into the open air after a meal; also from acids. HEARTBURN, HICCOUGH, ACIDITY, FLATULENCE—frequent and violent vomiting of food, mucus, or bile, or ineffectual efforts to vomit. *Distention and fulness* in the epigastrium, with excessive tenderness to the touch; a feeling of tightness of the clothes round the upper part of the waist; CRAMPS IN THE STOMACH; CONSTIPATION; reddish urine, with brick-dust coloured sediment; sleep unrefreshing, restless, either from suffering or otherwise, with disagreeable dreams, and drowsiness in the morning. See *Administration*, page 96.

One of the most distinctive indications for the employment of this remedy in preference to the next mentioned, is the temperament, which is restless, irritable, lively, and choleric. A disposition to *Hemorrhoids* is also a good indication.

For *Pulsatilla* we have nearly the same range of dyspeptic symptoms, with the difference that it is particularly adapted for females, children, individuals with light hair and a marked predisposition to purulent exudations of the cartilage at the edge of the eyelids, or to "styes," and for mild or phlegmatic dispositions. Amongst the characteristics, we more frequently find a *want* of thirst than thirst; a repugnance to fat and rich meat, and *suffering* after *taking pork and pastry;* a great difficulty in keeping the hands and feet sufficiently warm; frequent and loose, or difficult and loose, or slow evacuations; hypochondriasis, hysteria. See *Administration*, page 96.

BRYONIA. HEADACHE, *burning* or *expansive*, particularly after drinking, attended with bewilderment of the head and vertigo; TONGUE dry, coated white and yellow; sometimes the aversion to food is so strong, that the patient cannot bear the smell of it; loss of appetite, alternately with unnatural hunger; craving for acid drinks; great thirst; *insipid*, *clammy*, putrid sweetish, or *bitter* taste in the mouth; ACIDITY and FLATULENCE, or *bitter* rising after every meal, or after partaking of milk. HICCOUGH, nausea, water-brash, *vomiting of food*, or bile, particularly at night; tenderness of epigastrium to the touch, sensation of swelling in the pit of the stomach; pressure, as if from a stone in the stomach, especially after a meal, or on walking; *sensation of burning* in the pit of the stomach, and especially when *moving*. Constipation; temper restless, irascible, and obstinate; also when want of exercise or anger are frequently the exciting cause of the derangement, or the means of aggravating the symptoms. This dyspepsia is more apt to manifest itself in summer, or in damp weather, and is frequently accompanied with chilliness. POTENCY 6-30.

CHAMOMILLA. HEADACHE, with sometimes *semi-lateral*, pulling, shooting, and beating in the head; fulness, *giddiness*, and *staggering* in the *morning* when getting up; oppressive heaviness, vertigo, and sensation of a bruise; *headache sometimes felt during sleep*, with obscuration of the EYES; and yellow colour of the whites; TONGUE dry and cracked, with frothy mucus; *excessive thirst and desire for cold drink; bitter taste* of the mouth and of *food; want of appetite* and *dislike to food.* ACIDITY or sour risings, regurgitation of food, nausea, vomiting of food, mucus, and *bile; acute oppressive pain in the region of the heart*, distention at the epigastrium, pit of the stomach, and upper part of the waist, chiefly after eating, and at night attended with inquietude and terror; burning pain in the pit of the stomach, uneasiness, and feeling of sinking in the stomach; CRAMPS IN THE STOMACH, especially when traceable to coffee; sometimes constipation, but generally *relaxation of the bowels.* This remedy is valuable in indigestion, brought on by a *fit of passion*, or suppressed perspiration. See *Administration*, p. 96.

IPECACUANHA. FACE pale and yellowish, tongue sometimes clean, at others coated white or yellow; aversion to food, and particularly to fat or to rich indigestible food, such as pork, pastry, &c., or dyspeptic suffering on partaking of such; vomiting of food, drink, mucus, or bile, sometimes after a meal; retching or easy vomiting, generally attended with coldness of the face and extremities, and sometimes alternating with watery diarrhœa; sensation of emptiness, flaccidity, and sensation of sinking at the stomach. Headaches attended with nausea and vomiting; shooting pains, with heaviness and painful pressure on the forehead. Both this and *Pulsatilla* are valuable remedies for indigestion in children, arising from imperfect mastication or improper food. See *Administration*, page 96.

IGNATIA may sometimes follow *Pulsatilla* to complete a cure, or even supersede it, when there is a tendency to constipation, and particularly in temperaments alternating from high to low spirits, or *vice versâ*; it is especially indicated when *grief* has been the inducing cause of dyspepsia, hysteria, and hypochondriasis. $\frac{000000}{30}$.

In chronic cases, these remedies, as indicated, are chiefly valuable in the commencement of treatment, and may be required to be followed by other remedies to complete the cure. Sulphur $\frac{000}{6}$ or $\frac{00}{30}$, or TINCTURE OF SULPHUR, especially useful after *Pulsatilla* and *Nux vomica,* in removing any symptoms that may remain. HEPAR SULPHURIS $\frac{000}{6}$, is a valuable remedy in some cases of dyspepsia, but particularly in those in which the patient has previously been taking *blue-pill* or any other mercurial preparation for a considerable time.

ACIDUM SULPHURICUM, $\frac{0000}{3}$. Dyspepsia arising from excessive study, drinking, or other excesses, with the following symptoms: great weakness of digestion; acrid, foul, putrid taste in the mouth, dry tongue, burning and smarting sensation in the throat, sometimes attended with pricking, especially at night, and so troublesome as to prevent sleep (*Pyrosis*); offensive breath, especially in the morning (*aphthæ*); renewal or aggravation of the symptoms from *drinking cold water;* all cold drinks appear to disagree, unless a little brandy or some other ardent spirits is added to them; accumulation of water; saliva in the mouth; flatulence; bitter risings; vomiting of a limpid fluid, or of food. It may here be remarked, that, in cases where *Nux vomica* seems indicated, but the disposition is of a morose or hypochondriacal turn, COCCULUS $\frac{000}{30}$ may be substituted with effect; when the indications for temperament are not sufficiently distinctive, *Cocculus, Nux vomica* and *Pulsatilla* may be advantageously alternated. Finally, CARBO VEGETABILIS $\frac{000}{30}$ will frequently remove any symptoms that may remain after *Nux vomica.*

CINCHONA $\frac{00}{6}$ is a valuable auxiliary in the treatment of this derangement, when there is impaired appetite with great weakness of digestion, which is more liable to be experienced on partaking of supper; flatulence; bitter taste; languor; hypochondriacal disposition; and particularly when we can trace it to debilitating losses of fluids, such as to *abstraction or loss of blood,* too great a drain upon the resources during lactation, prolonged use of aperient medicines, &c., also disorders arising from abuse of tea, or from residing in impure atmospheres, and especially such as are overloaded with the exhalations of decayed vegetable matter.

Natrum c. may follow *Nux v.*, *Bryonia*, or *Cinchona*, with advantage, when a degree of weakness of digestion remains.

In *chronic* cases, this disorder sometimes takes a critical turn, vomiting becomes excessive, everything taken is returned from the stomach, the skin is hot and dry, the patient becomes emaciated, and the countenance cadaverous. Here, it need hardly be said, the aid of the experienced physician is required,—it will, therefore, be sufficient to intimate, that *Arsenicum* and *Lachesis* will in such cases tend much to invigorate the sinking energies, and even,—with the occasional aid of *Lycopodium*, *Veratrum*, *Baryta*, *Phosphorus*, *Conium*, or some one or other of the above-mentioned remedies, where necessary,—eventually effect a cure, provided the inroads of organic lesions have not already placed the unfortunate sufferer beyond the reach of art.

Accessory Treatment and Diet. In no other class of disorders is it more requisite to adhere strictly to dietetic regulations than in those where there is derangement in the digestive system, whether functional or organic: the patient so affected should, therefore, as closely as possible, regulate his regimen by the rules laid down at the commencement of this treatise, carefully avoiding, moreover, all such articles as he may find disagree with him, even if they appertain to the aliments allowed. He should generally abstain from soups, and every thing that has a tendency to distend the stomach, such as taking large quantities of warm liquids; he should not indulge his appetite to its full extent, avoid late hours, unnecessary exposure, severe mental exertion or anxiety, take sufficient exercise in the open air, and, as much as possible, keep his mind from dwelling upon his complaint, or on gloomy subjects.

WANT OF APPETITE. *Apepsia. Anorexia.*

Want of appetite being a concomitant symptom of many diseases, is treated in this treatise as such when present; but we now propose to look upon it as one of the *leading* symptoms of indigestion, and as such, deserving a particular notice. It may, as in the case of dyspepsia, in a great variety of cases be considered as attributable to an ill-regulated regimen, imperfect mastication of food, sedentary habits, and the neglect of taking sufficient exercise.

In many instances, removing the exciting cause will cure this disorder. Sufferers from this inconvenience should carefully avoid creating an artificial appetite, or partaking of the smallest quantity of food till a healthy call from nature proves that the former has assimilated; the habit of taking tea, and even, as the expression is, "making a meal of it," within a couple of hours after removing from the dinner table, is a frequent cause of apepsia and dyspepsia.

Another cause is the habit of drinking frequently, or very copiously during meals, and thereby attenuating the saliva and gastric juice, and rendering them less fitted for the purpose of digestion.

Other causes are the customs of sleeping after dinner, partaking of heavy suppers before retiring to rest, and indulgence in fermented, vinous or spirituous liquors, or in tea or coffee, particularly the latter.

An alteration in the hours of meals, and avoiding too long fasts between them, will frequently remove this affection.

In other cases, early rising, great attention to diet, avoiding rich or highly seasoned food, together with the daily use of pure, cold water,—drinking a tumblerful an hour or so before breakfast, three or four hours after dinner, and again about the hour of retiring to rest,—will suffice to restore the weakened digestive functions to a normal condition.

When, however, we cannot trace this disorder to any of the above, or some other probable cause, when every attention to regimen, and even an alteration of diet according to individual peculiarities or idiosyncrasy has failed to produce any good effect, we generally find the *want of appetite* accompanied with *other* symptoms of derangement of the digestive functions, which may prove useful in aiding us to select a proper remedy to restore the natural tone of the stomach; this will be found among the medicines most useful in DYSPEPSIA and CARDIALGIA: namely, *Nux vomica*, *Chamomilla*, *Pulsatilla*, *Cinchona*, *Ipecacuanha*, *Antimonium crudum*, *Bryonia*, *arnica*, *Hepar sulphuris*, *Lachesis*, *Sulphur*, and *Calcarea*.

Administration, the same as in Dyspepsia, (page 96,) which see.

Nux vomica is the principal remedy when the *want of appetite* can be traced to late hours, the habitual use of wine and coffee, sedentary and studious habits,—also when the following symptoms are present: dryness of mouth, tongue coated white with cracks or slimy mucus in the mouth, agustia, pyrosis, or inspidity of aliments, particularly meat, accumulation of water in the mouth, *aversion to food*, costiveness or constipation, confusion in the head or giddiness, as if the results of intoxication, amnesia, and difficulty of fixing the mind to a train of application, weight in the occiput, tinnitus aurium, heaviness and aching in the limbs, uneasiness, and a feeling of working or dragging of the tendons in the lower extremities, or cramps, restlessness, and general irritability of disposition,—symptoms aggravated in the morning. (p. 96.)

Chamomilla is frequently found useful after *Nux vomica*, when, although considerable benefit has been derived, the whole train of symptoms are not removed. The following are its particular indication: restless sleep, sensation of fulness and aching in the head, heat and redness of the face, a degree of fever, and tongue thickly coated, yellowish, rough and cracked, (anorexia and greenish diarrhœa,) general sensibility of the nervous system. This remedy is especially called for when a bitter taste in the mouth (or vomiting of bile, or of greenish mucus) ensues after eating. (*Administ.* p. 96.)

Pulsatilla. This remedy is specific in the affections arising from partaking of *over-rich* or *greasy food*, or *pork*, or *pastry*, or of aliments causing *flatulence*, such as vegetables, or of food in the preparation of which rancid butter or lard has been used. The more immediate indications are: whitish tongue with cracks, bitter, salt, or foul taste in the mouth, sliminess of the mouth, scraping roughness or acidity at the pharynx, bitter eructations, *aversion to warm food or to meat*, butter, and all rich food; *loss of taste;* distention of the abdomen, and particularly a feeling of tension under the false ribs, borborygmus, retarded or difficult defecation or diarrhœa, drawing in the limbs resembling that presentment in ague, exacerbation of symptoms in the evening in contradistinction to *Nux vomi a*, which is generally in the morning. This remedy is well adapted to the mild lymphatic temperament, and also when there is a peculiar sensibility, with a dislike to conversation, and valuable when imperfect mastication is the cause of the affection. Finally, in cases where there is a marked aversion to tobacco, even when accustomed to its use. Moreover, this remedy will be frequently found of benefit in some cases where *Chamomilla* has only temporarily relieved; but should a considerable degree of nervousness, or even irritability, remain after *Pulsatilla*, *Nux vomica* may be had recourse to. (See *Administ.* p. 96.)

CINCHONA in *anorexia* occurring during foggy weather when the air is charged with unwholesome vapours, or in the vicinity of marshy lands. The following are its indications: a sensation of constant satiety, with *general indifference to food*, and adypsia; tongue cracked or loaded with yellow or white coating; sensation of sinking and fluttering in the epigastrium (particularly when this symptom can be traced to the effects of tea); eructation after eating; desire for *highly-seasoned food, acids, pepper, and other condiments;* general weakness, with inclination to assume the recumbent posture, and inability to remain long in one position; uncomfortable feeling of dry heat, or shivering and sensitiveness in the open air; retarded or interrupted sleep; general feeling of uneasiness, with moroseness and peevishness. (*Adm.* p. 96.)

IPECACUANHA is indicated by the following symptoms: Nausea or vomiting, *without* foulness of the tongue, with *dislike to food.* Tobacco—even to smokers—has a nauseous taste, and causes vomiting. This remedy is also useful when the impaired appetite has arisen from *bolting* the food, particularly in the cases of children, and may be followed by *Pulsatilla*, when only partial relief has been obtained. (p. 96.)

ANTIMONIUM CRUDUM, in cases where a great disposition to nausea and vomiting with foul tongue exists; *anorexia*, dryness of the mouth with great thirst, particularly during the *night;* accumulation of phlegm in the throat with continual attempts to clear the throat; frequent rising soon after meals, of the food last partaken of; pain or disagreeable fulness at the epigastrium, frequently with sensibility to external pressure. In cases of recent standing with the above symptoms it is very speedily efficacious; and when relief does not quickly follow, the next mentioned remedy should be had recourse to.

Bryonia in recent derangement of the stomach with *anorexia*. When we find thirst more during the day than through the night, with a sensation of dryness in the throat, extending down the œsophagus; chilliness; *yellow*, dark-brown, or white coated, cracked tongue, with constipation. (p. 96.)

Arnica. This remedy is valuable when the *loss of appetite* has arisen from sitting up at night, watching at a sick bed; from not having devoted a sufficient number of hours to the period of rest; or from intense mental exertion, or from provocation or excitement. When from these causes the nervous system is powerfully affected; tongue coated yellow; taste foul, bitter, or sour, or nauseous or chalybeate, with offensive smell from the mouth; with rising of the food or eructations of the taste or smell of rotten eggs;* aversion to smoking and *desire for acids;* sensation of fulness in the scrobiculus after meals, with inclination to vomit; distention of the abdomen, with pinching colic, relieved by doubling up the body, and renewed by drinking the smallest quantity of wine; passing off and then coming on, with inclination to evacuate the bowels; general irritability and impossibility of fixing the mind upon any subject; inclination to remain lying down, which relieves a heavy stupifying headache, which the least motion or even conversation increases. (See *Administration*, p. 96.)

Hepar sulphuris is useful in *chronic* cases of *want of appetite*, with indigestion from the *slightest cause*, even with the most careful observance of diet. It is indicated by desire for high-seasoned dishes, acids, and wine; nausea, even inclination to vomit, particularly in the morning; and constipation, frequently with colic. This remedy is one of our

* (*Tartarus emet.*, *Sulphur*, *Valerian*, *Sepia*, *Stannum*, also cover the *latter* symptoms): the practitioner will therefore do well to bear the said remedies in mind when this particular symptom is a prominent one, and does not yield to *Arnica*.

chief antidotes to *Mercurius*, and consequently one best adapted to those affections arising from long-continued use of Calomel.

Administration. One grain of the third trituration in six dessert-spoonfuls of water, one daily, fasting. In other cases, it will be found more beneficial to give a globule or two of the sixth in a little water, and not to repeat the dose until five or ten days.*

Lachesis is a valuable remedy to follow *Hepar sulphuris* in obstinate cases, particularly when long continued constipation is complained of, and the symptoms have always been aggravated by *acid* drinks, &c.; in the latter case *Arsenicum* is also useful, and may sometimes precede *Lachesis* with advantage.

Administration. $^{0}\frac{0}{6}{}^{0}$ in the same manner as *Hepar sulphuris*.

In addition to the two last-mentioned remedies we may observe, that in the same class of cases, *Belladonna*, *Mercurius*, *Sulphur* and *Calcarea* may be used with considerable advantage, when the former remedies have only afforded partial relief.

Acidum sulphuricum is a useful remedy in cases of impaired appetite, with *weakness of digestion*, arising from habitual excess in the use of ardent spirits, or from debilitating loss of fluids, such as blood, &c., or in consequence of excessive study,—with the following symptoms: acrid or putrid taste, dry tongue, burning and smarting sensation in the gullet resembling heartburn; offensive breath, especially in the morning (aphthæ); disagreeable sensation of *pricking* in the throat, frequently occurring during the night, and disturbing sleep. In other cases, the practitioner or student may consult the subjoined remedies in the Materia Medica with advantage, either as applicable to the treatment of this affection or dyspepsia and cardialgia. *Sepia*, *Colchicum*, *Ferrum*, *Silicea*, *Ruta*, *Ammon. c.*, *Rhus*, *Aurum*, *Baryta c.*, *Acid. nitr.*, *Kali c.*, *Natr. m.* and *c.*, *Graphitis*, *Hyoscyamus*, *Ignatia*, *Staphysagria*,

* Vide note, p. 21.

Kreosotum, Petroleum, Anacardium, Causticum, Drosera, N. mosch., Capsicum. (See *Administration*, p. 96.)

DERANGEMENT OF THE STOMACH, ERUCTATIONS, &c.

Under this head we intend treating of a disorder which may arise in individuals of a generally unimpaired digestion—the characteristics of *eructations* will assist to indicate the remedy for persons subject to this unpleasant affection.

The ordinary causes of this derangement are: hurried, imperfect mastication; an overloaded stomach; fat, greasy, indigestible or tainted food, flatulent vegetables, ices, stimulants, &c., and are so well known that it is hardly necessary here to enter upon them, particularly as they will be more specially noted under the different medicines.

THERAPEUTICS. When the symptoms of approaching stomachic derangement declare themselves immediately, or a few hours after a repast, a little strong black coffee is frequently a sufficient restorative.

Should, however, this fail to relieve, and sick headache and inclination to vomit be present, we should assist nature by tickling the fauces with a feather, and by giving tepid water to drink until the stomach has completely evacuated its contents. Should, however, on the following morning, symptoms of deranged digestion continue, such as nausea, inclination to vomit, or vomiting, and disagreeable or offensive eructations, we should administer ANTIMONIUM CRUDUM $^{0}\frac{0}{6}{}^{0}$ in a little water, one of our most useful remedies in this affection, and which rarely fails to at least afford some relief. It is also peculiarly indicated when the affection has arisen from drinking sour or impure wine; or when, in addition to the symptoms of disordered stomach, a degree of *fever* returns every second day.

IPECACUANHA $^{0}\frac{0}{6}{}^{0}$. When a *rash* has been thrown out, from the effects of a disordered stomach, attended with anxiety, *oppressed breathing*, and sickness, this remedy will, in most cases, effect speedy relief;—but should the difficulty of breathing, or a degree of nausea or other uneasiness continue, BRYONIA should be exhibited.

BRYONIA $^{0}\frac{0}{6}{}^{0}$. In addition to the usefulness of this remedy in the foregoing instance, it is also very serviceable when the following symptoms are present: bitter eructations; *fever*, alternately with coldness and shivering; or redness of the face, heat in the head, and thirst with coldness and shivering; also where diarrhœa or constipation and peevishness or excessive irritability are present.

ARSENICUM $^{0}\frac{0}{6}{}^{0}$, acrid and bitter eructations with nausea and vomiting; also dry tongue, excessive thirst, salt taste in the mouth, and burning or violent pressure in the stomach, with diarrhœa or colic, and griping in the hypogastrium, particularly when arising from the effects of an *ice* which had been partaken of when warm, or from fruit, stale vegetables, or from *acids*. It may in many cases be advantageously followed by *Carbo vegetabilis*, which see.

NUX VOMICA $^{0}\frac{0}{6}{}^{0}$, offensive eructations, constipation, and confused headache, particularly if arising from previous intoxication, or even slight over-indulgence in *wine or other* stimulants; when possible, it should be taken the same night; as, taken in the morning, although eventually relieving, it frequently causes an aggravation for a few hours.

ARNICA $^{0}\frac{0}{6}{}^{0}$. Eructations resembling rotten eggs.*

PULSATILLA $^{0}\frac{0}{6}{}^{0}$, next to *Antimonium crudum*, the most important remedy in recent cases of deranged digestion, with eructations of ingesta, tongue foul and covered with mucus: chilliness and lowness of spirits; and also when a *rash* has been thrown out in consequence of the derangement. This remedy is, moreover, almost specific when the disturbance has arisen from the effects of rich food, such as *pork* or pastry, or even tainted meat, or from the effects of *ices*, *cold fruits*, or *crude vegetables*, *acid wine*, &c. (*Arsenicum* may follow *Pulsatilla*, if the latter do not effectually relieve.)

ACONITE $^{0}\frac{0}{6}{}^{0}$. When the affection owes its origin to par-

* See also note, p. 105.

taking of sour beer, vinegar, or other acids, particularly when we find oppressive pain in the stomach, great heat in the head, nausea, or actual vomiting of mucus, or even of blood.

HEPAR SULPHURIS $\frac{000}{6}$. When the digestion is naturally weak, and sour vomiting, attended with burning in the throat, colic and diarrhœa, is liable to ensue from the slightest error of diet, and particularly when anything of an acid quality has been partaken of. (*Lachesis* is often of great service here in alternation with *Hepar sulphuris*, at intervals of a week or so.)

CARBO VEGETABILIS $\frac{000}{12}$, although last mentioned, is not one of the least valuable remedies in this affection, and is often found particularly useful after *Pulsatilla*, *Arsenicum*, or *Nux vomica*, in removing any symptoms that may remain; it is, moreover, particularly useful where great susceptibility to the influence of the atmosphere, particularly to cold, exists at the same time; or in sufferings arising from abuse of *wine*, *ices*, salt; further, in derangement of the stomach arising from having partaken of game, or fish which has been too long kept, or meat which has been recooked while in a state of fermentation, as is liable to occur in warm weather;—in the latter instances, *Carbo v.* is to be preferred to any other medicine, and will rarely fail to afford relief; if any disagreeable symptoms remain, *Cinchona* $\frac{3}{3}$, may be administered in a little water, and followed, if required, by *Pulsatilla* $\frac{3}{6}$ in the same manner;—finally, this remedy is peculiarly valuable in obstinate and chronic cases of deranged digestion, when annoyance or inconvenience is felt after every meal, even amounting to nausea and vomiting attended with excessive flatulency, and where the pit of the stomach is tender on pressure.*

ADMINISTRATION of the medicines. A single dose, as above noted, is ordinarily all required; when, however, vomiting and other severe symptoms declare themselves, it may be better to dissolve four or five globules in eight or ten teaspoonfuls of

* A small quantity of finely powdered charcoal in a little good French brandy will be found an equally efficacious mode of administering this remedy as a corrective against any unpleasant effect arising from having partaken of tainted meat or fish.

water, and give one from time to time, according to the exigency of the case.

FLATULENCY. *Flatus, Tympanitis intestinalis.*

This affection, and the sufferings it entails, are generally found in individuals of weak digestion, and many also suffer from it immediately on taking cold in the abdomen or feet; it is also, as well known, a common result of errors in diet, and the too frequent indulgence in vegetables and fruits: In corpulent individuals the sufferings arising from this complaint, such as difficulty of breathing, palpitation of the heart, trembling of the limbs, confusion of the head, and swelling of the face, especially in hypochondriacal subjects, are most distressing. However, with proper attention to regimen, and suitable medical treatment, it is rarely very difficult to remove.

As an accompaniment of deranged digestion, it has also been noticed under Dyspepsia.

Against this complaint the most careful preservatives are: avoiding cold, exposure in cold damp weather, very cold drinks, or distending the stomach with a large quantity of warm fluid, particularly strong tea or coffee; each patient should also study his own digestion, and carefully refrain from partaking of any species of aliment which experience has found liable to produce flatulency. Sedentary habits also should be avoided, and a proper portion of the day devoted to exercise in the open air.

Therapeutics. In the treatment of this affection, the following medicines have been found most frequently called for: *Cinchona, Arsenicum, Nux vomica, Pulsatilla, Carbo vegetabilis, Colchicum, Belladonna, Colocynth,* and *Tincture of Sulphur.* Of these, *Nux vomica* and *Pulsatilla* are most frequently required.

Administration. In *recent* cases, six globules of the third potency may be given, dissolved in an ounce of water, a dessert-spoonful every half hour till relief ensues; after which a dose of a couple of globules every four or five days or so, to counteract the tendency to this affection. *

* Vide note, p. 21.

Cinchona $\frac{000}{6}$. When the affection can be traced to tea or warm drinks, an hour or two after a hearty meal, by which the process of indigestion has been interrupted; or to debility, loss of humours from venesection, or the continued use of purgatives; or to deranged digestion arising from flatulent food, with painful tension and *distention of the abdomen;* or when, on the occasional expulsion of flatus, a sensation of tension is felt in the umbilical region; another indication for this remedy is where coldness or shuddering is experienced after drinking.

Arsenicum $\frac{00}{6}$ where the last-mentioned symptom has not been relieved by the foregoing medicine.

Nux vom. $\frac{000}{6}$. In cases where the flatulence is attended with sensation of pressure at the pit of the stomach, causing dyspnœa and a feeling as if the clothing were too tight, or a sensation of pressure as from a stone, particularly when the affection arises from an habitual use of coffee, or sedentary habits.

Pulsatilla $\frac{000000}{6}$, when the affection has arisen from having eaten of rich or greasy food, after which a copious draught of water has been partaken of, and the abdomen is swollen with a pain as from a bruise, with borborygmus. *Carbo vegetabilis* is one of the most important remedies after the foregoing in chronic cases, and particularly when the inconvenience arises after partaking of the smallest morsel of food.

Colchicum $\frac{000000}{6}$, when from a considerable accumulation of wind the abdomen is extremely distended, or as it might be expressed, inflated, amounting almost to tympanites, and sounds *like a drum on striking it with the hand*—without any marked pain, but with heat and difficulty of respiration. (This remedy is often peculiarly efficacious when the derangement is attributable to vegetable food.)

Belladonna $\frac{000}{3}$. In cases of flatulent obstruction, in which the transverse section of the colon is the particular seat of the accumulated flatus, and becomes protruded like a pad, this remedy should be administered; it may be followed by *Colocynth*, when the relief obtained is only temporary, or when, from the manner in which the patient traces the course of his uncomfortable feelings, there is every reason to conclude that the flatulent distention and obstruction occupy the entire extent of the *colon*.

When the flatulence occurs very frequently, in fact, where a marked predisposition to it exists, we must have recourse to TINCTURE OF SULPHUR $\frac{000}{30}$, or one drop of the 30th potency.

Although I have pointed out the remedies best suited to the cases of this affection most ordinarily occurring, and have also treated of the same subject under DYSPEPSIA and COLIC, to which the reader is referred, I still think it advisable to add a few medicines which bear particularly upon this disorder, and deserve a careful study. They are: *Lycopodium, Cocculus, Natrum, Natrum muriaticum, Zincum foliatum, Magnetis polus arctus, Agnus castus, Ferrum, Graphitis.*

SPASMS OF THE STOMACH.

Gastrodynia, Cardialgia, Gastralgia.

DIAGNOSIS. Contractive and spasmodic or gnawing pains at the epigastrium, extending to the chest and back, attended with anxiety, nausea, eructation or vomiting, with faintness and coldness of the extremities; the patient is sometimes relieved by emission of ascending flatus, and when complicated with pyrosis, by a discharge of a quantity of limpid fluid; occasionally headache and constipation are present. In some cases the pain is very slight, but there is always more or less, and a degree of anxiety, with nausea, increased by taking food; it seems generally to arise from an abnormal state of the nerves of the stomach, and is frequently accompanied by a disease of the liver, spleen, or pancreas, or even by scirrhus of the stomach or duodenum. Although the real seat and nature of this disorder may be somewhat obscure, yet upon one point we may rest perfectly satisfied, that, even where it exists as a primary and idiopathic disease, the digestive function rarely fails to be considerably impaired during its progress. The disease is a frequent attendant on gout; and it very rarely occurs before the age of puberty. The paroxysms last for a longer or shorter time, and return in many instances periodically, and may be brought on by partaking of improper articles of diet, or in severe cases, by any solid food whatsoever.

The chief articles to be avoided by an individual suffering from this malady are—crude, uncooked vegetable substances, such as salads, cheese, new bread, sweetmeats, cherries, nuts, olives, and roasted chesnuts; and stimulants of all kinds, whether tea, coffee, alcoholic or fermented drinks.

The CAUSES are: long fasting between meals, very hot or cold drinks, and habitual use of ardent spirits, of indigestible food, worms, and in some instances, perhaps, exposure to cold or damp weather.

It is a more frequent affection of the female than the male sex, frequently occurring after the cessation of the usual monthly discharge, or from any interruption of its usual course: in such instances it is frequently accompanied with hysteria, syncope, and may pass on to vomiting of blood.

Notwithstanding the usually intractable nature of this affection, is has been treated with marked success by the method about to be pointed out.

THERAPEUTICS. *Nux vomica* is the principal, and in most cases, the most appropriate remedy against spasms of the stomach, and particularly in cases where this affection can be attributed to the long-continued use of strong coffee, or to an excessive indulgence in spirituous liquors; it is, moreover, of essential service in many cases of the same disorder which have arisen after the suppression of chronic or hæmorrhoidal discharges, or when the party affected is liable to fits of hysteria or hypochondriasis. The following are the immediate symptoms which call for the administration of this medicine: *Constriction, pressure, squeezing*, or *spasm* in the stomach, accompanied with the sensation as if the clothes were *too tight at the waist*, or as if flatus were pent up in the hypochondria. This sensation, as well as the pains before mentioned, become generally increased *after a meal, or after partaking of coffee;* in addition to which, a feeling of depression or constriction is experienced at the chest, which, in many cases, extends to between the shoulders and the lower part of the back. Frequently also nausea, accumulation of clear water in the mouth, or risings of sour bitter fluids, attended with a sensation of burning in the throat and gullet (pyrosis); sour or putrid taste in the mouth, vomiting of ingesta, flatulent distention of the bowels, *constipation*, aching in the forehead, palpitation of the heart, and anxiety. When these symptoms are liable to be excited by a fit of passion, or become aggravated *in the morning*, or when the patient is occasionally awakened out of his sleep by the spasmodic attack, this remedy is still more certainly indicated.

ADMINISTRATION. $\frac{00}{6}$ in a dessert-spoonful of water, and repeated in six hours if necessary; or in chronic cases with a constant pain, six globules of the same potency may be dissolved in four dessert-spoonfuls of water, and a dose taken every evening until finished. Of this, as of all the other medicines, we may administer a dose from two to four hours before an expected paroxysm, when the Cardialgia returns periodically, or when from some imprudence in diet we have reason to apprehend an attack. This precaution, if it fails altogether to check it, will often greatly modify it. Should *Nux vomica* merely afford a temporary benefit, followed by renewed aggravation, and in cases where the disorder returns again after it has been for a time suppressed by *Nux*, we should repeat that remedy; and if it then fail to afford relief, *Carbo vegetabilis* will generally complete the cure. Should this fail, particularly where the affection is traceable to the suppression of some chronic eruption, Tincture of SULPHUR ought to be administered. This medicine, as well as *Pulsatilla* and *Sepia*, whose value in such cases we shall notice under their several heads, is particularly useful in gastrodynia in females, arising from any disturbance of the menstrual function. Vide note, p. 21.

ADMINISTRATION. Of the *Carbo vegetabilis* we may dissolve $\frac{000000}{12}$ in eight teaspoonfuls of water, and give one morning and evening until finished. Of the *Tincture of Sulphur* $\frac{000000}{6}$ in the same manner.

In some cases also, where no improvement results from the exhibition of *Nux vomica*, the following should be consulted: *Chamomilla*, *Belladonna*, *Cocculus*, *Ipecacuanha*, *Pulsatilla*, *Sepia*, *Ignatia amara*, *Cinchona*, *Staphysagria*, *Stannum*, *Bryonia*, *Platina*, *Senega*, *Ratanhia*, and *Arnica montana*. Of course, also, a preference should be given from the first to that medicine whose symptoms approach most closely to those under which the patient is suffering.

Chamomilla $^{0}\frac{0}{3}{}^{0}$. For the employment of this remedy the principal indications are: *pressure, as if from a stone in the pit of the stomach*, or painful *pressure* at the *præcordial region*, as if the heart would be *crushed;* flatulent *distention* at the same part, as also of the hypochondria and abdomen, with shortness of breath, anxiety, and throbbing headache: *Mitigation* of the above symptoms *on partaking of coffee*, a distinguishing mark between the indications of this remedy and those of Nux vomica; on the other hand, as in the case of the latter, it is also indicated when the symptoms, as described, are liable to be brought on by a fit of passion.

Colocynth is more efficacious than *Cham.* in the latter case, and especially when the fit of passion is accompanied by indignation. In obstinate cases, where Chamomilla fails, notwithstanding the apparent similarity of the symptoms, Belladonna $^{0}\frac{0}{6}{}^{0}$ ought to be substituted for it: also when we meet gnawing pressure, or spasmodic tension in the pit of the stomach, *relieved on bending backwards and holding in the breath;* further, spasms of the stomach, which recurs daily during dinner, or else pain of so *violent a nature as to deprive the patient of consciousness. Carbo v.* may be preferred to *Belladonna*, however, when the most prominent symptom remaining consists of a sense of aching and pressure at the pit of the stomach and the præcordial region, causing a sensation as if the heart were about to be crushed. (See *Chamomilla.*)

Cocculus $^{00}\frac{0}{6}{}^{00}$, in many cases of this complaint are particularly indicated, when in addition to the usual symptoms there are constipation and constrictive pains over the entire abdomen, with flatulency and accumulation of water in the mouth, and alleviation of the sufferings on the recurrence of the latter symptoms.

Ipecacuanha $^{0}\frac{0}{3}{}^{0}$, is also useful in cases of this affection, when the paroxysms are accompanied with nausea, vomiting, dull darting pains in the pit of the stomach, and sensation of *excessive uneasiness* in the same region.

Pulsatilla $^{0}\frac{0}{6}{}^{0}$. In cases with shooting pains in the stomach, *which are aggravated by movement, and particularly by making a false step.* Pulsatilla is also one of the most appropriate remedies when the attacks are followed by vomiting, or accompanied by violent tension and squeezing, or throbbing and sensation of anxiety about the pit of the stomach, increase of pain after eating, or more particularly a feeling of pressure and pinching after dinner, with a relaxed state of the bowels, or a disposition thereto. Disposition to hysteria or hypochondriasis. It is, as well as *Sulphur* and *Sepia*, called for in cases of this affection, arising from suppressed menstruation. When *Puls.* does not afford much relief, the desired result is often attainable through *Ignatia.*

SEPIA $\frac{0}{1}\frac{0}{2}$. Gastrodynia arising from suppressed or difficult menstruation, and may in general cases advantageously follow *Pulsatilla :* it is indicated by most of the sufferings that arise, taking place after a meal, by pressure in the stomach as from a stone, and by a *burning pain* in the epigastrium and scrobiculus: by restoring singly, or in conjunction with *Pulsatilla* and *Sulphur*, the menstrual flux, it frequently removes the cardialgia and hysteria consequent upon this derangement, or at least places the affection in such a position that it is easily cured by some other medicine, closely corresponding to the remaining symptoms.

IGNATIA AMARA $0\frac{0}{1}\frac{0}{2}0$ is indicated under nearly similar circumstances as *Puls.*, with the exception of the state of the bowels, the Ignatia being more appropriate to cases attended with costiveness, and where the inclination to vomit is absent, or when the affection has been caused by grief, anxiety, etc., or occurs in hysterical or hypochondriacal individuals.

CINCHONA $0\frac{0}{6}0$ is of great service in most cases of spasms of the stomach with general weakness, arising from loss of humours, the result of *bloodletting*, or repeated hemorrhages, abuse of emetics or *aperients, too long continued suckling*, &c.; and is further indicated by great weakness of digestion, distention and uncomfortable weight, pressure, or pains in the stomach after eating, so that the patient feels much easier when fasting; these latter are the more immediate indications for the employment of this medicine. (Nux v. and Carbo v. may follow Cinchona, should the latter not remove all these symptoms.)

STAPHYSAGRIA $0\frac{0}{6}0$. This is useful in some cases of this complaint, and is particularly applicable when there is acute pressive tension and squeezing about the pit of the stomach, which sometimes obstruct the breathing, *but which is relieved by bending the body forward.* When the pain partakes of a marked tensive character, and *extends to the region of the navel,* with sensibility of the region of the stomach on external pressure, shortness of breath, anxiety, and nausea, STANNUM $\frac{0\,0}{12}$ will be found more appropriate.

BRYONIA $\frac{0\,0\,0}{12}$. This medicine is more particularly adapted to the milder cases of cardialgia, with *painful pressure,* or a feeling of *disagreeable fulness* in the stomach after a meal, which occasionally becomes converted into a feeling of constriction, cutting or pinching, and is *relieved by eructation* and *external pressure.* This remedy is moreover still more clearly indicated when the symptoms are generally accompanied with severe headache or painful compression in various parts of the head, and particularly at the temples, which are liable to be excited whenever any article of diet disagrees in the slightest degree; increase of the sufferings by movement; habitual costiveness.

PLATINA $\frac{0\,0}{30}$. *Spasms of the stomach* in females, occurring particularly at the *monthly period,* (*Chamomilla, Pulsatilla, Nux v.,* and *Cocculus,* are equally efficacious at such periods when the symptoms are as indicated under these remedies,) and especially when the catamenia at the same time are generally *very copious,* and of too *long duration.*

SENEGA $^{0}\frac{0}{6}{}^{0}$ will be found efficacious in cases with painful pressure and burning in the stomach, especially at night.

RATANHIA $^{0}\frac{0}{6}{}^{0}$. Spasms of the stomach, or painful constrictive pain, relieved by eructation, with loss of appetite, hiccough, distention of the abdomen, costiveness, and frequent micturition.

ARNICA MONTANA $^{000}\frac{0}{6}{}^{00}$, in spasms or pains in the stomach which have originated in the effects of a strain, or from a *blow,* &c., will be found specific. It is, however, also an excellent remedy when there is a sense of *pressure* as from a stone, or of fulness in the stomach and scrobiculus, *constrictive* pain in the stomach and in the *præcordial region,* shooting pain in the pit of the stomach, with painful pressure or aching, extending to the back, and tightness of the chest, increased by eating, drinking, and external pressure.

Bismuthum $^{0}\frac{0}{6}{}^{0}$. Cardialgia, with tenderness on pressure at the pit of the stomach in hysterical females. This remedy is further often of great service in some of the most obstinate cases, particularly when there is a sensation of great weight or pressure, with indescribable pain and uneasiness in the stomach.

Arsenic. Periodic pains in the stomach of a burning character, and with acrid, sour eructations, vomiting of ingesta, or of mucus, even of blood; anorexia, extreme debility, emaciation.

Lycopodium $\frac{0\,0}{12}$. Squeezing or compressive pains proceeding from each extremity of the stomach, with flatulent distention; want of appetite; pains in the back and loins, (constipation); exacerbation of the symptoms in the *open air*, after a meal or in the morning. Cardialgia in lymphatic females, with too copious catamenia.

Lachesis $\frac{0\,0}{12}$. Spasms of the stomach, particularly in persons addicted to excessive indulgence in wine or ardent spirits, relieved by partaking of food; flatulence, constipation, numbness, and paralytic weakness of the extremities.

Sulphur $\frac{0\,0}{6}$. Frequently an indispensable remedy in chronic cases, attended with heartburn; aggravation of the pains after a meal; constipation, hemorrhoids.

Calcarea $\frac{0\,0}{18}$. In obstinate cases, occurring in individuals who are habitually addicted to the abuse of wine or ardent spirits, *Calc.* will generally be found of great service, especially after the previous employment of *Nux v.*, *Lach.* and *Sulph.* It is further a valuable remedy in the cases of plethoric females subject to nasal hemorrhage, or to excessively copious menstruation; and is *generally* indicated when the paroxysms of pain come on usually at night, or *after a meal;* in which latter instance vomiting sometimes results, or nausea and acidity, with painful sensibility or pressure at the epigastric region; constipation, hemorrhoids, or chronic looseness of the bowels.

Administration. In most cases these medicines may be exhibited in the same manner as already noted under *Carbo vegetabilis* and *Sulphur*. (See also remarks upon *Nux vomica.*)

In severe cases, six globules of the potency named may be dissolved in eight dessert-spoonfuls of water, and one given every two, four, or six hours, according to the results obtained; for example, in individuals of delicate organization it may sometimes be needful to give a less number of globules, and to select a higher potency, the thirtieth.*

These are the principal remedies to be employed against the ordinary cases of Cardialgia; † but in some cases may be called for: *Sanguin.*, *Graph.*, *Gratiol.*, *Magn.*, *Nitr. sp.*, *Sil.*, *Stann.*, *Stront.*, *Am. c.*, *Cupr.*, *Daph.*, *Kali c.*, *Euphorb.*, *Kreos.*, *Natr.*, *Natr. m.*, *Asaf.* In hysterical or hypochondriacal subjects: *Ign.*, *Nux v.*, *Calc.*, *Grat.*, *Cocc.*, *Stann.*, *Bism.*, *Digit.*, &c.

HEARTBURN. *Black-water. Water-brash. Pyrosis.*

This is not an affection of the organ, which its name would imply, but a painful or uneasy sensation of *heat* or *acrimony* about the pit of the stomach, sometimes extending upwards. It is frequently accompanied with anxiety, nausea, and vomiting; or a violent gnawing spasmodic pain in the region of the stomach, from which the patient experiences no relief until he succeeds in ejecting a quantity of limpid fluid. The remedies required for the treatment of the disorder are the same as those mentioned under Dyspepsia, Flatulence, Spasm of the Stomach, according to symptoms: of which, *Nux v.*, *Puls.*, *Sulphur*, *Acid. sulphuricum*, *Carbo v.*, *Cinchona*, or *Calcarea* will be found the most appropriate in ordinary cases. (See the aforesaid derangements for particular indications.)

VOMITING OF BLOOD. *Hæmatemesis.*

Diagnosis. Blood evacuated by vomiting, sometimes pure, (generally venous,) of a dark colour, but sometimes of a bright red; it is occasionally mixed with bile, food, &c.; the quantity varies; blood is occasionally discharged in coagula by stool.

Premonitory symptoms. Weight, pressure, fulness or tensive

* Vide note, p. 21.

† Vide Dyspepsia, p. 95.

pain or spasm in the hypogastric or hypochondriacal regions; griping and colic; burning heat in the region of the stomach; anxiety, particularly on partaking of food or drink, or on pressure on the stomach; saltish taste in the mouth; impaired appetite and nausea; giddiness, syncope, cold perspiration; sometimes also an intermittent pulsation is perceptible at the scrobiculus.

Some only of the preceding symptoms may be present previous to the attack, and others during its course when very severe, or frequently renewed. We often find wild delirium or wandering, accompanied with spasms and a gradually increasing weakness, and remission of pulse with frequent syncope.

The most frequent causes of this affection are the sudden suppression of any sanguineous discharge, and the consequent determination of blood to the stomach; it is consequently apt to declare itself after a stoppage of the hæmorrhoidal flux, and is a very common affection in females, from the suppression or cessation of the catamenia; in which case, as before remarked under that affection, it is frequently preceded by CARDIALGIA. Other causes are: scirrhus of the stomach, internal lesions or injury of that organ from swallowing sharp substances, or from worms; poisons, drastic purgatives, or emetic drugs, external contusion, obstruction of important viscera, or a change in the constituent principles of the blood itself; the direct cause is the bursting of some of the vessels of the stomach.

The dangers arising from the use of *powerful astringents* are, inflammation or subsequent induration of the stomach, or putrid gastric fever.

THERAPEUTICS. Although it is unlikely that any one, not properly qualified, would think of treating a severe case of this affection, unless compelled to do so from the difficulty of obtaining medical advice, yet it may be advisable to point out such remedies as experience has proved to be most serviceable in it as ordinarily met with, — premising, however, that when it arises from any organic disease, of the existence of which the experienced practitioner can alone determine, a different course may be necessary.

When it occurs in females from the non-appearance or suppression of the monthly discharge, or from its final cessation, see articles CHLOROSIS, AMENORRHŒA, CESSATIO MENSIUM; from worms, see HELMINTHIASIS; poisonous substances, see POISONS; disease of the spleen, consult SPLENITIS.

We may now proceed to the consideration of the remedies above alluded to.

ACONITUM. When the premonitory symptoms above given declare themselves, and particularly when a considerable degree of fever precedes the attack.

ADMINISTRATION. $00\frac{00}{6}00$ in an ounce of water, giving a dessert-spoonful, repeating in half an hour, and then every hour till the fever abates; in this mode, if taken in time, we may often, by calming the circulation, prevent an attack.

NUX VOMICA. In a decidedly plethoric constitution with a marked (venous) stomachic or *abdominal congestion*, and tendency to constipation; particularly when arising from suppression of hemorrhoids, or of the menstrual flux, or from indulgence in vinous, spirituous, or fermented liquors, and still further indicated by irritability of temper.

ADMINISTRATION. $\frac{00}{6}$ in a teaspoonful of water, repeated in from three to twelve hours, according to the exigencies of the case.

PULSATILLA. The value of this remedy is noticed in the diseases of females above mentioned; it is also in many cases found more suitable than *Nux vomica* for males when of lymphatic temperament and mild disposition. Some of the best indications for this medicine will be found under DYSPEPSIA, CARDIALGIA, and DERANGEMENT OF THE STOMACH. ADMINISTRATION the same as *Nux vomica*.

CINCHONA. When a quantity of blood has been already vomited, this remedy, from its power of restoring the energy of the system after debilitating losses, is clearly indicated; it should also be chosen when the patient has had a severe attack of hæmatemesis, which has ceased of itself, but still left great weakness.

ADMINISTRATION. $\frac{000}{6}$ in about a teaspoonful of water, after which, if a slight aggravation ensue, we must wait quietly until it passes off; and while improvement continues progressing, refrain from repeating; and after forty-eight to seventy-two hours, we may give a second dose; but if no marked alteration of any kind declare itself, or if the disease advance, we may repeat it from four to six hours, the same dose.

ARNICA. One of our most important remedies in severe cases, and especially when occurring in individuals of a robust constitution, of a sanguine temperament and choleric disposition. It is further indicated when the patient complains of pains, resembling the results of a contusion, in all the extremities.

ADMINISTRATION. Six globules of the third potency in an ounce of water, a dessert-spoonful every three hours, desisting if a medicinal action declare itself, and lengthening the intervals according to the amelioration that takes place. In mild attacks, $\frac{00}{6}$ in a little water, repeated every six or even every twelve hours, have been found sufficient.

TINCTURE OF SULPHUR is useful in strumous habits, or when the affection has arisen from suppressed hæmorrhoids; its value, also, in cases of abnormal menstruation, will be pointed out in the proper place.

ADMINISTRATION. $\frac{0000}{6}$, in four dessert-spoonfuls of water, one morning and evening for two days, and if no severe symptoms direct our attention to another remedy, it should be allowed to continue its action for a week or fortnight, as long as a gradual improvement is going on; in fact, in such constitutions we should take every opportunity between the intervals of the attacks, of giving a dose or two of this medicine, should no other better calculated to combat this tendency appear to merit a preference.

The following remedies also deserve a careful study: *Phosphorus, Belladonna, Arsenicum, Lycopodium,* (may be ranked next to *Nux v.* in cases arising from *abdominal congestion,*) and *Hyoscyamus,* (which, with *Belladonna,* is particularly useful in cases with *Spasmodic* action,) *Lycopodium, Arsenicum, Phosphorus* and *Secale cornutum* (Schirrus.) Finally, *Carbo vegetabilis, Millefolium, Cantharides, Calcarea carbonica, Natr. muriaticum, Zincum* and *Causticum,* under peculiar circumstances, and as tending to eradicate the predisposition to such affections.

The application of dry cupping-glasses to the abdomen and under the ribs, or of a cloth which has been dipped in moderately cold water, to the lower region of the abdomen, sometimes form useful auxiliaries in arresting the hemorrhage. See also *Hemorrhage* from the *Lungs*, under HEMOPTYSIS.

DIET. The rules already given under DYSPEPSIA should be observed, but with still greater strictness; no solid food must be partaken of; all drinks should be cold; animal jellies, preparations of milk, light puddings, and broths, merely tepid, may be allowed in cases where the patient may require such nourishment; but nothing more must be taken than is absolutely necessary for that purpose; immediately after an attack, no food should be given for some hours, and then very cautiously and in small quantity. It is evident that, in such cases, absolute rest, both mental and bodily, is essentially requisite.

CONSTIPATION. COSTIVENESS. OBSTIPATION.

Obstructio Alvi.

We have now to treat of an affection which so frequently baffles the skill of the practitioners of the old school; their leading cause of failure is their ignorance of the great curative principle, and consequent proceeding upon a system opposed to the operations of nature. This affection is generally sympathetic with some other derangement of the organism, and, consequently, in our treatment of different diseases, we have had frequent occasion to allude to it. One of the leading causes of aggravation and excessive obstinacy in the *Constipation*, most closely approaching to an idiopathic form, is the practice of flying to aperient medicines on the slightest appearance of costiveness, under the absurd idea that *keeping the bowels open* is a species of panacea against disease of every description. Many mothers are so possessed with this idea, that they are continually administering physic to their children, without the slightest apparent call for it, and thus lay the foundation of dyspepsia and other visceral derangements in after-life. Many a slight case of costiveness which, if left to nature, would have disappeared of itself, leaving no ill consequences, has, by an ill-judged administration of aperients, been converted into obstinate *Constipation*, embittering existence and predisposing the constitution to a variety of diseases in after-life. To prevent misconception upon this point, we may remark that we by no means undervalue a regular state of the bowels; but when costiveness shows itself, we happily possess remedies calculated to restore the balance of the system; and in obstinate cases do not content ourselves with simply alleviating the symptoms, but mainly direct our attention to the permanent removal of the affection.

Many of the principal causes of this disorder, besides that mentioned, are the same with those particularized under INDIGESTION or DYSPEPSIA.

THERAPEUTICS. In trivial cases it will be found sufficient to pay proper attention to diet, to avoid too dry or indigestible food, masticate properly, to partake of meat only once a day, and to take sufficient exercise in the open air.* Should this course not have the desired effect, we must choose one or more of the following remedies: namely, *Opium, Alumina, Bryonia, Nux vomica, Pulsatilla, Platina, Natrum muriaticum, Plumbum metallicum,* or *Carbonicum, Sulphur, Lachesis, Veratrum, Lycopodium, Sepia, Veratrum, Silicea.*

OPIUM is chiefly to be selected in recent cases when Constipation is not habitual, but is also, like *Nux v.*, and other remedies, serviceable in cases of a more chronic character when arising from *sedentary habits.* In *old people*, it is generally more useful than *Bryonia* and *Lachesis*, although these and the other remedies must be borne in mind and administered when called for by the nature of the symptoms. The more immediate indications for *Opium* are: want of power to relieve the bowels, with a feeling of constriction in ano; pulsation and sense of weight in the abdomen, dull, heavy pain in the stomach, parched mouth, and want of appetite, *determination of blood to the head*, with redness of the face and headache.

* See also the concluding remarks of this Chapter.

ADMINISTRATION. $\frac{00}{3}$, in a little water, repeated in twelve hours if no benefit result. (Vide note, p. 21.)

ALUMINA. Constipation from an apparent absence of peristaltic motion; fæces hard, dry, broken, evacuated with considerable exertion of the abdominal muscles and forcing, and sometimes streaked with blood; constipation from *travelling*.

ADMINISTRATION. Same as *Nux v.*

BRYONIA is especially useful in constipation occurring in *warm weather*, and in persons of dark complexion and an irritable or obstinate disposition, with a tendency to be easily chilled and subject to rheumatism; it is further indicated when constipation arises from *disordered stomach*, and is attended with determination of *blood to the head, and headache*.

ADMINISTRATION. $\frac{00}{30}$, in a little water, repeated in twenty-four hours, even if partial relief ensue. In chronic cases, two globules be taken daily for a week or so until benefit result, or a change ensue which may render the selection of another remedy, appropriate to the modified symptoms, necessary.

NUX VOMICA. This remedy is particularly useful when constipation results from too heavy a meal, indigestible food, and stimulating liquids; or in chronic cases arising from long-continued indulgence in vinous, fermented, or spirituous drinks, or coffee, or from sedentary habits or excessive study. It is peculiarly adapted to persons of irascible and lively temper, with *determination of blood to the head, and headache*, unfitness for exercise, disturbed sleep, and a feeling of general oppression or heaviness; frequent and ineffectual efforts to relieve the bowels, attended with sensation of stricture and sometimes frequent, painful and difficult emission of urine. It is, as remarked under *Dyspepsia*, particularly indicated for individuals subject to hemorrhoids.

ADMINISTRATION. $\frac{000}{6}$, taken in a little water towards evening. In chronic cases $\frac{000000}{30}$, in six teaspoonfuls of water, one each night at bed time; or $\frac{000}{30}$ repeated every four to eight days. (Vide note, p. 21.)

PULSATILLA has nearly the same indications as *Nux vomica*, with the characteristic distinction of temperament before noted under Dyspepsia. In recent cases, it is particularly indicated when the obstruction has arisen from indigestion brought about by rich or greasy food, and when it is accompanied with moroseness and shivering.

ADMINISTRATION. $\frac{000}{6}$ or $\frac{000000}{12}$ in the same manner as *Nux v.*

PLATINA is a useful remedy when constipation has been brought about by travelling, when *Opium* has failed, or especially when the constriction is attended with straining.

ADMINISTRATION. $\frac{000}{6}$, $\frac{000000}{30}$, in the same manner as *Pulsatilla.*

PLUMBUM METALLICUM or CARBONICUM. Obstinate constipation, with ineffectual efforts; painful retraction and constriction of the anus; or evacuation of tenacious, hard, bullet-shaped fæces.

ADMINISTRATION. Same as *Nux vomica.*

NATRUM MURIATICUM. $\frac{0000}{6}$ or $\frac{00}{30}$. This remedy will sometimes be found efficacious when many others have failed to relieve, particularly in chronic and extremely obstinate cases.

ADMINISTRATION. Same as *Nux vomica,* or, in chronic cases, four globules of the 30th in a teaspoonful of water every four or five days until relief is obtained, or another remedy called for by an alteration in the symptoms.

SULPHUR is one of the best remedies in the relief of *habitual constipation,* and particularly when hemorrhoids are present, or a disposition to them exists; frequent inclination to go to stool, but without the desired result.

ADMINISTRATION. $\frac{000000}{30}$ in six dessert-spoonfuls of water. One to be taken morning and evening until finished; or in the same manner as described under *Natrum muriaticum.*

VERATRUM. Constipation, chiefly from inactivity of the rectum, with heat and dryness of skin, determination of blood to the head and lateral headache.

ADMINISTRATION. Same as *Sulphur.*

LACHESIS. Obstinate *constipation,* after *Nux v.,* in those who habitually take wine rather freely, attended with flatulent distention after meals and ineffectual efforts to eructate.

ADMINISTRATION. Same as *Nux vomica.*

SEPIA: May frequently be taken with advantage in *chronic constipation* after *Nux* and *Sulphur;* this remedy is, moreover, particularly well adapted for females in whom there is an irregularity or obstruction of the menstrual flux; constipation in individuals subject to rheumatism; hard conglomerate bullet-shaped fæces. (ADMINISTRATION. See *Sulphur.*)

SILICEA. When constipation is accompanied with *colic,* impaired appetite, and thirst; and the stools are hard, knotty and passed with great difficulty; tenesmus. (*Conium* is occasionally useful in completing the cure after *Silicea.*

ADMINISTRATION. See *Sulphur.*

LYCOPODIUM. *Chronic constipation* with ebullition and determination to the head; *flatulence,* sense *of weight* in the *lower part of the bowels.*

ADMINISTRATION. Same as *Sulphur.*

In *Constipation* with indurated fæces, formed into hard balls (*scybalæ*), *Plumb., Magn. m., Sep., Ruta, Verb.,* also *Nux v., Op.,* Veratr., *Sulph.,* &c.; and several other remedies in obstinate cases, the treatment of which, however, requires experience and a good knowledge of disease, and of the *Materia Medica.* In all cases of an obstinate or chronic nature, recourse may occasionally be had to an enema or lavement of tepid water, as a temporary mode of relief, until the medicine has effected the desired result. The drinking of a tumblerful of cold water* night and morning, and the partaking of a due proportion of fruit, bread, and vegetables along with meat at dinner, combined with early rising and daily exercise, (not violent so as to cause suffering,) will be found useful auxiliaries in promoting a regular action of the bowels. Constipation in alternation with diarrhœa, *Nux v., Lach., Rhus, Antim. c., Ruta, Bryonia, Opium* and *Phosphorus. Constipation* in aged per-

* We would suggest as an important adjuvant in many cases, the pouring of a stream of cold water, or the fall of a shower bath, on the lower third of the abdomen, or sitting in a cold hip bath for five minutes, every morning on rising, until the natural habit is restored, when it should be omitted, and only resumed on a repetition of the trouble.

sons: *Op.*, *Aur. m.*, *Natr. m.*, or *Verat.*, *Bry.*, *Lach.* *Baryt. c.*, *Ruta*, &c.

PILES. HEMORRHOIDS.

Diagnosis. Varices, or effusion of blood in the cellular tissue of the rectum, either within or without the anus, (internal or external piles;) or protrusion and filling of one or more of the inner foldings of the same intestine, and with or without bleeding, (open or blind piles,) preceded or accompanied by pains in the back, sacrum, and abdomen; sensation of itching, pricking, tickling, burning, or pressing at the rectum, sometimes extending to the adjacent parts, with, in general, constipation and not unfrequently derangements of the urinary functions.

The predisposing cause is attributable to a constitutional taint; among the exciting causes are habitual costiveness, severe exertion on horseback, prolapsus, use of drastic medicines, stimulating diet, the use of vinous, alcoholic, and fermented drinks, and coffee, and suppression of long continued discharges, sedentary habits, &c.

During the treatment of this affection it is of the utmost importance to attend strictly to the homeopathic rules for diet. *Strong or heating drinks*, such as *wines*, *coffee*, *tea*, and *stimulating* or *highly-seasoned food* of all kinds are particularly to be avoided. Sedentary habits and the use of soft cushions or chairs materially tend to aggravate the affection. The painful practice amongst surgeons of removing the hemorrhoidal excrescences by means of the knife or ligature, is much to be deprecated; for, independent of the danger not unfrequently attending the operation, it may occasion serious consequences by metastasis of the congestion, to some of the noble viscera; and besides that in a great number of cases it wholly fails, and the disease returns, and sometimes in an aggravated form.

Therapeutics. The medicines most used in this affection are *Aconitum*, *Nux vomica*, *Sulphur*, *Lycopodium*, *Arsenicum*

Belladonna, Hepar sulphuris, Pulsatilla, Platina, Ignatia, Antimonium crudum, and *Cinchona.*

Administration, as follows, except where particularly specified to the contrary: Six globules of the potency marked after each medicine, in six dessert-spoonfuls of water, giving one morning and evening until finished, and in ordinary cases allowing this exhibition to continue its action for a week or ten days. (Vide note, p. 21.)

Aconite, although not specific in its curative action, is useful in allaying pain when considerable and distressing inflammation exists, and may in such cases precede the administration of each of the following medicines, which are among the principal remedial agents in this disease.

Administration. $\frac{000}{6}$ in six teaspoonfuls of water, one every six hours, until the inflammation abates; twenty-four to forty-eight hours after which we may have recourse to one of the other remedies mentioned.

Nux vomica $\frac{000}{30}$, as we have before had occasion to remark, is a most valuable remedy in this affection; it is equally efficacious against both descriptions; it is particularly indicated for individuals who lead a sedentary life, or who indulge in the use of coffee or stimulating liquids, and for females during pregnancy. When hemorrhoids are present, attended with shooting, burning, or itching pains, colic, shooting and jerking pain, as if from bruises in the loins, rendering it difficult to rise or walk in an erect position, and when they are accompanied by constipation and sometimes painful and difficult urination, and the other symptoms described under Indigestion or Dyspepsia.

Sulphur $\frac{000}{30}$, may follow the administration of *Nux v.*, and an alternation at intervals of from a week to ten days of these remedies, frequently effects a cure in cases of long standing.

Arsenicum $\frac{00}{30}$. Hemorrhoids accompanied by *burning* and *shooting* pains, heat and agitation, and sometimes prostration of strength.

Belladonna $\frac{00}{30}$. Moist hemorrhoids, with an insufferable pain in the sacral region, as if the back would break or be rent asunder; difficulty in voiding urine.

Hepar sulphuris may follow *Belladonna* should that medicine fail to, or only partially relieve these symptoms.

Administration. Half a grain of the third trituration in six dessert-spoonfuls of water, one every six hours until finished.

Rhus toxicodendron $\frac{000}{6}$. When the violent pain mentioned under *Belladonna* still continues severe, and particularly if relieved by motion.

Capsicum $\frac{000}{12}$. When a burning sensation exists, attended with considerable itching and diarrhœa.

Pulsatilla $\frac{000}{12}$. Discharge of blood and mucus during stool, and at other times with painful smarting and sensation of excoriation in the hemorrhoids, pains in the back, pallid countenance and disposition to fainting.

Platina $\frac{00}{30}$, when there is frequent inclination to go to stool, followed by a very scanty and difficult evacuation, *succeeded by general shuddering and a feeling of weakness in the abdomen;* frequent creeping, itching and piercing at the anus, particularly in the evening; violent dull pinching in the lower intestine, discharge of blood during stool, and at other times.

Lycopodium $\frac{00}{30}$. An important remedy in chronic hemorrhoidal affections, particularly when there is congestion to the head, with giddiness and headache, flatulent distention of the abdomen, constipation, severe burning, itching, and pricking pains in ano, with painful protrusion of the hemorrhoids, and sometimes prolapsus ani after a motion; acrid discharge from the hemorrhoids; prurient eruption around the anus.

Ignatia $\frac{000}{12}$. Itching and creeping, also sensation of constriction and excoriation in the anus, and prickings extending deep into the lower intestine; discharge of blood or of bloody mucus, and rumbling noise in the abdomen, and protrusion of the lower intestine, accompanied with acute pain.

Antimonium crudum $\frac{000}{12}$. Discharge of mucus and of blood at every stool, *followed by severe colic* and pain in the hemorrhoids, with throbbing, itching, and *burning* at the anus, and discharge of viscous acrid moisture, *particularly at night;* frequent determination to the head, with bleeding at the nose;

stiffness in the back, shooting pains in the loins, burning and rheumatic pains in the limbs, flatulence, and constipation.

Colocynth. In cases of hemorrhoids, attended with excessive, almost insupportable colic, this is a most efficient remedy.

Administration. $^{0}_{6}{}^{0}$, in a teaspoonful of water, repeated every two or three hours, or oftener if necessary, until relief is obtained; in chronic cases, with less intense pain, it may be taken as described at the commencement of this Chapter, p. 128.

When the discharge of blood from piles amounts to *hemorrhage*, a dose or two of *Aconitum* may be given in the first place, followed by *Ipecacuanha*, if improvement do not speedily follow; again, if *Ipecacuanha* does not arrest or diminish the discharge in a few minutes, *Sulphur* must be administered, and followed in turn by *Aconitum;* if, nothwithstanding the employment of these remedies, the hemorrhage does not cease, *Belladonna* should be given, and then *Calcarea*.* Administration. A few globules of the third or sixth potency in a teaspoonful of water. When the hemorrhage abates under the action of any of the remedies, the dose must not be repeated until the improvement ceases, and the bleeding threatens to return; but should the medicine which previously relieved be found to have lost its effect on repetition, the next in rotation must be had recourse to.

Cinchona is valuable either as an immediate remedy to support the patient when there has been much loss of blood, or afterwards against consequent debility.

These are the principal remedies to be employed in the treatment of ordinary cases of hemorrhoids; and when judiciously selected, will be certain to afford the desired relief, provided the patient is careful to adhere strictly to the rules laid down in the introductory remarks to this affection. In severe cases of long standing, much patience and perseverance are required before the disease can be permanently removed.

* C. Hering's Hausarzt.

Against hemorrhoids with mucous discharge (*blennorrhœa intestini recti*), *Mercurius*, *Helleborus niger*, *Colchicum*, and *Spigelia*.

PROTRUSION OF THE INTESTINES.

Prolapsus Ani.

By this term is understood the protrusion of a portion of the mucous membrane of the lower intestine: it is of much more frequent occurrence in children than adults, and takes place during *straining* when at stool, or when urinating. The reduction of the protruded portion of intestine is easily effected by gentle pressure with the thumbs, or thumb and forefinger, which have previously been dipped in oil.

THERAPEUTICS. The principal remedies for removing the tendency to this affection are: *Ignatia*, *Nux vomica*, *Mercurius*, and *Sulphur*.

ADMINISTRATION. The same as in hemorrhoids; in children under ten years of age, one to two globules, in the quantity of water stated.

IGNATIA $\frac{6}{12}$, is particularly efficacious in mild or sensitive temperaments, attended with constipation.

NUX VOMICA $\frac{6}{30}$, is indicated for persons of irritable or lively disposition, and addicted to high and stimulating diet, with a tendency to hemorrhoids and constipation.

MERCURIUS $\frac{6}{6}$, is particularly suited for children, in whom the disease is attended with hardness and swelling of the abdomen, and where the straining is excessive.

SULPHUR is one of the best remedies for the permanent removal of the disease.

ADMINISTRATION. $\frac{00}{30}$ repeated in five or six days.

Calcarea, *Lycopodium*, and *Sepia* may be found necessary in some obstinate cases, after *Sulph.*, administered in a similar manner as described for that remedy. In other cases, *Plumbum*, *Arsenicum*, *Mezereum*, *Natrum m.*, *Colchicum*, *Ruta*, *Theridion*, and *Magnes Artificialis* have been found efficacious.

COLIC. *Enteralgia.*

Diagnosis. Griping, tearing, gnawing, or shooting pain in the bowels, chiefly confined to the region of the navel, generally attended with a painful distention of the abdomen, with spasmodic contraction, and sometimes accompanied with vomiting and costiveness, or diarrhœa.

The general exciting causes of this complaint are: acid fruits and indigestible substances; cold from wet feet, drinking cold beverages when heated, constipation, worms, &c. It is frequently also a concomitant symptom of some other derangement, but occurs equally often as the primary disease. We shall here content ourselves with giving the symptoms under the medicines, without entering upon the different varieties of this affection. One of the distinctive characteristics between this malady and internal inflammation, is the pain being somewhat relieved by pressure.

Therapeutics. The principal remedies in its treatment are: *Nux vomica*, *Pulsatilla*, *Chamomilla*, *Belladonna*, *Cocculus*, and *Coffea.*

Administration. Four globules at the potency named, dissolved in six dessert-spoonfuls of water, one to be taken every hour, or half hour, until relief is obtained, and afterwards a dose given every four or five days, to combat the disposition to this affection when such exists.

Nux vomica $\frac{0000}{6}$ is a valuable remedy in either flatulent or hemorrhoidal* colic, or colic arising from a chill, and is particularly indicated when there is a sensation of *fulness and tightness* at the upper part of the waist; deep-seated or cutting pains in the abdomen, with *acute and hard, pressive, and forcing-down* sensation, compelling the sufferer to bend double; violent cutting pains in the hypogastrium; confused headache, with occasional loss of consciousness; respiration short and difficult; flatulence, aggravation of the pains on the slight-

* See Hemorrhoids.

est motion, generally disappearing when at rest; violent pain in the loins, and sensation of internal heat and obstruction; *constipation*, coldness and numbness in the hands and feet during the paroxysm; at the monthly period in females, when we find weight or violent deep-seated aching pain in the abdomen, and aching in the sacral region; dragging pains extending to the thigh; aching and creeping sensation in the same part when sitting; painful pressure towards the rectum.

Pulsatilla $\frac{0000}{3}$ is more useful in the affection occurring in females, either during the catamenia or at other times, when coming on periodically in the evening during cold, damp weather; also when there are present a disagreeable *tightness and distention* of the abdomen and the upper part of the waist; pulsation in the pit of the stomach, *aggravation of the suffering when at rest or in the evening*, attended with *shivering, which increases* with the pains, and is mitigated by motion; severe bruising pains in the loins, especially when rising up; when it has arisen from overloading the stomach, or from rich greasy food, with inclination to vomit, *flatulence*, diarrhœa, paleness of the face, livid circle round the eyes, and headache; also in hemorrhoidal colic, with fulness of the veins of the hands and forehead, restlessness, anxiety, and sleeplessness.

Chamomilla $\frac{0000}{3}$. Bilious colic; colic in females during the menstrual flux. The following are the principal indications: sensation as if the intestines were gathered into a ball, and as if the abdomen were empty, with *tearing* and *drawing* pains, attended with excessive anxiety and restlessness; *distention under the lower ribs and in the pit of the stomach;* incarcerated flatulency, sometimes nausea, *bitter vomiting*, followed by desire to relieve the bowels, and *bilious diarrhœa;* livid circles round the eyes, alternate paleness and redness of the face; the pains come on particularly at night, at other times early in the morning, or after a meal. This remedy, as before stated, is particularly adapted for children of irritable temperaments, and is extremely serviceable in all cases in which a fit of *passion* has been the exciting cause of the sufferings. It is also useful when colic has arisen from cold in the feet, or checked perspiration. Although in most instances

Chamomilla is of itself sufficient, it has been sometimes found useful to precede it by a dose of *Aconite*. (*Colocynth* is often useful after *Chamomilla*, when the latter has only produced partial relief.)

BELLADONNA $\frac{0000}{6}$. Flatulent colic when there is *protrusion of the transverse section of the great intestine*, which becomes distended like a *pad*, attended with colic-like pain, doubling up of the body, which is relieved by pressure on the part; also severe bearing-down pains, aggravated by motion; at other times there is a sensation as if the above swelling had been removed downwards, deep into the abdomen, with feeling of bearing-down of the whole intestines; also in menstrual colic, with *spasmodic constrictions* in the abdomen, with burning pain lower down or in the small of the back; or pain under the ribs, as if *a number of nails were holding the intestines*. The symptoms are also attended with a liquid or puriform species of diarrhœa, and swelling of the veins of the head; the pains are sometimes so violent as almost to deprive the patient of reason.

COCCULUS $\frac{0000}{6}$ is indicated (*menstrual* or flatulent colic) when there are severe constrictive or *spasmodic* pains in the *lower part of the abdomen*; great flatulence, fulness, and distention of the entire abdomen, with nausea and difficulty of breathing; also when there is a sensation of emptiness, tearing and burning pains in the intestines, sometimes with squeezing, tearing and pulling pains, excessive anguish and nervous excitement and constipation.

COLOCYNTH $\frac{0000}{6}$. In the majority of violent and obstinate cases, we find this a valuable remedy; it is indicated when the pains are excessively violent, and of a *constrictive* or *spasmodic* character, or resembles stabbing and *cutting, as if from knives*; sometimes a sensation of clawing and pinching, tenderness of the abdomen, with a pain as from a blow; or *distention* of the abdomen; at other times a sense of emptiness is experienced, cramps and shivering, or tearing pains in the legs; during the continuance of the attack, excessive restlessness, agitation, and tossing about from the violence of the pain: when the pains come on, they continue without any apparent intermission;

after their disappearance, a sensation of bruising remains, and the sufferer feels as though the intestines were held together by thin threads, likely to break from the slightest motion. Both this remedy and *Chamomilla* are particularly efficacious in the so-called bilious colic, being indicated by the diarrhœa and bilious vomiting attending it, and in cases where passion has been the exciting causes. *Colocynth* is more particularly useful in the case of adults, or where the fit of anger is attended with indignation.

Sulphur $\frac{0000}{6}$ may follow either *Chamomilla* or *Colocynth* in cases of *bilious* colic where only partial relief has been obtained; or of *flatulent* colic after *Nux v.; Carbo v.; Cocculus*, or *Chamomilla ;* and hemorrhoidal after *Nux v. or Carbo v.*

Arsenicum $\frac{0000}{6}$ in colic arising from disordered stomach, with nausea, vomiting; diarrhœa, with green or yellow evacuation, violent gripings, headache, paleness of the face, and blue marks round the eyes; accession of the pains particularly during the night, or after eating or drinking.

Coffea $\frac{0000}{3}$ is valuable when we have to deal with colic with excessive pains, attended with great agitation, anxiety, and tossing about, grinding of the teeth, convulsions, suffocative, oppressive despair, acidity, coldness of the body and extremities. It is also useful in some kinds of menstrual colic, with a sensation as if the abdomen were being rent asunder; or with fulness and pressure in the abdomen and violent spasm which extend to the chest. Cutting pains in the intestines as if divided by a knife. The pains present so violent, as almost to drive the patient to distraction, and cause him to bend double and draw up his limbs; violent spasms in all his members.

Bryonia, colic with constipation, tension in the abdomen, and flow of saliva like salivation.

In cases of colic arising suddenly from indigestible food, a cup of black coffee, without milk or sugar, will frequently afford relief, by causing the stomach to free itself from the cause of annoyance; in instances where that article has not been made one of ordinary beverage. When from Constipation, Silicea is an excellent remedy, and sometimes *Conium*. See Constipation. For colic arising from worms, see Worms.

LOOSENESS OF THE BOWELS. *Diarrhœa.*

DIAGNOSIS. Fluid discharge from the intestines in increased quantity.

This affection is simply an increase of the peristaltic action of the intestinal canal, and is so well known under its different forms, that I shall simply allude to the principal exciting causes, and then proceed to the treatment.

The exciting causes are acid, indigestible food, a check of perspiration, sudden changes of temperature, the prolonged use of powerful purgatives, which, although still more frequently the cause of constipation, nevertheless, by producing irritation of the intestinal canal, also predispose to attacks of this derangement, worms, etc.

Sometimes diarrhœa is a salutary crisis, as remarked under fevers; here again the homœopathic treatment assists nature, and while it abridges the duration of the affection, and thereby obviates future debility, does not rashly check its course.

THERAPEUTICS. The principal remedies in this affection are *Dulcamara, Bryonia, Cinchona, Ferrum aceticum, Chamomilla, Rheum, Mercurius, Pulsatilla, Nux vomica, Arsenicum, Antimonium crudum, Rhus toxicodendron, Opium, Sulphur, Calcarea, Acidum phosphoricum*, and *Phosphorus.*

ADMINISTRATION. In recent cases, six globules of the sixth potency may be dissolved in about an ounce of water, and a dessert-spoonful after each motion until benefit results;—in the case of children, half the quantity, administered in teaspoonfuls. In chronic cases it will *generally* be sufficient to administer the dose night and morning, or only once a day, and even only once in four or five days or longer, according to the effects produced.*

DULCAMARA $\frac{000000}{6}$, should be administered in diarrhœa occurring in summer from cold, probably from wet feet or exposure to rain. Particular indications for its exhibitions are

* Vide note, p. 21.

when the diarrhœa is attended with colic, or cutting pain, chiefly in the region of the naval; when the evacuations are liquid, *slimy* and *yellow*, generally coming on at night, and attended with nausea or vomiting; want of appetite and great thirst; paleness of the countenance and lassitude.

BRYONIA. In cases of diarrhœa arising from the before-mentioned causes, and with many of the symptoms noted under *Dulcamara*, when this medicine has failed to afford the required relief in six or eight hours, it should be given, particularly if the looseness is liable to be aggravated after a meal, and any portions of undigested food are present in the motion; looseness after partaking of *milk: in diarrhœa occurring during hot weather*, when we cannot trace the causes to any errors of diet, requiring other remedies; this medicine is also indicated, and particularly so in the following instances: Diarrhœa from checked perspiration or being overheated; *cold drinks*—a chill from remaining in any cold exposed situation, or in draughts—or from biting, easterly winds. When this affection has been produced by passion, particularly in individuals of what physiologists denominate a bilious temperament, it is most useful—if any symptoms remain after *Chamomilla*, which in such cases deserve a preference. It may also be remarked, that the diarrhœa arising from drinking impure water when heated has frequently found relief in this medicine. When the water is strongly impregnated with vegetable substances, it may be advantageously followed by *Cinchona*. This is a case which seldom occurs, but knowing that it does occasionally, particularly with sportsmen on moors, and in marshy ground, it has been judged advisable to add these remarks. (*Antimonium* is sometimes required to complete the cure, after the previous exhibition of *Bryonia.*) See *Administration*, p. 137.

CINCHONA. Looseness, in consequence of indigestion, particularly if in consequence of partaking of fruit or flatulent food, such as vegetables; evacuations are very profuse, and sometimes attended with but little pain, and when the discharge comes on immediately after *partaking of food, or at night*, evacuations liquid and *brownish*, sometimes containing portions of *undigested* food; it is, in some instances, also indicated, when considerable spasmodic or colic-like pain is present, with flatulence, want of appetite, thirst, and great weakness; it is also valuable after improper treatment of this affection, when considerable debility remains. See *Administration*, p. 137.

Ferrum aceticum may be advantageously given in alternation with *Cinchona* at intervals of twelve hours, when the evacuations are partly composed of *undigested* food* and pass without pain; or this remedy may be administered alone, when the diarrhœa is unattended with pain, and there is paleness of the face, weakness of the eyes, pains in the back and anus; with great weakness of digestion. See *Administration*, p. 137.

Chamomilla $\frac{0}{6}$, is a remedy, as already stated elsewhere, particularly useful in children, either at the time of teething, or at a more advanced period, when the affection has been excited by checked perspiration; it is further particularly indicated, when the evacuations are *watery*, *bilious*,† *green*, *yellow*, or *slimy*, or of a fetor resembling rotten eggs; when there are *fulness at the pit of the stomach*, severe colic or spasm, pain in the abdomen, distention and hardness of the abdomen, bitter taste in the mouth, foul tongue, thirst, want of appetite, *bilious vomiting* and flatulency in infants, attended with restlessness and screaming, and drawing up of the limbs towards the stomach; in cases of adults, $\frac{00}{3}$. *Sulphur* is frequently useful in completing the cure when the pains or colic has been removed by *Chamomilla*. See *Administration*, p. 137.

Rheum $\frac{000}{3}$, when the symptoms, in a great measure, resemble *Chamomilla*, but the pain is not so violent, and the evacuations have a *sour* smell; paleness of the face is also an indication for this medicine. (See *Diarrhœa in children*.)

Mercurius $\frac{000000}{6}$. When the diarrhœa arises from a *chill*, and the motions are copious, *watery*, *slimy*, frothy, bilious, or *greenish*, or streaked with blood, and cause a smarting or burning sensation on being evacuated; also when there is painful *straining* before, during, and after evacuation; severe cutting pains; moreover, nausea and eructation, *cold perspiration*,

* See also *Arsen.*, *Merc.*, *Bryonia*, *Phosph.*, *Lachesis*.

† Diarrhœa biliosa.

trembling or shivering, and shuddering, great lassitude, and disposition to syncope; diarrhœa with ingesta.

PULSATILLA. One of the best remedies in *simple looseness* or diarrhœa arising from *errors of diet*, such as indulgence in *acids, fruits*, or rich indigestible food, attended with foul tongue and other *dyspeptic* symptoms. (See INDIGESTION.) Another remarkable indication for this remedy is one evacuation differing from another in colour. See *Administration*, p. 137.

IPECACUANHA $\frac{0000}{3}$. Looseness arising from indigestion, particularly if caused by imperfect mastication, attended with nausea and vomiting; paleness of the face, (see also *Arsen.*,) *weakness*, and desire to retain the recumbent posture (in the case of children). When *Ipecacuanha* does not appear to afford much relief, *Pulsatilla* ought to be had recourse to in the space of from 12 to 24 hours, after the last dose of *Ipecacuanha:* when, in the case of children, the motions have a very sour smell, *Rheum* is to be preferred to *Pulsatilla*, from whatever cause the attack may have arisen.

NUX VOMICA. *Scanty* evacuations or motions, consisting of slime and blood, attended with straining and *great weakness*, flatulency, and violent cutting pains in the region of the navel; for some of the accompanying symptoms the reader is requested to study the indications given under this remedy, in INDIGESTION. See *Administration*, p. 137.

ARSENICUM. Autumnal diarrhœa, or looseness arising from errors in diet, *acids, fruits, cold drinks, ices*, or from a *chill*, &c., the characteristic symptoms for its employment are *watery, slimy, greenish*, or *brownish corrosive, burning evacuations*, with *violent colic, excessive thirst, emaciation*, and *great weakness;* and when more liable to come on at night or after *eating* or *drinking*.—(*Vid.* the further indications for this important remedy in Part III., under BOWEL COMPLAINTS IN CHILDREN.)* See *Administration*, p. 137.

ANTIMONIUM CRUDUM. Also in cases arising from *disordered stomach*, with white tongue, loss of appetite, eructations

* When *Arsenicum* does not answer our expectations, *Veratrum* should be substituted; the latter remedy is, moreover, for the most part to be preferred when the disease appears to have arisen from atmospheric causes.

and nausea; diarrhœa alternating with constipation. (See article upon this affection.) See *Administration*, p. 137.

Rhus toxicodendron. Lumpy or pap-like diarrhœa, coming on only at night, preceded by colic, which disappears after each evacuation. See *Administration*, p. 137.

Opium $\frac{0000}{3}$. Diarrhœa arising from *fright* or from *cold*, followed, if required, by *Dulcamara* in the latter case. For other indications, *vide* Mental Emotions.

Lachesis. Diarrhœa from acid drinks, or sour unripe fruits, with severe griping; diarrhœa with ingesta.

Sulphur $\frac{000}{6}$. Is a most valuable remedy in diarrhœa, particularly during the night, occurring in strumous habits, or in very obstinate cases. In adults predisposed to hemorrhoids, or in children, when the diarrhœa is attended with excoriation and papular eruptions, it is particularly efficacious; also in cases where the slightest cold brings on a relapse or an attack; or when *milk* disagrees and causes a looseness.

Calcarea $\frac{0000}{6}$. May be had recourse to after *Sulphur*.

Acidum phosphoricum. In obstinate cases, with portions of undigested food in the evacuations; or occasional involuntary evacuations.

Phosphorus $\frac{0000}{6}$. In *chronic, painless diarrhœa*, with *gradual* prostration of strength; diarrhœa with ingesta.

Diet. Acids or acidulous wines, beer, coffee, strong tea, and fruits, whether raw or cooked, should be carefully avoided. Solid food proscribed as tending to keep up the intestinal irritation; and gruel, fresh milk in moderation, broths, and light mucilaginous food substituted.

DYSENTERY. *Dysenteria.*

Diagnosis. Constant urgency to evacuate the bowels, tenesmus, violent pains in the abdomen, a greater or less degree of fever, and stools of mucus or blood, or both.

It may appear suddenly, but is frequently preceded some time by loss of appetite, costiveness, flatulency, nausea or slight vomiting, with chills followed by heat of skin and accelerated pulse, then dull abdominal pains and increased evacuations; after a time no fæces are discharged, but white mucus, which may afterwards change to blood (*bloody flux*); stools, particularly when fever is present, very frequent and fetid; if not checked in time, the disease may terminate in ulceration or gangrene, or the patient may sink from exhaustion.

This affection is very frequently complicated with rheumatic pains, which will be noticed under the different remedies, as an additional indication for their employment. The exciting causes are, checked perspiration, particularly in warm weather; low or marshy situations, local irritations, such as worms, scybala, &c., and suppression of hemorrhoids, metastases, and sometimes, in infants, difficult dentition.

THERAPEUTICS. The principal remedies found useful in treatment are *Aconitum, Chamomilla, Pulsatilla, Ipecacuanha, Colocynth, Mercurius vivus, Arsenicum album, Carbo vegetabilis, Nux vomica, Cinchona,* and *Sulphur,* Staphys., Sepia, etc.

ACONITUM. This remedy is peculiarly adapted to the fever frequently present, and in young and plethoric patients is generally required in the commencement or in the course of the disease. It is indicated by full and hard pulse; severe pains, generally in one spot; abdomen tense and painful when touched, denoting the commencement of inflammation; also valuable when we find pains resembling rheumatism in different parts of the body, with shivering, or excessive heat and thirst.

ADMINISTRATION. As in INFLAMMATORY FEVER, which see.

CHAMOMILLA. If after the administration of *Aconite,* we still find violent heat and thirst, rheumatic pains in the head, and constant agitation and tossing. This remedy is also useful when this disease seems to take for its proximate cause gastric impurities formed in the primæ viæ; or when it has arisen from exposure to a cool atmosphere when in a state of perspiration. When we find foul tongue with clammy, bitter taste in the mouth, bilious stools, and before tenesmus declare itself, this evidently points out the remedy as more useful in the first or diarrhœal stage; it may be followed by *Pulsatilla,* when the symptoms given under that remedy present themselves.

ADMINISTRATION $\frac{0000}{3}$, in a little water, repeated every six hours, until improvement takes place, or indications for another remedy present themselves.*

PULSATILLA, when the *gastric* symptoms noted under *Chamomilla* are present, but the stools consist entirely of *mucus* striated with blood. (*Dysenteria pituitosa.*)

ADMINISTRATION, same as *Chamomilla,* but at the sixth potency.

The three remedies, above mentioned, are also valuable in dysentery arising from cold, or what is commonly denominated rheumatic catarrhal dysentery, *Rheumatismus Intestinorum.*

IPECACUANHA. This remedy is serviceable when the dysenteric affection seems fairly established; when the stool consists of slimy matter containing white flocks, followed by evacuations of sanguinolent mucus.

ADMINISTRATION, same as *Chamomilla.*

COLOCYNTH. In cases attended with *violent colic* and excessive distention of the abdomen, shivering with chills, apparently extending from the abdomen over the whole body, excessive agitation and restlessness, tongue coated white; slimy, and sometimes bloody evacuations; it is sometimes found useful to follow *Ipecacuanha* or *Mercurius.*†

ADMINISTRATION. $\frac{000000}{6}$, in six teaspoonsful of water, one every hour until improvement declares itself, when the intervals between the doses may be lengthened.‡

MERCURIUS VIVUS in the red dysentery or BLOODY FLUX,

* Vide note, p. 21.

† A successful procedure in our practice has been the *alternate* administration of *Colocynth* and *Mercury* for very many forms of dysentery. The general indications permitting, we have given the first trituration of the *Colocynth apple* (rubbed dry with Sugar of Milk) every two, three, four or more hours *during the day,* and *Mercury at evening* or *during the night.* In some cases, however, where the griping pains and tenesmus were intense, we have alternated the *Colocynth* and *Mercury* during the night, at such intervals as the urgency of symptoms demanded.

After a favourable impression from these drugs, the disease sometimes remaining stationary, especially during the autumn or prevalence of febrile miasms, we have found a dose or two of *Colchicum* to awaken anew the susceptibility of the system to the above or other indicated remedies.—ED.

‡ Vide note, page 21.

when we find *severe tenesmus* or *straining*, with evacuation, merely of a little mucus, sometimes succeeded by or accompanied with protrusion of a portion of the intestine and increased discharge of pure blood, or of *putrid, corrosive, greenish*, yellowish, or frothy mucus, intermixed with blood, and sometimes followed by the evacuation of small hard substances (scybala) after much straining; burning in ano; severe griping and lancinating pain *before, during*, and even after the motions; increased urgency to stool after each evacuation.*

In cases with the above symptoms, *Mercurius* may almost be considered a specific, or will at all events prove so efficacious a remedy, that any remaining symptoms will, in general, be removed with facility, either by means of *Colocynth, Acidum phosphoricum, Acidum nitricum*, (the two latter especially in the event of a continuance of the sanguineous stools,) or any of the other remedies which may seem more appropriate according to the indications for their employment, as given in this chapter.

Administration. A grain of the third trituration in an ounce of water, a dessert-spoonful every three hours until the symptoms are mitigated, when the intervals may be lengthened.

Bryonia is frequently called for in those cases in which it has been found necessary to administer *Aconite* at the commencement of the disease; but is more particularly indicated when the attack has occurred during the heat of summer from the effects of a chill, and is attended with typhoid fever of the inflammatory form; with loose evacuations of a brownish colour and putrid odour, occasionally containing lumps of coagulated mucus resembling undigested substances, or also small hard lumps or balls, (scybalous fæcal matter) with griping during, and burning in ano after the act of evacuating, aching pains in the limbs, aggravated by movement. When the disease has attained an advanced stage, and the accompanying fever is of a low typhoid type, the patient much exhausted and distressed with severe rheumatic or aching pains in the loins and extremities when reclining or sitting still, and the stools of a slimy,

* *Mercurius sublimatus corrosivus* is sometimes more speedily efficacious than *Mercurius vivus* or *Merc. solubulis* against the above symptoms.

frothy, white, gelatinous, or sanguineous nature, passed involuntarily at night in bed: Rhus not unfrequently gives a favourable turn to the disorder.

Administration of *Bryonia* and *Rhus*. Six globules of the third potency in about half an ounce of water, a teaspoonful every two hours until an alteration is effected.

Arsenicum. Dysentery of epidemic or contagious origin with fever of a typhoid or putrid type:* dysentery arising from exposure to noxious exhalations in marshy situations, &c.

This remedy may, however, be selected in all cases, from whatever cause arising, *when great weakness* and even *prostration* exists from the commencement, with *burning* pain in evacuating the bowels, *thirst and aggravations of the sufferings after drinking;* or, on the contrary, adipsia:—also when the disease threatens to assume the ulcerative or gangrenous character—characterized by previous severe pains, particularly burning, which suddenly cease; hypocratic expression of countenance; rapid sinking of the vital energies; pulse small and intermittent; coldness of the extremities; highly offensive, putrid, and cadaverous smelling evacuations, both of fæces and urine; unconscious passing of stools; offensive breath and petechiæ in different parts of the body.

Administration. Six globules of the third potency in an ounce of water, a dessert spoonful every two, three, or six hours, according to the urgency of the case, carefully watching the effects, and shortening or lengthening the intervals accordingly.

Carbo vegetabilis is a most useful remedy in these desperate cases, when the breath is cold, the pulse almost imperceptible, and the patient complains of severe burning pains: its indications closely resemble those of *Arsenicum*, with the exception of the thirst, and the aggravation caused by drinking. It may be given with benefit when that remedy has failed, or only partially relieved, and in this, as in other affections, many instances might be cited where a judicious alternation of these

* Dysenteria putrida.

two remedies has effected benefit—where neither of them might have been singly adequate to the exigency of the case.

Administration. Six globules of the sixth or twelfth potency exhibited in the same manner as *Arsenicum.*

Nux vomica. When *Arsenicum* has diminished these symptoms and warded off the danger, but we find that the fæces still retain a highly putrid odour; also at any period during the course of the disease, when the following symptoms are present: —Frequent *scanty evacuations* of mucus or sanguineous mucus, and occasionally small, compact, hard fæces (scybala) attended with violent cutting or griping pains in the region of the navel; borborygmus, pains in the loins, tenesmus, burning or sensation of excoriation in the anus, and sometimes protrusion of the intestine; great heat and excessive thirst.

Administration. Same as *Pulsatilla.*

Cinchona. In cases where the disease has an endemic character, occurring in marshy countries, and in many cases when a state of putridity remains in the fæces after the administration of the remedies above mentioned.

Administration. Same as *Chamomilla.*

Cantharides. Sanguineous stools mixed with whitish mucus or solid substances like false membranes; strangury.*

Administration. Six globules of the third in an ounce of water, a dessert-spoonful every four or six hours.

Sulphur. When the more marked symptoms are ameliorated by the use of the foregoing remedies, but the Dysentery still continues obstinate, and especially when the disease occurs in subjects who have previously been long affected with hemorrhoids; or when it has from time to time been subdued, and afterwards returned with greater or less violence; or even when the apparently best selected remedial agents have failed to check its course. It will frequently be found most efficacious in all these cases, since when this occurs we may suspect some latent constitutional cause is baffling our efforts.

* *Colchicum autumnale* is preferable to *Cantharides* when the symptoms are as described, and the disorder rages epidemically during the autumnal season.

In the instance first noted by its removal, the affection is terminated; in the second, the predisposition to a return of the attack is obviated; and in the third, the constitutional taint alluded to being controlled, the organism becomes susceptible to the specific action of the other medicaments.

ADMINISTRATION. $\frac{0}{6}{}^{0}$, in a little water, repeated at first every twelve hours until an effect is produced, then discontinued for a time and allowed to act.

In conclusion it must not be omitted to add, that when the disease is of long standing, and has become, so to speak, habitual, a cure is often effected by means of *Phosphorus*.

ADMINISTRATION. Two globules of the third potency in a little water daily, until a favourable change sets in.*

Rules of Conduct and Diet. In this affection it is of great importance to keep up a moderate degree of warmth around the abdomen, which is best obtained by flannel worn outside the linen.

During the course of treatment cold drinks are to be avoided, barely sufficient nutriment to keep up the strength of the patient allowed; and the more severe the inflammatory symptoms, the more strict must be the abstinence. No solids should on any account be given; but the diet should consist principally of mucilaginous or demulcent fluids, such as thin barley-water and gruel; in comparatively mild cases, weak chicken-broth or beef-tea, at the discretion of the physician, may be allowed. Even after convalescence this course of diet should be for a short time observed, especially when the disease is raging in an epidemic form, and a return to the usual diet *gradually* brought about. Wine and alcohol are absolute poisons in this affection.

Having thus given the best mode of treatment for this disease, ordinarily so fatal, we may remark that in a great majority of cases, the homœopathic method checks it at its commencement, without allowing it to assume the more frightful forms portrayed in the instructions of its treatment; and it passes

* Vide note, page 21.

off leaving the patient in sound health; in the most violent cases where it has already made head, and seems approaching a fatal termination, it may almost be said to be the only system which offers a *chance* of salvation to the sufferer; and in strumous constitutions, where, under the old mode of procedure, the results are commonly so unfortunate, it gently mitigates the violence of the symptoms, and safely conducts the patient through his perils.

Suppressed Dysentery. When the dysenteric evacuations have been suddenly checked by allopathic means, and a violent inflammatory or spasmodic action declare itself, such as severe pains, anxiety, dyspnœa, nausea, and empty retchings, or distention and tenderness of the abdomen; suppression both of fæces and urine; coldness of the face, tongue, and extremities; breath also cold; with *spasms* of various kinds in different parts of the body, which are renewed by any exertion, either of speech or movement—the following remedies will be found useful:

ACONITUM. Against any inflammatory symptoms that may present themselves, to be repeated according to the rule already given until relief follow.*

CUPRUM ACETICUM. When spasms or cold sweats predominate.

ADMINISTRATION. $\frac{0\,0}{6}$, in a little water, repeated in three to six hours, according to the effect produced.

BELLADONNA, against inflammatory colic, or if symptoms of abdominal inflammation set in, see article ENTERITIS, and also COLIC, and administer accordingly.

COLOCYNTH. Violent colic and distention of the abdomen, see COLIC.

VERATRUM ALBUM. Coldness of the body and extremities, and *retching*.

ADMINISTRATION. Six globules of the sixth potency in an ounce of water, a dessert-spoonful every two to six hours.

CARBO VEGETABILIS in extreme cases, with scarcely perceptible pulse, and cold breath.

* Vide note, p. 21.

Administration, as already given in the foregoing article. The use of clysters of warm water has in many instances been found serviceable in promoting an evacuation of the bowels, and bringing back the suppressed discharge.

When the patient has escaped the serious consequences above noticed, chronic complaints frequently are the result of Suppressed Dysentery; the most frequent are Dropsy, Paralysis, and Rheumatism.

CHOLERA.

By the term Cholera Morbus was formerly understood a disease attended with nausea, griping, purging, and vomiting, generally prevalent towards our summer months, and at the season when fruit was plentiful. But it has now become a generic term, under which are included two varieties—the Cholera Morbus, properly so called, and the Asiatic Cholera.

Diagnosis. The first named, sometimes called the Sporadic Cholera, generally commences with a sudden feeling of nausea and griping, followed by purging and vomiting; in severe cases accompanied with coldness of the body, particularly the extremities, and anxious and hurried breathings, excessive thirst, a feeling of cramping in the legs, sometimes in the arms, with spasmodic contractions of the abdominal muscles, shrinking of the features, and a hollow expression about the eyes; pulse weak, sometimes scarcely perceptible; thin, watery, and fetid, or bilious evacuations, sometimes with dark bilious vomiting, anxiety, and tenesmus.

Causes. The most frequent are worms, gall-stones, indigestible substances, fruits, or crude vegetables, alterations in temperature, moist or marshy situations, or damp weather, dentition, or parturition.

Therapeutics. In the treatment of Cholera in its sporadic form, (i. e., when the disease arises from occasional causes, such as cold, fatigue, &c.,) the following remedies will be found to be the most efficacious: *Cham.*, *Ipecac.*, *Nux v.*, *Veratrum album*, *Arsenicum album*, *Cinchona*, *and Pulsatilla*.

Chamomilla is almost specific when the attack has been

excited by a *chill* or a *fit of passion*, or great dread of being attacked during the prevalence of the disease.

The following are the symptoms which particularly indicate its employment: acute colic-like pains, or heavy *pressure* in the region of the navel, sometimes extending to the heart, with excessive anguish; bilious diarrhœa, cramps in the calves of the legs; tongue coated yellow, and sometimes vomiting of acid matter.

ADMINISTRATION. A few globules of the third potency to half an ounce of water, a teaspoonful every two to six hours, according to circumstances. (Vide note, p. 21.)

IPECACUANHA may be administered after the above, should the attacks of *vomiting* become more prominent; or it may be selected from the *commencement*, should *vomiting predominate*, or at least assume as marked a character in the complaint as the diarrhœa. Other indications are sensations of weakness, or softness, (flaccidity,) coldness in the face and limbs, sense of shivering in the abdomen; slight cramps in the calves of the legs, and in the fingers and toes. (Nux v. after *Ipec.*, when anxiety, pain in the abdominal parts, frequent small evacuations and tenesmus, frontal headaches, horripilation with internal chills.)

ADMINISTRATION. Same as CHAMOMILLA.

VERATRUM ALBUM. Should the disease increase, notwithstanding the administration of the preceding remedy, and assume the following characteristics, *violent vomiting with severe diarrhœa, excessive weakness, and cramps in the calves of the legs;* eyes hollow or sunken, countenance pale, and expressive of *acute suffering* and *intense anguish;* coldness of the breath and tongue, *excruciating pain in the region of the navel*, tenderness of the abdomen when touched; dragging pains and cramps in the fingers, shrivelled appearance of the skin on the palms of the hands. This is also one of the best remedies in both varieties of this disease.

ADMINISTRATION. Six globules of the third potency in a teaspoonful of water, repeated in half an hour or even less, should there be no change of any kind for the better; or one or two drops of the third tincture may be added to an ounce of water, a dessert-spoonful every half, one, or two hours, according to the severity of the symptoms; when amelioration has taken place, lengthening the intervals.

Arsenicum is useful when this malady assumes a severe character from the beginning, but it is more particularly indicated when the disease is attended with *rapid prostration of strength, insatiable thirst*, excessive anxiety, loss of articulation, with fear of approaching death, *burning sensation* in the region of the stomach, almost constant discharge from the bowels, or *renewal* of the discharge on every occasion that the desire for drink is gratified; suppression of urine or scanty micturition, followed by a burning sensation; *violent and painful vomiting, tongue and lips dry, cracked and blueish, or black;* hollow cheeks, pointed nose, pulse almost imperceptible, or *small, weak, intermittent*, and trembling; severe spasms in the fingers and toes; *clammy perspiration.*

Administration. Six globules of the sixth potency in a teaspoonful of water, to be repeated, in the same manner and under the same conditions as described for *veratrum.*

Cinchona is chiefly most useful against the weakness which remains after cholera, but is also serviceable occasionally during the course of the disease, particularly when there is vomiting of ingesta, and frequent watery and brownish evacuations containing particles of indigested food; also when there is oppression at the chest with eructations which afford temporary relief; severe pressure in the abdomen, especially after partaking of the smallest portion of food; great exhaustion, sometimes amounting to fainting. This remedy is particularly marked when the disease has been excited by indigestible substances, such as unripe fruit, &c., or by inhabiting a marshy situation.

Administration. $\frac{000}{3}$, repeated every four, six, or twelve hours according to circumstances, until amelioration result.

Pulsatilla, in mild cases, cases where there is *mucous* diarrhœa and dyspeptic symptoms. It is also useful when the disease has been excited by the use of indigestible articles of diet. (Vide Diarrhœa and Indigestion.)

Administration. $\frac{000}{6}$, repeated every four hours, until a favourable change takes place.

ASIATIC CHOLERA. This disease generally commences with vertigo, headache and singing in the ears, a sensation of flatulence in the stomach, griping pains, and a feeling of weight and oppression in the region of the heart.

In some, but not all cases of Asiatic Cholera, we find the lips, nails, and sometimes the whole skin of a blue colour, but in almost every instance the frame loses its power of generating heat; the pulse and pulsation of the heart are almost unfelt, circulation of the blood becomes stagnant.

Patients who have escaped through the second stage are frequently carried off by a typhoid fever in the third.

When the premonitory symptoms of this disease, as above noted, exhibit themselves, its complete development is *frequently prevented*, by the administration of the SATURATED SOLUTION OF CAMPHOR, one part of Camphor to twenty of spirits of wine.

ADMINISTRATION. One or two drops of the above every five minutes in a teaspoonful of cold water, until a cessation or amelioration of the symptoms take place, when the intervals between the repetition of the dose may be lengthened to every two, then every four or six hours.

In many cases also we may succeed in checking the disease at its commencement by *Ipec.* and *Nux v.*, or the remedies already mentioned under Sporadic Cholera, p. 150, administering, however, more frequently, say every hour at first. But when Cholera sets in in all its frightful forms, we should have immediate recourse to VERATRUM.

ADMINISTRATION. A few globules of the third in a teaspoonful of water every quarter of an hour: should no improvement set in after several doses, and the cramps change to *spasms* and *convulsions*, with spasmodic constriction of the chest, which obstructs respiration, CUPRUM must be had recourse to in the same manner as described for *Veratrum*. ARSENICUM should be alternated with *Veratrum*, when an intense *burning sensation* is experienced in the stomach and bowels, with extreme prostration of strength, great thirst, etc. (Vid. Indications, page 150.)

CARBO VEGETABILIS may often be given with advantage

when the patient is reduced to a state of almost complete asphyxia, *with scarcely perceptible pulse;* or when, on the cessation of vomiting, diarrhœa, and cramps or convulsions, congestion to the head and chest ensues, with oppressed breathing, coldness of the breath, and redness or lividity of the face, (which is covered with clammy sweat,) and lethargy :—Should the pulse become stronger under the action of *Carb. v.*, but the pain, vomiting, cramps, etc., return, *Veratrum* must again be had recourse to.

PHOSPHORUS (followed by ACIDUM PHOSPHORICUM, should *great clamminess* of the *tongue supervene*) is particularly useful in cases of *diarrhœa*, which are so liable to occur during the prevalence of cholera, and which, if neglected, are but too prone to pass on rapidly to confirmed cholera.

ADMINISTRATION. A few globules of the third potency every four or six hours.*

PHOSPHORUS is further indicated in the course of *congestion "in the chest"* during the *course of the disease;*—finally, it is one of the *most serviceable* remedies against the *obstinate diarrhœa* which sometimes remains after an attack. In conclusion, it may be added that a few doses of CANTHARIDES, 3, will be found useful when there is great irritation and pain in the bladder. *Rhus*, *Bryonia*, etc., when TYPHUS FEVER results (vide Typhus). *Belladonna*, followed, if required, by *Opium* and *Lachesis*, when there is CONGESTION OF THE BRAIN. *Aconite*, *Phosphorus*, *Bryonia*, *Belladonna*, etc., in the event of CONGESTION TO THE CHEST; and *Aconite*, followed by *Nux v.*, *Bryonia*, or *Mercurius*, etc., when the stomach and intestines become the seat of congestion (vide Congestion to the Abdomen.)

SECALE CORNUTUM is very useful in cases of *colourless diarrhœa*, with pains in the extremities remaining on the cessation of the vomiting, but is also valuable after *Veratrum* and *Cuprum*, when the *cramps* or *convulsions* do not yield to these remedies. *Cinchona* against the *weakness*,—and *Sulphur* and *Phosphorus* are two of the most important remedies against irritation or weakness in the alimentary canal, characterized

* Vide note, p. 21.

by frequent attacks of or nearly continual *looseness* occurring after cholera. The foregoing, then, are the principal remedies employed by homœopathists in cholera, and when the treatment is had recourse to from the commencement, it generally yields without difficulty; the disease rarely passing into the second stage, and almost never into the third.

The best preservatives against infection are *Veratrum*, *Cuprum*, and *Camphor;* an occasional dose of the preparation mentioned under the latter medicine, at page 152, has frequently been found sufficient to ward off an attack; it is more particularly during the *first stage* of the *disease itself*, however, under whatever form it sets in, that the greatest reliance is to be placed on this remedy. *Veratrum* and *Cuprum* are the prophylactics which have been employed with the greatest success. One drop of the tincture at the third dilution, or a few globules of the same potency of each medicine, may be taken alternately every third day, in a little water, fasting; avoiding, moreover, excesses of all kinds, late hours, exposure to night air, and melancholy thoughts, or fear, which are all strongly predisposing causes to attacks of this malady. When the disease happens to break out, notwithstanding these precautions, it is almost invariably in the *mildest* form. It may also be remarked, that during the prevalence of this affection the clothing should be sufficient to preserve the body at an equable temperature, and care taken to avoid chills or checked perspiration, or *cold* and *wet feet;* those who are affected with considerable perspiration in their feet should change their stockings at least once daily; a flannel bandage worn round the abdomen is also a useful precaution, and it should not be hastily laid aside when the danger seems to have passed away; also constant exercise should be taken during the day in the open air. Adherence to the homœopathic rules is a sufficient dietetic guide; raw vegetables and cold fruits, for example, melons, should be carefully abstained from, and even the more wholesome varieties and all cooked vegetables, except potatoes, be used in extreme moderation; pure beer and non-acid wines are not objectionable for individuals not attacked with the same limitation. It may appear almost supererogatory to observe that purity of air and thorough ventilation is highly necessary.

Accessory Treatment. The patient should be kept in a room of a warm temperature, the bed should be heated by artificial means, and bottles of hot water applied to the feet if necessary. The observance of this rule greatly facilitates the action of the medicine employed; anything which might disturb the equanimity of the sufferer, such as noise or contradiction, should be carefully avoided, and his spirits should be sustained as much as possible. Cold water is the best drink, but the patient should not be allowed to take too much at a time; the occasional administration of a small piece of ice, if possible, is often attended with benefit; and injections of iced water are sometimes serviceable in relieving the colic and cramps in the intestines. During the convalescence following this disease we must be careful not to indulge the patient to the full extent of his appetite.

Remarks. When this disease is raging as an epidemic, we not unfrequently find individuals suffering under many symptoms bearing a marked resemblance to those of cholera, but with constipation instead of diarrhœa, and retching in place of vomiting; this affection being closely analogous to *Suppressed Dysentery*, the reader will find the treatment under that head, article Dysentery.

CHOLERINE.

This affection being merely *diarrhœa*, occurring during the prevalence of cholera without any of the more severe symptoms of the disease, consult that article for its treatment.

LIVER COMPLAINT.

This disease is divided into the Acute and Chronic; the latter generally goes by the name of Liver Complaint, although a careful diagnosis will generally discover that the real disease is in the stomach and intestines; however, in many cases the liver itself becomes much affected from this cause, and in itself deserves considerable attention.

When the disease has been for a long time unchecked, and the inflammation becomes deeply seated in the substance of the liver, an abscess frequently forms, bursting either externally or internally; in the latter case not unseldom proving critical, or bringing on hectic fever.

ACUTE INFLAMMATION OF THE LIVER. *Hepatitis.*

This disease is much more common in tropical climes than with us. There, a high mode of living, exposure to heavy dews or damps in the evening, and the powerful rays of the sun by day, are among its principal exciting caüses; but it may also arise from violent mental emotions, the use of stimulating or alcoholic drinks, suddenly suppressed evacuations, strong emetics or purgatives, the use of mercury, gall-stones, external lesions, or injury of the brain.

Diagnosis. This differs according to the seat of the inflammation, when on the outer surface or convex side the symptoms closely resemble those of pleuritis; there is generally a violent pain in the right hypochondrium, sometimes resembling stitches, at others burning—shooting to the sternum, the right scapula, and point of the shoulder, and even affecting the right foot, with sensation of numbness or tingling in the arm of the same side, the pain increased by inspiration; a short dry cough, and the symptoms of inflammatory fever; bowels irregular, generally constipated, and evacuations in most instances of an unnatural colour.

In this form the patient can only lie on the *left* side.

When the seat of inflammation is on the inner or concave side of the liver, the pain is much less, and the patient complains rather of a sensation of pressure than actual pain, but the whole biliary system is much more affected. The eyes and countenance become yellow, and sometimes complete jaundice declares itself; the urine is orange coloured, the evacuations mostly hard and generally of a whitish or gray colour. We also find bitter taste in the mouth, vomiting, and considerable distress—the patient can only lie on the right side. Inflammatory fever is also present in this form, and in both, the right hypochondrium, on examination, will usually be found hot, tumefied, and painful on pressure.

Inflammation of the liver, unless well treated, is apt to assume the chronic form; it may also end in suppuration externally, or internally by a communication either with the lungs or intestinal canal, or by a vomica in the substance of the organ itself; in indurations or other alterations of structure, in gangrene, or in the formation of adhesions.

The disease may terminate by resolution, critical metastases, hemorrhoids, diarrhœa, epistaxes, or cutaneous, particularly erysipelatous eruptions.

THERAPEUTICS. The following remedies are those most required in its treatment:

Aconitum*, *Belladonna*, *Mercurius*, *Lachesis*, *Bryonia alba*, *Chamomilla*, *Nux vomica*, *Pulsatilla, and ***Sulphur***.

ACONITE is especially indicated in the commencement of the attack, and may always precede the other remedies, *when* there is violent inflammatory fever, attended with insupportable *shooting* pains in the region of the liver, with tossing, restlessness, and great anxiety and anguish.

ADMINISTRATION. $\frac{000000}{3}$ in an ounce of water, a dessert-spoonful every three hours. (Vide note, p. 21.)

BELLADONNA may be advantageously administered after *Aconite* has subdued the preceding symptoms, or from the commencement, when the following indications present themselves: oppressive pains in the region of the liver, which extend to the chest and shoulders; distention of the pit of the stomach, sometimes extending across the epigastrium, producing a sensation of tension, with difficult and anxious respiration; determination of blood to the head, with cloudiness and giddiness, sometimes causing faintness; great thirst, tossing about at night and sleeplessness.

ADMINISTRATION. Six globules of the third potency to an ounce of water, a dessert-spoonful every three or six hours, according to the violence of the attack; being careful, if a marked medicinal action declare itself, to allow it to pass off before repeating the medicine, and also to lengthen the intervals according to the amelioration produced.

When *Belladonna* fails to remove the whole of these symptoms, we frequently find that MERCURIUS will have the desired effect; this medicament is *too well known* as an *allopathic* remedy in the cure of this disease, and *the consequences produced by its abuse are frequently so great, as to render the disease almost incurable. It is generally administered, even when not indicated, until its marked pathogenetic symptoms declare themselves, and consequently the patient, in addition to the original malady, has frequently to contend with a medicinal disease.* The following are some of the principal indications for its employment:

Painful sensations in the region of the liver, with *shooting*, burning, or *oppressive* pains, not allowing the patient to lie long on the right side, sometimes augmented by movement of the body or part affected; bitter taste in the mouth, want of appetite, thirst, and continual shivering, sometimes followed by sweating, but without relief, with well marked yellow colour of the skin and eyes; also when there are enlargement and induration of the liver, or where we have reason to suppose the formation of matter. (Also, *Ars.*, *Hep. s.*, or Silic. The alternate employment of *Bell.* and *Bry.*; when the liver remained tumid and painful after the removal of the fever: *Phos.* and Bry.; when dull pain with dispepsia: *Carb. v.* and Bry.; when eructation, constipation, jaundice: *Carb. v.* and *Nux v.* in alternation.)

ADMINISTRATION. A grain of the 3d trituration to an ounce of water, a dessert-spoonful every three to six hours, according to results, and with the precaution specified under *Belladonna.*

LACHESIS. In subacute cases, or in those in which *Belladonna* or *Mercurius* have merely afforded partial relief, *Lachesis* is often of great service. It may also be administered with advantage alternately with the said remedies in obstinate cases occurring in drunkards. (*Administration*, see *Puls.*, 159.)

BRYONIA, when the pains in the region of the liver are mostly shooting, or consist of an obtuse pressure, with tension and burning, increased by touch, coughing, or respiration, and especially during inspiration; also much exacerbated by movement; also when the symptoms are attended with violent spasmodic oppression of the chest; rapid and anxious respiration, bitter taste in the mouth, tongue coated yellow; *constipation* present.

ADMINISTRATION. Same as *Belladonna.*

CHAMOMILLA, when there are pressive pains, pressure in the stomach, oppression of the chest, and a sensation of tightness under the ribs; *yellow colour of the skin*, pains *not* aggravated by motion, &c.; tongue foul and yellow, bitter taste in the mouth; *paroxysms of great anxiety. Chamomilla* is also almost a specific when the above symptoms have been brought on by a fit of passion.

ADMINISTRATION. Same as *Bryonia.*

NUX VOMICA is particularly indicated when the pains are shooting and pulsative, and attended with excessive tenderness at the region of the liver to the touch, pressure in the epigastrium and under the ribs, with shortness of breath; constipation; also when enlargement and induration occur; and in the chronic form, when there are marked symptoms of gastric derangement. (Vide *Nux vomica*, art. INDIGESTION.)

ADMINISTRATION. Same as *Bryonia.*

PULSATILLA. Sensation of tension in the region of the liver, and pressure or dull pain in the epigastric region; oppression at the chest, bitter taste, yellow tongue, nausea; *loose*, greenish, and slimy stools; excessive *anxiety*, especially towards evening or during the night.

ADMINISTRATION. Six globules of the sixth in an ounce of water, a dessert-spoonful every six hours.

SULPHUR is valuable to follow any of the preceding medicines, which, although apparently indicated, does not speedily declare a decided action, or when the disease continues, although in a diminished degree; it is particularly efficacious after *Nux vomica*, to combat the sequelæ of the disease

ADMINISTRATION. When to assist the action of the medicines, a single dose $\frac{0}{6}{}^{0}$ in a teaspoonful of water may be given, and followed by the remedy judged most appropriate to the case in the space of six or twelve hours, according to circumstances; when employed to combat the sequelæ of the disease, four globules at the same potency may be dissolved in four dessert-spoonfuls of water, and one exhibited morning and evening, and so on until relief is obtained, or another remedy is called for by an alteration in the symptoms.

Diet. The same as under Fevers, modified according to the violence of the disease.

LIVER COMPLAINT, OR CHRONIC INFLAMMATION OF THE LIVER. *Hepatitis Chronica.*

In this form of the disease we find many of the foregoing symptoms, but in a modified degree; further, a continued pain or uneasiness in the right side seldom leaves the patient, who gradually falls off in flesh and loses strength; and there is not unfrequently present an occasional cough with expectoration; sometimes considerable perceptible enlargement of the liver, either continual or returning periodically, with a number of dyspeptic symptoms; high coloured or red urine, yellow tinge of the skin and eyes, occasional febrile symptoms; the pulse, except during these attacks, generally quick but regular.

Nux vomica $\frac{00}{30}$ and Sulphur $\frac{00}{30}$ are two of the principal remedies in this affection, which, however, frequently requires a careful discriminative treatment, and all the acumen of the practised physician, to conduct it to a happy issue.

For the indications of these remedies, see Acute Inflammation of the Liver.

Administration. As in Indigestion, which see; under which also will be found directions for the regulation of Diet.

Carduus marianus. This remedy is indicated by most of the symptoms which have been described under *Bryonia* and *Nux v.* in the preceding chapter, but it is more particularly called for when there is bitter taste, with dull pain or occasional shooting or pricking in the right hypochondrium, increased by inspiration, yellow hue of the skin; short dry cough, or cough with expectoration of mucus streaked with blood; slight feverishness.

Aurum, Hepar s., Lycopodium, Magn. m., Natrum, Silex, Cinchona, Alumina, and *Calcarea,* have also been found useful in particular cases.

JAUNDICE. *Icterus.*

DIAGNOSIS. Yellow colour, varying in shade from a pale saffron to a dark-brown yellow, first in the eyes, then extending over the surface of the whole body; hard whitish fæces; orange-coloured urine; symptoms of deranged digestion, sometimes tensive pain or pressure in the region of the liver.

In severe cases even the perspiration will impart a yellow hue to the patient's linen.

The disease frequently declares itself without being plainly referable to any exciting cause; the principal are affections of the liver, indigestion, poisonous substances, taking cold, powerful mental emotions, emetics, or drastic purgatives or internal obstructions, such as gall-stones, or even worms obstructing the biliary duct.

Among the predisposing causes may be enumerated a too sedentary or irregular mode of life, indulgence in spirituous liquors, or a frequent use of aperients.

It may also be remarked that this disease frequently assumes the intermittent type.

Jaundice is not of itself to be considered as a dangerous disorder, but rather as an indication of some internal derangement, which, if neglected, may entail serious consequences, for example, dropsy, hectic fever, or general atrophy.

MERCURIUS and CINCHONA are two of the best remedies in the treatment of this disorder, particularly the former; but in cases when the patient has suffered from the abuses of that mineral substance, we give a preference to *Cinchona*, especially when we can trace the disease to have arisen from partaking of indigestible substances, or where it appears in an intermittent form.

In cases which have been excited by a fit of passion, as we have before noted—no unfrequent cause—we should have recourse to CHAMOMILLA, or NUX-VOMICA, should the bowels be confined, or alternately confined and relaxed.

Nux-vomica is also indicated when sedentary habits, over-study, or indulgence in spirituous liquors, appear to be the predisposing, or partly the exciting causes.

PULSATILLA. Lassitude, great weakness and anxiety especially towards evening, obtuse pressure, but sometimes also pricking or shooting pain in the region of the liver, extending occasionally upwards towards the right shoulder; whitish stools.

DIGITALIS. A most important remedy in many cases of this disease; the following are the principal indications for its employment: nausea, retching, or vomiting; tongue clean, or coated white; *pressure at the pit of the stomach and region of the liver;* sluggish state of the bowels, with *white, gray,* or *clay-coloured evacuations,* alternate heat and chills. (Icterus Spasmod. s. Spast.)

AURUM is frequently an excellent remedy in obstinate cases after *Pulsatilla,* when the disorder occurs in young females.

ADMINISTRATION.* In general cases, four globules at the sixth potency, in four dessert-spoonfuls of water, one exhibited morning and evening; in cases of very young children we may substitute one for four globules in the same quantity of water. (See remarks upon this subject in Introduction to Part III.)

Should Jaundice be accompanied with symptoms of inflammation, and pain and pressure in the hepatic region, see ACUTE INFLAMMATION OF THE LIVER; and that accordingly in the majority of such cases, *Aconite,* followed if needful by *Belladonna, Mercurius,* or *Chamomilla,* as best indicated, will be found of essential service.

In very obstinate icterus the alternation of *Sulphur, Hepar sulphuris, Lachesis,* and *Acid. nitricum,* has been found successful; but as these cases frequently arise from obstructions, atony, or a spasmodic or irritable state, they require considerable skill and discrimination in their treatment.

INFLAMMATION OF THE SPLEEN.

Splenitis.

DIAGNOSIS. Sharp pressing or shooting pains in the region of the spleen; in most cases a high degree of fever, with

* Vide note, p. 21.

general derangement; sometimes enlargement and tumefaction; and when very severe, hematemesis.

It declares sometimes in hot seasons, when it is not unfrequently mistaken for other affections. It may, however, arise in individuals of delicate constitutions, or in children when exposed to the influence of marsh miasms, particularly when to that cause has been added insufficient clothing, want of exercise, of proper nutriment, and long-continued mental disquietude.

The value of *Cinchona* in this malady and the power it displays of developing an affection closely similar, affords a beautiful exemplification of the truth of the homœopathic law.

From our very imperfect knowledge of the physiology of this viscus and its relation to the other organs, this disease, except when it presents itself in the tangible form above mentioned, is extremely difficult to diagnose. Its best characteristics are tenderness or sensibility on pressure in the splenic region, with general debility; paleness of the complexion, bloodless appearance of the conjunctiva, languid circulation, and tendency of the extremities to become cold.

THERAPEUTICS. The chief remedies in this affection are *Cinchona* and *Arsenicum,* which are useful not only in its treatment, but against the tendency to dropsy, which not unfrequently develops itself; this can but rarely occur, however, where the proceedings of the physician are guided by the homœopathic law, inasmuch as the very remedies employed to combat the disease itself, are the surest preventives against such a result.

The other medicines most frequently required are *Aconitum, Arnica montana, Nux vomica,* and *Bryonia alba.*

ACONITUM. Against the fever generally present, if the disease be severe.

ADMINISTRATION.* $\frac{000000}{3}$ to an ounce of water, administering one dessert-spoonful every half hour, hour, or four hours, according to the exigency of the case.

CINCHONA. When the inflammatory symptoms have abated, or if no fever of any moment existed from the commence-

* Vide note, p. 21.

ment, particularly if the disease owes its origin to marsh miasm, or if the accompanying fever present an intermittent type, in which case it should be administered during the *Apyrexia.* Moreover, if impaired appetite and general derangement be present, see this medicine under APEPSIA. Also, if the patient have been weakened by *hematemesis,* or *diarrhœa,* (see these articles.

ADMINISTRATION. In general cases we may dissolve $\frac{000}{6}$ in four dessert spoonfuls of water, and give a dose morning and evening, and so on until improvement results.

ARSENICUM, also useful where the disease assumes an intermittent character, or is complicated with that affection, (see *Cinchona,* and this remedy, in INTERMITTENT FEVER.) And further, when the patient complains of a violent *burning* pain in the region of the spleen, and a constant pulsation at the scrobiculus, attended with great anxiety; also watery or sanguineous diarrhœa, and burning at the anus; *excessive weakness,* and œdema of the feet.

ADMINISTRATION, same as *Cinchona.* In some cases it has been found advantageous to alternate these two remedies, giving a dose of the medicine selected morning and evening, allowing an action of one, two, or three days, according to circumstances, and then exhibiting the other in the same manner.

ARNICA, indicated by pressing pain in the left hypochondrium, causing dyspnœa, and when the vomiting of blood is very severe. ***Rhus*** is useful when severe corporal exertion has produced the disease.

ADMINISTRATION. $\frac{00}{6}$, in a teaspoonful of water, repeated in six hours, if necessary; but when the vomiting of blood is present, exhibit as under ***Hematemesis.***

NUX VOMICA is chiefly indicated by the symptoms of deranged digestion, constipation, &c, which remain after the more threatening symptoms are removed.

ADMINISTRATION. $\frac{000}{6}$ in a little water, at night, repeated every twenty-four hours while necessary.

BRYONIA is found useful in milder cases, where an aching, shooting pain is in the splenetic region, which is much aggravated by the slightest movement, or when the patient complains of a constant stitch in the side, or the left hypochondriac region, and general gastric derangement with constipation exists.

Administration. $\frac{0}{6}^{0}$, in a little water, repeated as the above until benefit results.

The preceding are the remedies which have been found most useful in the treatment of the disease in the acute form. Chronic enlargement and indurations of the spleen require a long and judicious course of treatment for removal, or even amelioration. I shall, therefore, briefly direct the attention of the reader to those remedies which have proved most successful in these instances—namely, *Sulphur*, *Calcarea carbonica*, and *Baryta carbonica* (particularly when the mesenteric glands have become affected), and further, *Lycopodium*, *Carbo vegetabilis*, *Plumbum*, *Ferrum*, *Mezereum*, *Platina*, *Stannum*.

INFLAMMATION OF THE STOMACH. *Gastritis*.

As there is some difference among medical authors as to the application of this term, it may be as well to state clearly the disease intended to be treated of in this place.

By gastritis is here meant inflammation of the mucous membrane of the stomach, which frequently involves the submucous tissue, and sometimes the muscular coat.

Diagnosis. Burning, pricking, or shooting pain in the gastric region, increased by pressure, inspiration or the passage of food. Swelling, considerable heat, and tension over the whole stomachic region, sometimes with pulsation; nausea, inclination to vomit, retching, vomiting, great thirst, increased or brought on by the smallest quantity of food or drink; sometimes with hydrophobic symptoms (*hydrophobia symptomatica*); soreness of the throat, with inflammation of the fauces; hiccough, sobbing, great restlessness, anxiety, and prostration of strength; coldness of the extremities; tongue generally red at the tip and round the edges, foul, rough at the centre and towards the root; frequently also syncope, violent spasms, convulsions, even tetanus; small, sometimes scarcely perceptible, and remittent pulse; sunken features, with expressions of anxiety, constipation, but frequently diarrhœa or alternations of these two states.

Death may ensue from gangrene, in which case the pains suddenly cease, the coldness of the extremities increases, and the pulse becomes scarcely perceptible and remittent; or from paralysis of the nervous system during the attacks of the spasms or syncope. When this disease has been improperly treated, if the patient has the good fortune to escape with life, it may pass into chronic inflammation, scirrhus, or ulceration of the stomach.

CAUSES. One of the most frequent is partaking of cold drinks or ice-water, when heated or during hot weather, and also acid or poisonous substances taken into the stomach; lesion from any rough-pointed body swallowed, external contusion, ardent spirits, suddenly checked secretions or evacuations, abuse of emetics, metastases.

THERAPEUTICS. The remedies which have been found the most useful in the homœopathic treatment of Gastritis, are: *Aconitum napollus, Belladonna, Ipecacuanha, Nux vomica, Antimonium crudum, Pulsatilla, Bryonia, Ranunculus bulbosus, Euphorbium, Cantharides, Hyoscyamus, Arsenicum.*

ACONITE $\frac{000}{3}$ is requisite in those cases in which synochal fever is developed,—and must be repeated until relief is obtained or an alteration in the symptoms calls for the selection of another remedy.*

IPECACUANHA $\frac{0000}{3}$ is useful when the vomiting is excessive, the epigastric region considerably distended, and the patient affected with great anxiety, restlessness and difficulty of breathing. *Antimonium crudum* $\frac{00}{6}$ may follow the former remedy, or be given in preference thereto, if the tongue be much loaded. *Bryonia* may be administered after any of the foregoing remedies, should they have afforded only partial relief, and particularly if the disorder has been excited by a chill from cold drinks when overheated.

NUX VOMICA $\frac{000}{3}$ is one of the most important remedies in Gastritis mucosa of drunkards, and in the same affection when occurring as a metastasis from suppressed hæmorrhoids;

* Vide note, p. 21.

finally, *Nux vomica* has been found efficacious after the previous administration of *Aconitum, Bryonia, Ipecacuanha,* and *Arsenicum* $\frac{0\,0}{6}$, when the disorder has been caused by a chill from drinking iced water when overheated. *Lachesis* and *Arsenicum* may, in some instances, be advantageously administered in alternation with *Nux v.*, in the idiopathic gastritis mucosa of drunkards.*

PULSATILLA $\frac{0\,0\,0}{3}$ has been recommended in the subacute form of gastritis, arising from the sudden suppression of some secretion, such as the menstrual flux, etc.; and also in cases proceeding from a chill in the stomach from ice, particularly after the previous employment of *Ipecacuanha* or *Arsenicum. Ranunculus bulbosus, Euphorbium,* and *Cantharides* have been recommended in the more violent forms of the disease, and especially when the *burning pain*, so commonly attendant on this disease, is well marked: When, however, in addition to the said symptom, there is *excessive prostration of strength;* thirst with violent vomiting immediately after drinking; small, quick, and occasionally intermittent pulse; anxiety, restlessness, and apparent sinking of the vital energies,—ARSENICUM must at once be had recourse to, whether the disease may have arisen from a chill in the stomach or any other cause, (excepting, of course, poisoning by that remedy, in which case the treatment to be followed will be found under the head of POISONS). The alternate administration of *Aconitum* with *Arsenicum* has been found useful in some cases; in others, *Veratrum* and *Arsenicum:* The former, at an earlier stage of the disorder, with accompanying inflammatory fever, and the latter where the *extremities have become cold*, the pulse small, features sunk and expressive of great anxiety; hiccough, thirst, vomiting on partaking of the smallest morsel of food, solid or liquid; extreme debility, and other symptoms mentioned in the diagnosis. In certain cases the attention of the practitioner may be directed to the following: BELLADONNA $\frac{0\,0\,0\,0}{3}$,—Inflammation of the fauces with redness of the tongue at the tip and margins; hydrophobia symptomatica. HYOSCYAMUS $\frac{0\,0}{3}$,—Stupor, or confu-

* *Opium* also may be included with advantage here.

sion of ideas with incoherent speech; convulsions, symptomatic hydrophobia. *Lachesis*, *Stramonium* and *Cantharides* may likewise prove useful in cases in which the latter symptom is present (see HYDROPHOBIA). Finally, *Colocynth*, *Mercurius vivus*, *Sulphur*, and *Chamomilla* may be mentioned as likely to prove serviceable auxiliary remedies in some instances. *Arnica* should be borne in mind, if the attack can be traced to lesion of the stomach from any rough or pointed substances having been swallowed, or also if from external contusion.

When the disease has passed into the chronic form, *Natrum m.*, *Lach.* and *Nux v.*, may be administered in alternation with great advantage: followed, if required, by *Lycop.*, *Colch.*, *Sulph.*, *Phosph.*, also the alternate employment of *Sulphur* and *Carb. v.*, &c. *Sep.*, *Plat.*, *Plumb.*, *Kali c.*, *Magn. c.*, *Rhus*. Vide CARDIALGIA (which chronic gastritis nearly resembles) and DYSPEPSIA.

INFLAMMATION OF THE BOWELS. *Enteritis.*

DIAGNOSIS. This disease is comparatively of rare occurrence in the idiopathic form, and appears much more frequently as a symptomatic affection, particularly in the course of some fevers—such as *low Nervous Fevers*, *Scarlet Fever*, *Measles*, &c.; also in all diseases attended with hectic fever.

It much more frequently occurs in the subacute or chronic than in the acute form. In the *acute* form of the disease, involving the submucous tissue and peritoneal coat, as well as the mucous membrane, the symptoms are usually as follows: Intense burning or pungent pain, generally in one spot of the abdomen, especially in the region of the navel, increased by the slightest pressure and by movement, with tightness, heat, and distention of the abdomen; sobbing, anxiety, and violent thirst, with aggravation of suffering from cold drinks; obstinate constipation; violent vomiting, first of slime and bile, and sometimes even of excrements (*Ileus miserere*); small and contracted pulse, inflammatory fever, flatulence, and frequently obstruction of urine.

In the subacute form of the disease, or in *simple enteritis mucosa*, the pain is often very slightly felt, in comparison with that which accompanies inflammation of the peritoneal coat, and generally consists of a diffused soreness over the abdomen, which is commonly, though not always, increased on pressure; but cold drinks or indigestible food almost invariably causes an aggravation of pain. The tongue is often red and smooth, though not invariably so; generally speaking, however, there is more or less redness at the tip and margins, however foul the centre may be. Loss of appetite, indigestion with nausea and vomiting, more or less prominent, according to the portion of the intestinal tube affected; being greater the nearer the seat of the inflammation is to the stomach. When the inferior parts are implicated (as is indicated by pain or soreness in the iliac regions and in the course of the colon), there is usually diarrhœa, the stools being frequently slimy and mixed with blood, in severe cases consisting of pure blood, particularly when the rectum is involved, in which case there is, moreover, considerable straining. The pulse is quick, the thirst sometimes excessive, with a greater or less degree of fever and *extreme languor*.

Unless resolution take place, it may terminate in induration of the intestines—laying the foundation of chronic constipation, suppuration, or gangrene.

The signs of approaching gangrene, or of its having set in, are the same as in gastritis, with the difference of situation.

Among its exciting causes are cold in the feet and abdomen, suppressed discharges, cathartics, worms, metastases, parturition, indigestible or highly stimulating food, prolonged use of acids, sour wine or beer, &c. The state of the atmosphere appears to have some share in producing it, from the circumstance that the disorder sometimes prevails almost as an epidemic.

THERAPEUTICS. *Arsenicum*, and where required, *Veratrum*, are the principal remedies in the first described variety of this disease, as well as in the severest forms of *gastritis*, to which latter, indeed, it bears a strong resemblance; but the treatment must necessarily be commenced with *Aconite* when the accompanying fever is intense, and the skin hot and parched. For the selection and administration of these two remedies, see GASTRITIS. *Opium* and *Plumbum* are the principal remedies against *Ileus Miserere*, as noticed in the Diagnosis. (See *Hernia.*)

In the subacute form of the complaint, a few doses of *Aconite* are often serviceable;—but as soon as the marked inflammatory symptoms have been subdued, one or more of the following remedies must be selected to complete the cure: *Belladonna, Mercurius, Acid. nitricum, Bryonia, Colocynth, Chamomilla, Nux v., Pulsatilla, China, Opium, Cantharides, Colchicum, Rhus, Phosphorus, Sulph., Silex.*

BELLADONNA.* Tongue *red* and *smooth*, or coated *white*, or *yellowish brown* in the centre with *intense redness of the tip* and *margins*, and inflammatory redness of the papillæ; skin hot and dry, *intense thirst*, with occasional delirium, especially at night; sensation of *soreness or of excoriation in the entire abdomen*, with tenderness on pressure, and sometimes considerable distention, particularly in the region of the arch or transverse section of the colon.

NUX VOMICA. *Redness* of the *margins* of the tongue, with yellow or *whitish* coating in the centre; sensation of *soreness*, with burning heat in the abdomen; loss of appetite; indigestion, with vomiting after partaking of food, and aggravation of the abdominal pain after drinking; flatulence, constipation, or constipation and looseness alternately; *scanty* watery stools, or stools consisting of a small quantity of mucus, sometimes tinged with blood, and attended with straining. This remedy is especially useful when the above symptoms have been caused by the sudden suppression of an *hemorrhoidal flux*, or from indigestible food, &c. *Sulphur* is frequently of great value in completing the cure after *Nux v.*

MERCURIUS is a most important remedy in this disease, even in the most serious cases, and especially after *Aconite* and *Belladonna*, or *Arsenicum*, should that remedy have been called for. The following are its principal indications: tongue

* The *alternation* of this remedy with *Mercurius*, the indication permitting, cannot be too strongly urged in this dangerous disease, especially when the symptoms are fearfully prominent.—ED.

very foul, coated *white* or dark brown; it is sometimes dry, but more frequently covered with thick mucus; *excessive thirst;* abdomen hard, tense, distended, and *very tender to the touch;* copious watery, bilious, and highly offensive stools; but more frequently there is constant urging to stool, followed, after *severe straining*, by the evacuation of a small quantity of mucus tinged with blood; at other times of pure blood in considerable quantity; extreme *prostration of strength*, chilliness and shivering, with tendency to sweating at night, which, however, brings little or no relief.

Acidum nitricum. The indications for this remedy are much the same as those described under the foregoing; it is therefore of great service in completing the cure when *Mercurius* has only produced partial relief. It is an invaluable medicine in *chronic* cases, attended with abdominal tenderness and *tenesmus*, and especially when the disorder occurs in individuals who have been previously subjected to an abuse of *Mercury* under allopathic treatment.

Bryonia. After the previous employment of *Aconite*, *Bryonia* is occasionally a useful remedy here, when the patient complains of severe headache, with constipation, and pain in the abdomen after meals; it is also indicated, however, when, after *Aconite*, there remains dark redness of the tongue, or whitish or *yellow* coated tongue, with parched mouth and considerable thirst; loose offensive evacuations, particularly after partaking of *food* or drink; nausea and vomiting after eating.

Pulsatilla. When the acute inflammatory symptoms of enteritis arising from the sudden suppression of some habitual discharge, such as the catamenia, or the hemorrhoidal flux, or occurring as a sequela of measles, have been subdued by *Aconite*, and the following symptoms remain: tongue loaded with a thick *white*, grayish, or yellow coating; *adipsia*, or, on the contrary, *excessive thirst*, deranged digestion, loss of appetite, with nausea and vomiting after partaking of a little nutriment; sensibility of the abdomen on pressure, or on every movement; flatulence.

COLOCYNTH. In cases where the large intestines are the seat of the inflammation, attended with *tympanitic distention of the abdomen*, soreness and sensibility to the touch; *tormina* and diarrhœa, with increase of pain followed by urgent desire to go to stool after *eating* or drinking; nausea, or vomiting of bilious matter; frequent discharge of flatus.

CHAMOMILLA. Is peculiarly well adapted to the treatment of the disorder as it is likely to occur in children, or in highly nervous and excitable females, who are extremely sensitive to pain, and complain loudly from trivial suffering; it is indicated, moreover, by a sensation of soreness in the abdomen, as if arising from internal excoriation or ulceration, accompanied with painful tenderness on slight pressure, and *slimy, whitish, watery*, or *greenish* or yellowish diarrhœa of an offensive odour.

CINCHONA. Is frequently useful after *Aconite* or any of the foregoing remedies, when there is a tympanitic distention of the abdomen; diarrhœa, aggravated after a meal, with undigested food in the evacuations; thirst, extreme weakness of digestion, and great debility.

CANTHARIS. In very serious cases, with discharge of pure blood at stool, and strangury; or in an advanced stage of the disorder, with evacuations of mucus and solid substances, like shreds of membrane, this remedy will frequently be found of considerable service.

COLCHICUM. Will also be found useful occasionally in advanced stages of the disorder, *with tympanitic distention of the abdomen*, diarrhœa, the stools consisting of *white* or transparent gelatinous mucus, or of blood mixed with substances resembling false membrane.

RHUS. When eruptions break out about the mouth, and there is redness of the tongue, with pain as if from soreness or ulceration in the abdomen, and tenderness on pressure; watery, slimy, frothy, or sanguineous stools; *low fever*, with nocturnal delirium. Rhus is chiefly used in symptomatic enteritis, such as frequently occurs in low *Nervous Fever*, which see.

The chronic stage of the complaint, which is chiefly characterized by fixed pain, fulness, or uneasiness and oppression in the lower part of the abdomen, *increased after meals* or after *cold drinks;* appetite impaired or capricious; *thirst*, particularly after dinner or at night; bowels constantly relaxed, or there is constipation alternately with diarrhœa; fetid and discoloured evacuations; skin hot, harsh, and of an unhealthy hue; pulse rather quick; tongue loaded, but red at the tip and margins,—or redness of the entire tongue, with large and elevated papillæ, especially at the root; emaciation, weakness, and languor. Here the foregoing remedies described for the acute and subacute variety, but more particularly ***Belladonna***, ***Nux v.***, ***Bryonia***, and ***Rhus***, together with ***Acidum nitricum***, ***Phosphorus***, ***Sulphur***, ***Silicea***, and ***Arsenicum***, will in most instances be found among the most serviceable.

ACIDUM NITRICUM. Is particularly indicated when there is thirst, attended with pains in the bowels or other uneasiness after drinking; impaired appetite, *tenderness of the abdomen*, fetid diarrhœa and *tenesmus;* greenish stools, with ingesta; skin dry and harsh during the day, sometimes with nocturnal sweats.

PHOSPHORUS. Soreness in the abdomen, with tenderness on pressure, and distressing distention after meals; obstinate diarrhœa, or constipation and diarrhœa alternately; stools containing ingesta; pulse rather quick and hard; weakness and emaciation.

SULPHUR. This remedy is one of the most useful in enteritis, arising from the suppression of some accustomed discharge, such as the hemorrhoidal, &c.; as also in cases arising from the driving inward of a tetter, or sudden healing up of an ulcer; tongue red, or loaded; thirst; pain, as from excoriation, in the abdomen, with tenderness on pressure; or fulness and uneasiness in the abdomen, increased by cold drinks or after meals; diminished or fastidious appetite, with aversion to meat; fetid diarrhœa, frequently containing ingesta; constipation, or constipation alternately with diarrhœa; flatulence; skin yellow or otherwise unhealthy looking, or dry and pealing, but often covered with perspiration at night, or towards morning; pulse quick and hard; emaciation, with considerable debility.

Silicea. When the disorder has been excited by the sudden suppression of the perspiration of the feet, or the rapid healing up of a chronic ulcer, *Silicea* is one of the most important remedies. The following symptoms are some of the more immediate indications for its selection: dryness of the mouth, loaded tongue, great thirst, with diminished appetite, and sometimes disgust at meat, or cooked and hot food, with desire for cold food and drinks; abdomen hard, *hot and tense*, and painful to the touch; constipation, or extremely fetid watery stools; borborygmus, especially on movement; skin dry and parched during the day, and covered with sweat towards morning; pulse quick and hard.

Arsenicum. Has already been noticed as the principal remedy in acute cases of a violent character; it is, moreover, a remedy of considerable service in some of the chronic varieties of enteritis, with a sensation as from excoriation, or of *burning heat* in the abdomen, attended with nausea, want of appetite, and *great thirst;* increase of pain after cold drink; borborygmus; diarrhœa, sometimes with ingesta; *fetid,* discoloured stools; skin parched, hard, and of a yellowish, unhealthy-looking hue; emaciation, with extreme debility.

Lachesis, Lycopodium, Natrum muriaticum, Secale cornutum, Hepar sulphuris, Sepia, Calcarea, Graphites, Carbo vegetabilis, Causticum, Antimonium crudum, and *Ipecacuanha,* may also be of considerable service in some cases—the two last named have occasionally been used with advantage after *Aconite* against the vomiting in acute cases. When we have reason to suspect worms as the cause of this affection, the patient must be treated accordingly. See Invermination, p. 181.

Administration of the Remedies. In the acute form of the disease, a few globules of the third potency of the remedy indicated may be added to an ounce of water, and a dessert-spoonful of the liquid given every three hours, lengthening the intervals as soon as improvement sets in. In the sub-acute and chronic form, the sixth, and in some cases the thirtieth, potency may be substituted for the third, and the doses administered at intervals of from six to twelve hours and upwards.*

Diet. In acute cases of inflammation, either of the stomach or bowels, the regimen must be placed under the same restrictions as described at page 17 (*Fever;*) and in sub-acute and chronic cases the food should be very light, and given in small quantities; raw fruit, green vegetables, and sometimes potatoes, must be strictly prohibited; the drink should consist solely of toast-water or barley-water, or the like.

INFLAMMATION OF THE PERITONEUM.

Peritonitis.

DIAGNOSIS. Painful tension and tumefaction of the abdomen with a sensibility to the touch even more acute than that in Enteritis; so much so that the patient cannot bear the pressure even of a sheet upon the abdomen; frequently constipation or ischuria, and the symptoms of enteritis.

CAUSES. General causes of inflammation, and moreover external injury, parturition, chill of the abdomen, and metastases.

THERAPEUTICS. In the first place it will generally be found beneficial to administer three or four doses of *Aconitum* at the third potency, exhibited at intervals of time varying according to the exigency of the case, until the fever and inflammation lower. This remedy has been found in many cases sufficient of itself to remove the affection, and in all it materially modifies its violence.

When the cause is external lesion, we should administer Arnica $\frac{0\,0}{6}$, and repeat it in twelve hours, and at the same time apply bandages wetted with a diluted tincture, as given under EXTERNAL INJURIES in cases of contusion.

Sometimes vomiting and other symptoms closely resembling those of enteritis are present, and frequently constipation and

* Vide note, p. 21.

ischuria; and other times merely the marked sensibility of the abdomen and tumefaction with gastric derangement; but, physiologically considered, these symptoms arising from the intensity and extent of the inflammation, and the sympathy of the other organs, our chief care must be to lower the inflammation, which being in a great measure brought under control by the medicine above noted, we will find considerable benefit from the employment of *Nux vomica* and *Mercurius* to combat any remaining symptoms.

NUX VOMICA. When there is *distention* of the abdomen with tendency to the predominance of gastric symptoms and ischuria.

ADMINISTRATION. $\frac{0}{6}{}^{0}$, repeated every six to twelve hours, according to the severity of the symptoms.

MERCURIUS is more particularly suited to the advanced stages of the disease, with weak, quick pulse, nocturnal sweats, and great weakness.

When the inflammation extends to the pleura, and the breathing becomes affected with acute shooting pain, we should have recourse to BRYONIA $^{0}\frac{0}{3}{}^{0}$, as described for Aconite. (See also PLEURITIS.)

When the peritoneal coat, or upper portions of the alimentary tube or of the stomach itself, becomes affected, evidenced by an increase in the intensity of the disease, the pain extending higher—vomiting, generally a rare symptom, becoming severe and continual—collapse of the features, small pulse, and a rapid sinking of the vital energies, closely resembling gastritis—we should have recourse to *Arsenicum*.

ADMINISTRATION. $\frac{0}{6}{}^{0}$, in a little water every four to six hours, until relief is obtained.

In cases where there are evidences of the brain being affected, *Belladonna* may be had recourse to. (See PHRENITIS.) In other instances *Cantharides, Chamomilla, Bryonia, Rhus, Lycopodium, Colocynth*, etc., may be found necessary.

As this is a disease whose care devolves more particularly upon the experienced professional man, I have contented myself with stating the remedies most likely to be called for in ordinary cases: in many instances the symptoms are so closely analogous to those which are met with in GASTRITIS, that most of the remedies which have been described applicable to the treatment of that disease will generally be found equally useful here.*

INFLAMMATION OF THE KIDNEYS.

Nephritis.

DIAGNOSIS. Pressing, pungent pain in the renal region, shooting along the urethra to the bladder, dysuria, strangury, and ischuria (when both kidneys are affected), hot and high-coloured or red-urine; drawing up, swelling, and pain of the testis on the affected side; numbness and spasms of the foot on the same side; nausea, vomiting, colic, and tenesmus; lying on the part affected and motion aggravate the pains.

CAUSES. Excessive use of stimulants; shocks of the body, falls, or strains, external injuries; long lying on the back, abuse of diuretics or cantharides, suppressed hemorrhoids or menstruation, metastases or calculi.

THERAPEUTICS. The principal remedies in this affection are, *Aconitum, Cantharides, Nux vomica, Pulsatilla, Belladonna, Hepar sulphuris, Cannabis, Mercurius, Arnica montana.*

ACONITE. In the inflammatory stage of this affection, this remedy should be administered in repeated doses, in the same manner as in Inflammatory Fever; after which, in the majority of cases,—

CANTHARIDES will be found most efficacious in the further treatment, and more particularly when the urine passes off in drops or is tinged with blood, or when micturition is exceedingly painful, with burning pain in the urethra, and when the general symptoms of shooting, cutting, and tearing pains in the loins and region of the kidneys are present, or even in cases of complete strangury.

* In PERITONITIS PUERPURALIS, *Aconitum, Ipecacuanha, Bryonia, Arsenicum, Veratrum, Chamomilla,* and *Pulsatilla* are the remedies which have chiefly been used; but some of the others which have been mentioned in the treatment of GASTRITIS may be found serviceable in particular cases.

Administration. Six or eight globules of third or sixth potency to an ounce of water, a dessert-spoonful every one, two, or three hours till benefit result.*

The proved value of this medicine when used homœopathically, in the cure of this painful disorder, is another of the many beautiful exemplifications of the truth of the homœopathic law; and its power of causing diseases of the urinary organs, even when applied in the form of a blister, is so well known, that in all medical works it has been noted as an exciting cause of this affection.

Nux vomica. When the affection can be traced to a suppression of a hemorrhoidal discharge, determination of blood to the abdomen, excess in wine or stimulants, and sedentary habits, and where we find constipation, feeling of faintness, nausea, vomiting, distention of the abdomen, drawing up of the testis and of the spermatic cord.

Pulsatilla. In females of phlegmatic temperament, when arising from irregular or suppressed menstruation.

Administration. $\frac{0}{6}^{0}$, of the last-mentioned remedies, repeated every twelve hours, while necessary.†

Belladonna. When shooting pains in the kidneys are present, extending to the bladder, —this medicine is further indicated when nephritis is accompanied with colic and cardialgia, heat and distention in the region of the kidneys, scanty micturition of an orange yellow or sometimes of a bright red, depositing red or whitish thick sediment; anxiety, restlessness, and periodical aggravation—constipation.

Administration. Same as *Cantharides.*

Hepar sulphuris is useful when we have reason to apprehend the formation of an abscess or the commencement of suppuration; here the diagnosis is difficult, and the professional student must be careful not to mistake the apparent alleviation of suffering for the subjugation of the disease. The following symptoms may serve as a guide in these cases: cessation of the acute pain; a sensation of throbbing and a sense of weight in the region of the kidneys; alternate chills and slight flushes of heat and copious perspiration.

* Vide note, p. 21. † Ibid.

ADMINISTRATION. A grain of the third trituration to an ounce of water, a dessert-spoonful every three or four hours, lengthening the intervals according to results.

MERCURIUS is also valuable in this stage, but more particularly when diarrhœa and tenesmus are present.

ADMINISTRATION. Same as *Hepar sulphuris*, at intervals of from six to twelve hours.

CANNABIS. When a dragging pain or sensation as if from excoriation is experienced, extending from the region of the kidneys down towards the groin, with painful urination.

ADMINISTRATION. Same as *Cantharides*, but at somewhat longer intervals.

COLCHICUM. When in addition to the usual symptoms of this disease there is *excessive nausea* with *tympanitic distention of the abdomen*, and painful and scanty emission of bright red urine.

ADMINISTRATION. Same as *Cantharides*.

When the disease has assumed a chronic form, and induration of the kidneys has taken place, *Mercurius* $\frac{00}{6}$, in a teaspoonful of water, will often be found useful, a dose once a week for three or four weeks, followed by *Aurum* $\frac{000}{6}$, a dose once a week, unless some marked indication call for the employment of another medicine.

In Nephritis arising from contusions or violent concussions of the body, *Arnica* is the principal remedy.

ADMINISTRATION. $\frac{00}{6}$, repeated in twelve hours, and a lotion applied externally. (See EXTERNAL INJURIES.)

In cases arising from the abuse of *Cantharides* in blistering, an occasional drop or so of the saturated solution of *Camphor* in a little water, and the inside of the thighs to be rubbed with the same preparation, twice a day, until relief is attained.

OBSERVATION. This disease sometimes arises from the presence of calculi in the kidneys; in which case the symptoms of fever do not occur until a considerable time after severe pain has been experienced; further, a numbness of the thigh, and a retraction of the testicle of the affected side, are considered as distinguishing marks of the existence of a calculus in the kidney or ureter:—Here the use of *Nociatiana rustica* has repeatedly been found an useful palliative, administered at a low potency $\frac{000}{3}$ every half hour. In conclusion, the following remedies, whose utility in various forms of nephritis or nephralgia, clinical observation has confirmed, may be pointed out as meriting the attention of the professional student: *Calc. c.*, *Lycop.*, *Capsicum*, *Phos.*, *Sepia*, *Uva ursi*, *Sarsap.*, *Kali c.*, and *Graphit.* In the event of suppuration: *Hep. s.*, *Ars.*, *Sulph.*, *Silic.*, *Kali n.*, *Sarsap.*

Patients suffering from Nephritis should strictly avoid wine, malt liquor, and spirits.

INFLAMMATION OF THE BLADDER. *Cystitis.*

Burning pain in the region of the vesica, with tension, heat, pain when touched, and external tumefaction; frequent and painful discharge of urine, or suppression, and generally tenesmus; fever, and sometimes vomiting, as in Nephritis. The causes closely resemble those of Nephritis, but it also occurs more frequently in parturition than the former affection.

Therapeutics. We should have recourse to **Aconitum**, as in Nephritis, when a considerable degree of inflammatory fever is present, followed by—

Cantharides, which here, as in the above-mentioned disease, is the leading remedy.

Nux vomica. When attributable to an indulgence in wine or spirituous liquors, this remedy, timeously administered, will in many instances check its further progress; also, when it results from suppressed hemorrhoids or dyspeptic derangements:—*Nux v.* may be followed, if required, by *Sulphur* and *Calcarea.* The two last named are well adapted to the treatment of the chronic form of the complaint.

Pulsatilla. Valuable in checking the development of the affection when arising from suppressed menstruation.*

* *Pulsatilla* is, moreover, serviceable in all cases, from whatever cause arising, when occurring in individuals of phlegmatic temperament, with the following symptoms: frequent desire to urinate, painful and scanty emission of slimy or sanguinolent urine, which deposits a purulent-looking sediment; burning and cutting pains in the hypogastrium, with external heat and tumefaction; suppression of urine.

HYOSCYAMUS. When difficult urination is present, but the disease is not far advanced, particularly when we have reason to suspect that this symptom arises from spasmodic constriction of the neck of the bladder, or when in fact it is more of a spasmodic than inflammatory character. Digitalis is also valuable, when in addition to the ischuria a constrictive pain is felt in the bladder. *Arsenicum* and *Carb. v.* have been found very serviceable in allaying the burning in the urethra during urination. When *Sulphur*, *Calcarea*, or any of the foregoing remedies have not succeeded in arresting it.

ADMINISTRATION of the first-named remedies, the same as in NEPHRITIS; *Hyoscyamus, Digitalis, Sulphur, Calcarea, Arsenicum* and *Carbo v.* in the same manner as *Nux.v.* and *Pulsatilla.* When this disease has arisen from the application of *Cantharides* as a blister in allopathic practice, *Camphor* must be administered as ascribed under NEPHRITIS.

When the disease arises from the presence of STONE or GRAVEL, the same remedies as those mentioned at the termination of the preceding chapter are the most useful.

INVERMINATION. WORMS. *Helminthiasis.*

The existence of worms in the intestinal canal, in the majority of cases, evidently arises from a peculiar constitutional taint, inducing a certain diseased state of the mucous or lining membrane and thereby giving rise to the formation of these parasites; and although no period of life is wholly exempt from their presence, yet infants and children appear to be much more subject to this affection than adults, on account of the predominance of nutrition at that age. Weakness of the digestive function, accumulation of mucus in the intestines, an ill-regulated diet, and a degree of moisture in the atmosphere, also favour their generation.

The three species most generally met with in the human subject are, the *ascaris*, *lumbricus*, and *tænia* or *tape-worm* ; of the latter there are two varieties,—the *solitary tape-worm*, composed of long and slender articulations, which has been known to exceed the length of thirty feet; and the *common tape-worm*, which varies from three to ten feet, seldom comes away entire, but in joints, which are considerably broader and thicker than those of the variety first mentioned.

The presence of worms, unless when passed, is not always easy of detection, since subacute inflammation of the mucous membrane from other causes will frequently present nearly the same range of symptoms; but here, (as in the treatment of many of the most serious acute diseases,) Homœopathy present two manifest advantages over the old system. In the first place, if acting upon the certainty of the existence of worms, we administer a remedy specific to the affection; in the next, when we are *uncertain* as to the true character of the complaint, and select a medicament *distinctly indicated by the united symptoms*, it will be found applicable to the affection, from whatever cause it arises; and a careful observance of the known pathogenetic powers of the remedies selected, will materially assist us in tracing the disease to its proper source.

Diagnosis. Worms, and especially *ascarides*, frequently exist in the intestines without occasioning any disturbance, and their presence is only known by their being observed in the evacuated fæces; but when the alimentary tube becomes irritated by them, a number of symptoms are developed, of which the following are the principal: Pallor and sickly appearance of the countenance, and sometimes flushing; livid circles round the eyes, dilated pupils, headache or vertigo, irregularity of appetite, fœtidity of breath, acrid eructations, occasional nausea and vomiting, foul tongue, tensive fulness of abdomen, with a sensation of gnawing and burning at particular parts of the intestines; hard and tumid belly; great thirst; discharge of mucus from the rectum, bladder, (and vagina;) heat and itching at the anus; slight febrile symptoms, and nocturnal wakefulness, with low spirits or irritability of temper, and gradual emaciation; we also generally notice an inflammatory redness of the nostrils, with great disposition to picking or boring at the nose, especially in children, with sudden screaming, when waking, and grinding of teeth. In addition to the above general symptoms of this affection, we frequently meet with severe colic-like pains, with slimy and bloody evacuations; involuntary discharge of saliva, especially when asleep; convulsions in children, and epileptic attacks, combined with cerebral affections in adults; inflammation of the bowels.

In *tænia*, in addition to the above, we find a sensation as of something rising into the left side of the throat, and then falling back; or a feeling of a lump on either side, with an undulatory motion; feeling of sugillation in the abdomen, creeping torpor and numbness in the fingers and toes.

THERAPEUTICS. *Acon., Ignat., Sulph., Calc. c., China, Ferr. m., Marum ver., Cina, Nux v., Merc., Valeriana, Spigel., Bellad., Sabad., Silic., Cicuta v., and Filix mas.* Of these, *Acon., Ferr., Ignat., Merc., Nux v., Valer., Marum v., Cina* and *Sulph. tinct.* are the most appropriate against Ascarides. *Cina, Nux v., China, Bellad., Merc., Spig.*, etc., against Lumbrici. And *Graph., Calc., Sabad., Frag. vesca,* or *Sulph., Merc., Calc.,* also *Carb. an., Carb. veg., Kali c., Magn. m., Natr., Phosph., Petrol., Plat., Tereb., Fil. mas., Punica gran., Stannum,* against tape-worm.

ACONITUM. When considerable febrile irritation exists with restlessness at night, fever, and irritability of temper, continual itching and burning at the anus, and at times a sense of crawling in the throat.

ADMINISTRATION.* $\frac{00}{6}$, to an infant $\frac{0}{12}$, in a little water, repeated in six hours if necessary; when it has lowered the fever we must have recourse to some other remedy.

IGNATIA AMARA, in most cases, which is also particularly indicated by spasmodic twitchings in one of the extremities or in individual muscles.

ADMINISTRATION. $\frac{000}{6}$ in four dessert-spoonfuls of water, one twice a day; for an infant $\frac{0}{12}$ in four teaspoonfuls, one night and morning.

SULPHUR, in case the annoyance still continues after the lapse of two or three days.

ADMINISTRATION. $\frac{000000}{6}$ in an ounce of water, a teaspoonful morning and evening until finished; for infants $\frac{00}{12}$ in the same manner.

CALCAREA CARBONICA and SILICEA may be administered in like manner, should no marked amelioration ensue; allowing an interval of about a week or ten days to elapse between the different remedies.

* Vide note, p. 21.

Ferrum metallicum, when there is frequent vomiting and accumulation of watery fluid in the mouth.

Administration. A grain of the third trituration to an ounce of water, a teaspoonful once a day; for infants $\frac{0\,0}{6}$ in the same manner.

This course of treatment, persevered in for a short time, has often proved successful in most obstinate cases, by purifying the constitution and restoring the mucous membrane to a healthy state. When *excessive* irritation is present, and does not appear to diminish readily under the action of the preceding remedy, we may give a drop of the tincture of *Urtica urens*, in a little water, or on a piece of loaf sugar, every night or morning for several successive days; and should this not relieve the annoyance, we may administer an enema of a dessert-spoonful of salt to a pint of water, of which from two to six fluid ounces, according to age, may be injected; if this act as a laxative, a mixture of vinegar and water in the proportion of one-fourth part of the former may be used.* After this palliative course of treatment, the course above mentioned may again be resumed should it appear necessary.

Cina. This is an eminently useful medicine in the case of worms, and is generally indicated where the following symptoms are met with: Frequent boring at the nose, great perverseness of temper, heat and irritation, constant inquietude and restlessness, with, in children, a desire for things which are rejected when offered; fits of crying when touched, paleness of face, with livid circle round the eyes; constant craving for food even after a meal, griping, distention, and hardness in the abdomen, with discharge of thread and round worms, and loose evacuations; occasionally, convulsive movements in the limbs, weakness and lassitude. This medicine is particularly indicated for Colic produced by worms.

Administration. Same as *Ignatia*.

Nux vomica is a valuable adjunct in cases of worms in which considerable derangement of the digestive function is present, with irritability of temper and constipation.

* Hering's Hausarzt.

ADMINISTRATION. $\frac{0\,0}{6}$ in a teaspoonful of water at bedtime, repeated in three or four days if called for.

MERCURIUS. When we find diarrhœa, distention of the abdomen, and hardness in the umbilical region, with increased secretion of saliva.

ADMINISTRATION. As *Ignatia.*

CHINA is appropriate when the symptoms are generally exacerbated at night, particularly the abdominal sufferings; or, when pressive aching pains are experienced below the umbilical region after every meal, and are attended with distention of the abdomen, pyrosis, pains in the epigastrium, and retching; also, when in addition to the foregoing, there is an over-excitability of the nervous system, with spasmodic twitchings of the muscles in various parts, tremulousness and debility. (*Valeriana* and *Veratrum* are also deserving of attention here.)

SPIGELIA in extreme cases, with colic, voracity, diarrhœa, and chilliness; or nausea in the morning.

ADMINISTRATION. As *Ignatia.*

BELLADONNA. Great nervous excitement; nocturnal delirium, with startings during sleep; tendency to be startled or frightened at the most trivial cause; also colic, headache, thirst, quick pulse, hot, dry skin; should these symptoms not yield to *Belladonna,* recourse must be had to *Lachesis,* or to *Silicea* should the febrile symptoms continue, and the patient affected be of a scrofulous diathesis.

ADMINISTRATION. Two globules of the sixth potency in a teaspoonful of water, until the febrile action is subdued.

CICUTA VIROSA. Worm colic with convulsions.

ADMINISTRATION. $\frac{0\,0}{6}$, in a little water, repeated in a few hours, if necessary. In severe cases, a drop of the third, in four dessert-spoonfuls of water, once every half hour.

The treatment of tænia, although similar to the above, has some modifications. In most cases we may give *Aconitum,* followed by *Cina,* after which considerable relief is often experienced; and then have recourse to FILIX MAS; when anything sweet disagrees with the patient, a drop of the third potency to an ounce of water; a teaspoonful twice a day, until finished :— also, *Punica granat.* has been employed with much success.

In chronic cases the following treatment has proved successful: *Nux vomica*, *Mercurius*, and *Sulphur*, each $\frac{00}{6}$, a single dose, alternated at intervals of from six to eight days. When any improvement takes place after the administration of any one of these remedies in particular, it will be well to repeat that medicine at the stated intervals, as long as it appears to do good, instead of going on to the next remedy in rotation.* Moreover, in this course of treatment, *Calcarea carbonica* $\frac{00}{6}$, may advantageously follow *Sulphur*, in scrofulous habits, at an interval of ten days. *Natrum muriaticum*, *Lycopodium*, *Graphites*, *Baryta*, or *Phosphorus*, have been found necessary to complete the cure in particular cases.

Regimen. The food ought to be wholesome and nutritious; meat, such as roast or boiled beef or mutton, once a day, in moderate quantity, and occasionally a light pudding; green fruits or vegetables must be strictly prohibited, and the utmost care should be taken to prevent children from eating raw herbs, roots, etc., which they are so prone to pick up in their rambles when not looked after. Plenty of exercise in the open air is of essential service, and must on no account be neglected.

* Vide note, p. 21.

DISEASES OF THE ORGANS

CONNECTED WITH

THE RESPIRATORY SYSTEM.

CATARRH, OR COMMON COLD,—CATARRHAL FEVER.

This term is given to an affection which consists of a mild degree of inflammation of the lining membrane of the nostrils, windpipe, and occasionally also of the ramifications of the latter; induced by exposure to sudden changes of temperature, or to a damp or chilly atmosphere with INSUFFICIENT CLOTHING, PARTICULARLY AS REGARDS CHILDREN. This complaint is characterized by slight fever, impaired appetite, obstruction of the nose, sneezing, unusual languor, pains in the head or in the back and extremities, and subsequently hoarseness or cough, generally preceded by transitory chills or shiverings; there is also a slight degree of wheezing and difficulty of breathing. When the disease is confined to the nose and sinuses it is termed A COLD IN THE HEAD; of which latter affection, and moreover, HOARSENESS and COUGH, I shall treat separately.

THERAPEUTICS. In many instances catarrh is carried off, or runs to a salutary termination, in a day or two; and this desirable result is frequently obtained by having *timely* recourse to the simple proceeding of remaining a little longer in bed, and encouraging a gentle sweat by drinking a *warm* demulcent fluid, such as gruel; bathing the feet and legs in warm water, at the temperature of about 98 to 100 degrees of

Fahrenheit, is also a useful auxiliary mode of restoring perspiration, but the patient should go to bed immediately afterwards. Very robust persons who are accustomed to be in the open air in all weathers, but who have caught cold after having overheated themselves, will frequently prevent any bad effects by drinking one or two glasses of cold water on going to bed; when, however, they have learned by experience that little benefit is to be derived therefrom, a few globules of *Carb. v.* or *Silicea* should be taken instead. A moderate degree of abstinence should, at the same time, be observed; veal or chicken broth, bread, sago, or semolino pudding, and such like, instead of the ordinary diet. The drink may consist of water-gruel, barley-water or toast-water. All strong liquors must be abstained from.

The following are the principal medicines to be employed in the majority of cases, when called for: *Nux v.*, *Cham.*, *Coffea*, *Bellad.*, *Bryonia*, *China*, *Dulcamara*, *Arnica*, *Merc.*, *Acidum phosph.*, *Sulph.*, *Calc.*, *Ipecac.*, *Arseni.*, *Silicia*, *Camphora*, and *Aconitum*.

ADMINISTRATION. Each medicine in a little water, at the dose specified; repeated in twelve hours, if required.*

NUX VOMICA $\frac{0\,0}{6}$ when the symptoms of common cold declare themselves, will often check the attack. It is also indicated by external pains in the head from the same cause. Tickling or scratching in the larynx, dry cough in the morning, also during the day, rarely during the night. In catarrhal fever, with disposition to chilliness. When convenient, it is preferable to administer this remedy towards evening.

CHAMOMILLA $\frac{0\,0}{6}$. In the treatment of children this medicine is generally preferable to *Nux vomica* in arresting the attack. It is (like *Belladonna*, *Bryonia*, *China*, *Dulcamara*, *Sulphur*, and *Silicea*) extremely valuable in restoring the suppressed perspiration, and removing the following symptoms: colic with pains in the head, ears, and teeth, thirst, ill humour, and impatience.

COFFEA CRUDA $\frac{0\,0\,0}{3}$. This remedy is indicated where there is excessive sensibility, fretfulness, and sleeplessness, with general pains, especially in young persons.

* Vide Note, p. 21.

Belladonna $\frac{0\,0}{6}$, when there is throbbing, bursting headache, attended with determination of blood to the head, increase of the pain from movement or exposure to cold air.

Bryonia $\frac{0\,0}{3}$. Headache, particularly at the temples, with aching pains in the limbs, much increased by the slightest movement.

Cinchona $\frac{0\,0}{3}$. Aching pains in the shoulder-blades, and in the extremities, increased by the slightest pressure on the affected parts, with great restlessness and constant desire to change the position of the limbs.

Dulcamara $\frac{0\,0}{6}$, when the pain is more of a passive or dull aching description, and felt only in particular parts of the head, with humming in the ears, and obtuseness of hearing; pains in the limbs, increased when at rest, and attended with a feeling of coldness, stiffness, and numbness; or when an offensive perspiration breaks out after an attack of cold; or when the affection has been brought on by suppressed perspiration, from exposure to cold and damp weather.

Arnica montana $\frac{0\,0}{6}$, when aching pains, or pains as if arising from a bruise, are felt in the limbs after exposure to cold, causing excessive restlessness and constant disposition to change the position of the affected parts, and increase of pain from the slightest touch or movement.

Mercurius $\frac{0\,0}{6}$, when the pains in the limbs and joints are accompanied with profuse sweating, which affords no relief; followed by *Dulcamara* should the sweat continue, and be of an offensive odour.

Acidum phosphoricum $\frac{0\,0}{6}$. Aching pains, relieved by movement.

Silicea $\frac{0\,0}{6}$. Pains in the limbs, colic and general derangement arising from suppressed perspiration, particularly in those who are subject to *sweating* at the feet.

Sulphur $\frac{0\,0}{6}$, in cases of swelling of the knee, or of the joints of the hand and fingers, from taking cold. It may, in many such cases, be followed by *Calcarea carbonica* in a week or ten days.

Ipecacuanha $\frac{0\,0}{3}$. Nausea and inclination to vomit, or *Dyspnœa*, almost amounting to suffocation, arising from having taken cold, followed by—

ARSENICUM $\frac{0}{6}^{0}$, should no amelioration declare itself in six or eight hours.

PULSATILLA. Useful in cold in the head with loss of taste and smell resulting from a chill, followed or preceded by *Belladonna*, should there be an uncomfortable sensation of heat in the eyes and head, and heat and smarting in the nose. Or by *Nux v*, should there be complete stuffing or dryness of the nose. (See CORYZA, p. 193.)

RHUS TOXICODENDRON, general indisposition from exposure to a thorough wetting when in a state of perspiration; followed by *Bryonia* in a few hours, if no improvement is experienced.

CAMPHORA,* when there is unusual weariness, heaviness, and general uneasiness, attended with *shivering*, and dryness or coldness of the skin, will generally succeed in preventing the development of an attack either of common cold or of influenza.

ADMINISTRATION. A drop of weak spirits of *Camphor* every two or three hours, until relief is obtained.

ACONITUM is usually called for in febrile attacks, provoked by cold,—when hot, dry skin is present,—and, when timely administered, will frequently prevent the affection from assuming a more serious form.

The remedies for any other effects arising from cold, will be found under the different heads, such as SORE-THROAT, DIARRHŒA, COUGH, HOARSENESS, etc.

Some individuals, particularly amongst those of the fair sex, are tormented with an extreme degree of susceptibility to cold; the best corrective to which is, to rub the *throat*, *chest*, and indeed the whole body, every morning with a wet towel, until a glow of heat is produced,—drying one part before another is commenced;—also to acquire a habit of going

* The happiest effects will speedily follow the administration of *Camphor* in incipient colds or influenzas, when, in addition to the indications recorded above, there are: tearful eyes, snuffling nose, hoarseness *and rough and sore sensation in the throat.* It seems also to predispose the system to accept more readily the impression of other remedies that may be subsequently required.

Our rule has been to administer a tablespoonful of weak Camphor-water, twice or thrice, at intervals of three, four, or six hours.—ED.

out *every day*, provided there is no inherent predisposition to pulmonary consumption; all *extremes*, either of heat or cold, should at the same time be avoided, and care taken, when the body is heated, to let it cool gradually:—When these means are not sufficient to remove the tendency to suffer from the slightest exposure to cold, the practitioner will find *Silicea, Carb. v.*, and *Calcarea*, administered at intervals of from two to three weeks, to have considerable power in removing this constitutional delicacy. In other cases, one or more of the following remedies must be had recourse to:—*Bryonia, Belladonna, Dulcamara, Nux v., China, Mercurius, Rhus, Chamomilla, Arsenicum, Lachesis, Rhododendron*, according to the character of the sufferings which are experienced after each exposure to the influence of the atmosphere.

HOARSENESS. *Raucitas.*

The seat of this affection is in the mucous membrane of the throat, (larynx,) which is extremely liable to be affected by the common causes of Catarrh; hence it is a frequent accompaniment of this disorder.

The remedies mentioned under Catarrh and Cough are those which are generally found most useful in this complaint. Amongst these, in cases of recent origin, the following deserve particular notice: namely, *Pulsatilla, Mercurius, Nux v., Capsicum, Rhus tox., Sambucus nigra, Chamomilla, Carbo vegetabilis, Drosera, Sulphur*, and *Hepar sulphuris.*

The indications for the employment of these medicines are as follow:

Pulsatilla $\frac{0000}{3}$. Almost complete aphonia, particularly when accompanied with loose cough, or thick yellow coryza.

Mercurius $0\frac{0}{6}00$. This remedy will be found useful in removing any symptoms remaining after the above, but is to be preferred should the hoarseness, from the commencement, be attended with thin coryza. And when a sensation of burning or tickling is complained of in the larynx, with the characteristic indication of *Mercurius*, namely, a disposition to *profuse sweating*, especially at night.

NUX VOMICA ${}^{0}\frac{0}{3}{}^{0}$. Hoarseness, accompanied with a dry, fatiguing cough, worse in the early hours of the morning, with dry obstruction of the nose.

CAPSICUM ${}^{0}\frac{0}{3}{}^{0}$. Hoarseness, and dry obstruction in the nose, attended with an unpleasant sensation of crawling and tickling in the nose; with a severe cough, worse towards evening; with pains in other parts of the body, such as the head and abdomen. It is also better suited than *Nux vomica* for individuals of a lymphatic temperament.

RHUS TOXICODENDRON $\frac{0\,0\,0\,0}{6}$. Hoarseness, accompanied with sensation of excoriation in the chest; oppressed breathing, with frequent and violent *sneezing*, unaccompanied by coryza, but occasionally by a great discharge of mucus from the nose during the attacks of sternutation.

SAMBUCUS NIGRA ${}^{0}\frac{0}{3}{}^{0}$. Hoarseness, with deep, hollow cough; oppression at the chest; frequent yawning; restlessness, and thirst.

CHAMOMILLA ${}^{0}\frac{0}{3}{}^{0}$. Hoarseness, with accumulation of mucus in the throat; cough worse at night, continuing even during sleep, and frequently with a degree of fever towards evening, and great irritability of temper. This remedy is frequently found specific in cases of children.

DROSERA $\frac{0\,0}{3\,0}$. Hoarseness, with very low, or deep and hollow voice.

CARBO VEGETABILIS $\frac{0\,0}{3\,0}$. Chronic hoarseness, worse in the morning and towards evening, with aggravation after talking.

SULPHUR $\frac{0\,0}{3\,0}$. Hoarseness, attended with roughness and scraping in the throat; and of great value in obstinate cases, where the voice is low, and nearly extinct; particularly in cold damp weather. (*Sulphur* is especially useful after *Puls.*)

HEPAR SULPHURIS ${}^{0}\frac{0\,0}{6}{}^{0}$. An admirable remedy in chronic hoarseness, particularly in individuals who have taken large quantities of mercurial preparations; otherwise CAUSTICUM is equally useful.*

* *Sulph. calcarea* and *Silicea* are most useful remedies in obstinate hoarseness attended with coryza.

Administration of the Remedies.* Dissolve the globules, at the potencies mentioned, in four dessert-spoonfuls of water, and exhibit one, morning and evening, for two days; or, in some cases, continue for three; being guided by the result. Of *Hepar s.*, half a grain, 3d trit., in the same manner.

When we find individuals in whom this affection occurs frequently at different seasons, or on the slightest exposure to cold or damp, we may naturally infer that there is a constitutional predisposition to chronic laryngitis, a malady requiring a judicious treatment by an experienced practitioner, as, if neglected, it may eventually end in

CHRONIC LARYNGITIS. PHTHISIS LARYNGEA.

Chronic Inflammation of the Larynx.

This is a comparatively rare disease, and, when present, there is generally a degree of ulceration. The following are its principal contents: pain in the larynx, and round the glottis; pain and difficulty in swallowing; hoarseness, and difficulty of respiration; frequent attacks of severe cough, with scanty and occasionally sanious expectoration; it sometimes ends in hectic fever, which carries the patient off.

The medicines to which we would particularly direct the attention of the practitioner in the treatment of this malady, are, *Hepar s.*, *Lachesis*, *Phosph.*, *Carbo veg.*, *Causticum*, *Acidum nitricum*, *Calcarea carb.*, *Arsenicum*, and *Spongia*.

Aconite with *Spongia*, and *Hepar sulph.*, and frequently also *Lach.*, are the most useful remedies in this disease in the *acute form*. (See also Croup.) *Administration*, see hoarseness.

The patient should, in both forms of this affection, adhere rigidly to dietetic rules, avoid unnecessary exposure, and enter as little as possible into conversation.

COLD IN THE HEAD. *Coryza.*

Diagnosis. This affection is a very general attendant upon Catarrh.

Therapeutics. When it is the leading symptom, or ex-

* See note, p. 21.

ists independently of those already mentioned, the best medicines for expediting its removal are *Nux vomica, Euphrasia, Pulsatilla, Chamomilla, Mercurius, Hepar sulphuris, Belladonna, Ammonium, Natrum,* and *Arsenicum, Lachesis, Silicea,* &c.

ADMINISTRATION. Three globules of the potencies named, to be dissolved in four teaspoonfuls of water, one to be taken morning and evening, unless otherwise specified.*

NUX VOMICA. Dry obstruction, especially, *during the night only,* with pressive heaviness in the forehead, and confusion in the head; heat in the face, increasing towards evening. If in combination with other *catarrhal* symptoms, see the indications already given for its exhibition under the several heads of CATARRH, HOARSENESS, and COUGH. This direction equally applies to the other medicaments here quoted.

ADMINISTRATION. Two globules of the sixth potency, to be dissolved in a teaspoonful of water, and taken towards bedtime; to be repeated the second day following; but should an alteration in the symptoms have taken place without any corresponding improvement, another remedy must be selected.

LYCOPODIUM $\frac{000}{12}$, will often be found efficacious after *Nux v.*, in obstinate cases of stuffing of the nose, particularly at night, rendering it necessary to sleep with the mouth open, which causes a disagreeable dryness without much thirst, confusion in the head, and burning pain in the forehead. This remedy is frequently more or less useful in colds in the head *of all kinds.*

ADMINISTRATION, same as *Nux v.*

PULSATILLA $\frac{000}{6}$. The discharge thick, fetid, greenish yellow, or mixed with clots of blood; loss of taste and smell, headaches, sneezing, chill, especially towards evening; disposition to weep, lowness of spirits, heaviness or confusion of the head in a warm room.

CHAMOMILLA $\frac{000}{3}$. The affection having risen from checked perspiration, acrid discharge from the nose, causing redness of the nostrils, and excoriation or soreness under the nose; chapped lips; *shivering, with thirst.*

MERCURIUS $\frac{000}{6}$. Dryness of the nose, with obstruction;

* Vide note, p. 21.

profuse discharge, producing excoriation, swelling or redness of the nose, pains in the head and face. This is a valuable remedy in the generality of *ordinary cases* of cold in the head, and particularly when the complaint is, as it were, epidemic.*

HEPAR SULPHURIS $\frac{000}{6}$. Chiefly when only one nostril is affected, or when headache is experienced, or the complaint renewed on each exposure to cold air; further, in most cases in which *Mercurius*, though apparently indicated, has produced little or no improvement.

BELLADONNA $\frac{000}{3}$, may follow the above, if required, but especially when the sense of smelling becomes variously affected, being at one time too acute, and another too dull.

AMMONIUM $\frac{00}{6}$. Stuffed nose, especially at night; swelling and painful sensibility of the nostrils; *dryness* of the nose.

NATRUM $\frac{00}{6}$. Cold in the head, renewed by the slightest chill, or exposure to a current of air; obstruction of the nose every second day.

LACHESIS $\frac{00}{12}$. *Swelling and soreness of the nose and nostrils, with copious watery secretion.*

ARSENICUM $\frac{00}{6}$. *Obstruction of the nose*, with, at the *same time*, discharge of thin, acrid, excoriating mucus, and burning heat in the nostrils, &c. *Suffering relieved by heat;* pain in the back, feeling of general debility, or prostration of strength. *Dulcamara* is useful when fresh obstructions arise from every trivial exposure to the air. *Ipecacuanha* may be had recourse to after *Arsenicum*, if the latter has only partially relieved.

GRAPHITES and also SILICEA are useful in all cases which are of frequent recurrence, and always of a most obstinate character.

CAMPHOR. In the premonitory stage of the complaint, with *shivering and headache*, the attack may frequently be checked by a drop or two of spirits of weak camphor.

Sulphur, *Calcarea*, *Graphitis*, *Silicea*, *Natrum*, and *Pulsatilla*, are the best remedies for removing extreme susceptibility

* When the secretion from the nose is excessive, and there is at the same time, confusion in the head with redness and soreness of the eyes and *eyelids*, and copious acrid or scalding lachrymation, *Euphrasia* should be prescribed.

to colds in the head.* Against the effects of a *suddenly* suppressed catarrh, the following are the most important remedies: *Aconite* against headache, followed by *Pulsatilla*, and then *Cinchona*, if the secretion does not return; difficulty of breathing, *Ipecacuanha*, followed, if required, by *Bryonia* and *Sulphur;* against hoarseness, cough, or disease in the respiratory organs, arising from a similar cause, see the remedies mentioned under these different heads.

COUGH. *Tussis.*

Diagnosis. Forced and audible respiration without fever; or a symptom in acute diseases, such as fever, pneumonia, or phthisis; either dry or accompanied with expectoration.

Cough, although not dangerous of itself, may become so, or form an important feature of other diseases. As a precursor of phthisis, it is too often neglected.

It may arise from an irritation of the air-passages or lungs; from cold or other causes, or from disease of the same organs, or be merely sympathetic or the consequence of derangements or other important viscera.

Therapeutics. The following are the medicines most useful in this affection: *Aconitum, Dulcamara, Bellad., Hyosc., Nux v., Pulsatilla, Ammonium carbonicum, Ammonium muriaticum, Chamomilla, Hepar sulphuris, Ignatia, Ipecacuanha, Mercurius, Carbo vegetabilis, Capsicum, Bryonia, Rhus toxicodendron, Arsenicum album, Drosera, Silicea, Lachesis, Causticum, Sulphur, Calcarea carbonica, Euphrasia, Sepia, Stannum, Verbascum, Arnica montana,* and *Squilla,* &c.

Aconitum $\frac{000}{3}$. Violent short cough, with *quick hard pulse* and *feverish heat;* pricking in the chest when coughing, or during inspiration. See *Bronchitis*, p. 225.

* In other cases this desirable result may be attained by the administration of *Mercurius, Hepar s.* and *Belladonna*, on each successive attack (when the symptoms resemble those which have been described under these remedies)—and failing these, *Silicea, Sulphur,* and *Calcarea;* and the other remedies mentioned above as useful in removing this susceptibility must be had recourse to.

DULCAMARA $^{\circ}\frac{\circ}{6}{}^{\circ}$. The following are indications for the selection of this remedy: moist cough, after exposure to wet, or cough with expectoration of bright-coloured blood; aggravation of the cough on movement or when out of doors; *alleviation* in the recumbent posture or when within doors.

BELLADONNA $^{\circ}\frac{\circ}{6}{}^{\circ}$. *Short, dry, barking,* (*spasmodic catarrhal,* or *nervous,*) *cough at night in bed,* and also during sleep, *renewed* by the slightest movement; dry cough day and night, with irritation or tickling in the pit of the throat, or sensation as if a foreign body were in the larynx, or as if dust had been inhaled; *spasmodic* cough, which scarcely allows time for *respiration.* Finally, this medicine is sometimes useful in cough with rattling of mucus in the chest, pricking in the sternum or in the hypochondria, and expectoration of thick white mucus, coming on especially after meals; *pains in the abdomen;* hoarseness, redness of the face, headache, sneezing after coughing, and pain in the nape of the neck.*

NUX VOMICA $^{\circ}\frac{\circ}{6}{}^{\circ}$. This is a valuable remedy in many cases either of catarrhal or nervous character, and is *particularly efficacious* where there is a *dry,* hoarse, fatiguing, and sometimes spasmodic cough, which occurs in an aggravated form in the MORNING, and occasionally also towards evening, and attacks more or less during the day, but relaxes again at night. When, however, it is occasionally supplanted by oppression at the chest, on lying down or on awaking during the night, accompanied with a feeling of heat, and dryness in the mouth, if there be any expectoration it consists merely of a *little mucus which is detached with great difficulty.* The cough is generally excited by a disagreeable *tickling* or scraping, with a feeling of roughness or rawness in the throat, sometimes attended with HOARSENESS and feeling of roughness in the chest, but more frequently with severe headache, or pain as if from a *blow or bruise in the epigastrium* and *hypochondria;* it is frequently aggravated after meals, or by movement, not un-

* *Hyoscyamus* frequently answers when *Belladonna* has only afforded partial relief, and may be preferred to the latter, when the nocturnal cough is mitigated for the time by sitting up in bed; also when there is mucus rattling in the throat. *Conium* in dry spasmodic cough, increased at night.

frequently also by reading or meditation, and is occasionally followed by vomiting.

Pulsatilla $^{0}\frac{0}{6}^{0}$. Severe shaking, catarrhal or nervous spasmodic cough, worse *towards evening* and *at night*, frequently followed by vomiting; sensation of *suffocation*, as if from the vapour of sulphur; increase of cough when in the recumbent posture; cough which is at first dry, then followed by *copious expectoration* of yellowish or whitish mucus, sometimes of a salt or bitter taste; or expectoration of mucus streaked with blood; wheezing or rattling of mucus in the chest; the paroxysms of coughing are frequently accompanied with soreness in the abdomen, as if from a bruise or blow, or painful shocks in the arms, shoulders, or back, and sometimes followed by a sensation as if the stomach became inverted from the violence of the cough; involuntary emission of urine when coughing; loose cough, with aching in the chest, hoarseness, cold in the head; excited by a sensation of scraping or of erosion in the throat; shivering.

Ammonium carbonicum $\frac{0\,0\,0}{3}$. *Dry, tickling, suffocating, cough*, in the morning, sometimes with fever, occurring during the prevalence of a cold, stormy, bleak, state of the atmosphere, and attended with a sensation of *heat or burning behind the sternum*, resembling that which is occasioned by drinking spirits; roughness of the voice; cold in the head.

Ammonium muriaticum $\frac{0\,0\,0}{3}$. This remedy is sometimes serviceable after the former when the cough sounds looser, yet is unattended with expectoration.

Chamomilla. Dry cough, excited by continual tickling or irritation in the larynx and chest, and increased by talking; the cough is most troublesome *during the night*, but also occurs during the day, particularly in the morning and towards evening; accumulation of tenacious mucus in the throat; wheezing in the chest; cough during sleep, sometimes accompanied with paroxysms, as of threatening suffocation; cough with scanty expectoration of tenacious bitter mucus. This medicine is well adapted to the treatment of coughs in children accompanied with more or less of the symptoms above described, or with hoarseness, cold in the head, dryness in the throat, and thirst; great fretfulness; fever towards evening; paroxysms of coughing after crying, or after a fit of passion.

HEPAR SULPHURIS $\frac{000}{6}$. Obstinate cases of violent *dry hoarse cough*, sometimes attended with a dread of suffocation, and ending in lachrymation. The attacks are frequently excited or aggravated on any part of the body being *exposed* or becoming cold from the *bed-clothes slipping* off, and are generally worse at night; also dry deep cough *excited* by a feeling of tightness in the chest, or by talking, stooping, or ascending stairs; hoarseness.

IGNATIA $\frac{000}{6}$. Shaking spasmodic cough, or *short hacking cough*, as if arising from the presence of dust or feather-down in the throat, which becomes aggravated the longer the paroxysms of coughing continues; dry cough with coryza, occurring both day and night. This remedy is further particularly efficacious when the attacks of coughing become *aggravated* after *eating*, or on lying *down at night*, or on rising in the *morning*, and when the sufferer is of a mild and placid temper, or subject to alternations of high and low spirits.

IPECACUANHA $\frac{000}{6}$. Catarrhal, nervous, or spasmodic cough, particularly at night, attended with painful shocks in the head and stomach, and followed by *nausea*, *retching*, and *vomiting;* or *dry cough*, arising from tickling in the throat; or *severe, shaking, spasmodic cough*, with oppressed breathing, almost amounting to suffocation. In the case of children, this remedy is frequently valuable when they appear to be threatened with *suffocation from the accumulation of mucus*, or where the paroxysm is so severe as scarcely to afford time for respiration, causing the face to assume a livid hue, and the frame to become quite rigid. (*Calc.* is often useful after *Ipec.*)

MERCURIUS $\frac{000}{6}$. *Catarrhal cough, with hoarseness, watery coryza, or with diarrhœa;* or dry cough, excited by irritation in the throat, or the upper part of the *chest*, which becomes particularly troublesome towards evening, and at night; sometimes with slight prickings in the chest when coughing or sneezing; excited or increased by *talking;* cough in children with discharge of blood from the nose, which coagulates as it flows, vomituritION, and headache; dry spasmodic cough, with retching after the paroxysms, and expectoration of blood.

CARBO VEGETABILIS $\frac{000}{30}$. Hollow cough excited by irritation, or a troublesome sensation of crawling in the throat, and attended with burning pain, and sensation as if from excoriation in the chest: catarrhal or nervous *spasmodic cough,* frequently followed by inclination to vomit or vomiting, occurring in paroxysms throughout the day; cough with *hoarseness,* especially towards evening, or *morning* and evening, increased by speaking. Chronic cough with expectoration of greenish mucus, or even of yellowish pus—or with expectoration of blood and *burning* sensations in the chest (a characteristic indication for this remedy as well as *Arsenicum.*)

CAPSICUM $\frac{000}{6}$. This remedy is frequently very efficacious in cases of cough occurring in individuals of the *lymphatic temperament.* It is particularly indicated when the paroxysms are more severe towards *evening* and at *night,* frequently attended with unsettled pains in various parts of the body, and bursting headache; also painful *pressure* and *aching* in the *throat* and *ears;* cough with offensive breath, and disagreeable taste in the mouth.

BRYONIA $\frac{000}{6}$. Catarrhal cough occurring in winter during the prevalence of frost and cold easterly winds, with aggravation of the fits of coughing on coming from the open air into a warm room. The following are the general indications for its employment: *dry cough excited* by constant *irritation in the throat,* or as if caused by vapour in the larynx and windpipe, with greatly accelerated respiration, as if it were impossible to obtain sufficient air; spasmodic, suffocating cough, *after partaking of food* or *drinks,* and also after midnight; cough with *prickings in the chest,* and violent bursting headache, especially at the temples, also with prickings in the pit of the stomach, or in the side: further, in loose cough with *yellowish expectoration* or slight spitting of blood, this remedy will frequently be found of great service; dry nervous cough.

RHUS TOXICODENDRON $\frac{000}{3}$. *Short, dry* cough, worse towards *evening* and *before midnight,* excited by *tickling in the chest*, attended with anxiety and shortness of breath; cough on waking in the morning, or short cough with *bitter taste* in the *mouth*, on lying down at night and on waking in the morning. Cough with expectoration of bright blood, with sensation of insipidity or exhaustion in the chest, or shooting pains in the chest and sides.

Arsenicum $\frac{000}{12}$, cough with oppression at the chest, and tenacious mucus in the *larynx* and chest; cough excited by a sensation of *dryness* and *burning* in the larynx. Dry *cough, chiefly in the evening after lying down*, often with difficult *respiration* and *fear of suffocation*, as if arising from inhaling the *vapour of sulphur;* dry cough, excited by eating or *drinking*, or *by ascending stairs*, or cough which arises *as soon as the open air is encountered; thin acrid coryza; sneezing; periodic* dry cough—nocturnal cough with general burning heat; cough with expectoration of sanguineous mucus; pulmonary catarrh in old people, also *Ipec., Tart. e., Baryt. c.;* or in alternation with *Arsenic.*

Drosera $\frac{000}{12}$, in many cases of *chronic cough with hoarseness;* or *deep, hollow cough*, with pain in the chest and under the ribs, alleviated by pressing the hand on the side, excited or aggravated by laughing; cough on lying down in the evening and during the night. Matutinal cough, with *bitter* and *nauseous expectoration;* dry *spasmodic* cough, aggravated at night, or towards evening, and frequently followed by vomiting of ingesta, or bleeding from the nose and mouth.

Silicea $\frac{00}{12}$. Cough with oppressed breathing on lying on the back, or cough attended with tightness and oppression at the chest as if something stopped the respiration while speaking or coughing. Fatiguing, or *deep hollow* cough, day and night, aggravated by *movement* or speaking, and sometimes attended with aching and pain as if from a bruise in the chest; *cough* with *copious expectoration of transparent mucus*, or of pus, sometimes streaked with blood; cough with asthmatic breathing and emaciation, with dread of suffocation at night; cough excited by a sensation as if a hair were on the tongue.

Lachesis $\frac{00}{12}$. Fatiguing cough excited by *dryness* or continual *tickling* in the *larynx* or chest; or by pain or tickling in the pit of the stomach or the epigastrium; also by the *slightest pressure* on the exterior of the throat; cough excited by talking, laughing, or reading aloud, or anything which may tend to increase the dryness or irritation in the throat; *short, dry, suffocating cough*, as if caused by the presence of a crumb of bread sticking in the throat, with ineffectual efforts to expectorate. Cough on rising from the recumbent posture, or attacks of cough always *after sleeping*, or on lying down to sleep; cough also *during the day*, or also at night during sleep, so that the patient is unconscious of it; continual hoarseness, with a sensation as if something were in the throat which could not be detached.

Causticum $\frac{000}{6}$. *Dry, hollow cough*, which even awakes one from sleep; short cough excited by tickling, crawling, or a feeling as if the throat were excoriated, or by talking and cold, attended at times with burning or a sensation of *soreness in the chest*, and rattling of mucus; pain in the hip, and occasionally involuntary discharge of urine when coughing.

Sulphur $\frac{000}{6}$. In some cases of chronic coughs, and particularly in *dry* cough, which disturbs the patient at night as well as during the day, the cough is frequently excited after partaking of food, or during a deep inspiration, and is generally attended with a sensation of spasmodic constriction in the chest, sometimes followed by inclination to vomit, or involuntary escape of urine, or pain as if from excoriation, or pricking pains in the chest; headache, pains in the chest, the abdomen, loins and hips; also, cough, with expectoration of thick, *whitish*, or yellowish mucus, or of a greenish yellow, fetid mucus, or *pus*, of a salt or sweetish taste; feverish cough with spitting of blood.

Calcarea carbonica $\frac{000}{6}$. Dry cough, aggravated towards evening, or at *night*, excited by *tickling* in the throat, or by a sensation as if there were a *feather down in the throat*; also, loose cough, with rattling of mucus in the chest, and expectoration of offensive *thick, yellow mucus*; anxiety.

Euphrasia $\frac{000}{6}$. Cough, with coryza and *lachrymation*; diurnal cough, with difficult expectoration of mucus; or matutinal cough, with copious expectoration, and oppressed breathing.

Sepia $\frac{000}{12}$. Cough with copious expectoration of mucus of a *saltish taste*, of a yellow or greenish colour; also dry *spasmodic* cough, particularly at *night*, or on first lying down, attended, in children, with crying, fits of choking, nausea, retching, and bilious vomiting. This remedy is especially adapted to individuals having a constitutional taint, such as the scrofulous, scorbutic, &c.; in chronic coughs, with thick, yellowish, greenish, or even *puriform* expectoration, with a putrid taste, it is a valuable remedy.

STANNUM $\frac{000}{6}$. Cough, with copious expectoration of a greenish yellow, of a *sweetish* or *saltish* taste, attended with great weakness and disposition to sweats; or dry shaking cough, worse at night or towards morning, excited or aggravated by speaking or laughing, and occasionally followed by vomiting of ingesta.

CINCHONA $\frac{000}{3}$. Paroxysms of cough as if excited by the vapour of sulphur, with whistling or rattling in the throat from mucus; expectoration difficult, consisting of clear tenacious mucus, sometimes streaked with blood; pains in the shoulders, or prickings in the chest and windpipe; cough, sometimes with bilious vomitings; cough after hemoptysis.

VERBASCUM $\frac{000}{6}$. This remedy is frequently of great service in children, though less frequently so than *Chamomilla.* Indications: dry, hoarse cough, worse towards evening and at night: occurring during sleep.

IODIUM $\frac{000}{3}$. Cough in *plethoric* children, with copious accumulation of mucus in the bronchi, and ineffectual efforts to expectorate.

PHOSPHORUS $\frac{000}{6}$. *Dry cough,* excited by *tickling* irritation in the throat or *chest,* or by laughing, talking, or drinking, or by cold air, and accompanied with pricking in the larynx; hoarseness, or pains in the chest as if from *excoriation;* cough with hoarseness, from fever and depression of spirits, sometimes with apprehensions of death; dry sounding cough, followed by expectoration of viscous or sanguineous mucus.

ARNICA $\frac{000}{6}$ is of great value in coughs, with bleeding from the nose and mouth; headache, pricking in the chest (pleurodynia), rheumatic pains in the loins and extremities, and soreness or pain, as from a bruise, in the chest and abdomen.

Squilla $^{0}\frac{0}{3}{}^{0}$. In short dry cough, excited by a full inspiration, or chronic cough, or catarrh with copious secretion of whitish viscous mucus, which is alternately expectorated with ease and difficulty, this remedy is useful.

Administration of the remedies. The dose mentioned after each medicine in a teaspoonful of water, repeated in from twenty-four to forty-eight hours, as required; in severe cases, six or eight globules in an ounce of water, a dessert-spoonful every three or four hours.*

These are the principal remedies to be had recourse to in this disorder; but in complicated cases we may have to call in the aid of other medicaments. In some obstinate, *nervous* coughs, occurring in highly irritable, nervous, and hysterical habits, which are generally *dry*, or attended with scanty and difficult expectoration, consisting of a little clear mucus, change of air will frequently readily effect a cure. For cough arising from Worms, see the remedies mentioned under that heading; or from teething, see Dentition. Stomach coughs, or coughs occurring in women during the last months of pregnancy, are to be relieved by the remedies mentioned under Dyspepsia. Unmedicated jujubes, or sugar candy, may be allowed occasionally, to moisten the throat or mouth, in cases of dry irritating coughs.

HOOPING-COUGH. *Tussis Convulsiva. Pertussis.*

This is *almost* peculiarly a disease of childhood, and one which few individuals escape during that period; it generally appears as an epidemic; and is, by the majority of physiologists, acknowledged to be communicable by contagion; we seldom find an instance of a person suffering a second time from its attacks.

Over many the affection passes lightly, but in the majority of cases it proves a distressing, and in some a fatal malady baffling all the ill-directed efforts of the allopathic physician to conduct it to a favourable termination.

Under the old practice, not only was a great deal of valuable

* Vide note, page 21.

time lost in endeavouring *to subdue inflammation* by antiphlogistic measures, but the patient's vital energies were weakened, and rendered less capable of contending with the disease, when it assumes the spasmodic type.

On the contrary, we have it in our power, by the administration of remedies *specific* to the affection, to check the inflammation at its outset, subdue the other distressing attendant symptoms, and shorten the duration of the complaint, without allowing it to leave after it any of those evil consequences, such as debility and emaciation, which oblige the patient to endure a tedious and protracted period of convalescence.

Diagnosis. Paroxysms of violent and convulsive expirations, in rapid succession, interrupted by long whistling inspirations, and in young subjects a loud shrill whoop, terminated by the expectoration of a quantity of mucus, or a fit of vomiting, after which the attack ceases for some time. If the case is severe, the features swell and become livid; blood escapes from the nose, mouth, and even from the ears. A complete cessation of respiration and almost suffocation takes place as if from spasm of the lungs, which lasts for minutes. The attacks return every three or four hours, more frequently in severe cases; the least excitement brings them on; they are more frequent and violent at night. Respiration is free during the intervals, and the patient in every respect healthy, except being weak.

Pathologists generally consider this disease under three stages: the distinction between the second and third is, however, not often very clearly marked.

The first or febrile stage commences with the symptoms of an ordinary catarrh, attended with slight fever, which gradually increases, the breathing becomes more difficult, and is accompanied with irritative cough and pains in the chest.

In the second or convulsive stage* the febrile activity disappears, and the characteristic cough and other symptoms of the disease develop themselves.

In the third or nervous stage there are longer intermissions

* The congestive and nervous of some authors.

between the paroxysms, but increased weakness from the duration of the cough.

Therapeutics. In the incipient, febrile, irritative, or catarrhal stage of the cough, the most appropriate remedies are to be found amongst those we have already pointed out in the treatment of Common Cough, and must be selected according to the indications there given, and administered in the same manner unless otherwise specified. By a careful selection of these remedies it is frequently possible to check the disorder in the first stage. Accordingly, the most suitable medicaments for this purpose are *Dulcamara*, *Pulsatilla*, *Mercurius*, *Belladonna*, *Hepar sulphuris*, *Chamomilla*, *Nux vomica*, *Arnica*, *Ipecacuanha*, *Aconite*, *Bryonia*, *and Phosphorus*.

Administration. See Cough, p. 204.

Dulcamara $\frac{000}{6}$. When the attack has apparently been excited by exposure to wet, (a thorough wetting,) the cough loose, with *copious and easy expectoration*.

Pulsatilla $\frac{000}{6}$. Cough loose, and accompanied with lachrymation, weakness of the eyes, sneezing, thick, discoloured coryza and slight hoarseness, and inclination to vomit after coughing; occasional diarrhœa, especially at night.

Mercurius $\frac{000}{6}$. Hoarseness, watery coryza, with soreness of the nostrils; dry fatiguing cough, generally occurring in two successive fits.

Belladonna $\frac{000}{6}$, is one of the most important remedies in the catarrhal stage of hooping-cough, when there is dry, hollow, or harsh and barking cough occasionally at night, or which becomes materially aggravated at that period. This medicine is also particularly well adapted to the angina or sore throat, which is not unfrequently concomitant at the commencement of the affection.

Hepar sulphuris. Cough worse at night, but looser than that indicating *Belladonna*. This medicine is also useful in forwarding the secretory process.

Administration. Half a grain of the trituration, at the third potency, to half an ounce of water, a dessert-spoonful twice a day.

Chamomilla $\frac{000}{3}$. Dry hoarse cough, or cough with difficult expectoration of tenacious mucus, followed by a feeling of soreness at the part from which the mucus seems to have been detached. The paroxysms of coughing are excited by an almost incessant irritation of the larynx, and in the upper part of the chest.

Nux vomica $\frac{000}{6}$, is of greater service when the cough approaches the second stage. It is indicated by the following symptoms: Dry, fatiguing cough, attended with vomiting, and occurring particularly from about midnight until morning, the paroxysms so protracted and violent as to produce apparent danger of suffocation, with blueness of the face, and occasionally bleeding from the mouth and nose. (Arnica is better adapted to this latter symptom when it occurs with a copious discharge of blood.)

Ipecacuanha $^{0}\frac{0}{6}{}^{0}$ is, like the former, of great value when the cough is attended with danger of suffocation, and each inspiration appears to excite a fresh fit of coughing. It is further indicated when the fits are attended with spasmodic stiffness of the body, and blueness of the face, great anxiety, and accumulation of mucus in the chest.

Aconite $\frac{000}{6}$ may be had recourse to from time to time, when marked febrile or inflammatory symptoms are present, bearing in mind, that its action is of short duration, and may be followed in a few hours by any other of the remedies which appear more particularly indicated.

The last mentioned remedy, *Bryonia* and *Phosphorus*, are chiefly called for when the cough threatens to become associated with inflammatory action in the lungs, &c.

Second or Convulsive Stage.—Therapeutics. *Drosera, Veratrum album, Cuprum aceticum, Arnica, Ferrum metallicum*, and *Conium maculatum*.*

Drosera is one of the principal remedies in the treatment of the disease when it has reached this stage; and in cases

* Acidum hydrocyanicum. In some cases we have had satisfactory results from the use of this acid. It is most indicated when the cough is violent, concussive, attended by rattling of mucus, suffocating respiration and ejection of blood from the mouth and nose.—Ed.

where the constitution has not been enfeebled by the transmission of hereditary weakness or other causes, it will speedily declare its beneficial effects, and materially shorten this trying and painful period of the disorder. The particular indications for the use of this medicine are, violent paroxysms of cough, occurring in such rapid succession as to threaten suffocation, and attended with the characteristic shrill sound during inspiration, and sometimes fever; after each fit of coughing, vomiting of food, or of stringy mucus; relief on moving about.

ADMINISTRATION. $\frac{0\,0\,0\,0}{6}$, in six teaspoonfuls of water, a teaspoonful after each severe paroxysm of coughing.*

VERATRUM ALBUM is indicated when the child has become *reduced* in strength and *emaciated;* or when it suffers from *cold sweats,* particularly on the forehead, with *excessive thirst, involuntary emission of urine, vomiting,* and other symptoms common to this stage; also pain in chest and inguinal region; slow fever.†

ADMINISTRATION. The same as *Drosera.*

CUPRUM ACETICUM. This has been found most useful in the nervous stage, *particularly when convulsions with loss of consciousness ensue after each paroxysm.* Also when we find vomiting after the attacks, and rattling of mucus in the chest, and wheezing at all times. In almost all cases a marked benefit has followed the employment of this remedy; sometimes it has been found sufficient of itself to cut short the disease, and in others, has so far modified it that other remedies which had before seemed to fail, have after its exhibition acted with the most marked effect, and completed the cure.‡

ADMINISTRATION. According to the formula already given in SCARLET FEVER, a dessert-spoonful after each paroxysm.

* Vide note, p. 21.

† *Carbo vegetabilis* is frequently useful in bringing this stage of the affection to an early and successful termination after the previous use of *Veratrum* or *Drosera,* or both of these important remedies; particularly when, notwithstanding the decrease of cough, the tendency to vomit still remains. (See also *Ferrum.*)

‡ *Cina* is also a useful remedy when there are convulsions, or *tetanic rigidity* of the whole body during or immediately after the fits of coughing, particularly in children affected with *worms.*

ARNICA is useful as an intermediate medicine when the *epistaxis* or *hemorrhage* from the mouth is considerable; and also in the affection itself when each paroxysm is succeeded by crying. (*Hepar s.* is also useful when the latter symptom follows a hoarse dry cough.)

ADMINISTRATION. In cases of hemorrhage, a drop of the tincture, at the second potency, and repeated after the next paroxysm if necessary. When indicated by the *nature of the attack*, $\frac{0\,0\,0\,0}{6}$, in six teaspoonfuls of water, one after each paroxysm.

FERRUM METALLICUM. This remedy will be found very useful as an intermediate when there is invariably vomiting of food on coughing soon after a meal.

ADMINISTRATION. A small quantity, say about a quarter of a grain of the *third trituration* in a dessert-spoonful of water once in twenty-four hours.

CONIUM. When the paroxysms occur particularly at *night*, and with great severity.

ADMINISTRATION. A globule of any potency, from the ninth to the thirtieth, in a teaspoonful of water, night and morning.

THIRD OR NERVOUS STAGE.—THERAPEUTICS. The same medicines as have already been given, according to the indications that present themselves. On the suppression of all the more serious symptoms, the remedies which have been recommended in the first stage are also useful in removing any catarrhal cough which may remain behind. Change of air is likewise beneficial.*

DIET. The diet must be light and of easy digestion; bread-pudding, semolino, and other light puddings of this description, provided the fever be not high, in which case, weak gruel, barley-water, and the like, must alone be allowed; when the more serious symptoms have been subdued, or in all mild cases, a little chicken broth, or beef tea, may be given; and so on, gradually increasing the amount of nutriment as the disease declines. The drinks to consist of toast-water or barley-water.

* In neglect or obstinate cases occurring in delicate constitutions, *Sulphuris Tinctura* and *Sepia* have been found useful. See also the remedies for coughs of a bad character under the head of COUGH.

CROUP. *Angina Membranacea.*

Angina perniciosa. Cynanche laryngea. Cynanche tracheitis. s. trachealis, &c., &c.

Diagnosis. Short, difficult, and hoarse respiration, accompanied by a shrill, whistling, squeaking, harsh, rattling, or metallic sound, with cough of the same character; the patient throws the head back; fever, and sometimes comatose state of the brain.

This well known disease is one that requires the promptest treatment to avert the danger. From the moment we are assured of the nature of the complaint, recourse must be had to the remedy most clearly indicated by the assemblage of the symptoms, so that not an instant be lost in arresting its further progress, since, if not skilfully kept in check, it sometimes runs to a fatal termination within twenty-four hours; although in the generality of cases, when such an event does take place, it happens about the fourth or fifth day.

Croup consists of a peculiar inflammation of the lining membrane of the windpipe, causing the secretion of a thick, viscid substance, generally opake, of about the consistency of the boiled white of an egg, which adheres to the interior of the windpipe, and takes the form of the parts it covers; when this, generally denominated the *false membrane*, has been allowed to form, the case becomes extremely critical.

That croup arises from inherent constitutional taint, is evident from the fact of some families having a peculiar tendency to this disorder. It particularly affects early childhood. The principal exciting causes seem to be, exposure to cold or damp, and derangement of the digestive functions, from a too nutritious or heating diet, too much animal food, or stimulants, such as wine or coffee. It seldom attacks adults, though we occasionally see exceptions to this rule, and is not unfrequently found in complication with other affections both of the lungs and windpipe.

The attack generally commences with the symptoms of a

common catarrh, such as cough, sneezing and hoarseness, with a greater or less degree of fever; in a day or two the cough changes its character, and becomes shrill and squeaking, or deep, hoarse, or sonorous, attended with a ringing sound during speaking and respiration, as if the air were passing through a metallic tube; as the disease progresses, the cough becomes more shrill, and when long continued, resembles the crowing of a young cock. There is seldom much expectoration, and when any matter comes up in coughing, it has a stringy appearance, resembling portions of a membrane. After inflammation has set in, considerable fever and restlessness continue, occasionally varying in intensity, but never wholly remitting; the countenance expresses great anxiety, and alternates from a red to a livid hue; the paroxysms are followed by a profuse and clammy perspiration of the whole body, more particularly of the head and face. When danger threatens, the pulse is hard, frequent, and occasionally intermittent; the breathing, particularly during inspiration, difficult and audible; the features become livid, and almost purple from the sense of suffocation; the head is thrown back; the cough assumes a veiled and husky tone; the voice sinks to a whisper; the eye has a dull, glassy, or dilated appearance, and the whole system seems in a state of utter prostration.

THERAPEUTICS. The medicines upon which the greatest reliance is to be placed in the treatment of this affection, are *Aconite, Cham., Bryon., Spongia, Hepar sulphuris,* and *Lachesis.*

ACONITE is called for during the *inflammatory* period of this dangerous disease with great febrile disturbance, burning heat, thirst, short dry cough, and hurried, laborious breathing. It may be exhibited as below specified, until these symptoms begin to abate. $\frac{0\,0\,0}{6}$, in six teaspoonfuls of water, one every half-hour to six hours, according to the violence of the fever. After *Aconite,* recourse must be had to—

SPONGIA, when there is a *hoarse, ringing, hollow,* and *squeaking* cough, with slow wheezing respiration, or *fits of choking,* with inability to breathe but with the head thrown back.

ADMINISTRATION. $^{0}\frac{0}{6}{}^{0}$, in six teaspoonfuls of water, one every half, or every one, two, or three hours, according to the intensity of the symptoms, and the effects produced by each dose.

HEPAR SULPHURIS. Either when the symptoms are partially subdued by *Spongia*, or when from the commencement the cough is *moist* or *loose*, with *accumulation of mucus in the respiratory organs*; or when, after *Aconite*, there remains a dry, deep, hollow cough with weak, *hoarse* voice, and more or less distressing oppression of breathing.*

ADMINISTRATION. One grain of the trituration, third potency, to an ounce of water, a dessert-spoonful every two hours, or oftener if required. It may also be advantageously alternated with *Spongia* at intervals of half an hour to an hour or more according to the severity of the case, and the effects produced; the administrator carefully noticing the effects of each medicine.†

PHOSPHORUS is preferable to *Spongia* when the inflammation threatens to extend to the air-passages and *lungs*, (PNEUMONIC CROUP,) or when the latter are implicated from the commencement, and may also be given in alternation with that medicine, or follow it; and may further, in some instances, be advantageously alternated with *Lachesis*.

LACHESIS $\frac{00}{12}$, in very serious and difficult cases, in which there is short dry cough with hoarseness: *great sensitiveness to the touch*, the *slightest pressure affecting almost to suffocation*; voice very low and hollow, with a sound like that of a person speaking through the nose; fainting; nausea; swooning; loss of sense; *rigidity of frame*; great prostration of strength, especially towards evening.

ADMINISTRATION. Six globules of the sixth in about an ounce of water, a teaspoonful every half-hour, hour, or two hours, according to the intensity of the symptoms, and their abatement.

After having subdued these threatening symptoms by the

* This remedy is of itself sufficient, in many instances, to arrest the progress of the disease, if administered as soon as the *incipient symptoms of the attack* are observed; but *Aconite*, *Hepar sulphuris* and *Spongia*, generally alternately, become necessary when the affection is more developed.

† Vide note, p. 21.

administration of the last-mentioned remedy, we may, if the disease is not wholly vanquished, again fall back upon *Spongia* or *Hepar sulphuris*, according to the indications given for those remedies.

There are other remedies which afford valuable assistance in the treatment of complicated attacks; but in truth it may be said, that in the *majority* of cases, under any circumstances, *Aconitum*, *Hepar sulphuris*, and *Spongia*, administered alternately, *are almost always sufficient to effect a cure* in a few hours.

It may, however, be mentioned, that *Tartarus emeticus* has been found valuable in some apparently hopeless cases arising from paralysis of the lungs; *Arsenicum*, *Sambucus*, and *Moschus*, in complications with Asthma Millari; and *Iodium* either alone in repeated doses, or alternately with *Aconite*, has been much recommended in obstinate cases, particularly when occurring in *plethoric* subjects. *Hepar sulphuris*, *Phosphorus*, and *Lycopodium*, have been recommended as useful against a predisposition to this affection.

[We are rejoiced to find that the subject of Croup has elicited so much attention from the profession during the few past years, and that some expedients have been proposed with a prospect of success in those fearful cases of *true membranous croup*, that have bid defiance, in the practice of every experienced Homœopathist, to the most renowned remedies of the school.

These medicines are AMMONIUM CAUSTICUM* (*Caustic ammonia*), BROMINIUM (*Bromine*,) and KALI BICHROMATUM (*Bichromate of potash*.) They have been urged principally in consequence of the correspondence of their pathogenetic effects with the pathological development of genuine croup, especially in regard to the transuded membrane. The *Vapour of chlorine*, on the testimony of Albers, has produced *true* croup symptoms, even to the formation of the membrane; but to what extent this gas may be made safely available, must be determined by subsequent careful experimentation.

* See note, p. 218.

According to the "Pressburgh physicians," the following are the characteristic expressions of

"CAUSTIC AMMONIA CROUP.

Deep, weak voice; fatiguing, interrupted speech. Increased secretion of mucus in the bronchia. Violent cough, with copious expectoration of mucus, especially after drinking.

Difficult, rattling, laboured breathing; stertorous breathing. Suffocative fits. Spasms of the chest."

"BROMINE CROUP.

Formation of pseudo membrane in the larynx and trachea.

Spasms in the larynx occasioning suffocation.

Cough with croup-sound, hoarse, wheezing, fatiguing, not permitting one to utter a word; accompanied with sneezing; with violent suffocative fits.

Respiration characterized by mucous rattling; wheezing; alternately slow and suffocative, and hurried and superficial; laboured; painful; oppressed; gasping for air.

Heat in the face.

Increased secretion of urine.

Pulse rather hard; slow at first, afterwards accelerated."

BICHROMATE OF POTASH-CROUP.

Dr. W. E. Payne, of Bath, Maine,* was induced to make trial of the Bichromate of Potash in croup, after reading Dr. Drysdale's "Summary of Pathological Appearances," produced by this drug, and contained in the British Journal of Homœopathy.

These appearances were:—"Respiratory apparatus.

"The air passages were constantly lined with a thick ropy muco-purulent fluid, when death was delayed beyond several days. In some instances the trachea was lined with a complete false membrane. The epiglottis, rima glottidis, trachea and bronchia, were, at different times, deeply injected. The lungs were generally healthy, and presented a remarkable contrast to the highly inflamed bronchia."

Also elsewhere in the same summary: "Elastic plugs of mucus in the nostrils."

* See note, p. 218.

Dr. Payne, relying on these croup-like developments, prescribed the Bichromate of Potash in two cases of croup successfully.

The first case presented the following phenomena, (those of an analogous case of croup that proved *fatal* under the usual remedies,) with this exception, "that the difficulty of breathing increased rather more rapidly, and the cough was rather more frequent."

"*Case* 1. Boy of two years; had enjoyed good health up to the time of this attack. A slight difficulty of breathing, when the mouth was closed, owing to one nostril being obstructed with a plug of mucus, was observable. Pulse irregular and intermittent. There was a slight elevation of the temperature of the skin. Otherwise the child appeared well. He was lively and playful. This state continued for three or four days without any perceptible change, except the appearance of a few small sores below the nostrils, which were somewhat moist. On the evening of the third or fourth day there was, evidently, a change or increase of the disease. The respiration, though not hard, could be heard distinctly in any part of the room when the child made a deep inspiration. This did not seem to proceed, as before, from the obstructed nostril, though this remained the same, but from some difficulty about the larynx. The child would frequently carry his hand to his throat and put his fingers into his mouth. On the following day the difficulty of breathing had evidently increased. On applying the ear to the neck, a whistling sound was apparent, like that which may be produced by the passage of air through a metallic tube. Voice hoarse. Cough not frequent, but hoarse, dry and barking or crowing. The child was restless, sleepless, and refused to drink, apparently because deglutition was painful. The tonsils and upper part of the larynx were red and swollen, and about the fauces was a small quantity of tenacious mucus. After the first day of invasion the child could swallow his drinks without difficulty, and was thirsty. As the disease progressed, the difficulty of breathing gradually increased, causing a strong action of the abdominal muscles, the muscles of the neck and shoulder-blades. The head was inclined backwards. The shrill whistling respiratory sound increased, together with a tearing sound like that produced by a saw running though a dry board. The cough was mostly dry, but occasionally sounded loose and rattling. It, however, grew less and less distinct, until towards the close of the disease it amounted to little more than a grunt. The child would be carried to and fro continually—not one moment would he allow his parents to sit with him. The breath became very offensive, and this offensiveness increased to an intolerant degree as the disease advanced. The plug of mucus remained in the nostril, but the herpetic sores gradually died away. The temperature of the skin was rather below than above the natural standard. During the last day or two of the disease the child was inclined to stupor. Though these symptoms gradually increased, yet there were occasional remissions;—the breathing became less difficult, and the whole general appearance of the child was much better; but this apparent giving way of the disease lasted only for a short time. The breathing could be heard often in the street."

Administration. *One* drop of the *sixth* dilution was mixed with half a tumblerful of rain water, and a tablespoonful of the liquid was given every *five* hours.

In this instance the Bichromate was not administered until eighteen hours after the commencement of the attack. During the use of this remedy, cold, wet linen was applied externally to the throat. After the difficult respiration became natural, *hoarseness* and a *barking cough* remained, which were subdued in three or four days by morning and evening doses of *Hepar sulphuris*.

Case 2. The second case, similar to the one detailed, was treated early in the course of the disease, without a consensual application of cold, wet linen to the throat, and recovered under the use of the Bichromate of Potash.

IODINE.

Dr. Koch, of Germany, commends *Iodine* as a most efficient agent against croup. As *Aconite* was employed alternately with this remedy in his thirteen successful cases, its specific power in his instances has been questioned. Dr. Tietze, who followed the experience of Dr. Koch, offers testimony in favour of *Iodine* in croup, and asserts that "it is only suitable in the treatment of croup as long as there is inflammation and exudation. When this latter process has stopped, *Iodine* probably ceases to have any good effect. *Hepar sulphuris* then appears to be in its place." *Iodine*, according to its pathogenesis, applies rather to a catarrhal than a membranous croup, but may hold a *preventive* place to *true* croup, as *Aconite*, *Spongia*, and *Hepar* have undoubtedly done in many instances, although Professor Ware deems the conversion of one form of croup into another impossible. Dr. Tietze states with apparent justice: "Although the symptoms which I have here described may not constitute real croup, yet everybody knows that they occurred under circumstances where croup must have been the inevitable consequence of this first attack, unless met in the outset by proper treatment."

Future observations of intelligent physicians will probably define these points, and especially the true position of *Iodine*. We add the following summary of the effects of IODINE by the "Pressburgh physicians."

"* The larynx is painful. (Vogel.)

* Pain in the larynx and expectoration of indurated mucus. (Hartlaub.)

* Pressure in the region of the larynx, as far as the fauces, as if those parts were swollen. (Jörg.)

* Aching and pricking pain in the region of the larynx and the sublingual glands, several attacks on one day. (Jörg.)

* Pressure in the throat inducing frequent hawking up of a quantity of tenacious mucus. (Hartlaub.)

* Contraction and heat in the throat. (Hartl.)

* Sore feeling in the throat and chest, while in bed, with wheezing in the throat and drawing pains in the lungs, which is felt regularly with the beats of the heart. (Hartl.)

* Inflammation of the trachea.

Roughness of the trachea the whole day.

Hoarseness. (Comdet.)

Hoarseness early in the morning.

* The asterisk indicates that these symptoms have been removed as well as produced by this drug.

Hoarseness for more than two weeks. (Hartl.)

The voice becomes deeper, and finally quite deep. (S. H.)

Sensation as if something were lodged in the larynx which he can bring up by hawking, the whole day and evening.

Intolerable titillation in the larynx, which can only be arrested by hawking and coughing, with accumulation of water in the mouth, early in the morning when in bed. (Gff.)

Expectoration of tenacious mucus, with pressure in the throat, as if something were lodged in it which he imagines he can swallow, early in the morning. (Hlb.)

Violent titillation in the throat, inducing a desire to cough. (S.)

Dry cough. (Matthey.)

Violent oppression of breathing. (Gölis.)

Asthma with pain during a deep inspiration; stronger, quicker beating of the heart, and smaller, more frequent pulse. (Jörg.)

* Asthma and arrest of breathing in the throat for a fortnight. (Hlb.)

Loss of breath. (Gärdner.)

Want of breath. (Neumann.)

Suffocative catarrh. (Orfila.)"

To the layman we cannot too strongly urge the necessity of promptly sending for a physician on the *first* threatenings of this frightful malady.

The physician will give close attention to the laryngeal wheezing or whizzing, and make a careful examination of the throat. The peculiar crowing tone of the larynx, and specks of coagulable lymph on the tonsils and in the throat, are sure indications of impending danger from TRUE CROUP.]—ED.

NOTE—1. Characteristics and Physiography of croup and its varieties. Arranged by a member of Homœopathic physicians in Pressburgh. Translated by Ch. J. Hempel, M.D. (*Hom. Exam.*, new series, vol. I., p. 438.) 2.—Bichromate of Potash in Membraneous Croup. By W. E. Payne, M.D., Bath, (Me.) (*Same Ex.*, vol. I., p. 343.) 3.—On croup. By John Peters, M. D., (*Same Exam.*, p. 187.) 4.—On the use of Iodine in croup, (*Same Ex.*, p. 75.) *These interesting papers, which have furnished the staple of our remarks on croup, deserve the careful perusal of physicians.*—ED.

INFLUENZA.

DIAGNOSIS. Catarrh appearing in an epidemic form, attended, in addition to the symptoms described at the commencement of the article, on COMMON COLD, with *extreme oppression and prostration of strength;* sleepiness, followed by shuddering and general chilliness; rheumatic pains in the head, back, and limbs; and slight redness of the eyes, painful pressure, and sensibility to light.

THERAPEUTICS. The principal medicine in the treatment of this affection is ARSENICUM, and in most cases, if not administered too late, it will be found specific.

The following are the characteristic indications for its employment: heaviness and rheumatic pain in the head; *profuse watery and corrosive discharge from the nose*, causing a disagreeable burning sensation in the nostrils; violent sneezing; shiverings and shuddering, with severe pains in the limbs; *oppression of the chest;* difficulty of breathing; thirst; anxiety; restlessness; GREAT PROSTRATION OF STRENGTH, with aggravation of suffering at night, or after a meal; inflammation of the eyes, with sensibility to light. These symptoms may be attended with deep *dry*, fatiguing cough, exacerbated in the evening, at night, or after drinking, or sensations of dryness and burning, with mucus in the throat, which is difficult to detach.

ADMINISTRATION. $\frac{0\,0}{6}$, in a little water, repeated every six to twenty-four hours, according to the greater or less severity of the attack, until improvement sets in.*

If this remedy be not sufficient to remove the disorder, we may have recourse to the following medicines: *Aconitum, Nux vomica, Causticum, Mercurius, Phosphorus, Belladonna, Pulsatilla, Camphor.*

ACONITUM. When the disorder assumes an inflammatory character, with quickness of pulse, dry hot skin, and short, harsh, shaking cough.

* Vide note, page 21.

Administration. $\frac{0\,0}{6}$, in a teaspoonful of water, repeated in from six to twelve hours as required.

Nux vomica. Obstruction of the nose, hoarse hollow cough, excited by tickling in the throat, and attended with severe headache, confusion in the head, giddiness, want of appetite, or sickness, thirst, aching pain in the lower part of the back, constipation, pain in the chest as if from excoriation.

Administration. $\frac{0\,0}{6}$, in a dessert-spoonful of water, repeated for two or three evenings successively.

Causticum will generally be found of great value, where Nux vomica has not produced the desired benefit, especially where the patient is of a lymphatic temperament. It is, however, more particularly indicated when there are aching pains in all the limbs increased by movement; facial pains; violent, dry cough, worse at night, with *pain in the chest* as from *excoriation;* constipation, disinclination for food; vomiting.

Administration. Same as *Nux v.*

Mercurius. *Dry* or *fluent coryza; pains in the* head, *face*, and *teeth;* sore throat; violent shaking cough, excited by irritation in the throat and chest; shivering or heat with profuse perspiration; aching in the bones and slimy bilious diarrhœa, attended with tenesmus.

Administration. $\frac{0\,0\,0\,0}{6}$, dissolved in four dessert-spoonfuls of water, one to be taken night and morning.

Phosphorus is frequently exceedingly useful after *Mercurius;* it is particularly indicated when there is excessive irritation in the larynx and bronchia, with alteration of the voice, and pain during articulation.

Administration. $\frac{0\,0\,0\,0}{6}$, the same as *Merc.*, but when the pulmonary symptoms give evidence of a greater degree of irritation, a few globules of the third potency may be dissolved in six dessert-spoonfuls of water, one to be taken every four hours.

Belladonna. Dry, spasmodic cough, aggravated towards night; sore throat, excessive headache, increased by talking, moving, or bright light; fixed look; confusion of ideas on closing the eyes.

Administration. $\frac{0\,0}{6}$, in a teaspoonful of water, to be repeated in twenty-four hours, if necessary.*

* Vide note, p. 21.

PULSATILLA. Loose cough day and night, exacerbated by lying down, thick offensive coryza, tendency to relaxation in the bowels, loss of appetite, foul tongue, disagreeable or insipid taste in the mouth.

ADMINISTRATION. $\frac{0}{6}{}^{0}$, in a dessert-spoonful of water, for three or four successive mornings, fasting.*

CAMPHORA. One or two drops of weak spirits of *Camphor* when taken at the commencement of the attack, and repeated until the chilliness or shivering begins to subside, will frequently check the further progress of the disease.

In a more advanced stage of the affection, with (laborious) asthmatic breathing, accumulation of mucus in the bronchi, and cold, dry skin, *Camphora* is further of considerable service.

Finally:—*Arnica* may be administered with advantage in some cases, particularly when pricking pains are experienced in the chest during inspiration (pseudo-pleurisy) with aching pains over the whole body, headache, and *hemorrhage from the nose; Ipecacuanha* after *Arsenicum* or any of the other remedies when there is *vomiting* or violent retching during or after each fit of coughing.

SENEGA. Tickling irritation and continual burning in the larynx or throat, with loud mucous râle, and fear of suffocation on lying down: *Stannum* in neglected or protracted cases with easy but excessive expectoration of mucus, and great weakness:—*Cinchona* may advantageously follow the last remedy when the expectoration has been diminished.

DETERMINATION OF BLOOD TO THE CHEST.

Congestio ad Pectus.

DIAGNOSIS. Sensation of great fulness, throbbing, weight, or pressure in the chest; and palpitation of the heart, attended with anxiety, short sighing respiration, and dyspnœa.

We find that the predisposition to affections of the chest and lungs is greater during the period preceding puberty, and for some years after, than at any other epoch of man's existence.

* Vide note, p. 21.

As remarked in the Diseases of Children in Infancy and during very early childhood, from the disproportion between the cerebral system and the other portions of the economy, the diseases which the physician has chiefly to combat are those arising from over-excitements of the nervous organization. In maturer years the tendency to abdominal congestion generally develops itself. This is easily explained by entering into the physiology of these different periods of human life; but as my object is rather the treatment of disease than the elucidation of these interesting points, I shall here content myself with briefly alluding to them.

There is no doubt, as already remarked, that a particular period of human life is peculiarly liable to chest affections, and, among others, to this disorder, but too frequently the precursor of other more serious maladies. Some constitutions, however, particularly those in which a hereditary phthisical taint exists, exhibit a marked predisposition to pectoral congestion. Amongst the most frequent causes of this predisposition being called into dangerous activity are, exposure to extremes of heat or cold; stimulants, such as alcoholic vinous, or fermented beverages, or coffee; the abuse of narcotic drugs; violent exercise, such as running, dancing, &c., or over-exertion even of the voice either in speaking or singing; sudden check of perspiration; cold or damp feet; sedentary habits; metastases; repercussed cutaneous eruption; or suppression of customary discharges, such as the catamenial and hemorrhoidal flux.

THERAPEUTICS. *Aconitum, Nux vomica, Ipecacuanha, Belladonna, Aurum foliatum, Mercurius, Pulsatilla, Spongia, Cinchona, Sulphur,* are the best remedies in general cases.

ACONITUM is especially indicated when there is *violent oppression* with *great heat* and *thirst*, palpitation of the heart, great anxiety, and shaking cough. It will be found particularly valuable for plethoric females of sedentary habits, who suffer considerably from congestion before and during the catamenia. In such cases it may be advantageously followed by *Mercurius*, to prevent a relapse. (In others by *Belladonna.*)

ADMINISTRATION. $\frac{000}{6}$, repeated in twenty-four hours if necessary, and the same symptoms continue. When the congestion runs high, it must be administered as in INFLAMMATORY FEVER, which see.

NUX VOMICA. When the affection has been developed by sedentary habits or by *habitual indulgence in the stimulants* already alluded to, or from *hemorrhoidal metastasis or suppression*, in such cases this remedy itself frequently effects a cure.

ADMINISTRATION. $\frac{6}{6}$, in the same number of dessert-spoonfuls of water, one each evening, at bedtime; adding thereto four or five drops of spirits of wine, to prevent its decomposition, and keeping the mixture protected from the air.

IPECACUANHA will frequently complete the cure, when Nux Vomica has not removed the whole of the symptoms.

ADMINISTRATION. $\frac{000}{3}$, in a little water, repeated every twenty-four hours until improvement results.

BELLADONNA. Oppression and throbbing at the chest, with shortness of breath and strong palpitation of the heart, extending into the head; short cough, chiefly at night; internal heat, and considerable thirst.

ADMINISTRATION. $\frac{00}{6}$, in a teaspoonful of water, daily until perceptible melioration arises, or an alteration of symptoms takes place which may call for another remedy.

AURUM. Extreme oppression of the chest, as if suffocation impended, sometimes with loss of consciousness and livid hue of countenance; palpitation of the heart; and excessive anguish.

DOSE. Half a grain of the third trituration, or a few globules of the sixth in half an ounce of water, a teaspoonful every four, six or twelve hours, according to circumstances.

MERCURIUS, as already remarked, is valuable after *Aconitum* on certain occasions, (see that remedy;) and also when there is burning heat and oppression at the chest, and frequent desire to take a deep inspiration; or, cough with expectoration streaked with blood, and palpitation of the heart.

ADMINISTRATION. $\frac{000}{6}$, in a teaspoonful of water, repeated in twelve hours, after which we may lengthen the interval, and only repeat again should a cessation of improvement take place; in many instances it may be exhibited in the same manner as *Nux vomica.*

Pulsatilla. Ebullition of blood in the chest with external heat; constriction in the chest with impeded respiration; palpitation of the heart; anxiety and aggravation of the symptoms towards evening, also when pectoral congestion has arisen in *phlegmatic* subjects from *hemorrhoidal suppression*, or in females from *stoppage of the menstrual flux.*

Administration. $\frac{00}{12}$, in a teaspoonful of water, repeated in twenty-four hours, if necessary, but in the majority of cases it may be administered in the same manner as given under *Nux vomica,* with a difference in time, taking a dose half an hour before breakfast.

Spongia tosta. When the symptoms are provoked by the slightest exertion or even movement, and are attended with anguish, sensation of threatened suffocation, nausea, prostration and fainting.

Administration. Same as *Aurum.*

Bryonia. Burning heat in the chest with a sensation of tightness, dyspnœa, and anxiety; palpitation of the heart; occasional prickings in the chest during inspiration.

Administration same as *Pulsatilla.*

Cinchona. When we can trace the affection to debilitating losses, with palpitation of the heart and oppressed breathing.

Administration. The same as *Pulsatilla.*

Sulphur. Ebullition of blood, weight, fulness, and pressure in the chest, aggravated by coughing, palpitation of the heart, dyspnœa, chiefly on lying down at night; it is also most serviceable in *suppressed hemorrhoids*, after *Nux vomica* or *Pulsatilla,* and after the latter remedy in checked catamenia.

Administration. $\frac{00}{6}$, repeated every five days until a marked alteration for the better take place, or the symptoms assume another form, calling for the employment of some other more appropriate remedy.

Phosphorus. In some obstinate cases this remedy is frequently successful in affording speedy relief, particularly when in addition to the more usual symptoms, shooting or pricking pains are frequently experienced on laughing, speaking, or walking quickly; palpitation of the heart, anxiety, sensation of heat extending from the chest into the throat.

ADMINISTRATION. A few globules of the third, night and morning, discontinuing as soon as decided relief is obtained.

Some one or more of the preceding remedies, if judiciously selected, and timely administered, will generally check the disease, and prevent it assuming a more dangerous form; for example, running into hemoptysis, phthisis, pneumonia, carditis, &c. The following, among others, have also been found useful in peculiar cases: *Rhus toxicodendron, Sepia, Natrum muriaticum, Phosphorus, Carbo vegetabilis, Acidum nitricum, Ammoniacum carbonicum,* and *Ferrum metallicum.*

INFLAMMATION OF THE MUCOUS MEMBRANE OF THE BRONCHIAL TUBES. COLD ON THE CHEST.

Bronchitis. Pulmonary catarrh.

This disease consists of a greater or less degree of inflammation of the mucous membrane of the bronchi, and is divided into acute and chronic. Of the former it is intended more particularly to treat. The disorder is of frequent occurrence, both as an idiopathic affection, and as a concomitant of measles, scarlatina, smallpox, hooping-cough, &c.

DIAGNOSIS OF ACUTE BRONCHITIS. Chilliness, succeeded by fever; hoarseness; difficulty of respiration; severe, frequent, and distressing cough, at first dry or with scanty expectoration of frothy or viscid mucus, which subsequently becomes copious and sometimes streaked with blood; constriction at the chest with a feeling of oppression; general weakness, foul tongue, and loss of appetite; rapid pulse, increase of the difficulty of respiration, which sometimes approaches to a feeling of suffocation; paleness of the lips, cadaverous and anxious countenance, loud wheezing, and on applying the ear to the chest, a louder sound than the natural respiration, either rattling, whistling, or droning, or harsh and broken, according to the advance of the disease.*

In the cases which terminate favourably, the first symptom of improvement which sets in is a greater freedom of breathing, with remission of the fever, and an alteration in the expectoration, which becomes thicker, whiter, and diminished in quantity. But when the disease takes an unfavourable turn, the difficulty of breathing increases, a state of excessive debility and collapse supervenes; the face becomes livid, the body covered with a cold and clammy sweat; the mucus accumulates rapidly in the bronchial tubes, and the cough, which has become feeble through the exhausted and sinking energies of the patient, is insufficient for its ejection; aeration of the blood in the cells of the lungs is prevented; cerebral symptoms declare themselves from impeded circulation, or the effect of unarterialized blood circulating in the brain, and the patient is carried off in a state of asphyxia.

In many, and the most dangerous cases of acute bronchitis, although a degree of oppression at the chest be present, no particular pain, heat of skin, nor fever, may exist: this is the most insidious form of the disease, in which it is but too frequently neglected until beyond the power of the physician's art; this occurs most frequently in children who may apparently be only troubled with a *slight wheezing*, of which scarcely any notice is taken or any medical aid called in, until suddenly suffocation threatens, or some organic lesion is produced, so that an affection which probably might have been easily subdued at the onset, is now beyond control.

The frequency of the disease in infancy and early life deserves a particular notice. It generally commences, as in adults, with the symptoms of a common catarrh; the breathing becomes quick and oppressed, and from the increased action of the diaphragm, the abdomen becomes prominent; both the shoulders and nostrils are in continual motion, but the

* Sibilant and sonorous rhonchi, in the early stage, and mucous or bubbling rhonchus when the secretion becomes increased, indicate both the nature and extent of the disease.

wheezing is often more marked than the difficulty of respiration, and on applying the ear to the chest, a mucous rattle is heard over almost every part; expectoration sometimes temporarily relieves, and occasionally the mucus is expelled from the air-passages by vomiting; the countenance is pale and anxious, and somewhat livid:—these symptoms are interrupted and relieved by occasional remissions, during which the child generally appears drowsy; but they return with additional severity, and, if not checked, an accession of extreme dyspnœa ensues, and death takes place from suffocation. When sore throat is also present, coughing produces considerable pain, and the child for that reason frequently endeavours to suppress it. There is also impaired appetite with thirst, although when the disease has advanced, it is found difficult to take a long draught, from its impeding respiration: this is very observable with children at the breast, who, after eagerly seizing the nipple, will bite it, and discontinue sucking, cry, and throw back the head, and after vomiting up the phlegm, continue for some time in that position.

In some cases, from the character of the voice and cough, bronchitis has been mistaken for croup.

The tubes of one lobe, or of one lung only, may be affected, but sometimes those of both lungs participate.

The exacerbation of suffering at night is a very remarkable symptom of this complaint.

The causes are the same as those of common catarrh.

Therapeutics. The remedies about to be pointed out as most appropriate in ordinary cases of this affection are: *Aconitum, Spongia, Belladonna, Nux vomica, Bryonia alba, Lachesis, Phosphorus, Pulsatilla, Mercurius, Cannabis, &c.*

Aconitum is the remedy upon which we must place our chief reliance in the inflammatory stage of the disease, and throughout its course, as long as a febrile character exists. Its more marked indications are *hot, dry skin, with strong, hard, and accelerated pulse;* hoarseness, with roughness of the voice; short, dry, and frequent cough, excited by tickling in the throat and chest; *obstructed respiration,* sibilant or sonorous rhonchus, anxiety, restlessness, headache, and thirst, with occasionally scanty expectoration of viscid mucus.

ADMINISTRATION. A few globules of the third potency, added to an ounce of water; a dessert-spoonful every three hours, until relief be obtained, after which we may either lengthen the intervals, or select some other remedy more appropriate to the symptoms present. It will also be found occasionally necessary to return to this remedy, as above remarked, during the course of the disease, particularly during the nocturnal febrile exacerbations.

SPONGIA is often of the greatest service after the previous administration of *Aconite*, when there still remains a considerable degree of inflammation in the bronchial tubes, especially the larger, with *sibilant or sonorous rhonchus;* and also at a more advanced stage of the disease, when the *mucous rhonchus* is distinctly audible; with hollow, dry cough day and night, but worse towards evening; or cough with scanty, viscid, ropy expectoration; heat in the chest, burning, tickling irritation in the larynx, quick, anxious, laborious respiration; hoarseness. (*Hepar s.* is sometimes useful after *Spongia* when the mucous rhonchus is predominant, the skin hot and dry, and the efforts to expectorate ineffectual.)

BELLADONNA. This remedy is useful when there is severe cephalalgia, materially aggravated by coughing: *oppression of the chest*, and constriction as if bound, with rattling of mucus in the bronchi; short, anxious, and rapid respiration; dry, fatiguing cough, especially at *night*, and thirst. Soreness of the throat, (see SORE THROAT.) *Sulphur* after *Belladonna.*

ADMINISTRATION. The same as *Aconite*, only at intervals of four, six, or twelve, instead of three hours.*

NUX VOMICA. Dyspnœa, with excessive *tightness of the chest*, particularly at night; hoarseness; dry cough, worse towards morning, attended with a sensation as from a blow, a bruise, in the epigastric or hypochondriac regions; cough with difficult and scanty expectoration of viscid mucus; dryness of the mouth and lips, thirst, constipation, peevishness.

ADMINISTRATION. The same as *Belladonna.*

* Vide note, p. 21.

Lachesis. *Oppression* at the chest, with short and hurried respiration, anxiety, and dejection; mucous *râle;* dry, fatiguing cough, sometimes followed by the expectoration of a little tenacious or *frothy mucus,* after much effort, occasionally streaked with blood; hoarseness.

Administration. Same as *Belladonna.*

Bryonia. Difficult and anxious respiration, with constant inclination to make a deep inspiration; hoarseness; headache; cough dry, attended with a sensation of burning, or cough with expectoration of viscid sputa; in some instances tinged with blood; *dryness of the mouth and lips,* excessive thirst. When, moreover, the respiration is impeded by shootings in the chest, and this infection threatens to become complicated with pleurisy, this remedy is still more particularly called for.

Administration. The same as *Aconite.*

Phosphorus. This important remedy is frequently of great utility in this affection when the more inflammatory symptoms have been subdued by *Aconite,* but the respiration continues much oppressed, accompanied with great anxiety, and heat in the chest; dry cough, excited by tickling in the throat or chest, aggravated by talking or laughing, and followed by expectoration of stringy mucus of a saltish taste: Further, when the disease has been neglected, or when, from the phenomena which present themselves at the commencement, we have reason to dread complication, or an extension of the inflammation to the substance of the lungs, which we generally recognise by crepitation and rusty sputa,—there will be additional reason for administering *Phosphorus.* (See Pneumonia.)

Pulsatilla. Respiration short, accelerated, and impeded, attended with rattling of mucus, heat in the chest, and anxiety; hoarseness; shaking cough, worse towards evening, at night, or in the morning, accompanied with considerable expectoration of tenacious, or thick, yellowish mucus, sometimes mixed with blood; *coryza* with copious discharge of *thick,* discoloured mucus.

Administration. Same as *Belladonna.*

SEPIA may be selected in preference to *Pulsatilla*, when the expectoration is *very copious*, though somewhat difficult, and of a *salt taste;* exacerbation of cough in the morning and towards evening,—followed by *Stann.*, if still profuse, but more easy, *greenish*, and less saline, or of a *sweetish* taste.

LYCOPODIUM. When the cough is materially worse at night, and attended with thirst, quickness of pulse, but moist skin or tendency to sweat; expectoration yellowish gray, and of a saltish taste; oppression at the chest.

MERCURIUS. This remedy may occasionally be found useful when the symptoms of bronchitis are found accompanied by excessive perspiration; when the cough is fatiguing, worse in the evening and at night, and excited by a tickling irritation, or sensation of dryness in the chest, with quick, short, oppressed breathing, and louder respiration than ordinary; hoarseness; *coryza* with watery, acrid discharge; swelling of nose. *Dulcamara* is occasionally serviceable after *Mercurius*, when there is a continuance of night sweats of an offensive odour.

ADMINISTRATION. $\frac{0}{6}$ in an ounce of water; a dessert-spoonful every four or six hours, until relief ensues.

CHAMOMILLA may also be mentioned as a useful remedy in cases of children, after the previous exhibition of *Aconite*, when a slight degree of whistling or sonorous rhonchus still remains; dry cough worse at night, occurring even during sleep. For further indications, see this remedy under the head of COUGH.

IPECACUANHA. Also very valuable in the case of children, but generally at a more advanced stage of the disorder, with mucous rhonchus in the chest, and when on coughing they are almost suffocated by the excessive secretion of mucus, and become livid in the face; shortness of breath, and perspiration on the forehead after each fit of coughing.—ADMINISTRATION. One globule every two hours until improvement results.

There are some other remedies which have been found of great value in the treatment of this affection, namely, *Tartarus emeticus*, *Arsenicum*, *Sulphur*, &c.

Tartarus emeticus is chiefly found useful in those extreme cases where the smaller tubes are clogged with mucus, and suffocation threatens; when the cough suddenly ceases, either from weakness or other causes.

Administration. A grain of the trituration at the second or third potency in four dessert-spoonfuls of water, one every quarter, every half, or every hour, according to the severity of the symptoms or the effects produced.

Arsenicum is occasionally of the utmost service in those unfavourable cases in which the pulse becomes very quick, feeble and intermitting, and the patient is reduced to a state of extreme debility and collapse.

Administration, $\frac{000}{30}$, in four teaspoonfuls of water, one to be given from time to time, as required.*

Sulphur is used in winding up a cure, and preventing the disease running on to the chronic form, or when the expectoration has increased in quantity and become whitish and less viscid. (Administration : see *Arsenicum.*)

For the benefit of the medical reader, I may add, that *Hepar sulphuris*, *Ammonium carbonicum*, *Cannabis*, *Bromium*, etc., may also be found useful in some particular cases. *Opium*, *Belladonna*, *Tart. em.*, and *Lachesis*, may be found serviceable against the symptoms of stupor which are so liable to set in in severe attacks of this disorder.

Diet. In the severe forms of bronchitis the diet to be observed should be the same as that mentioned under fever; but when the febrile and inflammatory symptoms have been *completely removed*, the patient should gradually return to a more nutritious diet, even though a considerable degree of cough and expectoration remain.

In the slighter forms of the complaint, spare diet, confinement to the house, in short, the simple measures laid down for the treatment of common colds in another part of this work, will frequently check or at all events materially shorten the attack. See also article Cough, in which further indications will be found for the selection of the remedies required in both varieties of bronchitis.

* Vide note, p. 21.

Chronic Bronchitis: *Bronchitis Chronica.* This complaint may be the result of the acute affection, or it may arise as a gradual and insidious inflammation of the mucus membrane of the bronchial tubes, or proceed from the inhalation of dust or other minute particles carried into the lungs; it may also be coeval with diseases of the heart, or declare itself after eruptive fevers. It differs from acute bronchitis chiefly in the greater mildness and longer duration of its symptoms, the continuance of which varies from several weeks or months to many years. It affects elderly persons more frequently than the young, but is of course liable to occur at all ages as the result of an acute attack, (although such a circumstance is comparatively of rare occurrence under proper homœopathic treatment,) the consecutive of measles, etc. A comparative exemption from cough, is frequently experienced during summer; but in winter, or in inclement springs, the patient is tormented with harassing cough, and copious viscid expectoration, especially in the morning, which in the severe forms of the disorder is peculiarly distressing. The expectorated matter in the chronic affection is of a different nature from that in the acute, being of a thicker consistence, and of a greenish or yellowish white colour; it is not unfrequently muco-purulent, and sometimes decidedly purulent, and occasionally streaked with blood, particularly in obstinate, inveterate cases. There is generally more or less dyspnœa, with acceleration of pulse after slight corporeal exertion; but in other respects the health may be good and continue so. In the more trying forms of the disorder, an aggravated state of all the symptoms enumerated is met with; moreover, where the sputa is of a purulent nature, hectic fever, extreme emaciation, nocturnal sweats, and occasional attacks of diarrhœa are frequent adjuncts; these latter are sometimes liable to cause the disease to be mistaken for tubercular consumption; but in the majority of cases, auscultation, percussion, together with a careful attention to the symptoms and the history of the case, enable us to form an accurate diagnosis between them.

In chronic bronchitis, the resonance of the chest is, on percussion, little if at all diminished. On applying the ear or stethoscope to the chest, the respiratory murmur is found to vary much in intensity, but is never permanently absent in any part of the chest, and is frequently *even puerile*. The mucous rhonchus in most of its varieties is heard in various parts of the chest at different times, and occasionally the whistling and sonorous rattles are discernible. When the dilatation of the bronchial tubes is considerable, as is not unfrequently the case in this affection, a loud bronchophony is heard which is with difficulty if at all to be distinguished from pectoriloquy, and a râle closely resembling a cavernous rattle is apparent in the vicinity of the dilated tube. The sound on percussion will, however, generally enable us to form the required distinction, the dulness of tone being not so great over a dilated tube, as it is in the vicinity of a vomica; the situation of the cavity of the two cases is, moreover, usually different: dilated bronchi being, as is well known, most frequently detected in the scapular, mammary, and lateral regions, and vomicæ in the subclavian and axillary regions. However, as before said, we must combine the history of the attack, the constitution of the patient, and the progress of emaciation, &c., with the symptoms to be heard by the ear after repeated examinations, in all doubtful cases, ere we come to a definite conclusion as to the exact nature of the case, where that is of material consequence; but as regards the prognosis, chronic bronchitis, with *purulent expectoration, dilated tubes* and *hectic fever*, has been truly considered to be nearly as formidable and serious a malady as phthisis itself, and hence ultimate recovery almost as doubtful.

As this is a disease which requires a long and judicious treatment for its removal, I shall content myself with a brief enumeration of the remedies hitherto found most useful in cases of this nature.

These are *Sulphur, Calcarea carbonica, Carbo vegetabilis, Pulsatilla, Hepar sulphuris, Phosphorus, Stannum, Sepia, Lycopodium, Natrum carbonicum, Natrum muriaticum, Baryta c., Lachesis, Causticum, Arsenicum, Silicea, Staphysagria, Kali carbonicum, Acidum nitricum*, and *Conium maculatum.*

See, however, the article COUGH, where indications for the selection of most of the above remedies will be met with.

INFLAMMATION OF THE LUNGS.

Pneumonia, Peripneumonia, Pneumonitis.

This disorder consists in an inflammation of the parenchyma of the lungs.

DIAGNOSIS. Shiverings and chills, followed by heat or fever; dyspnœa; respiration short and hurried; cough, short, dry, continuous, and distressing at the commencement, afterwards attended with scanty expectoration of viscid, lumpy, and extremely tenacious mucus, generally intermixed with brick-dust sputa, (giving it a rusty colour,)* but occasionally of a bright red; cough at every deep inspiration, or on every attempt to speak; interrupted speech, or a pause after every articulation; abdominal respiration, sometimes a dull pain in the chest, but more frequently rather a tightness than pain; pulse variable, generally full and strong and quick; but when the inflammation has run high,—hard, wiry, and greatly accelerated; tongue parched and dark coloured. The patient generally, in severe cases, lies upon his back.

In the first stage of many cases, when not marked by complication with bronchitis, on application of the stethoscope or the ear to the chest, the *crepitous râle* may be heard; but the sound on percussion only slightly impaired. As the inflammation gains ground, and the substance of the lung becomes altered in structure,† *bronchial* or *tubular* respiration is perceptible, with louder respiratory murmur than natural, in the sound parts of the lung, particularly in severe attacks; also bronchophony may be present; and the tone elicited by

* This rusty or sanguinolent hue being intimately combined, not in streaks: It apppears usually about the second or third day, and is a characteristic indication of the presence of the disease in question; at the same time, it must be borne in mind, that its absence is by no means a certain criterion of the non-existence of inflammation of the lungs.

† Second stage, or that of *hepatization.*

percussion more or less dull according to the seat of the structural derangement, but rarely so complete or extensive as in pleuritis with copious liquid effusion.

In the latter stages of the complaint, the face frequently becomes patched with red, and sometimes livid; and the prostration of strength is excessive.*

I have remarked that the pulse was variable, inasmuch as it has been frequently the fashion to lay too much stress upon that symptom; but the disease may run on to a fatal termination without it being beyond the natural standard. Neither is a hot dry skin a sure criterion, inasmuch as in the congestive form of this disease from the determination of the blood to the lungs, the surface of the body is almost invariably cold. Such are the general symptoms of pure Pneumonia, but in severe cases it is often found combined with pleurisy, when the pains of the chest are intense, and mostly of an acute shooting character. Bronchitis is another and still more frequent complication.

Therapeutics. *Aconite, Bryonia alba, Phosphorus, Tartarus emeticus. Rhus toxicodendron, Belladonna.*

Aconite $\frac{000}{3}$. In the stage of simple inflammatory congestion with severe inflammatory fever, whether or not accompanied or followed by severe shooting pains in the chest, this remedy is unquestionably of great service.

Administration. The same as in Inflammatory Fever.

Bryonia is generally the best remedy to follow *Aconite*, when the more severe febrile symptoms have been lowered by that medicine; or from the commencement, when the following indications present themselves: cough, attended with expectoration of viscid or tenacious mucus, of a brick-dust colour, oppression at the thorax, and acute shooting pain in the chest and sides, or rheumatic pains in the pleura, and pectoral muscles, or in the extremities, with increase of pain on move-

* In the third or suppurative stage of the disorder, the tubular respiration and vocal resonance commonly disappear, and a gurgling mucous râle is occasionally substituted. The expectoration becomes muco-purulent, or converted into a brown serous fluid; and the vital energies generally sink rapidly.

ment; foul tongue and constipation. A complication with pleurisy, pleuro-pneumonia, indicated by increased dullness on percussion, and in some instances a double-sounding voice, central bronchial respiration, and bronchophony, is often an additional reason for the selection of this remedy. (See also PLEURITIS.)

ADMINISTRATION. One drop of the tincture at the third potency, in about an ounce of water, a dessert-spoonful to be administered every four, six or eight hours, or a few globules of the third in a dessert-spoonful of water, repeated at similar intervals, according to the severity of the case.*

PHOSPHORUS. This remedy has been lately almost exclusively employed by Dr. Fleischmann,† of Vienna, in almost every stage of pneumonia under what form soever it presents itself, and with the most marked success, even when extensive hepatization has taken place. Although the homœopathic treatment hitherto adopted with *Aconitum*, *Bryonia*, &c., has proved eminently successful, yet this remedy, which seems to have such a specific influence over this serious disease, deserves a more extensive trial.‡

ADMINISTRATION. A drop of the tincture at the third potency, added to four dessert-spoonfuls of water, one in four hours, lengthening the intervals according to the effects produced.

TARTARUS EMETICUS is chiefly valuable in promoting resolution after hepatization has taken place, which is indicated by the greater or less degree of dulness on percussion, the bronchial or tubular respiration, and the peculiar pectoral sounds given by the voice, and may be had recourse to when

* Vide note, p. 21.

† Dr. Fleischmann's preparation is made with 10 drops to the 100, administered at the third to the sixth potency, from four to eight drops, in from two to four ounces of distilled water, a spoonful three to six times a day. Hygæa, vol. viii.

‡ It sometimes happens that, notwithstanding the early employment of this medicine, the physical signs of this disease *appear* to advance uninterruptedly, and it is only from unequivocal symptoms of improvement in other respects, that we feel encouraged to persevere with the remedy, and thereby obtain the most satisfactory and triumphant results.

the preceding remedy has not completely effected this desirable object.

ADMINISTRATION. One grain of the second potency in an ounce of water, a dessert-spoonful three times a day.

TINCTURE SULPHURIS may deserve a preference to the last-mentioned remedy in similar cases, in strumous habits, also where hepatization has advanced to some extent, and where *Phosphorus* may have only relieved; also where there is complication with pleurisy, and obstinate constipation. In obstinate or *chronic* cases, *Lachesis* and *Lycopodium* have been found very useful after, or in alternation with *Sulphur*.

ADMINISTRATION. A few globules of the third or sixth potency in a teaspoonful of water repeated in from six to twelve hours, according to circumstances,—if an improvement ensue, allowing the medicine to continue its action.

The preceding are the principal remedies used in the majority of cases of this disease; but the following also have been found excellent auxiliaries in some instances, and merit attention.

Belladonna, where the fever has returned, after having been apparently subdued by *Aconite*, and the difficulty of breathing and pain continue, particularly when the pain seems more at the sternum; the sputa tinged with blood and difficult of expectoration, the cheeks flushed, lips and tongue dry and scorched, leaving heat of the skin and incessant thirst.

Acidum nitricum has been of service in some cases, where, after *Aconite*, a cessation of pain has taken place with increase of fever.

Squilla has been recommended as useful in forwarding the crisis: further, in pneumonia accompanied with gastric symptoms, and where the expectoration is copious, or in cases which have previously been treated by venesection, and *China* has not proved sufficient to rouse the sinking energies.

Mercurius, when the fever has been lowered by the employment of *Aconite*, but pain and difficulty of breathing remain, *copious nocturnal sweats* exhaust the patient's strength, and the pulse is small and quick; also where there is prominent bronchitic complication:—In the latter instance *Capsicum*,

Nux v., *Pulsatilla* and *Bryonia*, have also proved efficacious: *Capsicum* particularly in the case of phlegmatic subjects; *Nux v.*, alternately with *Phosphorus*, especially in the case of drunkards; and *Pulsatilla* in chlorotic females. The indications for *Bryonia* have already been given. *Cannabis* has also been found useful in this frequent complication, and in one or two cases where there was disease of the heart and large vessels, with greenish vomiting and delirium.

Arnica $\frac{000}{3}$. Against effusion into the air-passages, with local congestions and hemoptysis.

Rhus tox. in the congestive stage of pneumonia, with restlessness, palpitation of the heart and redness of the face. But with diarrhœa and clammy sweats, *Arsenic*.

When inflammatory symptoms have been subdued, but the expectoration presents a muco-purulent appearance, and there is great prostration with nocturnal sweats, *Lycopodium* $\frac{00}{30}$ has been found very efficacious.

Lachesis $\frac{00}{30}$ has proved beneficial sometimes in alternation with *Arsen.* and *China*, in those almost hopeless cases which threaten to turn to gangrene of the lungs, (with fetid breath and sputa.)

Phosph., *Kali*, and *Lycop.*, $\frac{00}{30}$, useful in pneumonia occurring in phthisical subjects. It may be useful to add a few words respecting the pectoral signs in this affection when progressing to resolution: if no hepatization have taken place, the crepitous râle, at first audible, becomes gradually less perceptible, and the natural respiration is heard, till at last the former wholly disappears; if the lung have already partly solidified, but the disease is approaching a cure, the crepitous râle is first heard, then gradually yields to the natural respiration; in fact, the disease, so to speak, runs its course back again.

Diet. It is scarcely necessary to remark, that during the inflammatory period, an almost total abstinence must be observed; even during convalescence there is caution required, and care must be taken not to allow the patient to over-indulge his returning appetite, as any error in this respect may entail troublesome consequences. The drinks may consist of water, toast-water, and sometimes whey, rice or barley-water, sweetened with a little sugar if desired.

PNEUMONIA NOTHA, OCCULTA.

This affection, which is usually most insiduous in each approach, is more frequently met with in old than in young or middle-aged subjects, and is liable to terminate in paralysis of the lungs. Sometimes the attack is preceded by a feeling of general prostration; or comes on like an attack of common cold, with cough and alternate heats and chills. The cough is generally loose from the commencement; the sputa white, yellow, slimy, and generally blood-streaked. There is great weight or oppression at the chest, with quick laborious breathing; pain only when taking a deep inspiration, and generally in a small circumscribed spot. All these symptoms are usually aggravated by any thing which calls for an increased play of the lungs, such as talking, or laughing loudly, ascending stairs, etc.; finally, particularly in the more severe attacks, lying upon either side becomes oppressive, so that the patient is generally found on his back. Pulse soft but quick, the cheeks slightly flushed, the skin moist and damp, and sometimes there is nocturnal sweating, which affords no relief; towards morning the febrile action subsides a little, and the patient feels generally somewhat easier. The voice is low and weak, sometimes dying away to a whisper. In the treatment of this affection, a dose or two of *Aconite* is occasionally required, when the fever runs rather high, but *Mercurius* is more frequently called for, even at the very commencement, and particularly when there is nocturnal sweating and moist or clammy skin during the day; after *Mercurius* has been administered with more or less benefit, *Belladonna* will generally be found useful, and especially when a short dry cough remains, attended with spasmodic constriction in the chest which impedes respiration, and causes an oppressive sensation of suffocation. If *Belladonna* does not complete the cure, and the cough is accompanied with sibilant or wheezing respiration, a dose of *Aconite* may be given, followed by *Chamomilla* and *Nux v.*, the latter especially when there is dry cough, or cough with difficult expectoration of a little slimy mucus, and excessive tension and oppression in the chest. In those cases in which *Mercurius* affords little relief, and the breathing continues quick and laborious, and the countenance is expressive of great anxiety, *Ipecacuanha* in repeated doses is frequently followed by satisfactory results; but should the extremities become cold, and the sensation of constriction in the chest, with extreme anxiety, increase, VERATRUM may be administered: on the other hand, if the paroxysms of threatening suffocation become more and more distressing and the patient appears sinking from exhaustion—

ARSENICUM $\frac{000}{30}$ must claim a preference, and will often succeed in restoring the expiring energies of the patient when the case has assumed a perfectly hopeless appearance.

It may be added, that *Arnica* $\frac{000}{3}$ has been found useful in some instances in the early stage of the disorder, when a bruised or beaten pain was experienced in the chest, the cough not very troublesome, but attended with blood-streaked slimy sputa; followed by *Pulsat.* $\frac{000}{3}$ when the expectoration became more considerable, with melioration of the pectoral symptoms. Some of the remedies mentioned under PNEUMONIA VERA, such as *Bryonia*, *Tartarus*, *Sulphur*, *Lycopodium*, &c. may also be found useful in this complaint under particular circumstances.

TYPHOID OR CONGESTIVE PNEUMONIA.

In this variety of pneumonia the local symptoms are usually very obscure, and the accompanying fever is of the typhoid kind; the pulse quick and very weak, the skin harsh, dry, or clammy, tongue brown and parched, and the urine of greatly diminished quantity and high coloured.

In *some* cases the following physical signs can be detected: dulness on percussion, and absence of respiratory murmur in the lower and back parts of the chest, and occasionally bronchophony and bronchial respiration when the central or middle portion of the lung is the part affected.*

The remedies which have been used with the most advantage

* *Phosphorus* deserves attention in such cases, particularly when there is bronchial respiration.

in typhoid pneumonia, are *Opium*, *Arnica*, *Veratrum*, *Arsenicum*.

OPIUM $\frac{000}{3}$. This remedy is generally the most appropriate as soon as the disease becomes clearly defined, and may be repeated once or twice, after which, if no change be effected, *Arnica* $\frac{000}{3}$ should be administered.

Should no improvement result from the foregoing remedies, *Veratrum* $\frac{000}{3}$ may be administered, particularly when there is clammy sweat on the forehead, with coldness of the extremities and great weakness, and the respiration unequal, laborious and rattling.

ARSENICUM $\frac{000}{6}$ may follow *Veratrum* if the prostration and rattling respiration increase, the pulse become irregular, and the tongue dark brown or black: the alternate administration of these two remedies every half hour, to every hour or two hours, according to the urgency of the symptoms, is frequently attended with the best results; in other cases, *Veratrum*, *Ipecacuanha* and *Arsenicum* answer better:—But when only temporary improvement results, a few globules of *Sulphur* may be administered; and then again *Veratrum* and *Arsenicum*, or *Veratrum*, *Ipecacuanha*, and *Arsenicum* alternately, or any one of these remedies alone from which any marked degree of improvement may previously have been observed to arise. *Bryonia*, *Rhus*, and *Senega* will be found useful in some cases. Some of the leading indications for the employment of the two former will be found under the head of NERVOUS FEVER, (which see.) *Senega* is chiefly serviceable when the lungs are loaded with mucus. *Belladonna* will be found serviceable when temporary blindness is complained of, and *Natrum m.* when the prostration of strength increases, notwithstanding the administration of *Arsenicum*, which is generally so valuable in such cases. When galling or excoriation (decubitus) has ensued from lying in bed, *Cinchona* and *Arsenicum* must be administered alternately; in milder cases, *Arnica* in the form of lotion (one part in ten) will frequently remove this evil. When symptoms of INCIPIENT PHTHISIS PULMONALIS supervene on pneumonia, *Sulphur* is one of the most important remedies; but will in most cases require to be followed by *Lycop.*, *Lachesis*, *Phosph.*, *Ammon. c.*; in others by *Kali c.*, *Acid. nitr.*, *Natrum m.*, *Calcarea*, *Hepar sulph.*, *Stannum*, *Pulsat.*, *Carbo v.*, *Silicea*, *Sepia*; and *Ferrum* and *Cinchona* as intermediate remedies. A proper knowledge of the *Materia Medica* is indispensable to facilitate the selection of these remedies.

INFLAMMATION OF THE PLEURA.

Pleurisy, Pleuritis.

Diagnosis. Severe pain in the side, like a stitch, or as from a stab, remaining in one circumscribed spot, interfering with breathing, and increased by inspiration; difficult and anxious respiration, but not so oppressed as in pneumonia and bronchitis; quick hard pulse; hot skin, particularly over the chest, or the seat of the disease; dry tongue; scanty and high-coloured urine; and occasionally cerebral symptoms. Position in bed, usually dorsal; and if the effusion be free and partial, a change to the sound side creates great uneasiness.

Pleurisy seems to consist in a peculiar inflammation in the pleura, with a disposition to effusion or to the secretion of plastic lymph; and the disease may run its whole course without any of the symptoms above given declaring themselves.

At the commencement of the disease there is *diminution of motion and respiratory murmur* from pain (subsequently these abnormal signs arise from *effusion*) and a *rubbing sound* is not unfrequently heard, generally about the centre of the chest, accompanying the pectoral movements. Soon after the outset of the inflammation, in the great number of cases, exudation ensues, and if not encysted, accumulates at the lowest part of the chest. When, in such instances, the quantity exuded is considerable, and the lung is not restrained by adhesions, that organ will be floated upwards to some extent, and a dull stroke-sound elicited from the parts *beneath it*, whilst the *upper* will be found unusually resonant.

As the fluid accumulates and ascends in the chest, the antecedent clearness of stroke-sound becomes impaired, as is more especially obvious on gentle percussion,—the breath-sound diminished, and respiration more impeded. When these latter abnormal symptoms are met with as high as the middle regions of the thorax, the vocal resonance there, and particularly anteriorly, becomes preternaturally distinct, and is changed to a small, sharp and tremulous note resembling the bleating of a goat, and hence termed œgophony; posteriorly the resonance partakes somewhat more of the character of bronchophony, from the greater caliber of the tubes at the root of the lung. Œgophony and all sound of the voice ceases at the affected side of the chest, as the liquid effusion increases, with exception of those portions where the lung may have been adherent, or at the space within an inch or two of the spine; percussion now gives an extremely dull sound from the lung being deprived of and rendered impermeable to air by compression, and the respiratory murmur is abolished or only heard in the interscapular and subclavicular region, particularly the former.

In those cases in which the effusion is very considerable, *enlargement of the affected side* takes place. This enlargement is generally discernible only during expiration at first, but as the exudation increases, the difference can readily be detected, during the entire performance of respiration. In attenuated subjects, the intercostal spaces will also be observed to have become prominent instead of presenting their natural depression. But should absorption be effected after such an enlargement, the state of matters is reversed, and the side which was previously enlarged becomes abnormally contracted —the result of atmospheric pressure, and unantagonized muscular action.

Displacement of organs adjoining the effusion, such as the heart, liver and mediastinum, is also an occasional result of extensive effusion.

On examining the sound side of the chest, in addition to the negative proofs of the absence of disease, an excess of the usual normal signs will also be perceived, indicated by an accelerated and deeper action, together with a greatly increased degree of respiratory murmur, resembling that of children, and hence denominated *puerile*. The signs of improvement and approaching recovery are marked by a diminution of pain, fever, dyspnœa and enlargement of the side; a return of the respiratory murmur, together with an increasing clearness of sound on percussion. When the result is fatal, death occasionally supervenes very rapidly from the compression of both lungs; but in most cases this event is more gradual and arises from atrophy of the lungs, as also affections of the heart, and consequent dropsy, caused by the efforts required to propel the blood through the compressed lung.

In *all* cases of pleurisy the whole of the above detailed symptoms are not to be deemed constant, or even *certain* diagnostic signs:

The absence of marked dulness on percussion, is not a conclusive test that effusion has not taken place. The greater or less degree of clearness of tone appears to depend upon the condition of the lung under the effusion, and the elasticity of the parietes that cover the latter. If the quantity of the effusion be very considerable, and the lung deprived of its air by compression, the sound on percussion is necessarily almost uniformly dull; but when the exudation is inconsiderable and the compression is not sufficient to deprive the lung of its air, the stroke-sound will be found to consist more of a *tympanitic* and frequently even a *louder* tone than the normal expanded lung. Subsequently, however, if the pressure be unrestrained, the lung will be deprived of its air, and the part formerly so resonant will then yield a dull sound. The auscultatory phenomena are in like manner naturally liable to be materially modified by circumstances. Much depends on the extent of the exudation, and upon the state of the lung on which it rests. If the lung still contain air, both voice and respiratory sound will be found indistinct or inaudible. If, from the extent of the effusion, or from the long continuance of the disorder, the portion of lung be entirely emptied of air, weak bronchophony and bronchial respiration will be discernible; but when the amount of effusion is very great, possibly filling the whole cavity of the pleura, no sound whatever will be audible.* On the other hand, when the quantity effused is inconsiderable, the normal sounds frequently remain unchanged. Again, the physical signs are liable to be further modified by old and close adhesions, arising from previous disease, which render the lung adherent to the walls of the chest. And upper lobes are the most subject to these adhesions; and in such cases the free portion of lung is pressed upwards by the subjacent effusion, against the superior part of the thorax. And although the lung may yet admit air, still, from the degree of compression to which its vesicular structure is subjected, both breath and stroke-sound will be bronchial, and loud bronchophony pervade the upper part of the affected side. The lower part of the chest from whence the lung has been separated or raised upwards by the effusion will necessarily give decided dullness on percussion.

Finally, it may be added that *ægophony*, although a frequent phenomenon in pleuritis, has no necessary connection with the presence of liquid in the pleural sac, and is consequently not to be held as an essential link in the chain of evidence in determining the existence of the disease.

The same may in a great measure be said of the intercepted vibration of the voice, usually felt by the hand when placed against the chest, for this, although a very useful and early *corroborative* indication of the accumulation of fluid in the cavity of the pleura, is yet liable to some exceptions both positive and negative.

The *rubbing sound* already referred to is an important sign; it is not so audible at the commencement of the attack as it is at a later period; when the effusion becomes more consistent, *then* it is rarely absent.

From what has been stated, it will be seen that some of the *preconceived characteristics* cannot, *individually* considered, be taken as conclusive indications of the existence of pleurisy. The *collective* physical signs, however, in the majority of cases, are far from equivocal, and are mainly to be depended on

* *Brit. Jour. of Homœopathy*, vol. 1, p. 42.

in forming the diagnosis. Pain is, with few exceptions, an invariable concomitant on pleurisy, and its presence and intensity has been found of great use, in combination with other signs, in estimating the amount as well as the *quality* of the effusion; for it has been found that the greater the quantity of *plastic* lymph it contains, proportionally greater will be the pain.* Great rapidity of effusion is also a frequent, though not an infallible source of extreme pain. The greater or minor degree of dyspnœa depends on the quantity and rapidity of the effusion, as well as the condition of the lungs; when both sides of the chest are the seat of effusion, the oppression is usually excessive. The fever is in like manner modified by the nature and extent of the exudation being generally slight or altogether absent when the quantity is trivial, slow, and not unfrequently intermittent when more extensive but of a serous character, and highly inflammatory when much plastic lymph is contained in the effusion.†

Cough is not an accompaniment of simple pleurisy; when present, there is either bronchitic or pneumonic complication, or the case may be one of hemorrhagic-pleuritis.

Therapeutics. The chief remedies are *Aconitum napellus*, *Bryonia alba*, *Sulphur*, *Belladonna*, (atropa), *Mercurius*, *Arsenicum*, *Arnica montana*, *Hepar sulphuris*, *Calcarea*, *Phosphorus*, *Lycopodium clavatum*, *Carbo vegetabilis et animalis*, *Cinchona officinalis*, *Digitalis purpurea*, *Kali carbonicum*, *Ipecacuanha* (cephaælis), *Helleborus niger*, *Sabadilla*, *Scilla maritima*.

Aconitum. Is an indispensable remedy in allaying *inflammatory fever* when attendant on pleurisy; and is in many cases, indeed, when timely administered, alone sufficient to cure the disease. It rarely fails to effect the desired results, in from six to eight hours; should it not do so in that space of time, another remedy must be selected. In most instances *Bryonia* will be the most appropriate, but we must not hesitate to select *Sulphur* in preference if called for, or indeed any other remedy that may seem more strikingly indicated.

* *Brit. Homœop. Journ.*, vol. 1, p. 44. † *Ibid.*

Administration. A few globules of the third potency every two hours; or one drop of the tincture at the third potency to an ounce of water, a dessert-spoonful every two to three hours.*

Bryonia alba should in general cases follow *Aconitum* when the fever has been somewhat allayed by that remedy. It is more particularly indicated, either in simple or complicated pleurisy, when the following symptoms are encountered at an early stage of the disease; aching, burning, but more especially *acute shooting pains* in the chest, much increased *during inspiration* or *on movement; dry cough,* or dry sounding cough, followed by expectoration of dirty yellow-coloured mucus streaked or tinged with blood, and attended with aggravation of pain; *oppressed and anxious* respiration; palpitation of the heart; dry, cracked, brown, or *yellow*-coated tongue; *bitter taste, nausea,* and occasionally *vomiting* of mucus, or of a bitter, bilious-looking fluid; aching or painful pressure at the scrobiculus and hypochondria; intense thirst, especially at *night;* constipation; head confused and heavy; giddiness on sitting up in bed; aching and shooting pains in the head, or pain as if the head would burst, particularly at the temples, with exacerbation on coughing, or moving; fiery, or bluish redness, and puffiness of the face; restless, disturbed sleep, frequent startings; nocturnal delirium, with alternations of comatose sleep; burning heat of the skin; occasionally, partial, clammy perspiration; pulse generally frequent, hard and small, but sometimes full, unequal, intermittent and weak; aching in the limbs. Lastly, when in connection with many of the above, the following symptoms are met with: dullness on percussion, particularly at the right mammary and scapular regions, with puerile respiration; cough on lying on the right *side,* or impossibility of lying otherwise *than on the back,—Bryonia* will rarely fail to render undeniable service, and can indeed with difficulty be dispensed with. (Vide *Sulphur.*)

Administration. The same as *Aconite,* but at intervals of from three to four hours.

* Vide note, p. 21.

SULPHUR may with advantage follow *Bryonia* when the pain mentioned has been removed by that medicine, and often completes the cure. It is also of value when the fever continues after the administration of *Aconite,* and may be administered without the previous employment of Aconitum, when the fever is not violent, yet we have reason to suspect recent effusion of plastic lymph. Again, when the affection has already been of *some days' duration* and is complicated with *pneumonia,* it is our chief stay in preventing solidification, or effecting resolution where that has already commenced, and may therefore generally be selected in preference to Bryonia, in such cases, unless the latter be otherwise strongly indicated, in which event a dose or two of that medicine previous to the employment of *Sulphur* may be found serviceable.

ADMINISTRATION. A globule or two of the third potency in a teaspoonful of water every two to three hours; or two drops of the tincture in three ounces of water, a tablespoonful every three hours; or in very severe cases every hour.

These three are the most important remedies in the greater number of cases of pleuritis, and are frequently found sufficient to effect a speedy cure. There are often occasions, however, in which it will be found necessary to select one or more of the under-mentioned remedies.*

MERCURIUS $^{0}\frac{0}{6}{}^{0}$. Has been found very useful in cases where the fever has been subdued, but pain and dyspnœa have not been relieved by Aconite, and the patient's strength is becoming exhausted by *copious nocturnal sweats.*

ARNICA MONTANA. Principally when pleuritis is caused by external injury; but also in other cases when the more *inflammatory* symptoms have been subdued by *Aconite,* etc.; and pain in the chest, with oppressed respiration, only remain; also to *promote absorption* when considerable effusion has taken place.

ADMINISTRATION. One drop of the tincture of the third potency to an ounce of water, a dessert-spoonful every three

* *Belladonna* has been recommended in cases where the fever returned, and pain and dyspnœa continued notwithstanding the employment of Aconite.—*Brit. Homœop. Jour.*, vol. i, p. 51.

or four hours; or two or three globules of the third, in a teaspoonful of water, at the same intervals, until the pain begins to yield and the breathing becomes freer, when the intervals between the doses must be lengthened or the medicine discontinued, and only resumed should the improvement proceed tardily; but if pain return, *Aconitum* must again be had recourse to, after which *Belladonna*, in repeated doses, is often extremely useful, if not sufficient to effect the desired end. In other cases, ***Bryonia*** or ***Sulphur*** will be seen to be more appropriate, and must be selected accordingly.

ARSENICUM $^{0}\frac{0}{6}{}^{0}$ is our main dependence in those serious cases where serous effusion to a *very great extent* has taken place, and where the respiration is painfully impeded and asthmatic, with extreme prostration of strength.

HEPAR SULPHURIS $^{0}\frac{0}{6}{}^{0}$ has been particularly recommended when the effusion is *plastic*, and the disease has been of *some duration*, (chronic plastic pleurisy,) or where, even at the commencement, there appears, from the pain, fever and dyspnœa, continuing with but slightly diminished severity after *Aconite*, every probability that the case will prove extremely obstinate and tenacious. Complication with pericarditis or bronchitis is an additional indication for the employment of *Hepar* under the above circumstances.

PHOSPHORUS.. From what has been said of this remedy in *Pneumonia*, it will readily be suggested that it may be useful in cases of complication of pleuritis therewith, and such it has repeatedly proved to be. In complications with bronchitis, and in that form of pleuritis which so frequently shows itself in phthisis pulmonalis, it has further been found of essential service. Vide PNEUMONIA and BRONCHITIS.

ADMINISTRATION. A few globules of the third, or a drop of the sixth, in a little water every three or four hours, or oftener if necessary, until the respiration becomes easier.

CARBO VEGETABILIS is a good remedy when pleuritis is complicated with chronic bronchitis; or at an advanced stage of the disorder, when the patient is much emaciated and hectic at night, presenting in short the usual symptoms of threatening purulent degeneration. It is also peculiarly useful against asthmatic sufferings resulting from an attack of pleurisy in the chronic cases.

Administration same as *Arsenicum*, except in the latter instance when it must be given at longer intervals.

Cinchona is chiefly useful after severe depletion, to restore the energies of the patient.

Administration. ${}^{0}\frac{0}{6}{}^{0}$ or $\frac{0\,0}{3\,0}{}^{0}$, repeated in twelve hours.

Lycopodium $\frac{0}{6}{}^{0}$ will be found serviceable in similar cases to those in which both *Arsenicum* and *Carbo vegetabilis* (or *animalis*) have been found applicable, also where there are considerable dropsical swellings and obstinate constipation.

Digitalis ${}^{0}\frac{0}{3}{}^{0}$ in lower potencies has proved useful in many cases of serous pleurisy with slow fever, small weak pulse, accelerated by the slightest movement; and coldness of the extremities with internal heat.* In conclusion, *Kali carbonicum* may be instanced as serviceable in pleuritis occurring in tuberculous subjects; and *Ipecacuanha* as a useful palliative against dyspnœa and convulsive cough in complications with bronchitis. *Helleborus niger* has been recommended in some cases of serous, and *Scilla* in plastic pleurisy, but they, as well as *Colchicum*, *Lachesis*, and some others which need not be mentioned here, require the test of further experience to corroborate even the little that has been adduced in their favour in the treatment of pleuritis.†

When either through neglect or otherwise, pleuritis has terminated in purulent degeneration, and become chronic, *Arsenicum*, *Carbo*, *Lycopodium*, *Hepar s.* and *Kali carbonicum*, will generally be found to be the remedies from which the greatest assistance is to be obtained where cure is at all practicable. Pains in the chest arising from adhesions or from thickening of the pleura, after an attack of pleuritis, are often

* Brit. Journ. of Homœopathy, No. 1, p. 53.

† *Rhus toxicodendron* has been strongly recommended in serous pleurisy :—When low, typhoid symptoms become apparent, the said remedy will deserve an additional claim on our attention. Typhoid appearances, and important complications of any kind, a bad habit of body, or indications of a purulent, sanious, or hemorrhagic effusion, are all to be held as unfavourable signs.

relieved by ***Ranunculus b., Euphorb., Mez., Nitr., Thuja***, may also be found serviceable. *Sulph., Sepia,* ***Kali c., Am. c.,*** *Lyc.*, and *Mezer.* are useful in chronic pleurisy.

DIET. The same rules are to be observed as in ***Pneumonia.***

PLEURODYNIA. SPURIOUS OR BASTARD PLEURISY. PSEUDO-PLEURITIS.

By these terms is here meant that painful affection usually referred to the intercostal muscles, which is productive of many of the symptoms described under true pleurisy, and is consequently liable to be mistaken for the said disease, particularly when attended with febrile excitement, as is frequently the case in hysterical females. The history of the commencement of the affection, together with the aid of auscultation and percussion, enable us to discriminate satisfactorily between the two diseases.

When therefore we have satisfied ourselves from the normal condition of the auscultatory phenomena, etc., that the case we have to deal with is one of pseudo-pleurisy, we must select a remedy from amongst the following: ***Arnica montana, Bryonia,*** *Nux v.,* ***Pulsatilla, Ranunculus bulbosus,*** *Sabadilla.*

In the majority of cases *Arnica* is the principal remedy, and is occasionally sufficient to effect a speedy cure after a single dose. In other instances, however, the disorder does not yield so readily, and one or more of the other remedies enumerated must be had recourse to.

BRYONIA. When the pain is of an *acute darting* description, as if from a sharp instrument running into the side, and is occasionally almost insupportable during *inspiration* or even the slightest movement of the body; and when the party affected is of a nervous or bilious temperament.

PULSATILLA. This remedy is frequently very useful in alternation with *Arnica;* it is more particularly indicated when the pain is occasionally of a *fugitive* character, moving from one part of the chest to another, becoming increased towards evening, and sometimes experienced more during expiration than inspiration. Temperament phlegmatic.

NUX VOMICA. Shooting pains in the hypochondria increased by the *respiratory movements* of the chest ; especially when the affection occurs in hypochondriacal subjects or in those who are addicted to indulgence in vinous or spirituous drinks. Temperament bilious or sanguine.

It is, moreover, one of the best remedies in this complaint; the characteristic indications are as follows, and show a marked resemblance to the symptoms which are so frequently met with in, and are in some respects peculiar to *pseudo-pleurisy;* stitch in the side, or shootings, with *painful sensibility of the external parts of the chest,* but particularly of the *intercostal spaces,* aggravated by any movement, and especially by taking a deep inspiration, yawning or stretching.

Ranunculus bulbosus. The value of this medicine in pains resulting from adhesions of the pleura has already been alluded to. (Vide Pleuritis.)

In acute pains in the chest of every description of a nervous character, depending upon an abnormally exalted sensibility of the *pleura,* this remedy is one of primary importance.

Sabadilla is also useful in this affection.

Administration of the remedies. In some cases a single dose of one or two globules of the 3d or 6th potency is sufficient to effect a cure; in others it will be found necessary to repeat the dose every six, twelve, or twenty-four hours, according to the severity of the attack, until relief is obtained. (See note, p. 21.)

SPITTING OF BLOOD. HEMORRHAGE FROM THE LUNGS.

Sputum Cruentum. Hæmorrhagia Pulmonum. Hæmoptysis.

Diagnosis. Expectoration of blood by coughing, in greater or less quantity, attended by symptoms more or less severe.

This disease presents itself in three varieties: first, by an effusion of blood from the mucous lining of the bronchial tubes; secondly, from congestion of the lungs, with engorgement of the parenchyma from effusions; and thirdly, the rupture of a blood-vessel in the tubercular cavity of the lungs during the course of phthisis pulmonalis. It is, however, proposed to deal generally with the subject, and to point out the different remedies found useful in the treatment, according to the symptoms present. We must be careful not to confound this disease with affections of the mouth or gums, or blood from the nose escaping through the posterior nares, and returned by the mouth. When from the chest, it is almost invariably attended with a sensation as if it came from a deep-seated source, is warm, generally tastes sweet, and there is frequently a simultaneous burning and painful sensation in the chest.

When the attack is preceded by well known premonitory symptoms, the party affected should refrain from loud or prolonged speaking, calling, singing, blowing wind instruments, violent exercise of the arms, running, ascending stairs, or in short any thing which is calculated to increase the respiratory action, or otherwise fatigue the chest.

When spitting of blood occurs in a robust and healthy person of sound constitution, it is not very dangerous; but when it attacks slender and delicate persons of weak lax fibre, it is more serious and difficult of removal. It is, however, chiefly when the patient has had a succession of severe attacks and the blood is discharged in large quantity, that the case may be considered dangerous.

The disease may present itself without any marked pains or difficulty of breathing, and pass off with no return of the attack; or be preceded by dry cough, oppression, or tightness at the chest, shivering, coldness of the extremities, great lassitude, and high pulse; and be accompanied by hacking or husky and distressing cough, anxiety, quick pulse, pale and livid countenance; cease and then return in a few hours, and be followed by difficulty of respiration and cough: in still more severe cases, when a marked tendency to phthisis exists, anxiety, oppression at the chest and febrile symptoms are more severe; pure blood is coughed up, and the paroxysms frequently return.

The rupture of a blood-vessel is a rare occurrence, although it sometimes occurs in phthisis. When a blood-vessel of any consequence, included in a tuberculous excavation, gives way, the result is generally fatal.

Causes. Indulgence in spirituous beverages, overheating the body by immoderate exertion, or too great external heat; blowing wind-instruments; contusion of the chest or back; falls; lesions of the lungs; breathing a vitiated atmosphere, or vapours charged with acrid substances; colds or coughs; violent mental emotions; diseased state of the lungs, whether from pneumonia or phthisis; a general strumous habit; suppressed menstrual, hemorrhoidal, or other discharges; or repercussed cutaneous eruptions.

Therapeutics. In by far the greater number of cases, the discharge or spitting of blood soon ceases of its own accord; the most important object therefore is to seek to *cure* the complaint when the hemorrhage has ceased, and thereby prevent returns or check development of organic disease of the lungs. The principal remedies in the treatment of this affection are ***Pulsatilla, Nux v., Bryonia, Sulphur, Arnica, Aconitum, Ipecacuanha, Acidum sulph., Arsenicum, Opium, Cinchona, Carbo, Ferrum met., Rhus, Phosphorus***, and *Sepia*. These are not only calculated to arrest the hemorrhage, but also to *prevent a relapse*, where that is practicable.

Administration. Unless otherwise specified, a drop of the tincture at the potency mentioned after each medicine, in an ounce of pure water, a teaspoonful every two, four, or six hours, or much oftener where apparently called for; but this being a disease in which considerable judgment and tact are required in the exhibition of the medicines, it is scarcely possible to give rules in this treatise applicable to all cases.*

Pulsatilla. In cases of females, arising from suppression of the monthly discharge, or in either sex, of a hemorrhoidal flux, particularly of leuco-phlegmatic temperament, and also in the other instances, with the following symptoms: expectoration of dark coagulated blood, attended with shivering, especially towards evening, or at night, and great anxiety; pain in the lower part of the chest; feeling of flaccidity in the epigastrium, and weakness. One drop of the Potency 6. (*Hæmoptysis vicaria.*)

Administration. When from the causes first mentioned,

* Vide note, p. 21.

if not particularly severe, $\frac{000}{6}$ repeated in twelve, or even twenty-four hours, and subsequently at much longer intervals, will be found sufficient; but in violent attacks the dose must be repeated every two to four hours, but discontinued as soon as improvement begins to set in. When in females, the menses do not return, notwithstanding the employment of *Pulsatilla, Cocculus, Sepia, Sulphur* or any other remedy better adapted to the entire case, should be selected; (vide *Chlorosis, Amenorrhœa*, or *Catamenia*, suppression of.)

BRYONIA is a good remedy in cases where the expectorated blood is excited by a tickling cough, and is often in a coagulated state; oppression at the chest, with frequent necessity to take a deep inspiration; anxiety and irascibility.

ADMINISTRATION. Same as *Nux vomica.*

NUX VOMICA $^{0}\frac{0}{3}{}^{0}$ is adapted to individuals of an irritable temper, in whom this affection owes its origin to a hemorrhoidal suppression, a fit of passion, or exposure to cold. It is further indicated by dry cough, which causes headache, with excessive tickling in the chest and exacerbation of the symptoms towards morning. (*Hæmoptysis vicaria.*)

ADMINISTRATION. In mild cases $\frac{000}{6}$, repeated in twenty-four hours; in severe, prescribed in the case of *Pulsatilla.* When *Nux v.* does not afford speedy relief, *Sulphur* will generally be found to succeed; but should any other remedy appear to be more appropriate, it should unhesitatingly be selected in preference.

RHUS $^{0}\frac{0}{3}{}^{0}$. When the blood expectorated is of a bright red, the mind much agitated, and the patient is irritable and rendered worse after the slightest vexation or contradiction.

ARNICA MONTANA $^{0}\frac{0}{3}{}^{0}$. Principally in cases arising from external lesion, such as a severe blow in the chest, or from lifting a heavy weight, or any other exertion, even blowing wind-instruments; but also in almost all cases, where the stethoscope detects effusion of blood into the parenchyma, attended with a sensation of constriction and burning in the chest, pain as from contusion in the scapular and dorsal region, and dyspnœa. Moreover, profuse expectoration of dark coloured blood or coagula, brought up without much exertion, or bright frothy blood, mixed with mucus and clots; sensation of tickling behind the sternum; general heat, great weakness and syncope. (*Aconite* $^{0}\frac{0}{3}^{0}$ is sometimes necessary before, or alternately with *Arnica*, &c.)

Acidum sulphuricum is frequently of service after *Arnica* when the cough continues, and brings on fresh bleeding.

Administration. One or two drops of the 6th in about a tumbler of water, a dessert-spoonful every hour or half hour.

In *severe cases* attended with manifest danger: *Aconitum, Ipecacuanha, Arsenicum, Opium*, and *Cinchona*, are the most useful, and must, as usual, be selected according to the prevailing symptoms. When one of these is insufficient to check the hemorrhage entirely, another must be chosen to meet the remaining symptoms.

Aconitum $\frac{0\,0\,0}{3}$ is often found most serviceable in warding off an attack by the great power it possesses in controlling the circulation, and is indicated previous to the paroxysm by the premonitory symptoms of shivering, with accelerated pulse, palpitation of the heart, a sensation of ebullition of blood in the chest, with burning and fulness in the same region; paleness and expression of anxiety in the face; great anguish and anxiety, aggravated by lying down, or *during the attack* when the expectoration is profuse, coming on in gushes, and excited by a slight dry cough. (*Hæmoptysis plethorica.*)

Ipecacuanha $^{0}\frac{0}{3}^{0}$, when a taste of blood remains in the mouth a few hours after the employment of *Aconite* was commenced, when there is frequent tussiculation, with nausea, weakness, and expectoration streaked with blood.

Arsenicum. When the *anxiety, anguish*, and palpitation of the heart increases, notwithstanding the administration of *Aconite;* and when, in addition, we find extreme restlessness and general dry burning heat. Potency 6. Two or three globules in a teaspoonful of water, repeated in two hours.*

The Administration of this remedy alternately with *Ipecacuanha* has been found to succeed in many instances when neither of them separately have been found sufficient to con-

* Vide note, p. 21

quer the disease. Giving an occasional dose of *Nux vomica* as soon as the hemorrhage has in a great measure been checked, to such individuals as have been in the habit of indulging in spirituous, vinous, or fermented liquors, or coffee. Should hemorrhage return after a temporary cessation, *Sulphur* may be administered, followed in turn by *Arnica* if the desired result be not thereby effected.

OPIUM $\frac{0\,0\,0}{3}$. Heat, dyspnœa, with sensation of burning heat at the region of the heart; coldness, particularly of the extremities; tremor in the arms; dry hollow cough, with expectoration of blood and frothy mucus, and sometimes also weakness of the voice; drowsiness, with sudden starts; aggravation of cough after swallowing. It will be found useful in the most serious cases, particularly in those addicted to *spirituous* liquors; in the latter case it is useful to follow it with *Nux v.*

CINCHONA $\frac{0\,0\,0}{3}$ or $\frac{0\,0}{6}{}^{0}$, as already mentioned in several places in this work, is one of our best remedies in restoring the vital energies of the patient after considerable loss of fluids, whether blood or other secretions; it is therefore particularly efficacious *after* a severe attack of this affection, but is also indicated *during* its course, when the spitting of blood takes place after a *violent* cough, or when there is a continual taste of blood in the mouth, or when we find shivering alternately with accesses of heat, frequent and short-lived perspirations; tremor, and confusion of vision, with a sensation of vacuity or lightness in the head, weakness and desire to remain constantly recumbent.

ADMINISTRATION. Same as *Pulsatilla*.

FERRUM METALLICUM. May be exhibited with advantage after the last mentioned, in severe cases, or may be preferred if the expectoration follows a *slight* cough, and is scanty, but consists of pure bright red blood, attended with pain between the scapulæ, with inability to remain long in a sitting posture: the patient feels the concomitant symptoms relieved by movement, but is speedily fatigued, especially by conversation. It may in some cases be advantageously alternated with *Cinchona*, *Carb v.*, *Arnica* and *Arsenicum*,—or *Sulphur* may be required to complete the cure in some cases.

ADMINISTRATION. One grain of the 3d potency.

SULPHUR. This remedy is frequently useful in completing the treatment after the administration of other medicines; and it is also particularly suitable for individuals disposed to hemorrhoidal affections, in derangement of the menstrual flux, or hemoptysis arising from suppressed cutaneous eruptions, such as scabies, &c. (*Hæmoptysis vicaria*, &c.)

ADMINISTRATION. $^{0}\frac{0}{6}{}^{0}$, in a little water, repeated in four to eight days, for three or four successive times, when administered as a remedy to complete the cure; but it may be given every four to six hours, or even oftener, when administered to check existing hemorrhage. In other instances, particularly in the case of those who have been given to excess in the use of stimulating beverages, *Nux v.* and *Arsenicum* may be advantageously administered in alternation with *Sulphur*, at intervals of five or ten days. (See note, p. 21.)

After hemoptysis has disappeared, besides having to guard against a relapse in which, as above stated, *Sulphur* is our chief auxiliary, we have to take every precaution lest inflammation arise in the part primarily affected, or the disease degenerate into PHTHISIS, which objects will sometimes be best attained by the administration of *Phosphorus* in combination with a strict observance of an antiphlogistic regimen, and the other rules about to be given for the conduct of the patients suffering from this affection.

The almost specific action of this medicine in changes of structure of the substance of the lungs, has been already commented upon under *Pneumonia;* it may also be remarked that it is, along with *Aconitum*, one of our chief remedies in hemorrhages from the lungs during the course of phthisis.

SEPIA $^{0}\frac{0}{6}{}^{0}$ is also useful in this affection occurring in PHTHISIS, but when it is rather to be looked upon as one of the general symptoms than forming a disease of itself; by its power over the uterine economy, it is also of great service in cases of hemoptysis, arising from derangements connected with that organ. (*Hæmoptysis phthisica et vicaria.*)

The following remedies may also be noted as worthy the attention of the practitioner in peculiar cases: *Belladonna*,

Bryonia, Carbo v., Hyoscyamus, Ignatia, Dulc., Cocculus, Crocus, Conium m., Lachesis, Acidum sulph., Acidum nitr., Ledum, Lycopod., Millefolium, Silicea., Staphysag., and *Cuprum m.*, etc.

DIET, etc. The rules given under HEMATEMESIS should be observed as regards regimen; both mind and body should be kept perfectly quiet; the patient should speak as little as possible, be kept in a semi-recumbent posture, or if his strength allow, sit upright.

PULMONARY CONSUMPTION. *Phthisis Pulmonalis.*

Short cough, which is either dry or accompanied by the expectoration of a frothy mucus, slight at the commencement, but more or less constant. Shortness of breath, and symptoms of gastric derangement, etc. Hectic fever by flushing of the face (often after a meal); night sweats. In the second stage, the cough is more severe at night; after meals or at times of excitement a circumscribed red patch still appears on each cheek, but at other times the colour of the cheek is faded. In the third, the tubercles are expectorated of cheese-like particles, mixed with pus, mucus, blood, etc. *Acon., Bryon., Bellad., Lach., Hep. s., Spongia, Phosph., Dulc., Puls., Arsen., Nux v., Hyosc., Silic., Calc. c., Carbo v., Acid. n.*, and *Sulph.*, are indicated in the first stage. In the second : *Acid. n., Silic., Kali c., Sulph., Calc. c., Natr. m., Merc., Lach., Phosph., Lycop., Carb. v., Samb., Hep. s., Spong., Chinch., Ferr., Conium, Zinc., Am. c., Lauroc., Graph., Nitr., Iod., Dros., Plumb.*, etc. In the third stage, the same remedies as the foregoing; also, *Guaiac., Sepia, Stann., Staphys., Acid. phos., Sanguin.* : see chapter on COUGH. When sweats are distressing: *Samb., Stann., Chinc., Phosph., Ars., Carb. v., Carb. a., Silic., Merc., Nitr., Lach., Sulph.* and *Lycop.* When diarrhœa predominates : *China., Ferr., Ars., Phosph., Acid. phos., Sepia* : see *Diarrhœa.* It requires a separate treatise to do justice to this disease, and therefore we refer to: *Consumption, treated homœopathically*, by *A. C. Becker, M. D.*

ADMINISTRATION. $\frac{000}{3}$, or $\frac{000}{6}$, or $\frac{00}{30}$. Vide Note, p. 21.

DERANGEMENTS

OF

THE CEREBRAL SYSTEM.

DETERMINATION OF BLOOD TO THE HEAD.

Congestio ad Caput.

This is an affection to which many individuals who lead a sedentary life are subject; intense mental application and habitual indulgence in the use of spirituous liquors, or other stimulating liquids, such as coffee, etc., are also frequent exciting causes, particularly in those who inherit a predisposition to the disorder.

Diagnosis. Fulness of the vessels of the head and neck, the pulsation of which the patient experiences through the entire frame; heat, redness, and turgidity of the face; repeated attacks of giddiness, particularly on sleeping, sitting in a warm, confined apartment, or an exposure to the rays of the sun when exercising in the open air; headache, generally above the orbits, and in the forehead, increased by stooping or coughing; disturbed, unrefreshing sleep; drowsiness during the day.

Therapeutics. *Aconitum napellus*, *Nux vomica*, *Belladonna*, *Opium*, *Coffea*, *Chamomilla*, *Ignatia*, *Arnica*, *Mercurius*, *Pulsatilla*, *Dulcamara*, *Cinch.*, *Sanguinaria canad.*, etc.

Aconitum. This is the principal remedy to commence with in all recent cases, and is alone sufficient speedily to remove the affection, particularly in children when fright and anger combined have been the exciting causes.

Administration. $^{0}\frac{0}{6}{}^{0}$, in a teaspoonful of water, repeated in six, twelve, or twenty-four hours, if necessary; for children, $\frac{0\,0}{1\,2}$ or $\frac{0\,0}{2\,4}$, in half an ounce of water, a teaspoonful every twelve hours until relief is obtained.

NUX VOMICA. As has already been repeatedly observed, this remedy is exceedingly efficacious in complaints arising from sedentary habits, intense study, or that much more culpable habit, the excessive indulgence in spirituous or vinous liquors, &c.; it is accordingly one of the most useful remedies in determination of blood to the head, induced by such causes; it is also very serviceable in cases arising from a violent fit of passion, and is more particularly indicated when we meet with the following symptoms: distention of the veins with violent pulsation in the head; heat and redness of the face; attacks of giddiness, violent headache, particularly in the forehead and over the orbits, aggravated by reflecting, or by any attempts at mental application, also by stooping or coughing; disturbed sleep; nervous excitability, and disposition to be angry at trifles; constipation. *Calcarea* after *Nux v.* in obstinate cases, in persons addicted to indulgence in spirituous liquors.

ADMINISTRATION. $\frac{000}{12}$, a teaspoonful of water, repeated in twenty-four hours, and again in the same manner after an interval of from three to five days, if required. *Calcarea* will frequently be found of signal benefit after *Nux vom.*, in obstinate cases occurring in persons addicted to indulgence in spirituous liquors.

BELLADONNA. After a previous administration of *Aconite*, when necessary, this is one of our most important remedies in the treatment of congestion to the head. Indications: great distention of the vessels of the head, attended with severe jerking burning pains in one half of the head, aggravated by the *slightest* movement or the least noise; by bright redness and bloatedness of the face, redness of the eyes, sparks before them, and sometimes dimness of vision; darkness before the eyes; diplopia; buzzing in the ears; attacks of fainting; somnolency.

ADMINISTRATION. $\frac{00}{6}$, in a teaspoonful of water, repeated in six, twelve, twenty-four hours, or at shorter or longer intervals, according to the greater or less severity of the symptoms, or the effects produced by the preceding dose.

OPIUM is of speedy service in cases arising from *fright;* but it is, moreover, a remedy of extreme value in the most serious cases of congestion, either arising suddenly from the effects of a draught of cold or iced water, especially when heated, with the following symptoms: vertigo, heaviness of the head, humming in the ears, dullness of hearing, *stupor;* also, when from constipation, or from the effects of a *debauch,* pressure in the forehead from within outwards, with redness and bloatedness of the face, great depression, fugitive heat; violent thirst; dryness of the mouth; acid regurgitations, nausea and vomiting.

ADMINISTRATION. A drop of the third potency in an ounce of water, a dessert-spoonful every hour, or every two to six hours, according to the urgency of the symptoms, and the effects produced; or a globule or two of the third or sixth in a teaspoonful of water at similar intervals.

COFFEA. In cases arising from excessive joy, this remedy will be found to exert a salutary influence; excessive and uncontrollable liveliness; great heaviness of the head, or aggravation of the sensations when speaking; sleeplessness.

ADMINISTRATION. $^{0}\frac{0}{3}{}^{0}$, repeated in twelve hours, if necessary.

CHAMOMILLA. Congestion caused by vexation, or a fit of passion, particularly in children, is speedily relieved by this remedy.

ADMINISTRATION. One or two globules of the sixth potency in a teaspoonful of water.

IGNATIA, when induced by a stifled vexation, or harrowing, concentrated grief.

ADMINISTRATION. $\frac{0}{6}{}^{0}$, in a teaspoonful of water daily, for about a week.

ARNICA. In cases arising from external violence, such as severe falls or contusions, followed by stupefaction, vertigo, sensation of pressure or coldness over a small circumscribed space; tendency to close the eyes; disposition to be frightened, and vomiting; the external and internal administration of *Arnica,* when timely had recourse to, will frequently be found specific. This remedy is, however, equally useful in other cases with the following symptoms: heat in the head with coldness of other parts of the body; sensation of obtuse pressure on the brain; painful burning or throbbing in the cranium; humming in the ears; vertigo, with confused vision, especially on assuming the erect posture after sitting for some time.

ADMINISTRATION. $\frac{00}{6}$, in a teaspoonful of water, repeated every twenty-four hours until relief is obtained, or a change in the symptoms calls for some other remedy; and a lotion of one part of the tincture to ten of water, applied to the injured part, in cases arising from external violence.

MERCURIUS. Congestion with sensation of fulness, or *as if the head were compressed by a band;* nocturnal *aggravation* with darting, piercing, tearing or burning pains; disposition to sweating. After *Arnica, Belladonna,* or *Opium, Mercurius* is frequently found serviceable in completing the cure.

ADMINISTRATION. Same as *Arnica.*

PULSATILLA. This remedy, as will be found stated in the proper place, is well adapted in many cases of congestion occurring in young girls at the critical age, or in all cases occurring in cold, lymphatic temperaments with the following symptoms: distressing semi-lateral pain in the head, particularly of a pressive character, or if the pain in the head commences at the occiput and extends to the root of the nose, or *invertedly.* Amelioration of the symptoms from exercise, or from pressing or binding the head; exacerbation while sitting; sense of weight in the head; vertigo; inclination to weep; anxiety; coldness, or shivering.

ADMINISTRATION. The same as described under *Arnica.*

LYCOPODIUM. Is a valuable remedy in some obstinate cases of congestion, attended with giddiness, ebullition, flatulence, anxiety, and habitual constipation.

DULCAMARA. Congestion attended with continual buzzing in the ears, dullness of hearing, and particularly when the affection has arisen from getting the feet wet, or from a chill in cold, damp weather.

ADMINISTRATION. $\frac{2}{6}$, in a teaspoonful of water, repeated in from twenty-four to thirty-six hours, if necessary.

SANGUINARIA CANADENSIS. Distention of the vessels, heaviness of the head, with fulness and aching as if the head would burst; pressure behind the orbits. The pains are chiefly in the forehead, sinciput and right side of the head.

CINCHONA. Congestion occurring after repeated blood-lettings, or hemorrhage in general, is generally relieved by this remedy.

ADMINISTRATION. $\frac{000}{6}$, in a teaspoonful of water, repeated in four days.

After the completed action of *Cinchona*, a dose or two of *Sulphur* and *Calcarea carbonica*, $\frac{00}{6}$, *at intervals of about a week*, will materially tend to strengthen the impaired constitution when *Cinchona* is not of itself sufficient to effect that desirable object.

Nux vomica, *Veratrum* and *Valerian* are also valuable remedies in particular cases arising from debilitating losses; the attention of the student or practitioner may also be directed to the following remedies: *Rhus toxicodendron*, *Bryonia alba*, *Cicuta virosa*, *Hepar sulphuris*, *Silicea*; the two latter, together with *Sulphur* and *Calcarea*, are more particularly adapted to the treatment of chronic cases. See *Dyspepsia* and *Apoplexy*.

In cases of *giddiness* simply, or when that is the prevailing symptom, the following remedies are amongst the most useful: MERCURIUS, when the giddiness comes on only in the *evening*, especially on assuming the erect posture; or in the morning on getting out of bed; and is attended with nausea, dimness of sight, heat, anxiety, and desire to lie down. NUX VOMICA. Giddiness during *mental application*, or *after a meal*, or when in the *recumbent posture*, particularly in nervous or bilious subjects; and in cases where *sedentary habits* or *dissipation* have given rise to the affection. PULSATILLA. Giddiness, especially on *looking upwards*, or when *sitting*, or at other times, such as during or after meals, when attended with *heaviness of the head*, buzzing in the ears, headache, and *paleness* of the face, sometimes alternating with heat; confusion of sight; lowness of spirits; nausea, and inclination to vomit; phlegmatic temperament. CINCHONA. Giddiness on elevating the head, or during *movement*, relieved by reclining. *Rhus*. Giddiness on lying down, but which becomes relieved after retaining the recumbent posture for some time, and then returns on assuming the erect posture, sometimes to such an extent as to occasion falling, attended with fear of dissolution; giddiness after a hearty meal. CHAMOMILLA. Giddiness on rising, with tendency to faint; giddiness during a meal; irritability. ARNICA. Violent giddiness during dinner or *after a hearty meal;* in the latter instance, *Nux v., Pulsatilla, Rhus,* or *Chamomilla,* are also very useful, and must be selected according as they may be otherwise indicated; but as such cases are frequently fraught with danger, experienced advice must be sought.—Giddiness on rising from the *recumbent posture,* or on *stooping. Aconitum,* followed by *Belladonna,* particularly if in addition to the foregoing symptoms there is frequently partial loss of consciousness, cloudiness of vision, giddiness from the motion of a carriage, sometimes with disposition to faint: *Hepar s.* followed by *Silicea,* should the former not suffice, or afford only a slight degree of improvement. SULPHUR often very serviceable after *Pulsatilla,* when the attacks are most liable to come on while *sitting;* or it may be selected in preference to the said remedy when the giddiness generally comes on whilst walking up a hill or ascending stairs; or at other times attended with nausea, fainting, or bleeding from the nose. *Lycopodium,* giddiness with tendency to congestion, accompanied with *flatulence,* headache, anxiety, and obstinate constipation. *Lachesis,* giddiness with absence of mind, or paleness of the face, nausea and vomiting; fainting, bleeding from the nose, particularly when the attacks come on chiefly in the morning on waking.

OPIUM, *threatening* vertigo with *confusion of ideas;* or decided giddiness, with *humming* in the ears, and clouded vision on *sitting up in bed,* which renders it necessary to lie down again; vertigo from *fright.*

CONIUM. *Violent giddiness,* with dread of falling to one side on looking *backwards.* Giddiness arising from disordered stomach, with nausea or vomiting. *Aconitum,* followed by *Antimonium crudum,* and subsequently *Pulsatilla* if necessary, from a continuance of the symptoms in a greater or less degree.

DIET. The homœopathic regimen already given in Introduction should be rigidly adhered to, and stimulants of all kinds carefully avoided; moreover, early rising, and daily exercise in the open air, should not be neglected; the use of the flesh brush in the evening is also of some service.

APOPLEXY. *Apoplexia.*

Diagnosis. Sudden or gradual loss of consciousness, sensation, and motion, with greater or less disturbance of the pulse and respiration.

Few diseases offer a greater number of varieties in form than the one above named; and there is scarcely a single classification of the many that eminent medical writers have given to the world, that is not more or less liable to objection.

It is also extremely difficult to diagnose clearly between the different varieties, the external symptoms not always bearing a uniform relation to the internal injury; thus all the indications of serous apoplexy may declare themselves from sanguineous extravasation; and it is not always possible to decide in apoplexy whether effusion or simply congestion of the vessels of the brain has taken place.

Premonitory Symptoms. Continued inclination to somnolence, heavy profound sleep with stertorous breathing, incubus, grinding of the teeth, shocks or cramps, a general feeling of heaviness or disinclination to the least exertion; frequent yawning and fatigue after the slightest exercise. A sense of weight and fulness, and pains in different parts of the head. Cephalalgia and megrim, or vertigo and fainting; pulsation of the temporal and carotid arteries, with swelling of the veins of the head and forehead; disturbance of the cerebral system evinced by loss of memory, forgetfulness of words and things, irritability of temper, or mildness and indifference, despondency and weeping; infiltration of the conjunctiva, dimness of vision, specks or motes before the eyes, or flashes of fire or sparks during darkness; acuteness of vision or diplopia, sometimes also the words in a line appear to run into one another; difficulty of opening or closing the eyes; noises, humming, singing, &c., in the ears; dulness of hearing, dryness of the nostrils, pinched appearance of the nose with unpleasant odour, sneezing and slight epistaxis; stammering, and indistinct enunciation; difficulty of deglutition, numbness or torpor, or pricking sensation in the extremities, with occasional partial attacks of paralysis in the face, distorting the features, and affecting the utterance, or in some of the muscles of the limbs, pains in the joints; weak or unsteady mode of progression, difficulty of micturition, &c.

THEIR TREATMENT. Against the preceding, Homœopathy possesses remedies by whose proper application the practitioner may, if consulted in time, succeed in warding off the attack of this dreaded malady.

The following are the medicines most appropriate to the treatment of the foregoing symptoms which are most generally called for in the treatment of the disease itself, or to Determination of Blood to the Head, (see that article:) *Aconitum, Belladonna, Nux vomica, Lachesis, Opium.*

ACONITUM. In all cases where there are evident symptoms of plethora, determination of blood to the head, characterized by redness and fulness of the face, distention of the veins of the forehead, quick full pulse, restlessness and anxiety.

ADMINISTRATION. $\frac{6}{6}$, dissolved in six teaspoonfuls of water, one every twelve hours.*

BELLADONNA. Should the symptoms of congestion not speedily yield to Aconite, or should only a partial degree of amelioration have taken place; or further, should the following symptoms present themselves: redness and bloatedness of the face, injection of the conjunctiva, violent beating of the carotid and temporal arteries, noises in the ears, darting pains in the head, with violent pressure at the forehead increased by movement, the least noise or bright light; or diplopia, and almost all the symptoms relative to the eyes already mentioned; dryness of the nose, with unpleasant smell and epistaxis; difficulty of deglutition; slight attacks of paralysis in the face; paralytic weakness or heaviness in the limbs.

* Vide note, p. 21.

ADMINISTRATION. $\frac{6}{12}$, in six teaspoonfuls of water, one every twenty-four hours, or every six or twelve in more alarming cases, taking care if the slightest symptoms of *medicinal aggravation* declare themselves, to discontinue the medicines for a time.*

NUX VOMICA is particularly suited to cases in which the apoplexy threatens individuals of sedentary habits addicted to the use of ardent spirits, or too great an indulgence in the pleasures of the table, and also when the following symptoms present themselves: *headache*, especially at the *right side*, with *vertigo*, confusion and humming in the ears, nausea, and inclination to vomit; drowsiness, feeling of languor with great disinclination to exertion, either mental or bodily; cramps of the limbs, especially at night, and weakness in the joints; constipation and dysuria, irritability of temper, aggravation of the symptoms in the morning, or after a meal, and also in the open air; bilious, sanguine, or nervous temperament.

ADMINISTRATION. The same as *Belladonna.*

OPIUM is a most important remedy in almost all severe attacks, but particularly in old people, when we find the following symptoms: marked congestion to the head, indicated by *stupor*, vertigo, heaviness in the head, and violent pressure in the forehead, singing in the ears, and obtuseness of hearing; sleeplessness or agitating dreams, or frequent and almost overpowering drowsiness during the day, redness of the face, and constipation; pulse slow, but full.

ADMINISTRATION. $\frac{6}{3}$, in the same manner as *Belladonna.*

LACHESIS is indicated by many of the same symptoms which have been enumerated under *Nux v.*, together with the following distinctive characteristics: frequent abstraction of mind, or vertigo with congestion, and aching pains in the *left* side of the head, and *lowness of spirits;* pulse weak, and slow.

When any of the symptoms before noticed present themselves, *is the proper time* to prevent the attack running on to apoplexy; sometimes the signs are so marked that we can have but little doubt of the result, unless timely precautions

* Vide note, p. 21.

are taken; at others, so slightly as to be almost imperceptible; and in others again, the attack comes on suddenly without any marked premonitory symptoms whatever. See *Congestio ad Caput*.

Apoplexy. A work of this nature is scarcely the place to enter upon the many varieties of this dangerous and complicated affection. Where so much depends upon the tact and promptness of the practitioner, to do the subject the justice it merits, would require almost a treatise of itself. I shall therefore content myself with quoting the leading indications of those remedies which have hitherto been chiefly recommended, or found most successful in the treatment of the disease itself.

Opium is held as a most important remedy in all cases of apoplexy when the disease has attained considerable height. It is, however, one of the best remedies to commence with, when the attack has arisen from excess in drinking, and the symptoms are as follows: slow, *stertorous breathing; red* and *bloated* face; heat of the face and head, which latter is also covered with sweat; *insensible* and dilated pupils; stupor; tetanic rigidity of the entire frame, or convulsive movements and trembling in the extremities; foaming at the mouth.

Nux v. has been found of great service in completing the cure after the previous use of the above remedy; but may also be administered at the commencement when the attack has occurred in an individual of *bilious* or *sanguine* temperament, and of irritable temper, in consequence of over-indulgence in vinous or spirituous liquors; or when the attack has resulted during or after a fit of passion, and the patient appears in a state of drowsiness approaching to stupor; the breathing stertorous; eyes dull and glassy; hanging of the lower jaw, with copious secretion of saliva; paralysis, particularly of the inferior extremities (paralysis paraplegica); hemiplegia.

Lachesis is also a valuable remedy in this disease, especially when ocurring in habitual drunkards; with drowsiness or loss of consciousness, *lividity of countenance*, convulsive movements or *tremour* in the extremities; or paralysis, especially of the *left* side; pulse weak and slow.

ARNICA. Apoplexy after too hearty a meal, with loss of consciousness (drowsiness or stupor); stertorous breathing; moaning or inarticulate muttering; *involuntary evacuations; paralysis of the extremities* (hemiplegia left side); pulse strong and full.

BELLADONNA. Lethargy, *loss of consciousness;* the patient lies speechless, with *the mouth drawn to one side;* convulsive movements of the limbs or facial muscles; hemiplegia, particularly of the right side; *dilated, immovable pupils;* red and bloated face.

PULSATILLA. Lethargy, loss of consciousness; bloatedness and bluish-red hue of the face, occurring after a full meal which has been hurriedly swallowed;* or sudden loss of the power of movement; palpitation of the heart; pulse almost entirely suppressed; respiration stertorous; temperament phlegmatic.

BARYTA CARBONICA. This remedy, like *Opium,* is peculiarly well adapted to the treatment of many of the affections of old people. It has accordingly, like the foregoing remedy, been found very serviceable when the serious affection at present under consideration is met with in patients of advanced age, particularly when the following symptoms are encountered: *Coma somnolentum,* with moaning and muttering; circumscribed redness of the cheeks; mouth drawn to the one side; *paralysis of the tongue,* or of the upper extremities; hemiplegia (right side); confusion of ideas; childish manners. The following remedies may also be pointed out as being worthy of the attention of the experienced homœopathic practitioner: *Stramonium, Hyoscyamus, Cocculus, Ipecacuanha, Ignatia, and Cuprum aceticum;* and in some cases, *Coffea cruda, Antimonium crudum, Conium maculatum, Digitalis, Mercurius,* and *Tartarus emeticus;* and in the paralysis resulting from apoplexy, *Belladonna, Baryta carbonica, Causticum, Nux vomica, Rhus, Silicea, Lycopodium, Graphites,*

* Ipecacuanha is equally indicated when the attack has arisen from such a cause, and may therefore be employed after, or in alternation with Pulsatilla, should the latter remedy not afford speedy relief.

Carb. v., *Oleand.*, *Bryonia*, *Cocculus*, *Plumbum*, *Stramonium*, *Stannum*, *Sulphur*, *Calcarea*, and *Zincum metallicum*.

I cannot conclude this article without giving expression to the gratification I, in common with the majority of the most eminent of my homœopathic medical brethren, feel at the gradually increasing distaste to bloodletting upon the part of our opponents. Many have renounced the use of the lancet altogether; and others, while they do not wholly discountenance its employment, surround the cases in which it ought to be had recourse to with so many restrictions as almost to amount to a prohibition. At all events, we may hope that the time has already arrived, at least for the more enlightened of our profession, when even those who still adhere to its employment in particular cases will not rashly prescribe bleeding in all instances of cerebral compression, where, if had recourse to before a reaction has set in, it may destroy the patient, either by his sinking under it, or by effusion, if that has not already taken place, or by increasing it if it has.*

INFLAMMATION OF THE BRAIN AND ITS TISSUES. BRAIN FEVER.

Phrenitis. Encephalitis.

Diagnosis. Coma, or constant delirium, or both, with signs of determination of blood to the head; fullness and redness of the face and eyes; beating of the carotid and temporal arteries; sometimes attempts to grasp the head.

When depending upon inflammation of the *tissues*, the pain is more acute than that arising from inflammation of the *substance* of the brain. Paralysis also more frequently accompanies the latter form.

In inflammation of the brain or of its membranes, the symptoms are exceedingly diversified; the extent and duration of the disease, the age, the sex, and constitution of the patient,

* Against *paralysis* resulting from apoplexy, the following remedies have principally been employed with advantage: *Nux v.*, *Cocculus*, *Belladonna*, *Stramonium*, *Zincum*, *Lachesis*, and *Sulphur*.

assist in giving to the affection a variety of character. Much assistance may be derived, in ascertaining whether the brain is affected or not, by examining the eyes and general expression of the countenance. The pupils in the first stages are commonly found more or less contracted, but as the disease advances, they often become dilated. Occasionally the attack is preceded by premonitory symptoms, such as *congestion of blood to the head*, attended with sensations of weight, or stupifying, pressive, constrictive, and sometimes shooting pains in the head. In some instances slight feverish symptoms are complained of, with ringing in the ears for about the space of a week; giddiness, and a sense of weight on the crown of the head; pulse rather quick, and the heat of the skin somewhat increased at night, attended with restlessness and a difficulty of lying long in one position; moreover, the patient is observed to be irritable and annoyed at trifles; anomalies in the mental powers may next be observed, such as obstupefaction, drowsiness, with slight delirium; or a high degree of excitement, in which the patient is affected by the slightest noise, and the eyes have a brilliant and animated expression, or are blood-shot, with fiery redness of the face, and violent delirium. According to the seat of the inflammation, or the constitution of the patient, the accompanying fever is of greater or less intensity; the pulse is very variable in the course of the same day; it may be regular, intermitting, quick and weak, or very slow and strong. A very slow or a very quick pulse generally indicates danger. The patient frequently complains of heat in the head, whereas the extremities are cold. When there is stupor, or a tendency to it, the eyes look heavy and void of all expression; vomiting sometimes takes place and proves very intractable; the stupor becomes more profound, convulsions appear, and death sooner or later ensues. The peculiar and delicate structure of the brain and its membranes in children renders them much more susceptible to the attacks of this serious disease, and great attention ought to be paid to the following symptoms: heaviness and tendency of the head to gravitate backwards, attended with pain, of which latter circumstance we are sometimes made aware, in very young children, by the little sufferer frequently raising its hands to the head; alternation of temper; intolerance of light; nausea, occasionally followed by vomiting; tendency to costiveness; drowsiness; wakefulness, or starting during sleep. Secondly, *continued boring of the head against the pillow;* a high state of excitement, in which the slightest noise, or rays of light, throws the child into a fit of screaming, or a state of discontentment; heavy sleep; great heat in the head; *redness* and swelling of the face, with perceptible throbbing in the vessels of the head and neck; great agitation, with continued tossing about, especially at night; eyes red, sparkling, convulsed, or fixed; pupils immoveable, and generally dilated.

CAUSES. Anything tending to irritate the brain, such as extremes of heat or cold; the abuse of ardent spirits; external injuries of the head; concussions from falls; mental emotions, or over-exertion of the faculties; excesses of all kinds; sanguineous congestion; metastases; contagious diseases; repressed eruptions, &c.

THERAPEUTICS. With regard to the treatment of this disease, we should have immediate recourse to ACONITE at the commencement of the attack, when the skin is *hot and dry,* and the pulse rapid, with the ordinary indications of pure *Inflammatory Fever*, which is especially liable to be the case in young plethoric subjects.

ADMINISTRATION. The same as in *Inflammatory Fever.* After which we may have recourse to any of the following remedies as indicated: namely, *Belladonna*, *Hyoscyamus*, *Opium*, *Stramonium*, and *Cuprum aceticum*.

BELLADONNA. This remedy seems to possess a certain specific influence over inflammation of the brain and its meninges; and is generally the one we should select when the following, among other symptoms, present themselves: *great heat of the head;* redness and bloatedness of the face; with *violent pulsation of the carotids; burying of the head in the pillow*, and increase of suffering at the *slightest* noise, with extreme sensibility *to light;* violent shooting and burning pains in the head; *eyes red and sparkling,* with protrusion or *wild expression;* contraction and dilatation of the pupils: *violent and furious delirium;* loss of consciousness; sometimes low muttering; convulsions, occasionally symptomatic hydrophobia; vomiting; involuntary evacuation of fæces and urine.

ADMINISTRATION. One drop of the tincture at the third potency in an ounce of water, a dessert-spoonful every three to six hours; or a globule or two of the third or sixth potency in a teaspoonful of water, at the intervals stated,—being guided by the intensity of the symptoms and the effects produced.*

BRYONIA. This remedy will frequently be found of great efficacy in children when *Aconite* and *Belladonna* have produced but trivial improvement, and the symptoms indicate a tendency to rapid effusion, in which case *Helleborus* may follow *Bryonia* if required. (Vide HYDROCEPHALUS.)

HYOSCYAMUS is appropriate when there is *drowsiness, loss of consciousness,* delirium about one's own affairs; inarticulate speech; tongue coated white, with frothy mucus about the lips; dilatation of the pupils; fixedness of the vision; skin dry and parched; redness of the face; and picking of the bed-clothes with the fingers.

ADMINISTRATION. Same as *Belladonna.*

OPIUM. When there is *lethargic sleep,* with *stertorous breathing; half open eyes* and confusion or giddiness after waking; sanguineous congestion; complete apathy and absence of complaint.

ADMINISTRATION. Two drops of the second or third potency in an ounce of water, of which we may give a dessert-spoonful every hour until relief takes place, unless some other more specific remedy be called for by some alteration in the symptoms.

STRAMONIUM, when there is starting or jerking in the limbs; sleep almost natural, followed by absence of mind after waking, but sometimes attended with moaning and tossing about; vision fixed, and the patient frequently appears in a

* Vide note, p. 21.

state of dread, and utters cries; redness of the face; feverish heat, with moisture of the skin; in many of the symptoms it bears a close resemblance to *Belladonna*, but with the exceptions of being indicated by signs of more spasmodic character, and exhibiting less acuteness of pain in the head.

ADMINISTRATION. Same as *Belladonna.*

CUPRUM ACETICUM. The value of this remedy in cases of repercussed exanthemata, and the consequences therefrom arising, has been already noticed under SCARLET FEVER; under which also some of the symptoms indicating its employment are commented upon; it is also called for in a peculiar *sensitive* rather than *inflammatory* or *irritable* state of the brain, which not unfrequently appears in children during the course of catarrhal fever or difficult dentition, of which affection the following are the symptoms:—At the commencement, crossness or fretfulness, or apathy and indifference; sleep disturbed and restless. As the disease gains ground, drowsiness, with inability to sleep; incapability of holding the head erect, and flushing of the face; dryness of the mouth without increase of thirst; disgust of food, nausea, even vomiting; torpor of the bowels, rarely diarrhœa; shudderings, followed by heat, occasional burning; seldom perspiration; pulse variable, generally rather accelerated and full; exacerbations and fever (synocha) towards and at night; subsultus tendinum, and grinding of the teeth during the exacerbations.

Belladonna, *Rhus*, *Lachesis*, and *Mercurius*, have also proved serviceable in cases arising from repercussed exanthemata.

ADMINISTRATION. As in SCARLET FEVER.

CINA is useful in irritation of the brain in children, apparently arising from helminthiasis.

ADMINISTRATION. As under WORMS, (which see.)

In chronic cases, *Sulphur*, *Helleborus niger*, *Arsenicum*, and *Lachesis*, are the most generally useful.

It may be added, that *Aconite* followed, if required, by *Belladonna*, *Camphora*, *Lachesis*, are the most appropriate remedies when the affection has arisen from exposure to the sun (*coup du soleil*).

Aconite, Bryonia, Arsenicum, Hyoscyamus, when resulting from a violent *chill* in the head. From suppressed otorrhœa, *Sulphur, Pulsatilla.* External injury, *Arnica, Belladonna, Mercurius.* Abuse of ardent spirits, *Opium, Lachesis.* And when from intense mental application, *Belladonna*, &c., according to the symptoms.

TETANUS.

This is a disease characterized by a general spastic rigidity of the muscles. Its varieties are TRISMUS, the lock-jaw, OPISTHOTONOS, which is the most common, when the body is drawn or bent backwards by the spasmodic contraction of the muscles, sometimes to such a degree that the occiput touches the heels. EMPROSTHOTONOS, when the body is bent forwards; a rare form of the disease. PLEUROSTHOTONOS, in which the body is bent to one side; a still more rare variety.

The disorder is chiefly occasioned either by exposure to cold (idiopathic tetanus), or arises from some irritation of the nerves resulting from local injury, particularly of tendinous parts, (traumatic tetanus.) It is of much more frequent occurrence in warm than in cold climates. In this and in other climates, the amputation of a limb, or the twitching of a nerve by a ligature, are not unfrequent sources of its occurrence. When it takes place in consequence of such a cause, or of any other external lesion, the symptoms *generally* set in about the eighth day, and sometimes later; but when it supervenes on exposure to cold, they usually declare themselves much earlier. In some cases, the attack comes on suddenly, and with extreme violence; but it more generally approaches in a gradual manner; a slight stiffness being at first experienced in the back part of the neck, together with an uneasy sensation at the root of the tongue, difficulty in performing the act of deglutition, and an oppressive tightness is complained of in the chest, with a pain at the inferior extremity of the sternum, or the scrobiculus cordis, extending into the back; the respiration is impeded; the countenance pale, pulse small, bowels constipated, and urine high coloured; a stiffness also takes place in the lower jaw, which ere long increases to such an extent, and compresses the jaws so closely and firmly, that the smallest opening is not admitted of, and the patient is now afflicted with what is termed lock-jaw. In some instances, the spasmodic contractions proceed no further; in others they return with great frequency and increased severity, and also extend to the arms, the abdominal muscles, the back and inferior extremities, so as to bend the body forcibly in one or other of the directions before stated. Finally, the arms, lower extremities, head, and trunk, become rigidly extended, from an equipoised spasmodic action of the flexor and extensor muscles. The tongue is also seized with spasms, and is not unfrequently injured by the teeth becoming clenched together, just as it happens to be convulsively darted out.

As the affection advances, the eyes become fixed and immovable, the whole countenance frightfully distorted, and expressive of extreme anguish, the pulse irregular, the strength completely exhausted, and a termination is put to the sufferings, generally about the fourth day in acute cases, by one concentrated spasm. In some cases the fatal termination is protracted considerably beyond the stated period.

The spasmodic action does not continue unremittingly, the muscular contractions occasionally admitting of some remission, but is generally immediately renewed as soon as the patient makes an effort to speak, drink, or change his posture.

THERAPEUTICS. The remedies which have chiefly been used in homœopathy in the treatment of this distressing disease are: *Belladonna, Stramonium, Cicuta virosa, Arnica, Opium, Hyoscyamus, Angustura, Rhus, Ignatia, Lachesis, Natrum muriaticum, Mercurius, Aconitum, Sulphur, Veratrum, Phosphorus, Camphor, Staphysagria, Moschus.*

BELLADONNA is one of the most important of these, particularly in idiopathic tetanus, properly so called, or in trismus; it has also proved useful in the traumatic variety, however, after the previous employment of *Arnica.* It is principally indicated when a sensation of *constriction* is experienced in the throat, and tightness at the chest, with grinding of the teeth, *spasmodic clenching of the jaws, distortion* of the mouth, foaming, obstructed deglutition, and renewal or exacerbation of the paroxysms on attempting to drink. In some cases of trismus, the alternate use of ***Belladonna*** and ***Lachesis***, or ***Belladonna, Angustura,*** and ***Cicuta virosa,*** have been found necessary; and of ***Belladonna, Lachesis, Hyoscyamus,*** and ***Stramonium*** in opisthotonos; or ***Opium, Rhus,*** and ***Belladonna.***

ARNICA MONTANA. In cases of traumatic tetanus, which is by far the most fatal variety, this remedy is, in most instances, the most appropriate to commence with, and should be used both internally and externally, in the form of an extremely weak lotion (about a teaspoonful or a drachm to a pint of water). Should symptoms of improvement not set in, in twenty-four to forty-eight hours, *Opium* and *Hyoscyamus* must be had recourse to. Any local irritation which may seem to have excited the disease must at the same time, if possible, be carefully removed.

OPIUM has proved extremely useful in some of the severest forms of opisthotonos arising from cold; but as above stated, it is also valuable in traumatic tetanus. (Likewise in tetanus from fright.)

Rhus and *Ignatia* have been found very efficacious in severe cases of opisthotonos, in which the body has been bent up in the form of an arch, and on some occasions with the back of the head touching the heels, when the complaint arose from terror.

MERCURIUS has frequently succeeded in curing inflammatory trismus, with swelling of the angle of the lower jaw, and tension of the muscles of the throat and neck, from cold.

These are a few *general* indications for the employment of the foregoing medicines. The following may also prove serviceable in various forms of tetanus: ***Aconitum, Sulphur, Veratrum, Phosphorus, Camphora, Staphysagria, Moschus, Bryonia, Nux platina, Ipecacuanha, Secale cornutum, Cannabis indica, Cantharides, Cicuta virosa, Cina, Rhus toxicodendron, Gratiola, Stannum;*** but considerable care must necessarily be bestowed on the selection of the proper remedy.

When, from the spasmodic clenching of the jaws, it is found impossible to introduce the medicine into the mouth, the effect of olfaction must be tried; it has also been found useful to moisten the lips and nostrils with the medicine dissolved or diluted in water; and in some cases, the administration of the remedy in the form of enema (a few drops of the third potency to an ounce or two of water) has been found very efficacious (See also HYDROPHOBIA, HYSTERIA, and MYELITIS.)

CUTANEOUS DISEASES.

ST. ANTHONY'S FIRE. ROSE.

Erysipelas.

Diagnosis. The first local symptoms are heat, tingling or pricking pains, with diffused swelling, tension, and deep redness of the affected part. This is, ere long, followed by pungent, burning, and sometimes tearing or shooting pain, which is aggravated by motion or pressure; the surface presents a shining appearance. On pressure, the redness disappears for a moment, but immediately returns on removing the finger. The constitutional symptoms vary according to the severity of the case; they generally consist of shiverings, succeeded by flushes of heat; sleepiness, wandering pains, dry tongue, nausea, oppression at the stomach, and headache; vesications sometimes arise on the affected parts, attended with increase of fever. (*Erysipelas bullosum.*) In a few days the redness changes into a yellowish hue. When the face is attacked, the features become much disfigured by the swellings, and delirium supervenes. The disease assumes a very serious aspect when it affects the face and scalp, and accordingly requires the utmost attention and discrimination in the treatment pursued.

The hair often falls off after a severe attack of erysipelas of the face.

Causes. Derangement of the digestive functions, exposure to cold or powerful mental emotions; occasionally it appears during menstruation; certain kinds of food also provoke it in some idiosyncrasies; for example, lobsters, oysters, or other shell-fish.

THERAPEUTICS. The principal remedies in the treatment of the ordinary forms of erysipelas are *Aconite*, *Belladonna*, *Bryonia*, *Pulsatilla*, *Rhus tox.*, *Arsenicum*, and *Lachesis*.

ACONITE, in case of *much fever*, or *hot*, *dry* skin.

ADMINISTRATION. $\frac{00}{6}$, repeated in from six to twelve hours if required, in slight cases; but even during the disease, if the fever runs high or assumes a synochal type, exhibit as under INFLAMMATORY FEVER, (which see.)

BELLADONNA, chiefly in *Erysipelas phlegmonodes*, but also in *œdematodes* and *erraticum*, when the redness expands in rays, and an acute shooting pain with heat and tingling is experienced in the affected part, which is aggravated by movement. Facial erysipelas, with burning heat, excessive swelling, so that the eyes are almost closed, violent headache, thirst, dry hot skin, restlessness, disturbed sleep, delirium.

In such instances, *Belladonna* is generally alone sufficient to effect a cure; but sometimes it will be found necessary to have recourse to *Lachesis* or *Rhus toxicodendron*, in alternation with *Belladonna*; or to *Hepar s.*, when the skin is smooth, looks less glassy and inflamed after the employment of Belladonna, but the heat, pain and swelling remain unaltered. (See *Rhus*.)

ADMINISTRATION. A few globules of the sixth, or even a drop of the tincture of the third potency, to an ounce of water, a dessert-spoonful every six hours. In mild cases $\frac{00}{6}$, repeated in twelve to twenty-four hours, if necessary.*

BRYONIA is frequently useful when the disorder affects the joints, and when the pain is exacerbated by the slightest movement. *Belladonna*, however, is equally appropriate in most affections of this nature. (*Sulphur* is sometimes required to complete the cure after *Bryonia*.)

ADMINISTRATION. Same as *Belladonna*.

PULSATILLA, when the hue of the skin is less intense, or of a bluish red, and the morbid spots frequently disappear from one place to reappear in another (*Erysipelas erraticum*).

* Vide note, page 21.

It is further indicated when the disease affects the internal and external ear, particularly in vesicular erysipelas, after *Rhus tox.* (*Belladonna* and *Rhus*, and, in some instances, *Graphites* are called for in fugitive or wandering erysipelas.)

ADMINISTRATION. $\frac{0\,0}{6}$, morning and evening, until symptoms of improvement result, or another remedy is called for.*

RHUS TOX. is our best remedy in vesicular erysipelas, and also appropriate in erysipelas with gradual but very extensive œdema, (*Erysipelas œdematodes*,) particularly when the disease has a tendency to extend itself to the brain and membranes, and the symptoms closely resemble those developed in Encephalitis. In some instances it is necessary to have recourse to *Belladonna* and *Hepar sulph.* to complete the cure,—or to *Belladonna* and *Rhus* alternately. (*Graphites* is also useful in some obstinate cases of vesicular erysipelas.)

It may also be remarked, that *Rhus* is especially suitable to erysipelas arising from particular kinds of food in certain idiosyncrasies; in other cases of this kind, however, *Pulsatilla* or *Bryonia* will be found equally serviceable, according to the symptoms and the temperament of the patient.

(ADMINISTRATION. $\frac{0\,0}{6}$, repeated in six or twelve hours, if necessary; and in severe cases, a drop of the tincture of the third potency o an ounce of water, one dessert-spoonful every four hours until benefit result, lengthening the intervals or ceasing to exhibit according to results.

NUX VOMICA. In erysipelas of the *knee* or *foot* with extremely painful bright red swelling; also successful in *pseudo-erysipelas*, in irritable subjects, particularly females. (ADMINISTRATION : see *Rhus tox.*)

ARSENICUM, when vesicles of a blackish hue, with a tendency to degenerate into gangrene, present themselves, (*Erysipelas gangrenosum*) ; still more clearly pointed out, if great prostration of strength be present. This medicine may also be advantageously alternated with *Carbo vegetabilis;* but as such cases fall especially within the province of the experienced homœopathic professional man, it will be needless to enter into the mode of administration, which must be regula-

* Vide note, p. 21.

ted by circumstances. *Lachesis* and *Rhus* are occasionally of great service after, or in alternation with *Arsenicum.*)

Cuprum aceticum. The value of this remedy, upon the testimony of Dr. Schmid, of Vienna, has been already noticed in repercussed eruptions, when a marked metastasis to the brain has taken place. See Scarlet Fever.

Sulphur and *Arsenic* are important remedies when erysipelas has terminated in ulceration. In some chronic forms of the complaint, *Acidum nitricum, Euphorbium, Sulphur, Graphites, Silicea,* (pseudo-erysipelas,) and *Hepar s.*, have been found serviceable. The alternate use of *Bellad.*, *Rhus,* and sometimes *Laches.* or *Crotal.*, has removed permanently, a disposition to erysipelas of the face. In Erysipelas Scroti, or Cancer Scroti, (*Chimney Sweeper's Cancer,*) *Arsenicum* is the most important remedy; *Rhus, Clematis* and *Lachesis* have also been recommended.

The greatest care must be observed to avoid the risk of taking cold even during convalescence; such an accident occurring during the disease is, as is well known, frequently attended with the most dangerous results. The troublesome itching so frequently attendant upon erysipelas, is often materially relieved by the application of wheaten starch, or flour of maize. In conclusion, I may be allowed to remark, that by the fortunate discovery of remedies perfectly homœopathic to most of the forms of erysipelas, we are now enabled to treat this affection with the same facility and certainty as we are other diseases curable by well-known specifics.

BOIL. *Furunculus. Abscessus nucleatus.*

Diagnosis. Round or rather cone-shaped hard elevations, of different sizes, slowly inflaming and suppurating, discharging matter generally at first tinged with blood, but still retaining a portion of morbidly-altered cellular tissue, which may form the nucleus of another after the first has healed.

Causes. A peculiar constitutional tendency; they are, however, frequently critical, as in gout, following acute fevers or eruptive diseases, and sometimes forming the termination of chronic exanthemata, such as itch, &c.

THERAPEUTICS. The following are the remedies most serviceable in this troublesome affection: *Arnica montana, Sulphur, Belladonna, Mercurius, Aconitum, and Hepar sulphuris.*

ARNICA is the best remedy in most cases of boils, and will frequently prevent their return; but in the majority of cases, *Sulphur* is necessary to eradicate the affection, which desirable result is best accomplished by the use of these two remedies at each attack, for two or three successive times. It sometimes happens, however, that the pain and constitutional disturbance is so great that it becomes necessary to have recourse to one or more of the subjoined remedies:

ADMINISTRATION. $\frac{0\,0}{6}$, repeated in three days, if necessary; in other cases, it may be found more advantageous to exhibit $\frac{0\,0\,0}{6}$ in three teaspoonfuls of water, taking one night and morning until finished.*

ACONITUM, when the boil presents an extremely inflammatory appearance, and the affection is accompanied with considerable fever and restlessness, is promptly efficacious in subduing these symptoms, and may precede a more specific remedy.

BELLADONNA, should the boil have an inflamed, fiery, or erysipelatous red appearance; or, moreover, should it, if situated upon the extremities, be associated with swelling and tenderness of the glands under the armpit, or upon the groin; dry, hot skin, thirst, headache.

ADMINISTRATION. Same as *Arnica.*

MERCURIUS. Should the *swelling* refuse to yield to that remedy after the inflammatory redness has been subdued.

ADMINISTRATION. The same as *Arnica.*

When matter has formed, HEPAR SULPHURIS will be found conducive to bringing the tumour to a head, and thereby curtailing suffering.

ADMINISTRATION. $\frac{0\,0}{6}$, repeated in from six to twelve hours, if necessary.

A tendency to frequent returns of this affection is, as already stated, often obviated by the repeated exhibition of *Arnica* and *Sulphur;* but when from some innate taint there are

* Vide note, page 21.

not found sufficient, this result is often attained by the employment of *Lycopod.*, *Nux-vom.*, *Phosphorus*, and *Acidum nitr.*

CARBUNCLE.

Anthrax. Furunculus Malignans. Pustula Nigra.

Diagnosis. A livid, bluish, or black spot, upon an extended surface, extremely painful, readily running to gangrene, and proving fatal from the extension of mortification. The disease is attended by headache, thirst, foul tongue, sickness, loathing of food, languor, jactitation, and sleeplessness.

Therapeutics. The best remedies in this affection are *Lachesis*, *Silicea*, and *Arsenicum album.*

Lachesis. When the anthrax presents a livid appearance, and is disposed to extend rapidly or to burrow.

Administration. $\frac{0\,0\,0\,0}{6}$, in four teaspoonfuls of water, twice a day, exhibiting at longer intervals, if improvement takes place.*

Silicea. When administered from the commencement in simple non-contagious carbuncle, is frequently found sufficient to effect a perfect cure.

Administration. $\frac{6}{30}$, in three dessert-spoonfuls of water, one daily,—to be repeated if required.

Arsenicum. When the carbuncle threatens to terminate in gangrene; it is also the most efficacious remedy when the disease has arisen from contagion.

Administration. A few globules of the sixth, or even a drop of the tincture, at the third potency, to an ounce of water, a dessert-spoonful every six, twelve, or twenty-four hours, according to the emergency of the case.

In some cases *Cinchona, Rhus tox.*, *Pulsa.* and *Silicea*, may be found serviceable in completing the cure, after *Arsen.*

CHILBLAINS. *Perniones.*

This affection is too well known to require any particular description; the exciting cause is exposure to transitions of

* Vide note, p. 21.

temperature, from cold to heat, and *vice versâ*, but their origin is more deeply seated; the feet are the part most generally attacked, but we frequently find the hands also suffer. When they burst, and become ulcerated, they constitute an exceedingly painful affection.

Severe suffering from chilblains is an indication of constitutional taint not to be neglected, and individuals so afflicted should place themselves under a proper course of treatment; for until the system is completely renovated, they are continually subject to their recurrence.

THERAPEUTICS. In the treatment of this affection, the following medicines will be found valuable:

Nux vomica, *Pulsatilla*, *Belladonna*, *Arnica*, *Chamomilla*, *Arsenicum*, and *Sulphur*.

NUX VOMICA $\frac{000}{6}$, is particularly indicated when the inflammation is of a bright red colour, with swelling, attended with *itching, increased by warmth*, and when the chilblains evince a tendency to burst.

PULSATILLA $\frac{000}{6}$, when the inflammation is of a livid hue, with itching and beating in the part affected, and when the suffering comes on or is exacerbated in the evening or towards midnight. (*Sulphur* is often very useful after *Pulsatilla.*)

BELLADONNA $\frac{00}{12}$, when the inflammation is of a bluish red (but lighter than that indicating *Pulsatilla*), and *very considerable*, attended with a creeping, tingling sensation.

ARNICA $\frac{000}{6}$,* when the swelling is hard, *shining*, and painful, attended with itching.

CHAMOMILLA $\frac{000}{3}$, when with the inflammation and itching, a burning sensation is present, followed by

ARSENICUM $\frac{00}{12}$, when the pains are excessively violent, attended with severe burning, or when the chilblain bursts, and becomes converted into an irritable sore, with a tendency to fester. *Arsenicum* may in some such cases be advantageously alternated with *Carbo vegetabilis* $\frac{00}{12}$.

* The Homœopathic or Arnica Court Plaster, of sufficient size to cover the chilblain, is frequently of great service in mitigating the suffering.—ED.

Sulphur $\frac{000}{6}$ is a valuable remedy when the inflammation and itching are very severe, and the affection has refused to yield to the foregoing.

Administration. Two or three globules at the potency given after each medicine, repeated every three days, if necessary, until benefit results, or some other remedy becomes indicated. In the instance of *Arnica* we may also apply a lotion in the proportion of one part of the mother-tincture to five of water.* In conclusion, the following remedies may also be consulted: *Acidum nitricum, Petroleum, Rhus toxicodendron, Bryonia, Ledum, Mercurius, Cinchona*, and *Secale cornutum.*

CORNS. *Clavi Pedis.*

That these troublesome excrescences not unfrequently arise from an inherent vice of constitution, is evident from the fact that many individuals who wear tight boots and shoes, which are unquestionably the principal excitant, escape them, while others, with every precaution, suffer severely. Such being the case, the main object must be, by a course of properly-selected internal remedies, to eradicate the predisposing cause; among which, *Antimonium crudum*, (externally as well as internally, as described under the head of Chilblains,) *Phosphorus, Rhus, Bryonia*, and *Ammonium Carbonicum, Lycopodium, Petroleum, Sepia, Acidum Phosphoricum*, and *Sulphur*, will be found useful. Great alleviation of suffering has, however, been found to result from bathing the feet in warm water, and then applying a very weak *Arnica*† lotion, (a drop or two of the tincture to an ounce of water,) after having previously pared down the corn carefully.

* The external application of the other remedies also, is frequently very serviceable; in which case we may dissolve a few globules, or a drop or two of the tincture of the same remedy that we are administering internally, in about an ounce or so of water, and bathe the chilblains with the lotion twice a day; in addition to this, it is sometimes advantageous to envelop the affected parts in a piece of linen which has been dipped in the lotion.

† The Arnica plaster may be applied to corns as to chilblains, and will often afford the greatest relief to those corns commonly called *soft*.—Ed.

While upon this subject, it may be remarked that NUX VOMICA has been found serviceable in cases of swelling and redness of the *heel*, resembling chilblains, attended with acute, burning, shooting pains, materially increased by the pressure of the boot or shoe, or by walking.

Arnica may be recommended as above, should not *Nux vomica* be found to relieve.

ABSCESS. LYMPHATIC TUMOURS AND DISEASE OF THE CONGLOBATE GLANDS.

Abscess. By this term is meant a collection of purulent matter, resulting from morbid action, contained in a sac or cyst of organized coagulating lymph, furnished with absorbent and secreting vessels.

Abscesses are divided into acute and chronic. The former is preceded by sensible inflammation in the affected part, which is soon followed by suppuration. The commencement of the suppurative process is evidenced by a change in the description of pain, which becomes more obscure and throbbing, the increase of swelling, and, when matter is formed, by the perceptible fluctuation when the abscess is not too deeply seated; lastly, particularly in idiopathic cases, when the formation of pus is in considerable quantity, the fever which attended the previous inflammation is lessened, and irregular chills or rigours supervene, succeeded in turn by heat and increase of fever.

When the abscess is mature, the tumour points, or presents a sort of conical shape, generally near the centre of the cutaneous surface; over this spot the skin assumes a reddish hue, becomes thin, and ere long gives way, and allows the contents of the cavity to escape.

The signs of the formation or existence of a chronic abscess, on the other hand, are in the generality of instances devoid of any apparent disorder, either local or constitutional, until it begins to approach the surface and form an external swelling. The secreted matter is unhealthy, thin, and serous, and contains substances resembling curds or flakes. When the pus is evacuated, and the air admitted into the cavity, inflammation of the cyst arises, and is productive of a salutary effect, if the abscess be small; but if it be large, great constitutional disturbance ensues; the cavity, instead of contracting and filling up under the process of healthy granulation or incarnation, goes on discharging copiously, and hectic fever is produced.

THERAPEUTICS. In acute abscesses we may apply poultices and warm unmedicated fomentations, and forward the suppurative process by the administration of *Hepar sul.* $\frac{3}{6}$, in repeated doses. The lancet is never necessary except when the pus, by its extensive diffusion or pressure, especially when seated under ligamentous or tendinous expansions, is liable to injure important parts; or when, from its situation, there is reason to apprehend its discharge into any of the cavities of the body.

When it is necessary to effect an artificial opening by means of the lancet, the incision ought to be made at the most depending point where this can be safely or readily accomplished; and when this is impracticable, in consequence of the great thickness of the parts between the purulent matter and skin, the most prominent or pointed part ought to be selected. When, on the other hand, this latter happens to be at the upper part of the abscess, the lancet must be laid aside, and the abscess allowed to open spontaneously, or, still better, through the instrumentality, or at all events the important aid, of *Hepar sulphuris*, *Silicea*, and *Lachesis*. The former two may frequently be administered in alternation with advantage; the latter is more particularly to be preferred when a considerable portion of the skin has been much distended, and presents a deep red or bluish appearance, or where its structure has been destroyed by the magnitude of the abscess. *Mercurius* is occasionally useful when there is induration.* The subsequent

* *Carbo a.* is equally serviceable here, and may follow Mercurius when that remedy fails to answer our expectations. Baryta is also useful in such cases, particularly when there is considerable surrounding swelling as well as induration, even after the opening of the abscess.

treatment is generally more easily conducted, and the healing of the cavity more speedily effected, when the matter has been evacuated by the aid of the appropriate medicine, instead of the lancet.

In chronic abscesses, it has usually been found most beneficial to make an outlet for the matter as early as possible, to prevent a large accumulation, and thereby avoid the consequent frightful constitutional disturbance which is so prone to occur in such cases, from the extent of the inflammation after the bursting of the abscess. The opening should be made near the base of the abscess, and merely be large enough to admit of the exit of the matter.

When this collection of matter is very extensive, it frequently accumulates again after having been evacuated; hence it has been recommended to heal up the opening immediately, and to make a new one again when necessary, but before the pus has accumulated in any considerable quantity.

When the matter has been withdrawn, a dose or two of *Mercurius* should be administered, followed by *Hepar sulph.*, *Silicea*, and sometimes also by *Calcarea*, and *Phosphorus*. *Silicea* and *Phosphorus* have been described as useful when atrophy or consumption resulted in consequence of chronic suppuration.

It may here be mentioned that, in LYMPHATIC TUMOURS, *Sulphur*, and in ENCYSTED, (whether steatomatous or otherwise,) *Calcarea* has been found very efficacious.* Further, that in enlargement and induration of the CONGLOBATE GLANDS situate in the neck, under the chin, and behind the ears, such as is usually met with in scrofulous habits,—*Mercurius* and *Dulcamara* are two of the most important remedies.† When

* *Graphites*, *Silicea*, *Hepar s.*, and *Sulphur*, *Causticum*, *Baryta c.*, *Carbo v.*, *Acidum nitricum*, *Lachesis*, or *Phosphorus*, &c., may be found useful in some cases.

† In old standing or obstinate cases of glandular enlargement and induration, *Baryta c.*, *Staphysagria*, *Carbo a. et v.*, *Hepar s.*, *Sulphur*, *Calcarea*, and *Silicea*; as also *Kali c.*, *Lycopodium*, *Iodium*, *Acidum nitricum*, *Bovista*, or *Belladonna*, etc., are remedies of great utility, and must be selected according to the general features of the case, when *Mercurius* and *Dulcamara* are found insufficient to discuss the swelling, etc.

suppuration or ulceration ensues, *Hepar sulphuris*, *Lachesis*, and *Silicea*, are more useful. These latter, particularly *Hepar sul.* and *Silicea*, together with *Sulphur* and *Calcarea*, in some cases, are moreover extremely useful in materially obliterating the unsightly scars which are so frequently met with in glandular swellings which have been neglected or improperly treated by means of stimulating embrocations, caustics, &c.

ITCH. *Scabies. Psora.*

This contagious, inflammatory affection of the skin, is characterized by an eruption of pointed vesicles, transparent at the summit, and filled with a viscid and serous fluid. These are subsequently intermixed with, or terminate in pustules. With the exception of the face, they appear on every part of the body, but much more frequently and abundantly about the wrists, between the fingers, and at the bend of the joints, &c., and are accompanied by incessant and almost insupportable itching, without fever.

THERAPEUTICS. *Sulphur* is unquestionably the most important remedy in this disorder, particularly at the commencement. In the less violent varieties of the malady, and in the purulent species, especially when confined to the fingers and wrists, it is indeed specific.

A dose of the remedy may, in such instances, be administered daily for a week or ten days, but discontinued as soon as signs of improvement set in. In some rather obstinate cases, that is, when, after a fortnight to three weeks, but little improvement has been effected, we shall find the treatment facilitated by the simultaneous employment of the remedy externally, at the *same potency* which we are administering it internally, (by adding a few globules, or a drop, to a couple of ounces of water, and applying the liquid as a lotion night and morning). A very speedy or a *sudden suppression* of the eruption is, on the other hand, not to be regarded as a cure, but as a driving in or repercussion of the eruption.

Against other varieties of the disorder, and in neglected cases, *Sulphur* is not sufficient to effect a cure, and we are hence, frequently, under the necessity of having recourse to *Mercurius*,

Carbo v., *Hepar s.*, *Causticum*, *Sepia*, *Veratrum*, *Lycopod.*, etc. as follows: *Mercurius*, when the eruption is accompanied by intolerable itching, especially on becoming warm in bed; looks dry and cracking, but consists of minute vesicles resembling papillæ, when not narrowly examined, which are slightly inflamed and bleed easily when scratched (*scabies papuliformis*). These little elevations or vesicles are sometimes intermixed with pustules, which on breaking form scabs. It is sometimes necessary to administer *Sulphur* in alternation with *Mercurius*, in this form of the complaint, at intervals of four or five days, until an improvement or change in the symptoms result:—

In the event of an amelioration, it is found useful to cease to administer the medicine as long as it continues; but if the improvement soon comes to a close, or a change occurs in the character of the eruption, another remedy must be prescribed; if the affection has retained the papular-looking form, and *Mercurius* alone has previously been administered, *Hepar s.* may be selected; but if both *Sulphur* and *Mercurius* have been employed, *Carbo v.* may be advantageously alternated with *Hepar*; and should any symptoms remain thereafter, *Sepia* or *Veratrum* will generally speedily remove them. When, however, we observe that pustules have made their appearance, and are found interspersed amongst the original elevations upon the epigastrium, or other parts, *Causticum* should be selected. In scabies papuliformis: *Mezer.* and *Silic.*

In the postular or humid variety (*scabies purulenta*), distinguished by distinct, prominent yellow pustules, having a moderately inflamed base, which are usually met with on the hands and feet, and subsequently, if unchecked, on the back, shoulders, arms, and thighs, about the axillæ, and near the knee- and elbow-joints,—*Sulphur*, as has been already stated, is the principal remedy; considerable benefit will nevertheless be obtained by giving *Lycopodium* in alternation with it. Should improvement ensue, and the eruption take on a drier aspect, *Mercurius* and *Carbo v.* will in most instances serve to complete the cure. But if no beneficial effect is produced after two or three repetitions of these remedies at intervals of four or five days, *Graphites* must be exhibited at short intervals for three or four successive times, lengthening the intervals at each repetition of the dose; and should no alteration be brought about soon after, *Mercurius* may be administered in the same manner.

When the pustules are large, they coalesce and form irregular blotches, which sometimes ulcerate to a greater or less extent; in such cases *Clematis* and *Rhus* will be found serviceable. When, on the other hand, the pustules assume a prominent and globular form of a yellowish or bluish colour, *Lachesis* has been found to be the most appropriate remedy.

In *Scabies lymphatica*, or watery itch, characterized by transparent vesicles of considerable size, without an inflamed base, much the same treatment may be pursued as has been described for the dry or papuliform variety; in some cases thereof, however, the alternate use of *Sulphur*, *Rhus*, and *Arsenicum*, is requisite. When *Scabies* has been materially altered in its character by the abuse of *Sulphur* in allopathic practice, *Mercurius*, *Causticum*,—*Rhus* and *Staphysagria*,—or *Acid. nitricum*, *Dulcamara*, *Calcarea*, and *Pulsatilla*, have been used with success. Finally, *Creasote* externally (largely diluted) and internally, has been recommended in some obstinate cases of *Scabies;* and *Sulphur*, *Arsenicum*, and *Carbo v.* in cases which have been suppressed or repercussed by powerful external applications. Should furunculi appear: *Silicea*.

WHITLOW. *Paronychia. Panaris.*

By this term is understood an abscess more or less deeply seated, forming about the end of the finger, attended with severe pain and considerable swelling; it has much tendency to reappear in individuals who have once suffered from its attacks, which clearly demonstrates the advantage of treating it as a constitutional, and not as a merely local affection; in so doing we may have recourse to the following medicines: *Mercurius*, *Hepar Sulphuris*, *Rhus*, *Sulphur*, and *Silicea*.

THERAPEUTICS. We may generally commence the treatment by MERCURIUS.

Administration $\frac{00}{6}$, repeated every twelve hours, until relief is obtained. But should the swelling not decrease after a few doses of *Mercurius*, or the pain become intense, recourse must be had to the alternate administration of *Silicea* and *Hepar s.**

Rhus is more particularly indicated when there is a considerable degree of *erysipelatous* inflammation.

Administration $\frac{00}{3}$, in the same manner as *Mercurius*.

Lachesis. In cases where the affected part is of a dark red or bluish hue, and the pains extremely violent, this remedy may be administered, followed by *Arsenicum* and *Carbo v.*, if an angry-looking, black, and painfully burning sore form on the affected finger.†

But we must have recourse to the alternate administration of Sulphur $\frac{00}{30}$, and Silicea $\frac{00}{30}$, at intervals of eight days each, in cases where a constant tendency to a recurrence of the complaint exists.‡ These remedies, particularly the latter, are the most appropriate in those severe cases in which the matter forms between the periosteum and bone, and when the latter has become diseased in consequence.

Magnetis Polus Articus. The application of the north pole of the magnet for a minute or two to the finger will often afford speedy relief when the pain is so intense as to be almost insupportable. A poultice is also somewhat soothing under such circumstances.

IRRITATION OR ITCHING OF THE SKIN. *Prurigo.*

This affection is usually an accompaniment of other diseases, and is to be treated accordingly; however, in some

These two remedies are moreover exceedingly serviceable in forwarding suppuration, and are therefore equally useful in rapidly bringing the abscess to maturity, and causing the discharge of the pus, when it is no longer possible to effect resolution; but when the matter is deep seated, and evacuation is not speedly obtained, the lancet must be employed.

† *Hering's Hausarzt.*

‡ *Hepar s.* and *Causticum* have likewise been recommended as useful for the attainment of this desirable end.

cases it declares itself in an idiopathic form, and is generally caused by scarcely perceptible colourless elevations under the cuticle; at other times, they are of a considerable size, soft and smooth, but without desquamation, or any peculiar eruptive appearance.

THERAPEUTICS. Against this extremely distressing irritation, SULPHUR is frequently the specific remedy, particularly when exacerbation ensues on the evening, or when the body is warm in bed; but in other and more ordinary cases, the following remedies will be found serviceable: *Ignatia amara, Pulsatilla, Mercurius, Rhus toxicodendron, Hepar sulphuris, Nux vomica*, or *Arsenicum album.*

IGNATIA AMARA. When the irritation is most severe, after going to bed, and resembles flea-bites all over the body, and after scratching,—which relieves—shifts readily from one part to another.

PULSATILLA. When the irritation comes on in the warmth of the bed, and is aggravated by scratching.

MERCURIUS. When the irritation continues through the whole night, and *Pulsatilla* proves insufficient; also in cases when the parts affected bleed readily after scratching. (*Sulphur* is sometimes useful every four or five days, in alternation with *Mercurius*, in such cases.)

RHUS TOXICODENDRON. When itching is accompanied by violent burning sensation, followed by

HEPAR SULPHURIS, if necessary, to complete the cure.

NUX VOMICA alternately with ARSENICUM, when the irritation or itching appears on undressing.

In obstinate cases of almost all kinds, *Sulphur*, followed by *Carbo v.*, will be found serviceable. *Lycopodium, Graphites, Silicea*, &c., may be called for in particular cases. *Opium* is often useful in the case of old people.

In Prurigo scroti, *Sulphur, Acidum nitricum, Dulcamara*, and *Rhododendron*, have chiefly been recommended.—Prurigo pudendi: *Sulphur, Sepia, Conium, Calcarea, Natrum m.*, and *Sulphur.*—P. ani: *Sepia, Acidum nitricum, Thuja, Mercurius, Sulphur*, as also *Kali c., Baryta c.*, and *Zincum.*

ADMINISTRATION $\frac{000}{30}$, in four dessert-spoonfuls of water, one daily; to be repeated, if necessary.* Of *Mercurius* and *Rhus toxicodendron* we may substitute the sixth for the thirtieth potency.

RINGWORM (HERPETIC OR VESICULAR.)

Herpes circinnatus. Herpes serpigo.

This affection generally occurs in children. It has been considered contagious from the circumstance of several children of one family, or at the same school, being sometimes attacked at the same time; but there is every reason to believe that this opinion is erroneous, from the circumstance of none of the other species of herpes being communicable by contact. When not complicated with another disease, it is not attended with any general constitutional derangement. The disorder is characterized by an eruption of small rings or circular bands, the vesicles only occupying the circumference; these are small, and have a red coloured base of greater or less intensity. About the third or fifth day the vesicles become turbid, and then discharge, when little brownish scabs form over them. The portions of skin within the circlets are usually healthy at first; but for the most part subsequently become rough, of a reddish hue, and scale off as the vesicular eruption dies away. The duration of the eruption frequently does not extend beyond a week or two, but when there is a series of consecutive rings on the face, neck, arms, and shoulders, as more frequently happens in warm climates (where the affection moreover assumes a more serious and obstinate character), or during hot weather in this country, it is necessarily protracted considerably beyond this period.

TREATMENT. In the majority of cases, the affection yields readily under the action of *Sepia*, of which from two to three globules of the sixth potency may be given in a little water, and the dose repeated on the fourth day, if required by any appearance of tardiness in the subsidence of the eruption, or should there be any indications of the formation of fresh rings.

* Vide note, p. 21.

In some obstinate cases, the alternate use of *Rhus* and *Sulph.* every four or five days is found necessary. *Calcarea* and *Causticum* have been recommended in others. All kinds of outward applications must be avoided.

RINGWORM OF THE SCALP. PUSTULAR RINGWORM.

Porrigo Scutulata. Tinea Capitis. Tinea Annularis. Favus Confertus.

This disease is still more popularly known than the above by the term of *ringworm* (or *ringworm of the scalp*). It is unquestionably of a highly contagious nature, being readily communicated among children who make use of the same comb and brush, or even towel, and is of long and uncertain continuance,—indeed there are few cutaneous affections which have more frequently baffled the unwearied efforts of practitioners than it has done; and it would have been well had *less* been attempted by those of the old-school in the way of treatment; for in but too many instances the so-called *cure* has proved worse than the disease.

Pustular ringworm commonly attacks children from the age of two years to the period of puberty; it is not confined to the scalp, but also appears on the neck, trunk, and extremities; when confined to the trunk, it proves by no means so obstinate and rebellious a disease as when located in the hairy scalp.

Diagnosis. The affection is characterized by circular red-coloured patches, on which appear numerous small yellowish points or pustules, which do not rise above the level of the skin, and are generally traversed in the centre by a hair. These pustules, which are much more thickly studded in the circumference than the centre of the circular patches, soon break and form thin scabs,* which frequently unite with the

* Sometimes cup-shaped, or concave (characteristic of *favus*), and at first of a tawny, but subsequently of a light yellow or whitish colour; when they crack and break up, they become reduced to a powder which looks like pulverized sulphur.

adjacent patches, and assume an extensive and irregular appearance, but commonly retain a somewhat circular shape. These incrustations become thick and hard by accumulation, and are detached from time to time in small pieces which bear a close resemblance to crumbling mortar. When the scabs are removed, the surface is left red and glossy, but studded with slightly elevated pimples, in some of which minute globules of matter appear in the course of a few days.

By these repetitions of the eruptions, the incrustations become thicker, the areas of the primary patches extend, and new ones are formed, so that the corresponding edges become blended, and frequently the whole head thus becomes affected. The circular character of the primary groups is still indicated, however, by the portions of arcs of a circle perceptible in the circumference of the larger incrustations. As the patches of clusters extend, the hair covering them usually becomes lighter in colour, and breaks off short, and as the process or scabbing is repeated, it is thrown out by the roots, and finally there remains only a narrow chaplet of hair round the head. If the hair follicles are destroyed, the baldness remains permanent.

Causes. The disease appears to originate spontaneously in children of scrofulous, flabby, or feeble and emaciated habit, if they be ill-fed, ill-lodged, uncleanly, and not sufficiently exercised; but it is chiefly propagated by contagion.

Therapeutics. It cannot be denied that, even under homœopathic treatment, the disease frequently proves extremely obstinate; but in many cases the difficulty experienced in effecting a cure arises from the previous treatment which the patient has undergone, or from the culpable conduct on the part of the parents or others in having allowed the disorder to pursue its course for a lengthened period, unchecked and utterly neglected, ere proper assistance is sought.

The following are the principal remedies employed in the homœopathic treatment:

Rhus, Arsenicum, Staphysagria, Hepar s., Lycopodium, Dulcamara, Bryonia, Phosphorus, Graphites, Baryta c., Calcarea, Oleander, Sulphur, &c.

The medicines must be selected according to the various changes which take place throughout the course of the disease; but as it would occupy much more space than would be warranted in a work like the present, to attempt to give directions calculated to meet every case, it will be necessary to give only a few of the general indications for some of the more important remedies, and merely to point out others as being worthy of attention in cases which do not yield to the ordinary remedies. While the patches are in an irritable and inflammatory condition, *Rhus* will usually be found the most appropriate remedy; the head should at the same time be regularly and gently sponged with tepid water twice a day, and a linen cap worn. Should a dry exfoliation and scabbing then ensue, *Sulphur* may be had recourse to; but if, on the other hand, an offensive discharge breaks out, attended by violent itching, without much redness, *Staphysagria* may be administered, and then again *Rhus*. If, notwithstanding the administration of these remedies, very little favourable progress is made, or if, on the contrary, the affection becomes rather worse, and the exudation takes on an acrimonious character, and is productive of an extension of the disorder, or of the formation of ulcers, *Arsenicum* must be exhibited; after the action of which, *Rhus* will frequently produce a satisfactory effect. These remedies may occasionally be applied externally also with good effect, by dissolving a few globules of the remedy used in a little water, and applying the liquid once or twice a day to the affected parts.

When the foregoing remedies are insufficient to effect a cure, which is unfortunately not a rare circumstance, particularly when strumous subjects are afflicted with the disease, the following remedies must be used:

Hepar s., when the eruption is not confined to the head, but also appear upon the forehead, face, and neck; when, moreover, the eyes and eyelids become inflamed and weakened, and soreness or ulceration breaks out on or behind the ears. In the latter case, *Baryta c.*, *Graphites* and *Oleander* are also useful.

Dulcamara, when the glands of the throat and neck are enlarged and indurated (or *Bryonia* when there is inflammation and tenderness of the said glands); after which *Staphysagria* may be administered, and then one or more of the remedies mentioned at the commencement, followed by *Baryta c.*

If these remedies prove ineffectual, *Sulphur*, *Graphites*, *Calcarea*, *Lycopodium*, *Phosphorus*, or *Oleander*, must be administered according to circumstances. In some cases, the alternate use of two or more will be found advantageous, such as *Sulphur* and *Calcarea*,—*Sulphur*, *Rhus*, and *Graphites*,—*Graphites* and *Lycopodium*,—*Graphites* and *Phosphorus*, and so on. When there is soreness of the ears in addition, *Hepar s.*, *Baryta c.*, *Graphites* and *Oleander* claim some preference. A dry, inert, and scaly appearance of the eruption chiefly requires *Sulphur* and *Calcarea*, but also *Hepar*, *Phosphorus*, *Rhus*, and *Arsenicum* or *Oleander*. A humid or moist-looking eruption: *Staphysagria*, *Rhus*, *Arsenicum*, *Lycopodium*, *Sulphur*, *Sepia*, and also: *Baryta c.*, *Calcarea c.*, *Graphites*, *Cicuta virosa*, and *Oleander*.

In the other varieties of scald-head, such as the *Porrigo lupinosa*,* *Porrigo furfurans*,† *Porrigo favosa*,‡ &c., the same

* Characterized by small, dry, circular scabs, of a yellowish white colour, having raised margins, and a central depression, like that on the seeds of the lupine. The incrustations are deeply set in the skin, to which their edges are firmly adherent.

† This variety commences with the eruption of small pustules containing a straw-coloured fluid, which soon discharge dry, and form thin laminated crusts, or scale-like exfoliations. This affection is confined to the scalp, and is attended with considerable itching and soreness, although there is but slight excoriation; the hair partially falls off, and occasionally becomes subsequently somewhat lighter in colour.

‡ Distinguished by the eruption of large, soft, straw-coloured pustules, generally somewhat flattened, possessing an irregular margin, and surrounded by a slight inflammatory redness. They are met with on other parts of the body as well as the scalp, and are accompanied by much itching. On breaking, these pustules discharge a viscid matter, which hardens into semi-transparent, greenish-yellow scales. The disease extends to the face, and eventually the ulceration spreads over the entire head, and from the continued discharge the hair and moist scabs become matted together. Pediculi are generated in large numbers, and aggravate the excessive irritation. The incrustations thicken into irregular masses, bearing some resemblance to honey-comb. The acrid exudation from the ulcerated patches on the scalp exhales an offensive and pungent vapour.

class of remedies are required as above enumerated; whilst against *Porrigo decalvans* (characterized chiefly by patches of baldness), *Graphites*, *Phosphorus*, *Baryta*, *Lycopodium*, and *Zincum*, have been found the most serviceable; but *Sulphur*, *Calcarea*, *Silicea*, &c., and most of the other aforesaid remedies, may be found indicated in particular cases. With regard to the administration of the remedies, it may be stated that at the commencement of the disorder, a dose may be given daily, or every second day, until symptoms of improvement make their appearance, in which case the medicine must be discontinued while the case progresses favourably, and only renewed when matters become stationary or the disorder threatens to extend itself. When no signs of improvement become perceptible, or when, on the contrary, the malady evidently seems to be getting gradually worse, notwithstanding the exhibition of two or three doses of a particular remedy, another must be selected according to the indications.

In cases of old standing, the intervals between the repetition of the dose must generally be lengthened, or a dose may be given daily for a week, and then a period of ten to twelve days, and even upwards, allowed to elapse before the medicine is repeated, or another remedy substituted.

Undeviating attention to cleanliness must be observed throughout the entire course of the complaint, and the homœopathic diet rules strictly adhered to in the majority of cases. The hair ought to be removed early in the disease.

ULCERS. *Ulcera.*

An ulcer may be the result of a wound, bruise, burn, or abscess; it may also arise from a bad condition of body, particularly when combined with sedentary habits, and gross or unwholesome living. In the latter case, its formation is preceded by a greater or less degree of pain, heat, redness, and swelling in the part. In many instances a little vesicle or pustule appears, which, on bursting, exposes a gap or breach in the skin. Sometimes there is at the commencement a single small excavation; at others, several contiguous ulcerated spots are observed, which speedily become blended together, and form a sore of considerable magnitude.

When no effort at cicatrization or healing is taking place, the ulcer always presents an excavation or hollow, the margins of which are red, sharp, sometimes thick, prominent, rounded, and callous, but often jagged and irregular. The surface of the ulcer at the same time presents a dirty white or yellowish colour, and is usually covered with, and discharges a thin watery humour or sanies, frequently tinged with blood, and sometimes so acrid as to inflame and corrode the skin. While the process of ulceration is extending, the edge of the adjacent skin is inflamed and painful; but as soon as a tendency to heal sets in, this ceases, and healthy granulations form, which present a florid colour, are of a firm consistence, and have a pointed shape resembling minute cones. The matter secreted is altered to a bland, thick, and whitish or cream-like fluid (healthy pus) not adherent to the granulating surface. These granulations do not rise higher than the surrounding skin, and when they have risen to the level of the latter, those at the margin of the ulcer become covered with a smooth thin bluish film, which is at first semi-transparent, but soon changes to an opaque on being converted into new skin.

Therapeutics. In the treatment of ulcers in general, the following are the most important remedies: *Arsenicum*, *Carbo v.*, *Lachesis*, *Mercurius*, *Sulphur*, *Silicea*, *Sepia*, *Lycopodium*.

Arsenicum is chiefly useful when the ulcer presents a livid aspect, or looks bloody, and bleeds at the slightest touch, and, instead of healthy pus, secretes an ichorous discharge mixed with blood; the edges of the sore are at the same time hard and irregular, and the patient complains of great pain, particularly of an intense *burning* description. *Carbo v.* is indicated under similar circumstances, and is therefore very useful in alternation with the former remedy, especially when the discharge from the ulcer is of a very offensive nature, and the burning pains are much exacerbated towards evening and during the night. When the ulcer is large, or seems disposed to extend rapidly, or when it is surrounded by numerous small ulcerations or pustules; further, when there is considerable swelling and discoloration of the surrounding parts, the leg presenting a mottled, dark-blue or purple aspect,—*Lachesis* forms a most important and eminently useful remedy.

Mercurius will usually be found very serviceable when the ulcer is deep, and secretes a thin and offensive discharge; but should healthy granulation not supervene on the filling up of the cavity under the action of *Mercurius: Sulphur* or *Silicea*, or both these remedies, must be prescribed alternately. When the discharge continues thin and offensive notwithstanding the employment of *Mercurius*, *Asafœtida* may be administered, provided *Arsenicum*, or some other remedy, does not merit a perference.

Sulphur is almost indispensable in nearly every case of long standing, and is frequently sufficient of itself to effect a cure in many chronic cases. It is more particularly indicated, however, when excessive itching, burning, or gnawing and smarting pains are experienced in the sore, and there is at the same time œdematous swelling, and reddish brown discoloration of the limb, when the ulcer is seated in the inferior extremities.

Silicea is another remedy of nearly equal importance to *Sulphur* in the treatment of chronic ulcers. It is accordingly of the utmost service in many cases when administered in alternation with that remedy, and in those of a very obstinate character, with *Sepia* and *Acidum nitricum*. The secretion of a thick and discoloured pus is a useful indication for *Silicea*. When the pus is of a deep yellow colour, the margins of the ulcer callous or inverted, and an intolerable itching, sometimes with pain of a burning description, is experienced at night in bed,—*Lycopodium* may be given with advantage; also in *superficial* chronic ulcers.

In administering the remedies, it is frequently sufficient to give a dose every eight or ten days; in other cases, it is found necessary to dissolve a few globules, or a drop or two of the tincture at the 6th, 12th, or 30th potency, in a pint or so of pure water, to which a tablespoonful of spirits of wine has been added, and order a tablespoonful to be taken daily.*

* Vide note, p. 21.

When the ulcer is inflamed or extremely painful, a soothing effect is often derived from the application of linen dipped in warm water; and if the ulcer be seated in the leg, the affected limb should be kept at rest, and not allowed to remain in a depending position. In others, and a still larger number of cases, the application of lint dipped in, and kept constantly wet with cold water, is more efficacious, especially when the ulcer presents a sharp, jagged, and undermined appearance, with no distinct formation of granulations, but exhibits a surface consisting of a whitish spongy substance, covered with a thin and acrid discharge, and bleeds on being dressed.

When, on the other hand, the granulations are sufficiently developed, but of a pale colour, and often large and flabby, with a smooth and glossy surface, the edges of the sourrounding skin being at the same time thick, prominent and rounded, the pus thin and watery, intermixed with flakes of coagulating lymph which adheres closely to the surface of the sore, but the pain trifling, and the sore comparatively insensible,—considerable assistance will generally be derived from the employment of a moderately tight and properly applied bandage.

The promotion of healthy granulation and cicatrization is, further, materially forwarded by the external employment of the same remedy which we are prescribing internally, (in the manner as described under the heading of CHILBLAINS); and in other cases, it will be found sufficient to keep the dressings constantly wet with cold water.

We must, however, never omit the internal administration of the appropriate remedy, otherwise the sore will be liable to break out again and again at longer or shorter intervals, though apparently healed up in a satisfactory manner, under the employment of external treatment alone.* In the treatment of healthy or healing ulcers, dry lint may be applied to

* In chronic indolent ulcers on the inferior extremities, such as are frequently met with in elderly persons, the treatment ought to be exclusively internal at the *commencement*, and the doses administered at intervals of a week and upwards.

the wound, and the dressing changed only once in forty-eight hours, when the secretion of pus is scanty, and not sufficient to moisten the lint in a shorter period.

Ulcers attended with, or arising from a varicose state of the veins, are usually very obstinate and difficult to heal, particularly when it is inconvenient or impossible for the affected party to remain at rest. Under such circumstances, it is essential that a properly fitting bandage or laced stocking should be worn. The best remedies calculated to effect a permanent cure are: *Arnica, Pulsatilla, Lachesis, Sulphur*, and *Silicea*; also *Arsenicum, Carbo v.*, and *Acid. phosphoricum.* The two first named, when given alternately about once a week, early in the disorder, are occasionally sufficient to effect a cure; but for the most part it is necessary to have recourse to the others, either to complete the cure or to prevent a relapse. The indications for their selection are, in this form of ulcer, much the same as already given in the treatment of ulcers in general. *Acidum phosphoricum* is extremely useful in cases with more or less lymphatic ulceration, particularly when the patient has previously been powerfully affected with mercury under allopathic treatment.

Acidum nitricum will prove of essential service after *Acid. phos.* if required.

Sepia, Arsenicum, Petroleum, Silicea, and *Sulphur*, are the most serviceable when proud flesh forms on the ulcers.

Against the following varieties of ulcers, most of the subjoined medicines have been found of the greatest utility.*

PHAGEDÆNIC. *Arsenicum, Silicea, Mezereum, Hepar s., Sulphur*; also *Conium, Acid. nitricum*, and *Ranunculus.*

SCROFULOUS. *Sulphur, Silicea, Calcarea, Lycopod., Carbo v., Arsenicum, Acid. mur., Baryta acet.*, and *Belladonna.*

PUTRID ULCERS, or those occurring in *Cachectic, Scorbutic* subjects. *Sulphur, Silicea, Arsenicum, Carbo v., Hepar s., Acidum muriaticum, Pulsatilla*, and, in some instances, *Ammon. c. et m.*

* The characteristic indications for many of the remedies will be found in Bœnninghausen's Manual of Homœopathic Therapeutics, by Chs. Hempel, M. D.

GANGRENOUS ULCERS. *Arsenicum*, *Lachesis*, *Cinchona*, *Silicea*, *Belladonna*, and *Conium*; also *Rhus toxicodendron*, *Secale cornutum*, and *Squilla*.

CARCINOMATOUS. *Arsenicum*, *Lachesis*, *Conium*, *Sulphur*, *Silicea*, *Diadema aranea*, *Mercurius*; also *Aurum*, *Staphysagria*, and *Hepar s*.

FISTULOUS. *Sulphur*, *Silicea*, *Calcarea*, *Lycopodium*, *Pulsatilla*, and *Antimon*.*

MERCURIAL. *Hepar s.*, *Acidum nitricum*, *Acidum phosphoricum*, *Aurum*, *Carbo vegetabilis*, *Sulphur*, *Silicea*, *Belladonna*, *Thuja*, *Sarsaparilla* and *Acid. fluor.* (especially about the ankle, with more or less implication of the bones).

SYPHILITIC. *Mercurius* chiefly, but also *Acid. nitricum*, to promote healthy granulation when the former is *insufficient*, or to combat mercurial complication when the patient has previously been subjected to injurious doses of that remedy. In other cases, *Lachesis* and *Thuja* are requisite to establish the cure.

It may be added here, that *Thuja* and *Acidum nitricum*, applied externally and internally, are the chief remedies against SYCOSIS. In some cases of this affection, however, *Mercurius* and *Sulphur*, alternately, or one or more of the following remedies: *Acidum phosph.*, *Cinnabar*, *Lycopodium*, *Euphrasia*, *Staphysagria*, and *Sabina*, will be found requisite.

* In *fistula in ano*: *Sulph.*, *Calc.*, *Silex*, *Caus.*, and *Puls.*, have chiefly been employed with success. In *fungous ulcers*: *Sulphur*, *Silicea*, *Calcarea*, *Graphites*, *Sepia*, *Staphysagria*, *Petroleum*, *Antimonium*, *Iodium*, *Thuja*, and *Acid. nitric.*; and in *fungus hæmatodes*: *Phosphorus*, *Thuja*, *Acid. nitr.*

GENERAL

DERANGEMENT OF THE SYSTEM.

GOUT. *Arthritis.*

This disease, particularly when it has assumed the chronic form, requires a long and discriminative course of treatment. The chief danger arises from its liability to transfer its seat from the part first attacked, to some of the principal internal organs, such as the head and stomach; in such instances it assumes a peculiarly critical character.

From some peculiar predisposition, it is often hereditary; until therefore this tendency is eradicated by a proper mode of treatment, where practicable, it is useless to expect a permanent cure.

Diagnosis. Pains in the joints, with inflammatory or chronic cold swelling, with symptoms of deranged digestion.

These signs, however, may only partially declare themselves, or be marked by some other chronic malady; indeed, there is scarcely any disease of that character with which it may not be complicated.

Prior to the attack, we generally find symptoms of general derangement of the digestive function, with slight access of fever; the veins of the feet become swollen, and a sense of numbness, cramps, or twitching, is present, with a deficiency of perspiration. When the attack comes on, which most frequently occurs in the evening or during the night, it is generally with a feeling of dislocation in the joints of the feet, and burning or severe scalding pain in the part attacked, more or less intense; after a time these sensations disappear, leaving the part red and tumefied; the fit occurs again at intervals, generally diminishing in intensity; in many instances, considerable fever is present.

Among the exciting causes of gout may be numbered the following: a luxurious mode of life; stimulating diet or drinks; sudden check of perspiration; mental emotions; sedulous application to studious pursuits, and neglect of taking proper exercise in the open air; and a use of aperient medicines and tonics. In plethoric habits, the gout shows a considerable inclination to shift its seat to the head, and in dyspeptic individuals to the stomach and intestines.

THERAPEUTICS. In general cases of this affection, the principal medicaments are *Aconite, Pulsatilla, Nux v.*, and *Bryonia.*

ACONITE in plethoric or corpulent habits, when there is considerable inflammatory fever, with hard and quick pulse.

ADMINISTRATION. $\frac{0\,0}{6}$ in a little water, repeated in six hours if necessary; in very severe cases exhibited as in INFLAMMATORY FEVER.

PULSATILLA, where the pains are of a shifting nature, exacerbated towards *evening or in bed,* with paralytic or torpid sensation in the part affected, and more particularly when the dyspeptic symptoms given under this medicine (see INDIGESTION or DYSPEPSIA) present themselves, and when the pain is relieved by uncovering the affected limb.

When, on the contrary, the pain is increased by uncovering, and relieved by warmth, the patient weak, depressed, and exhausted, *Arsenicum* will be found of material service in affording relief. Pains worse at night, with restlessness and constant necessity to change the position of the extremities; pale and anxious or haggard countenance, are generally relieved by *Ferrum,* or *Ferrum* and *Rhus* in alternation; and in other cases by *Cin.*, especially when there is sensibility to the touch, and aggravation of the sufferings from the most trivial pressure or blow.

ADMINISTRATION. $\frac{0\,0}{6}$ repeated in from six to twenty-four hours, according to results.*

NUX VOMICA, when the pains are *worse towards the morning;* a paralytic and torpid sensation, with *cramps and throbbings in the muscles;* and moreover, when in addition to other

* Vide note, page 21

dyspeptic symptoms, we find constipation and hemorrhoids, or inclination to that affection, and an irritable or choleric temperament; furthermore, when indulgence in wine or fermented liquors has been the inducing cause.

Administration. Same as *Pulsatilla.*

Bryonia, where the pains are *increased by the slightest motion;* aggravation of suffering at night; coldness and shivering, with general perspiration or fever. For the dyspeptic symptoms present, see article *indigestion*, p. 95.

Administration. *Same as Pulsatilla.*

Each of the medicines here mentioned may successfully follow *Aconite*, when the febrile symptoms have been in some measure brought under by the administration of that remedy.

In chronic cases, the applicability of the following medicines should be consulted: *Argent., Lycopodium, Aurum, Sulphur, Calcarea carb., Colocynth, Hepar sulph., Colchicum, Phosphorus, Conium, Daphne, Kali c., Causticum, Guajacum, Iodium, Rhododendron,* and *Manganum.* Also, as intermediate remedies,—*Arnica, Ledum palustre,* and *Sabina.*

In ARTHRITIS VAGA the following remedies have been recommended in addition to *Pulsatilla: Nux v., Arnica, Manganum, Nux moschata:* and also *Rhododendron, Plumbum, Daphne,* and *Asafœtida.*

ARTHRITIC NODOSITIES. *Caustic., Lycopod., Aurum, Ledum, Graphites, Rhododend., Calcarea, Sepia, Staphysagria.* As also, *Agnus, Antimon., Bryonia, Phosph., Sabina, Zincum.* ARTHRITIC CONTRACTIONS are sometimes benefited by *Sulphur, Causticum, Bryonia, Rhus, Guajacum:* —or, *Colocynth, Silicea, Calcarea,* &c. *Arthritis* occurring in individuals whose occupations compel them to work in the water, is chiefly to be relieved by *Calcarea, Pulsatilla, Sarsaparilla,* and *Sulphur.*—And in some cases by *Arsenic, Dulcamara, Antimonium, Nux moschata* and *Rhus.*—*Nux v.* is one of the most important remedies against the precursory symptoms of gout; and *Belladonna* against recent *metastasis.* In CHIRAGRA: *Nux v., Bry., Lyc., Cocc., Ant., Agn., Rhod., Sulph., Lach., Led.,* &c., are the most generally appropriate remedies. And in PODAGRA: *Arnica, Sabina, Ledum;* in many cases are equally important; *Bry.*, *Sulph.*, *Calc.*, *Cocc.*, *Am. c.* and *muriat.*, *Ambr.*, *Lyc.*, &c.

RHEUMATISM. *Rheumatismus.*

Diagnosis. Pains in the muscular or membranous structure, generally with swelling of the adjacent cellular tissue, with slight redness and increased generation of heat, caused by taking cold.

This disease is of two kinds, the *Acute* and *Chronic;* the former is accompanied by fever, preceded by restlessness; heat alternating with chills; thirst; coldness of the limbs and extremities; constipation and accelerated pulse, followed by pains in the large joints, generally shifting their situation, leaving redness, swelling, and tenderness, of the parts affected; it is also frequently attended with excessive perspiration and weakness. In the latter, or Chronic Rheumatism, the swelling of the parts, except in very severe cases, is commonly less perceptible; sometimes there is present a feeling of general stiffness or numbness, with little or no fever.

Other symptoms incidental to this complaint, we shall notice more particularly under the head of the different medicaments more efficacious in the treatment. The principal exciting causes are damp, chill, or a sudden check of perspiration. People who have resided long in a tropical climate or have been subject to continual exposure to cold or wet, are very liable to suffer from rheumatism in the chronic form.

Therapeutics. In the treatment of this affection, the following medicaments have been found particularly useful: *Aconitum, Belladonna, Bryonia, Chamomilla, Nux vomica, Mercurius, Pulsatilla, Rhus toxicodendron,* &c.

Aconitum when we find high fever, dry heat, thirst, and redness of the cheeks; excessive *shooting or tearing pains,* extremely violent at night; occasionally redness or shining swelling of the parts affected; aggravation of pains by the touch; excessive irascibility of temper.

ADMINISTRATION. $\frac{0\,0}{6}$ in a little water, repeated every six hours, until the fever is lowered; in *very severe* cases exhibited as in INFLAMMATORY FEVER, which see.

BELLADONNA is useful when the pains are of a shooting or burning description, principally in the joints, aggravated by movement, and worse at night; when the parts attacked are much swollen, very red, and shining, and particularly when there is fever, with determination of blood to the head, with throbbing of the vessels of that part, and redness of the face, heat of skin, thirst, sleeplessness, pain.

ADMINISTRATION. $\frac{0\,0}{6}$ in a little water, repeated every twelve or twenty-four hours, according to circumstances.*

BRYONIA may follow *Aconite*, or the preceding medicine, with great benefit, or be administered independently. The following are the more prominent symptoms: severe shooting pains, much increased by motion of the affected part, or by a cold draught of air; swelling of the joints of the upper and lower extremities; headache, gastric derangements, and constipation; pains aggravated at night, or particularly on the slightest irritation; irascibility and perverseness of temper; the pains seem situated more in the muscles, and particularly about the joints, than in the bones.

ADMINISTRATION. Same as *Belladonna*. In general cases it is advisable to repeat the medicine in twenty-four hours.

CHAMOMILLA when we find dragging or tearing pains, with a sensation of numbness or of *paralysis* in the parts affected, feverishness; great agitation and tossing; desire to remain lying down; perspiration; exacerbation of suffering at night, with temporary relief from sitting up in bed, or frequent changing of posture. Aching pains all over on awaking in the morning, and chilliness during the day.

ADMINISTRATION. $\frac{0\,0}{3}$, in the same manner as *Belladonna*.

NUX VOMICA $\frac{0\,0}{6}$, when there are, sensation of numbness, paralysis, or tightness in the parts affected, with cramps and palpitation of the muscles; pains of a dragging description, chiefly confined to the joints, trunk of the body, back, loins,

* Vide note, p. 21.

and chest, aggravated by cold; gastric derangement; constipation; irritability of temper. *Cocc.* and *Ignat.* after *Nux.*

ADMINISTRATION. Same as *Belladonna.*

MERCURIUS is indicated in cases where the pains are increased by the warmth of the bed, or exposure to damp or cold air, aggravated at night, and *especially towards morning;* also where there is considerable puffy swelling of the parts affected. This medicine is particularly useful when the pains seem seated in the bones or joints; *profuse perspiration without alleviation of suffering,* is also a good indication for its employment. (*Lachesis* is often efficacious when *Mercurius* fails to relieve the foregoing symptoms.)

ADMINISTRATION. Same as *Belladonna.*

PULSATILLA $\frac{00}{12}$, is useful in *shifting* rheumatic pains, particularly if attended with a sense of torpor or paralysis, relieved by exposure to cool air, worse at night or in the evening.

ADMINISTRATION. Same as *Belladonna.*

RHUS TOXICODENDRON $\frac{00}{6}$, is indicated when there are: Sensation of torpor, dullness, and crawling, with feeling of *paralytic weakness or trembling of the extremities* when attempting to move them; sensation of bruising or of laceration, as if the flesh were torn from the bones, or as of scraping of the bones; *pains worse during rest,* relieved by motion; inflammatory or shining redness in the joints, with stiffness, and sometimes a darting pain when handled; aggravation of suffering in cold or damp weather. This remedy may sometimes follow *Bryonia* with considerable advantage. *Ferrum* is sometimes useful in alternation with *Rhus,* particularly when the pains are relieved by frequently shifting the position of the limbs.

COLCHICUM. Rheumatism, with gastric derangement and slight fever during the prevalence of cold, damp weather.

ADMINISTRATION. Same as *Belladonna.*

Obstinate cases of rheumatism frequently require a long, careful, and discriminative treatment. In some cases much benefit will be obtained from repeated doses of *Sulphur;* in others, *Calcarea,* particularly when the pains are increased at every change of the weather. *Hepar sulphuris* and *La-*

chesis alternately have been recommended in the severest kinds of acute rheumatism. *Colocynth* is frequently useful against the stiffness which remains. In the event of a sudden metastasis to the chest, attended with oppressed respiration, palpitation of the heart, and excessive agitation, *Aconitum* should be immediately administered in repeated doses until relief is obtained; but should improvement only prove temporary, *Sulphur* and *Pulsatilla* have been recommended to be given in alternation. *Belladonna* and *Bryonia* may also be of service in dangerous results of this kind. When the heart becomes implicated in acute rheumatism or rheumatic fever, (*endocarditis rheumatica,*) *Bellad.* $\frac{000}{3}$, in repeated doses, is a useful remedy if timely administered; and may in some cases be advantageously employed in alternation with *Acon.*, and followed by *Spigelia* $\frac{000}{3}$ and *Digitalis* $\frac{000}{3}$; also *Arsenicum.*

These remedies, together with *Cannabis, Arsenicum, Lachesis,* in some instances are the most valuable in the treatment of idiopathic ENDOCARDITIS OR CARDITIS.

For CHRONIC RHEUMATISM, the following are the principal remedies: *Sulph., Lycop., Caust., Hepar, Lach., Phos., Veratr., Clem.* When the pains are aggravated or excited by the slightest chill,—*Aconite, Calc., Bry., Dulc., Merc., Sulph., Acid. phos.*, will generally be found the best from which to select a remedy. When the attacks are excited by unfavourable weather,—*Calc., Rhus, Dulc., Rhod., Verat.*, or *Lycop., Carb. v., Lach., Hepar, Mang., Nux m.* And when every change of weather brings on a relapse,—*Calc., Silicea, Sulph., Dulc., Merc., Lach., Rhus*, and *Veratrum*, are usually the most useful.

For rheumatism arising from a chill in the water, or from cold, moist weather,—*Calcarea, Nux m., Sarsaparilla,* or *Sulph., Dulc., Carb. v.*

Rheumatism with paralytic weakness,—*Arnica, Ferrum, China,* &c.

Against unsettled or shifting or rheumatic pains, in addition to *Pulsatilla: Arnica, Bryonia, Nux m.*, and in some instances *Rhus, Rhodo., Daphne, Mang., Plumb.*, or *Crocus, Valeriana* and *Asafoet.*

Rheumatism from congelation,—*Arsenicum, Bryonia, Nux moschata,* chiefly.

LUMBAGO.

DIAGNOSIS. Violent pain of a rheumatic character in the lumbar region, either periodical or permanent, frequently accompanied with a considerable degree of fever.

THERAPEUTICS. The medicines most valuable in its treatment are: *Aconite, Bryonia, Nux vomica, Rhus toxicodendron, Belladonna, Pulsatilla,* and *Mercurius.*

ADMINISTRATION and POTENCIES of the remedies. Same as in RHEUMATISM, which see.

ACONITE may be given at the commencement if much fever declare itself.

BRYONIA where the pains in the back are of a severe pressive description, constraining the individual to walk in a stooping position; aggravated by the slightest motion, or draught of cold air, and attended with a general sensation of chilliness.

NUX VOMICA is particularly indicated when the pains resemble those *produced by a bruise*, or by excessive *fatigue;* also when they are much increased by *motion* and *turning in bed* at night, and attended with considerable weakness; and moreover, when irritability of temper and constipation are present.

This is a valuable medicine in chronic cases, and may follow *Bryonia* in acute lumbago with considerable advantage.

RHUS TOXICODENDRON may be exhibited when the same indications as those given under the preceding medicine are present, with the distinction of the pains being *aggravated by rest.* It is also a useful remedy in chronic cases.

BELLADONNA, when the pains are deeply seated, causing a sensation of heaviness, gnawing, or stiffness; it may follow *Aconite* with considerable benefit, when slight inflammatory symptoms are present.

PULSATILLA, when the pains, resembling those mentioned under NUX VOMICA, are moreover attended with sensation of constriction; it is particularly indicated, as remarked in other parts of this work, for females, or individuals of mild, sensitive, or phlegmatic temperaments.

MERCURIUS, when the pains are much of the same description as those given under NUX VOMICA, but considerably aggravated at night, incapacitating the sufferer from taking rest. (See also *Rheumatism.*)

INFLAMMATION OF THE PSOAS MUSCLE.

Psoitis.

DIAGNOSIS. Pain in the renal region, hip, and downwards to the leg. The limb can neither be stretched nor drawn upwards without pain; in walking, there is hobbling in the gait, with the body inclined forward; turning in bed, or lifting any weight, increases the pain. Occasionally, but seldom, we find swelling of the psoas muscle and in the region of the groin; it in some measure resembles NEPHRITIS, from which, however, it is distinguishable by the absence of disturbances of the urinary system, etc.

This disease is generally more painful than dangerous; it may, however, prove fatal from matter forming and discharging itself internally into the cavity of the abdomen, but more frequently abscesses open in the groins, anus, perinæum, or thighs; it may also produce caries.

THERAPEUTICS. The remedies given under LUMBAGO and RHEUMATISM (which see) are equally useful in most cases of this disorder; however, as there is generally a greater degree of fever present than in that affection, *Aconitum*, followed by *Belladonna*, should generally form the commencement of our treatment.

The following may be mentioned in addition:

COLOCYNTH, when there is a feeling of contraction in the psoas muscles when walking, and the disease is more of a chronic nature.

ADMINISTRATION $\frac{00}{6}$, repeated in from twelve to twenty-four hours, according to circumstances.*

* Vide note, p. 21.

When shiverings or rigours are complained of, followed by a sensation of throbbing, and increase of pain in the affected part, and we have reason to apprehend incipient suppuration, we may exhibit *Staphysagria* in repeated doses, followed by *Silicea* or *Hepar*, to bring the abscess to a head as quickly as possible, and thereby relieve the sufferings of the patient.

In by far the greater number of cases of *Psoas* or *Lumbar abscess*, however, we have no premonitory symptoms which might lead us to anticipate such a disease, and are but too often unaware of the existence of the disorder until an external tumour is formed. (See Chronic Abscess.)

When the bones have become affected, or when abscess has arisen from diseased vertebræ, *Silicea* may be productive of all the benefit we can look for in so serious a state of matters.

Staphysagria may follow the above when a discharge of a peculiarly offensive sanies takes place.

Aurum, Asafœtida, Argentum, Plumbum, or *Sulphur* may also prove of service in the latter form of lumbar abscess.

SCIATICA.

Diagnosis. Pain in the region of the hip-joint, which frequently extends to the knee and foot, following the course of the sciatic nerve. It often interferes with the motion of the foot, causing stiffness and contraction.

Therapeutics. The remedies are *Aconitum, Arsenicum, Chamomilla, Ignatia, Nux vomica, Pulsatilla, Colocynth* and *Rhus toxicodendron.*

Aconitum. When considerable constitutional disturbance attended with fever is present.

Administration. $\frac{0}{6}{}^{0}$ in a little water, repeated every six hours till the fever is lowered.

Arsenicum. When burning pains are complained of, or sometimes a sensation of coldness in the affected part—acute dragging pains in the hips with great restlessness, obliging patient to move the limb frequently in order to obtain relief, occasional intermission of suffering, or periodical return; great weakness and inclination to lie down—mitigation from the application of external heat. It is also useful in those cases of marasmus or emaciation arising from a long continuance of want of rest, the result of pain, and from derangement of the digestive system.

Administration. $\frac{00}{6}$, repeated in from twelve to twenty-four hours.*

Chamomilla. More particularly indicated when the pains are frequent at night, attended with excessive sensibility and irritability of fibre; sensation of torpor in the affected parts.

Administration. $\frac{00}{3}$, in the same manner as *Arsenicum.*

Ignatia. When the pains are of an incisive nature, particularly on moving the limb, and more especially when occurring in individuals of a mild, melancholic temperament, or in dispositions disposed to alternations of extremely high and low spirits.

Administration. Same as *Arsenicum.*

Nux vomica. When the pain becomes aggravated towards morning, and is attended with a sensation of stiffness and contraction so as to interfere with the motion of the foot, and also a sensation of paralysis or torpor and chilliness in the parts affected, and particularly in individuals of an irritable temperament.

Administration. Same as *Arsenicum.*

Pulsatilla. When the pains are aggravated towards evening, and during the night, or when seated, but somewhat relieved in the open air; this remedy is best adapted for an individual of mild disposition and leuco-phlegmatic temperament.

Administration. Same as *Arsenicum.*

Colocynth is an important remedy in this distressing disease. It has been found of the greatest service in cases where the right leg was affected, and the pains liable to be excited, or much aggravated by a fit of anger or indignation.

Rhus. This medicament is more peculiarly indicated when the pains are aggravated by rest, relieved by motion, or by

* Vide note, p. 21.

warmth; with disposition to melancholy or an unaccountable feeling of dread.

Veratrum, *Staphysagria*, *Manganum*, *Mezereum*, *Hepar s.*, *Sepia*, *Phosphorus*, *Ruta*, *Kali c.*, *Conium*, etc., may also be found useful in particular cases of this complaint, or *Neuralgia* generally. (See also the remedies described for the treatment of rheumatic pains, art. RHEUMATISM.)

ADMINISTRATION. Same as *Chamomilla*.

PAIN IN THE HIP. HIP-GOUT. RHEUMATISM IN THE HIP.

Coxalgia, Coxagra. Ischias.

DIAGNOSIS. A pain in the hip-joint dependent upon a true gouty inflammation, almost universally of an acute description, the pain is extremely violent, and extends from the hip-joint to the neighbouring aponeurosis, the periosteum, and the adjacent ligaments; consequently, sometimes reaches upwards to the back or downwards to the thigh, rendering motion excessively painful, either in walking, rising up, sitting down, or turning in bed. When the pain is not deeply seated, there is generally absence of either swelling or redness.

This species of gout usually assumes the irritable character, runs its course quickly, and forms an active local inflammation, which very rapidly terminates in suppuration when unchecked. It occurs more frequently in the male than in the female subject.

When suppuration supervenes, the pain becomes more obtuse, pressing and throbbing; the inflammatory fever assumes the suppurative character (*febris suppuratoria*), indicated by shivering and shuddering, alternating with heat, to which a number of other sufferings become united, such as swelling, pains in the knee, limping, luxatio spontanea, &c.

THERAPEUTICS. The following remedies have been found most effective in the treatment: *Mercurius*, *Rhus toxicodendron*,

Arsenicum, *Aconitum*, *Belladonna*, *Chamomilla*, *Pulsatilla*, *Hepar sulphuris*, *Colocynth*, etc.

MERCURIUS is a useful remedy when the disease is attended with halting in the gait, and sharp, cutting, tearing, and burning pains, which are materially aggravated at night and during every movement, and are usually attended with profuse nocturnal sweating; also where exudation threatens or is present.

ADMINISTRATION. A grain of the third trituration in an ounce of water, a dessert-spoonful exhibited morning and evening, and continued as long as advantage appears to result from its employment.*

RHUS TOXICODENDRON. When darting, tearing, or dragging pains are experienced in the hip-joint, attended with tension and stiffness in the muscles, aggravated or chiefly present during rest. Also painful sensibility of the joint when arising from the sitting posture.

ADMINISTRATION $\frac{000000}{3}$, in six dessert-spoonfuls of water, one every twelve hours until relief is experienced.

ACONITUM. When the affection is attended with marked febrile symptoms, or considerable inflammation of the joint itself exists from the commencement.

ADMINISTRATION $\frac{6}{6}$, in six dessert-spoonfuls of water, one every two, four, or six hours, until the above symptoms are relieved.

BELLADONNA is particularly indicated in the inflammatory stage when attended with a marked redness of the skin, and considerable pain on the slightest movement, with lameness; in such instances it may advantageously precede *Mercurius*.

ADMINISTRATION $\frac{6}{6}$, in the same manner as *Rhus tox.*

CHAMOMILLA $^{0}\frac{0}{3}{}^{0}$, in recent cases, with pain at night in bed.

PULSATILLA is occasionally found serviceable in mild cases of this disorder, partaking of a rheumatic character, when the patient complains of *wrenching* pains in the hip-joint, which are aggravated towards night, and even when in a state of rest. (*Acid. nitr.* is sometimes useful after *Puls.*)

ADMINISTRATION $\frac{6}{6}$, in six teaspoonfuls of water, one daily.

* Vide note, p. 21.

Hepar sulphuris is chiefly useful in case of exudation, and may in such instances follow *Mercurius* with some advantage.

Administration. A grain of the trituration at the third potency in an ounce of water, a dessert-spoonful every three or six hours, according to the result.

Colocynth $^{0}\frac{0}{3}{}^{0}$ is a useful remedy in subacute or chronic cases, when the pain is constant, and of a squeezing description, accompanied by a sensation as if the entire joint were tightly and painfully bound; also when the attacks are liable to be brought on or excited by a fit of passion, indignation, or mortification.

Arsenicum. Pain or shoots along the interior of the affected limb like a hot stream, increased by every movement or change of temperature; paleness of the face, oppression at the chest, attacks of faintness.

The following remedies have also been found useful in many cases: *Sulphur, Silicea, Graphites, Bryonia alba, Calcarea carbonica, Digitalis, Argentum, Arsenicum, Acidum nitricum, Creosotum, Asafœtida, Aurum foliatum, Cantharides, Lachesis, Chamomilla, Staphysagria, Nux vomica, Acidum phosphoricum, Sepia,* and *Calcarea phosphorata.* (See also the following article on Hip-disease, and that on Rheumatism where indications for some of the above mentioned will be found.)

HIP-DISEASE. *Morbus Coxarius.*

Diagnosis. Chronic inflammation of the bones composing the hip-joint (particularly the acetabulum), frequently commencing only with pain or uneasiness in the knee of the limb attacked, or a slight weakness of the part affected, attended with limping; afterwards emaciation, and elongation of the limb itself takes place, and as the complaint progresses, a severe fixed pain is felt behind the trochanter major, increased by pressure on the front of the acetabulum, extending down to the knee, ankle, and foot, which is accompanied with feverish symptoms, restlessness, and flattening of that part of the nates which is generally fullest and roundest, depression of the crest of the ileum, and distortion of the spine.

This complaint is most frequently met with in children, but no age, sex, or condition of life, is exempt from its attacks;

it is peculiarly insidious in its approach, the pain and uneasiness in the knee above mentioned being frequently the first symptoms denoting its presence; hence it is not unfrequently mistaken for some complaint of that joint, by inattentive or inexperienced practitioners; a most deplorable oversight, since it is only in the incipient period of the disease that a favourable prognosis can be given; if no appropriate relief be timely administered, matter forms within the joint, the acetabulum and sometimes the head of the femur become destroyed by caries, luxation upwards and outwards takes place, and the limb, which had previously been preternaturally elongated, now becomes contracted and shortened; the sufferer is then either destroyed by excessive constitutional irritation, or recovers with an anchylosed joint.

Causes. An inherent constitutional taint, such as scrofula, is no doubt the principal predisposing cause; but it is generally attributed to external violence, or exposure to damp or cold, lying down upon damp grass in summer, or some other exposure to cold or damp.

Therapeutics. *Mercurius* and *Belladonna* are our principal remedial agents, but we may also find occasion to have recourse, in some cases, to the following, namely: *Rhus tox.*, *Colocynth*, *Sulphur*, *Silicea*, *Calcarea phosph.*, *Pulsatilla*, *Sepia*, and *Staphysagria;* also the first-named medicines.

Mercurius. This remedy is of itself sometimes found to act as a specific in the early and curable stage of the disease; it is more particularly indicated when the patient is of a scrofulous diathesis and sallow complexion, and when no pain is complained of, but the disease is insidiously advancing.

Administration. A grain of the trituration at the third potency to an ounce of water; a dessert-spoonful night and morning, carefully watching the effect, and discontinuing the medicine when any alteration in the symptoms becomes perceptible; afterwards either returning to its exhibition, or selecting another medicament, according to the result.

Belladonna is more especially called for in the inflammatory stage, when the patient evidences *considerable pain.*

Administration. A drop of the tincture at the sixth potency to an ounce of water, exhibited in the same manner as *Mercurius*. In some cases it may be found advantageous to alternate these remedies according to the symptoms that present themselves.

Rhus toxicodendron. Darting or dragging or tearing pains in the hip-joint, accompanied with tension or stiffness of the muscles, most painful when in a state of rest; and severe pain on arising from a sitting posture.

Administration. A drop of the tincture at the third potency, exhibited in the same manner as *Belladonna*.

Colocynth has been found of much value in this disorder, either after *Bellad.* and *Merc.*, or in preference to these medicines when, from the commencement, the hip-joint is described to feel as if firmly and painfully bound by an iron clasp, with pain extending down the limb, and stiffness in the knee-joint.

Sulphur is called for in chronic cases, particularly when arising from a scrofulous or psoric metastasis.

Administration $\frac{6}{6}$, in six dessert-spoonfuls of water daily.

In cases of abscess or caries in this disease, *Silicea* and *Calcarea phosphorata* may be pointed out.

The following remedies are likewise deserving of attention in the treatment of this serious malady: *Calcarea, Bryonia, Hepar s.*, *Acidum phosphoricum, Phosphor*, and *Lachesis*.

In affections of the Knee-joint, *Silicea* forms one of the most important remedies, particularly when the disease begins in the synovial membrane. *Acid. nitr.*, *Aurum*, *Acid. phosph.*, *Lycopodium*, *Lachesis*, *Sulphur*, or *Calcarea*, have, in addition to *Silicea*, been found useful in inflammation of the synovial membrane of the joints, in consequence of the effects of *Mercury;* and *Rhus*, *Bryonia*, *Lycop.*, *Nux v.*, *China*, or *Sulphur*, when as a result of gout or rheumatism *Sulphur* and *Calcarea* have chiefly been recommended in lymphatic or scrofulous enlargement of the knee; but also the following in some cases: *Silicea*, *Lycop.*, *Arsenic.*, *Iodium*, and *Arnica*.

In the event of suppuration: *Silicea*, *Merc.*, *Hepar s.;* and in that of serous infiltration: *Silicea* and *Sulph.;* or *Calcarea*, *Merc.*, *Iodium*. In glazed or shining, white, soft or doughy swellings of the knee: *Pulsat.*; also in soft, colourless swellings of the knee, whether painful or otherwise. Sometimes the alternate employment of *Iodium* and *Pulsat.* is required, especially in strumous habits. When the swelling is red, painful: *Bryonia*, or *Bryon.* and *Iodium* in alternation, in scrofulous subjects.

DETERMINATION OF BLOOD TO THE ABDOMEN.

Congestio viscerum abdominis. Congestio ad abdomen.

This derangement is characterized by a disagreeable or painful sensation of weight, heat, and burning, with hardness and tension in the lower portion of the abdomen.

Nux vomica is one of the most frequent sources of relief in those who lead a sedentary life, or are much addicted to over-indulgence in the pleasures of the table, and particularly when the following symptoms are complained of: hardness, tension, and fixed pain in the abdomen, sense of great weakness or prostration, rendering it difficult or almost impossible to walk about; constipation, with pain in the loins, spirits oppressed and irritable.

Administration, $\frac{000}{30}$, in a teaspoonful of water, repeated in four days.

Sulphur will frequently be found serviceable in completing the cure after the above, or it may be selected in preference in cases of long standing, when we meet with the following indications: dull pains, and disagreeable sensation of distention in the abdomen, constipation, tendency to obstinate hemorrhoidal attacks, extreme dejection.

Administration. $\frac{000}{30}$, repeated every five or six days until improvement results, or an alteration in the symptoms calls for the employment of some other remedy.

Carbo vegetabilis may be selected when the symptoms are accompanied with excessive flatulency, and will frequently be found of great service in some obstinate cases when alternated with the two preceding remedies.

Administration. $\frac{000}{30}$, in three dessert-spoonfuls of water; a dessert-spoonful daily; repeated in the same manner four or five days after.

Arsenicum will also be found useful, especially when there is a disposition to diarrhœa with *extreme weakness:* or—

Capsicum, when these symptoms occur in individuals of a lymphatic temperament.

The two latter remedies may be administered in the same manner as is described under *Carbo vegetabilis.*

Sepia is often of much utility in the case of females, particularly when the symptoms are analogous to those described under *Sulphur.*

Administration. Same as *Sulphur.*

In particular cases, the following will also be found useful: *Pulsatilla, Belladonna, Mercurius, Bryonia, Lycopodium, Chamomilla, Rhus toxicodendron, Veratrum.* In consulting the articles on Dyspepsia, and Hemorrhoids, the reader will find further assistance in the selection of the above remedies.

Daily exercise in the open air, together with a careful attention to regimen, must be observed by those who are afflicted with this affection.

ACUTE INFLAMMATION OF THE EYES.

Ophthalmia.

Diagnosis. Superficial bright scarlet redness, pain, and heat of the eye, generally with marked sensibility to the action of light; either with dryness or an increased secretion of ophthalmic humours. When severe, accompanied by cephalalgia, febrile symptoms, and increased intolerance of light, particularly when the entire eyeball (*Ophthalmitis*) or the sclerotic coat is affected (*Sclerotitis*), in which latter case, moreover, the redness presents a pink appearance.

This affection may arise from a variety of causes, such as exposure to extreme light, the strong heat of a fire, particularly after coming out of an extremely cold atmosphere, external injuries, or cold.

Therapeutics. The following remedies are those most generally required in the treatment of this affection, according to the form in which it presents itself, namely: *Aconitum, Belladonna, Nux vomica, Cinchona, Digitalis, Euphrasia, Ignatia, Arnica montana, Pulsatilla, Mercurius*, and *Sulphur.*

Aconitum. Valuable at the commencement of the treatment, in general cases of non-catarrhal inflammation; but even in a simple inflammation of the conjunctiva or simple catarrhal ophthalmia, should the *inflammation be considerable and attended with fever.*

Administration $\frac{0}{6}^{0}$, repeated in from six to twelve hours, until the inflammation is lowered.

Belladonna, if great sensibility to light remains. Also in *Acute, Arthritic, Rheumatic,* and even *Scrofulous* ophthalmia, when the following symptoms present themselves: redness in the conjunctiva, margin of the eyelids, and corner of the eyes, with a swollen and tumid appearance; or redness of the sclerotica, with *intolerance* of, and pain increased by light; great sensibility of the eyes and eyelids; aching pains above and around the orbits, or pains which penetrate deeply into the orbits and head, with aggravation on moving the eyes; flashes of light, sparks or darkness before the eyes, with extreme dimness of vision *towards evening;* objects appearing reversed or *double;* moreover, when there are the following catarrhal symptoms: severe cold in the head, with acrid discharge, causing excoriation, and sometimes an eruption of pimples under the nose, and on or about the lips; periodical return of short, dry, barking, spasmodic cough, *aggravated towards night,* and severe headache. (*Mercurius* and *Hepar s.* are often required to complete the cure after the employment of *Belladonna.*)

Administration $\frac{0}{6}^{0}$, in a little water, repeated every six, twelve or twenty-four hours, according to the severity of the affection.*

Nux vomica. In *catarrhal, arthritic,* or *rheumatic* inflammation of the eye, when there are burning, *pressive,* or aching pains, feeling as of sand in the eye, with *stiffness, smarting,*

* Vide note, p. 21.

tickling, and itching; foul tongue, and other symptoms of disordered stomach; slight fever in the morning and towards evening; irritable temper; pressure on the eyes and eyeballs on attempting to open them; redness of the canthi; the eye streaked, blood-shot, and swollen, with adhesion of the eyelids; sensibility to light; briny lachrymation; affection worse towards morning. *Nux v.* and *Pulsatilla,* are two of the most useful remedies in simple inflammation of the conjunctivà, particularly at the commencement of the attack; but *Sulphur* is often required to complete the cure.

ADMINISTRATION. $\frac{00}{6}$, in a little water, repeated in twenty-four hours, or sooner if required.*

CINCHONA. When the inflammation is less intense, but the motion of the eye painful, and the sensation before noted as of sand in the eye, with the distinction of the affection, *exacerbation towards evening;* when the pains are of a burning or pressive nature, with headache in the forehead, as if arising from a *suppression of the nasal discharge.*

ADMINISTRATION. Same as *Nux vomica.*

ARSENICUM chiefly in *catarrhal* and *scrofulous* ophthalmia, when there exists a violent *burning* pain, or pains of so severe a description as almost to drive the patient distracted; specks and ulcers on the cornea.

ADMINISTRATION. Same as *Nux vomica.*

EUPHRASIA. For the exhibition of this medicine, the particular indications are: white of the eye much inflamed and of a pink or rose colour (*Sclerotitis*)*;* painful *pressure* and smarting in the eyes; *profuse and acrid flow of tears,* excited or increased by exposure to cold; copious secretion of mucus, sometimes sanguinolent; or bright redness of the conjunctiva, with distention of the veins; minute pustules on different parts of the conjunctiva; white opaque specks on the cornea; excessive intolerance of light (scrofulous inflammation of the conjunctiva); severe cold in the head, with *profuse fluent nasal discharge; violent* headache, and aggravation of the symptoms towards evening.

* Vide note, p. 21.

Administration. Same as *Nux vomica.*

Ignatia may be administered with advantage when there is pressure in the eyes, profuse flow of tears, great intolerance of light, but with *little* or *no* perceptible *redness* of the eyeball; severe coryza; in *catarrhal, rheumatic* or *scrofulous* inflammation.

Administration. Same as *Nux vomica.*

Pulsatilla. Aching, or *burning* and *smarting* irritation in the eye as if from the insertion of sand under the lids, with scarlet redness of the eyes and eyelids, and copious secretion of mucus, disordered stomach, foul tongue, and chilliness towards evening, followed by febrile heat; or pricking, shooting, piercing pains in the eye, with bright redness of the eyes, and profuse lachrymation, especially on looking at the light, or on going into the open air, and generally of a scalding or acrid nature; or, on the other hand, excessive dryness of the eyelids, especially in the evening, with nocturnal agglutination; *photophobia;* swelling of the lids; aggravation of the symptoms towards evening; sensitiveness with disposition to weep. (*Ferrum* is occasionally very serviceable after *Pulsatilla*, especially in scrofulous ophthalmy; at other times, *Sulphur* is preferable.)

Administration. Same as *Nux v.*

Mercurius. In many cases of catarrhal, *rheumatic*, and *scrofulous ophthalmia*, as also in *iritis*, this medicine is frequently to be employed with advantage. Its ordinary indications are: lancinating pains, or painful and irritating pressure as if from sand, especially on reading, or otherwise fatiguing the eyes, but also when at rest in bed; pricking and itching in the eyes, particularly in the open air; rose-coloured redness of the eye (sclerotitis), with injection of the veins; profuse lachrymation; great sensibility to light, but especially that of the fire or candle; vesicles and pustules on the sclerotica: ulcers on the cornea; *pustules* and *scabs round the eyes,* and *at the margins of the eyelids;* cloudiness of the sight; violent pains in the orbit and forehead; renewal of the inflammation on the slightest exposure to cold. (*Hepar s.* or *Sulphur* is frequently required after *Mercurius.*)

SULPHUR is an important remedy in inflammation of all kinds, whether catarrhal, rheumatic, or scrofulous, when of an obstinate or inveterate character. It is, however, more particularly indicated by the following symptoms: *pressure, smarting*, and *burning* as if from sand; itching in the eyes or eyelids; dimness of sight, with dusky appearance of *specks, vesicles* or *pustules* and *ulcers* on the *cornea;* pustules or granular elevations in the eyelids, and scabs round the orbits; inflammation of the *iris*, with irregularity of the pupil; *copious lachrymation*, and *excessive photophobia*, and aggravation or suffering on moving the eyes; painful *dryness* of the eyes, especially within doors; contraction of the eyelids; imperfect vision, with scintillations; cephalalgia, and violent pains in the orbit, etc.

Chronic cases of this affection frequently require a long and careful course of constitutional treatment to effect a perfect cure; one of our best remedial agents for this end is *Hepar sulphuris*, which is also of great service in acute attacks after *Bella.* or *Merc.*, in individuals predisposed to this affection. Among the other medicines which may be consulted with advantage in *catarrhal, rheumatic*, or even *scrofulous* ophthalmia, are: *Sulphur*, *Calcarea carbonica*, or *Causticum*, *Graphites*, *Sepia*, *Spigelia*, *Acidum sulphuricum*, *Petroleum*, *Lachesis*, *Acidum nitricum*, *Ferrum metallicum*, *Colocynth*, etc.

If the inflammation arise from external injury, caused by a blow, or the entrance of any foreign body in the eye, we may exhibit *Aconitum*, and follow it in about twelve or sixteen hours with ARNICA $\frac{00}{6}$, bathing the eye occasionally at the same time with a lotion of *Arnica;* five drops of the tincture to an ounce of water; and should the said treatment not suffice to effect a cure, *Sulphur* must be had recourse to, followed, if called for, by *Calcarea*, or any other remedy which may appear better indicated. Finally, the following may be pointed out as being eminently useful, or worthy of attention, in the varieties of ophthalmia enumerated.

For CATARRHAL OPHTHALMIA, in addition to those above mentioned: *Chamom.*, *Hepar sulph.*, *Lycopodium.*

RHEUMATIC (*Sclerotitis :*) *Bryonia, Chamomilla, Rhus,* and *Veratrum; Lycopodium, Spigelia ;** in addition to those described under the heading of INFLAMMATION OF THE EYE.

SCROFULOUS : *Arsenicum, Conium, Hepar s., Sulphur,* and *Calcarea*; also *Dulcamara, Causticum, Ferrum, Graphites, Sepia, Petroleum ;* or *Aurum, Baryta c. et m., Lycopodium, Cannabis, Chamomilla, Digitalis, Iodium, Mercurius Corrosivus,*† *Magnesia, Natrum m.,* in conjunction with those which have been alluded to as suitable to this variety of the disease at the commencement of this article.

SYPHILITIC : *Mercurius* and *Acidum nitricum* chiefly; in some cases, *Aurum, Lachesis, Sulphur, Bellad.*

SYCOSIS : *Thuj. Acidum nitr.*, and sometimes *Merc.*

GONORRHŒAL : *Pulsatilla* chiefly ; also *Tussilago pet.*

ABUSE OF MERCURY under previous allopathic treatment : *Hepar sulphuris, Acid nitricum, Sulphur, Pulsatilla,* and in some cases *Belladonna, Lachesis, Staphysagria, Lycopodium, Thuja, or Cinchona.*

FUNGUS HÆMATODES : *Thuja, Carbo a.*, and *Phosph.*‡

IRITIS ARTHRITICA : *Cocculus, Staphysagria, Conium, Lycopodium, Calcarea, Nux v., Bryonia.*

IRITIS MERCURIALIS : *Hepar s., Acid. nitr., Lach.*

In ULCERATION OF THE CORNEA, the following remedies have hitherto been employed with the most satisfactory results : *Arsenic., Euphrasia, Sulphur, Lachesis, Calcarea, Bellad., Mercur., Hepar sulph., Silicea,* and *Natrum m.*

SPECKS ON THE CORNEA, or OPACITY of the same : *Belladonna, Euphrasia, Sulphur, Calcarea, Hepar sulphuris, Pulsatilla ;* as also : *Arsenicum, Acid. nitricum, Cannabis, Magnesia, Aurum, Lycopodium, Silicea, Sepia.*

* *Spigelia* is specific in a large number of cases of arthritic and rheumatic ophthalmia. *Aconit.* is required in the first place. *Sulphur,* preceded by or alternated with *Acon.*, is of nearly equal efficacy in some instances.

† Efficacious in the acute scrofulous ophthalmia, with ulceration of the cornea and disposition to staphyloma, hypopyon, etc.

‡ For the description of the cure of an interesting case of fungus hæmatodes of the eye, vide *Brit. Journ. of Homœopathy,* No. 2.

CATARACT. The remedies which have chiefly been described as efficacious in this affection of the eye are: *Sulphur, Silicea, Cannabis, Caustic., Conium, Magnesia, Phosph.*, etc.*

STRABISMUS: In addition to the ordinary simple mechanical remedies, great assistance has been derived from, and in other instances the cure solely effected by, *Belladonna* and *Hyoscyamus*, when the affection was not of too long standing.

FISTULA LACHRYMALIS. The following remedies have been employed with success in this affection: *Petrol., Silicea, Stannum, Calcarea, Pulsatilla, Sulphur, Lach., Acid fluor.*

WEEPING or WATERY EYE (*involuntary flow of tears.*) When this affection proceeds from an obstruction of the lachrymal duct, it must be treated by the remedies above enumerated; but when it merely consists in a relaxed condition of the glandular apparatus of the eye, with a superabundant secretion of tears, (*epiphora,*) the subjoined remedies have been found successful: *Euphrasia, Spigelia, Paris.* In other cases, a selection may be made from amongst the following: *Puls., Sulph., Euphorb., Clematis, Sepia, Merc., Ferrum, Ledum, Graphites, Phosph., Lycopod., Silicea, Acid. sulph., Thuja, Petrol., Rhus, Verat., Sabad, Digitalis, Nux v.*, etc.

ÆGYLOPS (*Anchylops*). Against this sore, which has its seat immediately under the internal angle of the eye: *Acid. nitr.* (See also FISTULA LACHRYMALIS, of which this affection is now commonly considered to be a mere modification, or only a certain stage.)

BLOOD-SHOT EYE. This derangement may arise from a blow or fall, the act of retching, vomiting, or violent coughing,

* *Aconitum* $\frac{000}{3}$ ought to be given immediately after surgical operations on the eye, and repeated as soon as any abnormal symptoms threaten to break out. In individuals of mild and easy disposition, with severe shooting pains in the temples, as also in the eyes: *Ignatia* Pains of a jerking or twitching description attended with vomiting and lienteria: *Azarum.* Burning pains with diarrhœa: *Arsenic.* Throbbing and jerking pains in the eyes: *Crocus.* Shooting pains from the temples, with loss of appetite: *Thuja.* When depression failed, but the lens broke in pieces under the operation, *Senega* promoted the absorption of the particles. When, on the completion of the cure, the sight was impaired by a false perception of colours, and particularly when every object appeared to be covered with blood, *Strontiana* was successful.

crying, etc. It presents a bright, scarlet appearance in most instances at the commencement, but usually assumes a livid hue at a subsequent period. The affection generally disappears of itself; but as it is liable to prove exceedingly obstinate occasionally, absorption is materially facilitated, and the unsightliness removed by the internal and *external* employment of ***Arnica.*** (See EXTERNAL INJURIES.) *Bellad.*, *Lachesis*, *Nux v.*, or *Cham.*, may be required in certain cases.)

Against HÆMORRHAGE FROM THE EYES: *Bellad.*, *Carbo veg.*, *Chamomilla*, *Nux vom.**

SHORT SIGHT. NEAR-SIGHTEDNESS. *Myopia.*

The medicines which have been employed with the greatest effect in this affection are: *Pulsatilla*, *Sulphur*, *Carbo v.*, *Acid. phosp.*, *Phosphorus*, *Conium*, *Acidum nitricum*, *Ammonium c.*, *Anacardium* and *Petroleum*; of which, *Pulsatilla* and *Sulphur* have proved the most serviceable when the affection occurred as a sequel of *ophthalmia*;—*Acidum phosph.*, when resulting from *typhus*, or from debilitating *loss of fluids*;—and *Carb. v.*, *Acid. nitr.* and *Sulphur*, when attributable to the effects of *mercurial* action.

Against *sudden* attacks of blindness: *Aconitum*, followed by *Mercurius*, *Sulphur* and *Silicea.* Against blindness towards evening, *Belladonna* is the principal remedy; in other cases, *Veratrum* will answer better. Should neither of these effect much improvement, *Hyoscyamus* may be administered.

SWELLING OF THE LIPS (*scrofulous*:) *Belladonna* and *Mercurius* are two of the most useful remedies in this affection when there is simultaneous retraction of the lip. If ulceration and incrustations accompany the disorder, *Belladonna*, *Mercurius*, *Hepar*, *Sulphur*, *Staphysagria*, *Silicea* and *Sepia.* If there be tumefaction simply, *Aurum*, *Mercurius*, *Bryonia*, *Belladonna*, *Hepar*, *Lachesis*, *Sulphur*, *and Calcarea.*

SCIRRHUS. Against indurations of this serious character, either in the face or lips: *Belladonna*, *Conium*, *Sulphur*, *Silicea*, *Carbo a. et v.*, *Phosphorus*, *Staphysagria* and *Magnesia m.*

* See Diseases of the eye, treated homœopathically. From the German, by A. C. Becker, M. D.

are chiefly to be recommended; and the following against *carcinomatous* ulcerations (both internally and externally): *Arsenicum, Lachesis, Clematis, Conium, Sulphur, Silicea, Acidum nitr., Arnica*, etc.

WARTS on the face. *Causticum*, and, in some cases, *Kali, Sepia, Dulcamara, Thuja, Acidum nitricum*, and *Sulphur*, are most useful. The employment of the knife or of caustic in such cases is highly improper, and often attended with the worst effects. Against these excrescences on the other parts of the body, such as the hands, etc., *Sulphur* and *Calcarea* form two of the best remedies in cases of long standing; *Causticum*, when large and painful; *Lycopodium*, when large, and intersected with deep clefts; when moist: *Thuja, Acid. nit.* and *Sabina* (externally and internally),—*Dulcamara, Natrum, Sepia* and *Rhus*, have also proved useful in some cases.

HORDEOLUM. *Stye.*

DIAGNOSIS. This is a little hard tumour appearing like a small dark-red boil, generally in the corner of the eye, or upon the eyelids, attended with severe inflammation, and frequently causing fever, considerable pain and suffering. It suppurates slowly and imperfectly, and has no tendency to burst spontaneously.

THERAPEUTICS. The two most valuable medicines in the treatment of this affection, are *Pulsatilla* and *Aconitum*.

PULSATILLA will, in most cases, suffice to remove the stye, if given on its first appearance.

ADMINISTRATION $^{0}\frac{0}{6}{}^{0}$, in four teaspoonfuls of water, one morning and evening. This medicine may be again exhibited whenever an attack threatens.

ACONITUM. When inflammation runs high, attended with great pain, fever, and restlessness.

ADMINISTRATION $^{0}\frac{0}{6}{}^{0}$, in four teaspoonfuls of water, one every six hours, until the inflammation is reduced; or, in some instances, *Staphysagria* may be found useful to complete a cure, particularly when the swelling degenerates into a hard white tumour; and in some scrofulous habits, in addition, *Arsenicum, Sulphur, Lycopodium*, etc.

LIPPITUDO (*bleareredness*): *Aconitum, Euphrasia, Mercur., Pulsat.* chiefly; also *Sulph., Calc., Phosph., Lycop., Sepia, Silic.*, etc.

Against BLEPHARITIS (*inflammation of the eyelids*): *Aconitum, Bellad., Hepar, Pulsatilla, Nux v., Chamomilla*, and *Euphrasia*, have chiefly been employed with the most success in the *acute* form of the complaint; and *Arsenicum, Sulphur, Calcarea, Antimonium, Cinchona*, etc., in the *chronic* variety.

In INFLAMMATION OF THE MARGINS OF THE EYELIDS, OF MEIBOMIAN GLANDS (*ophthalmia tarsi*): *Bellad., Merc., Hepar, Euphras., Nux v., Pulsat., Cham.*, etc.

CATARRHAL INFLAMMATION OF THE EYELIDS (*inflammation of the conjunctiva palpebrarum*): *Arsenicum, Mercurius, Hepar*, chiefly.

When the *external* surface of the eyelid is inflamed, *Aconitum, Belladonna, Hepar sulphuris*, and *Sulphur*, are more particularly called for.

INFLAMMATION OF THE EARS, AND EARACHE.

Otitis. Otalgia.

OTITIS. DIAGNOSIS. Violent, frequently insupportable pain in the ear, with sensibility, and even inflammation of the meatus auditorius externus, and greater or less fever.

The pain, when excessive, communicating with the whole head, may bring on delirium, or even inflammation of the brain.

OTALGIA may exist either as the effect of otitis again, or, if neglected, may pass on to inflammation; in many cases again, it may arise by sympathy from toothache, or declare itself as a purely neuralgic affection.

THERAPEUTICS. The medicaments applicable to the majority of cases of these troublesome and painful disorders, are: *Mercurius, Pulsatilla, Belladonna, Nux vomica, Arnica, Dulcamara*, and *Chamomilla, Hepar, Cinchona, Sulphur*, etc.

ADMINISTRATION. Six globules at the potency specified under each medicine, in an ounce of water, a dessert-spoonful every half hour to six hours and upwards, according to results, carefully watching the effect of each exhibition. (See remarks upon this important point in INTRODUCTION, article ADMINISTRATION AND REPETITION OF THE MEDICINES.)

MERCURIUS $\frac{000000}{6}$. When the pain is attended with a sensation of coldness in the ears, and *exacerbation of suffering in the warmth of the bed ;* shooting or tensive pains in the internal ear, extending to the cheeks and teeth; inflammation and induration of the ear, with soreness of the orifice, and discharge; swelling of the glands. When *Mercurius* affords only partial relief, a dose of *Hepar s.* will often subdue the remaining symptoms; but if a purulent discharge continue, accompanied by humming in the ear, and pricking pains, *Sulphur* will generally be found requisite.

PULSATILLA $\frac{000000}{3}$, is a most valuable remedy in this affection. It is particularly indicated *when the external ear* is much affected, and appears inflamed and swollen; with heat, shooting and tensive excoriating pain internally; moisture in the ear, or somewhat copious discharge. This medicament is particularly useful in cases of females, and in individuals of chilly habit.

BELLADONNA $\frac{000000}{3}$, when *determination of blood to the head,* with redness of the face, exists; with digging, boring, *tearing or shooting pains extending to the throat, and extreme sensibility to the slightest noise ;* when the pains are more severe internally; also when the brain partakes of the inflammation, and delirium is present. (*Hepar* is sometimes required after *Belladonna* to complete the cure in obstinate cases, when the inflammation has ended in suppuration.)

NUX VOMICA $\frac{000000}{3}$. When the pains are of a *tearing, shooting* nature, extending to the forehead, temples, and bones of the face, worse towards morning; dryness of the ear; and particularly when the affection occurs in persons of a lively, choleric disposition.

ARNICA $\frac{000000}{3}$, in individuals of nervous, excitable temperament, subject to be attacked from slight causes; also, when great sensibility to noise is present. (*Cinchona* is often useful after *Arnica,* especially when the pains are aggravated by lying on, or touching the affected ear. In other cases, *Sulphur* will be found more efficacious, particularly when the sensibility is excessive.

DULCAMARA $\frac{0\,0\,0\,0\,0\,0}{6}$, when the affection has arisen from a chill or wetting, will, in many cases, prove sufficient for its removal; it is also indicated when the pains increase at night, and are attended with nausea.

CAMOMILLA $\frac{0\,0\,0\,0\,0\,0}{3}$, when there are *stabbing* pains in the ear, as from knives; great sensibility to noise, or even to music; extreme sensitiveness, susceptibility, and irritability.

Against *humming* or *buzzing* in the ears, *Nux v.* will be found serviceable in recent cases, when the annoyance is worse in the morning; *Pulsatilla* when in the evening; *Dulcamara* when at night; or *Mercurius* when accompanied by sweating. *China*, *Carbo v.*, and *Acidum nitricum* when the affection occurs in individuals who have taken mercury in large quantities. In chronic cases, *Aurum*, *Petroleum*, and *Causticum*, etc., have been found useful; the last-named remedy, particularly when there is great sensibility to cold, and tendency to suffer from rheumatic pains in the limbs.

OTORRHŒA. When this disorder results from acute inflammation of the ear: *Pulsatilla*, *Sulphur*, and *Mercurius*, are the principal remedies.

CATARRHAL or MUCOUS OTORRHŒA. *Belladonna*, *Mercurius*, *Pulsatilla*, and *Sulphur*, chiefly.

PURULENT OTORRHŒA. *Mercurius*, *Pulsatilla*, *Sulphur*, *Belladonna*, *and Hepar*,—or *Silicea*, *Calcarea*, *Causticum*, *Acid. nitricum*, *Asafœtida*, *Lachesis*, *Petroleum*, etc. When the discharge is offensive, *Causticum*, *Hepar*, *Aurum*, *Carbo v.*, *Sulphur*, and *Silicea*.

SANGUINEOUS OTORRHŒA. *Mercurius*, *Pulsatilla*, and *Silicea*,—also *Lachesis* and *Cicuta*, etc. When the disorder has arisen from the abuse of mercury: *Hepar s.*, *Acid. nitricum*, *Aurum*, *Asafœtida*, *Sulphur*, and *Silicea*, have proved the most useful; and when over-doses of sulphur appear to have given rise to it, *Pulsatilla* and *Mercurius*.

When we have reason to apprehend caries of the ossicula auditoria: *Silicea*, *Sulphur*, *Aurum*, and *Natrum m.*, are the remedies from which we may hope to obtain the most assistance,

Against the effects of suppressed otorrhœa: *Belladonna*,

Pulsatilla, and *Mercurius;* and, in some cases, *Nux v.*, *Bryonia* or *Dulcamara*, may be selected, according to circumstances. *Belladonna* and *Bryonia* chiefly when there is fever, headache, or unequivocal signs of cerebral irritation; *Mercurius, Belladonna*, and *Pulsatilla*, followed, if required, by *Sulphur*, *Calcarea* and *Hepar*, when the glands of the neck or the parotids become tumefied. When *orchitis* results: *Pulsatilla* and *Nux v.* or *Mercurius.*

In DYSECOIA or DEAFNESS, the following remedies have chiefly been employed with the most success: *Pulsatilla, Mercurius, Sulphur, Calcarea, Causticum, Graphites, Ledum, Acid. nitricum, Phosphorus, Petroleum, Ammonium c.*, etc.

For CONGESTIVE DEAFNESS: *Belladonna, Hyoscyamus, Sulphur, Silicea, Mercurius, Graphites, Phosphorus*, etc., have more particularly been recommended.

NERVOUS DEAFNESS: *Causticum, Petroleum, Phosphorus, Acid. phosphoricum*, etc.

CATARRHAL or RHEUMATIC DEAFNESS: *Mercur., Pulsat., Arsenic., Bellad., Ledum*, or *Sulph., Calcarea, Hepar, Lachesis, Acid. nitr., Chamomilla*, and *Coffea.*

DEAFNESS from the *repercussion* of chronic *eruptions: Sulphur* and *Antimonium;*—or, *Causticum, Graphites*, etc. When deafness results as a sequel of measles, *Pulsatilla* is one of the most useful remedies; in other cases, *Carbo v.* will be found requisite.

When after SCARLATINA: *Belladonna* and *Hepar.*

SMALLPOX: *Mercurius* and *Sulphur.*

DEAFNESS from the abuse of *Mercury* is generally capable of being removed, or materially relieved, by *Acidum nitr., Staphysagria, Asafœtida*, or *Aurum; Hepar s., Sulphuris, Petroleum* or *Sulphur.* When the disorder is attributable to hypertrophy of the amygdalæ: *Aurum, Mercurius, Acid. nitricum*, and *Staphysagria*, have principally been recommended. When in consequence of fevers, or other disorders, particularly of a nervous character: *Phosphorus, Acid. phosphoric., Veratrum*, and *Arnica;* and when occurring as a result of a suddenly checked discharge from the nose or ears: *Hepar, Lachesis*, and *Ledum;*—as also: *Belladonna, Mercurius*, and *Pulsatilla*, have generally been found the most appropriate.

BLEEDING OF THE NOSE.

Epistaxis.

Bleeding at the nose often appears at the termination of many diseases, such as fevers, epilepsy, etc., and is in such instances salutary; it also frequently relieves or cures headache, vertigo, etc., and ought therefore not to be interfered with, unless it be excessive, last too long, recur too frequently, or take place under a debilitated state of the system. The attack is frequently preceded by a degree of quickness of the pulse, flushing of the face, throbbing in the temporal arteries, confusion or dimness of sight, heat and itching in the nostrils, and other signs of congestion.

The remedies usually required are: *Aconitum, Arnica montana, Belladonna, Bryonia, Cinchona, Pulsatilla, Mercurius, Rhus toxicodendron, Secale cornutum ;* or *Carbo vegetabilis, Graphites, Causticum, Magnes artificialis, Ammonium muriaticum, Ferrum, Kali Sepia, Sulphur, Calcarea, Acidum nitricum, Baryta, Bovista, Crocus, Conium, Cina,* etc.

When the bleeding is excessive, *Acon., Arn., Bellad., Cin., Merc., Puls., Rhus., or Sec.*, are the most useful.

When the hemorrhage arises from *congestion in the head,* a preference may be given to *Acon., Bellad., Cin., Crocus, Con.*, or to *Graph., Rhus., Chamom., Alum.*, etc.

When from being *overheated,* or in consequence of indulging to excess in *spirituous liquors,* etc., *Nux vomica,* or *Acon., Bellad., Bryonia, Thuja.*

EPISTAXIS in females who have *too scanty catamenia : Puls., Graph., Caustic., Sep.*, or *Sec.* In those, on the contrary, who have *too copious* a menstrual discharge : *Acon., Calc., Croc., Sabina.*

In *debilitated subjects,* or those who have previously been exhausted by loss of humours, *Chin.* chiefly, or *Sec.* and *Ac. nitricum.*

In consequence of *physical exertion, Rhus,* or *Arnica* principally.

In consequence of a *blow* or *contusion, Arnica.*

Bleeding from the nose in children, arising from worms: *Cina* or *Merc.*

At every attack of CORYZA: *Pulsatilla* or *Arsenicum.*

When nasal hemorrhage is liable to occur from the most trivial cause: *Sulphur*, *Silicea*, *Sepia*, *Calcarea*, and *Carbo v.*, and in some cases, *Graphites* and *Lycopodium* are the best remedies to eradicate the constitutional tendency.

The following are characteristic indications for some of the above remedies.

Aconitum $\frac{000}{3}$. Prolonged or violent bleeding at the nose, in plethoric subjects, with a considerable degree of fever, flushing of the face, pulsation of the temporal and carotid arteries, or general fulness of the vessels of the head.

Belladonna $\frac{000}{3}$. Frequently of the greatest service, after, or in alternation with the above remedy, but also when there is bleeding from the nose at night, *which awakens the patient from sleep*, and sometimes returns in the morning; bleeding from the nose from being overheated. (See Bryonia and Rhus.)

Bryonia $\frac{000}{3}$. Bleeding from the nose, chiefly in the morning, or *at night during sleep*, causing the patient to awake; epistaxis from suppressed menstruation; bleeding of the nose from overheating during warm weather, obstinate or irritable disposition.

Mercurius $\frac{00}{6}$. Bleeding of the nose *during sleep*, or while coughing, with speedy coagulation, so that the blood hangs in clots at the nostrils; bleeding from the nose, preceded by tightness round the head, as if it were bound.

Carbo v. $\frac{00}{6}$. Bleeding at the nose *during the night*, with ebullition of blood; violent nasal hemorrhage in the *morning* while in bed, followed by pain in the chest; discharge of a few drops of blood from the nose every forenoon; excessive bleeding from the nose several times a day, particularly after *stooping*, or after every exertion, preceded and followed by great paleness of the face. (See Rhus.)

Graphites $\frac{00}{6}$. Bleeding of the nose towards night, with heat in the face, preceded by determination of blood to the head in the after-part of the day, particularly in females who have *scanty catamenia.* (See Pulsatilla and Causticum.)

PULSATILLA $\frac{000}{3}$. Hemorrhage from the nose every afternoon, evening, or before midnight, especially in females with suppressed or scanty catamenia, or in those of a mild and placid disposition.

CAUSTICUM ${}^{0}\frac{0}{6}{}^{0}$. *Violent bleeding* at the nose, chiefly in females in whom the menstrual flux is extremely scanty.

MAGNES. ARTIFICIALIS. Bleeding from the nose, particularly in the *afternoon*, preceded by aching and weight or pressure at the forehead; protracted bleeding after blowing the nose.

ARNICA ${}^{0}\frac{0}{3}{}^{0}$. In addition to being the principal medicine in violent nasal hemorrhage from external injury, or from great physical exertion, is, moreover, an important remedy in all cases in which the hemorrhage is preceded by itching in the nose and forehead; and when the nose feels hot, and the blood discharged is red and liquid.

RHUS ${}^{0}\frac{0}{3}{}^{0}$. Bleeding of the nose from physical exertion, such as *lifting a heavy weight*, or, when blowing the nose, spitting, etc., or nasal hemorrhage, which becomes aggravated or renewed on *stooping, or during the night.*

FERRUM $\frac{00}{6}$. Nasal hemorrhage in debilitated subjects, with excessive paleness of the face. (Especially after *China.*)

SEPIA $\frac{00}{6}$. Frequent attacks of hemorrhage from the nose, with pale or sallow complexion, especially in females with obstructed catamenia. *Sulphur*, either alone or in alternation with *Sepia*, and sometimes *Carbo vegetabilis*, *Graphites*, and *Lycopodium*, is of great service in removing a susceptibility to bleeding of the nose. (See also the remedies enumerated under *nasal hemorrhage from the most trivial cause.*)

NUX V. $\frac{00}{3}$. Bleeding of the nose, especially in the *morning*, from overheating, or after drinking wine, etc., or in habitual drunkards. (*Lachesis* and *Calcarea carbonica* are sometimes requisite here, in addition to *Nux v.*)

DULCAMARA ${}^{0}\frac{0}{3}{}^{0}$. Bleeding at the nose after getting the feet wet; flow of hot, clear blood from the nose.

CROCUS ${}^{0}\frac{0}{3}{}^{0}$. Discharge of dark coloured, thick or viscous blood from the nose, particularly in females who menstruate too copiously, sometimes followed by fainting.

MOSCHUS $^{0}_{3}{}^{0}$. Frequently serviceable when the nasal hemorrhage occurs in nervous, hysterical females.

AMMONIUM C. Bleeding from the nose after a meal.

SILICEA. Nasal hemorrhage in scrofulous subjects.

When the hemorrhage is of an active kind, the patient should be placed in the erect posture, and kept cool and quiet for some time afterwards. The diet in all cases must be low, and unstimulating.

When there is reason to fear suffocation from the bleeding continuing inwardly, and getting into the throat, as is liable to happen in extremely debilitated subjects, in whom little or no reaction appears to follow the administration of the remedies, the anterior and posterior outlets from the nose may be plugged; the latter by passing threads up the nostrils, and bringing them out at the mouth, then securing pieces of sponge, or small rolls of lint to the ends; after this, the threads should be drawn back, and tied sufficiently tight so as to bring the plugs somewhat firmly against the orifices.

Sprinkling or dashing cold water on the face; exposing the face to a current of cold air; placing the feet or hands in warm water; applying a wet cloth round the abdomen, and even dipping the head into a pail of iced water, or salt and water, are amongst the best of the popular means, or occasional auxiliary modes of stopping an excessive or prolonged discharge of blood from the nose.

With regard to the administration of the remedies, the repetition of the dose, if called for, must depend upon the greater or less degree of the severity of the attack. We ought to be in no hurry to repeat in the majority of cases. (See also what has been said on this matter in the INTRODUCTION.)

SWELLING OF THE NOSE.

The remedies for this, as well as all other maladies, must be selected according to the cause, where known. Thus, if the affection has arisen from a *contusion*, *Arnica* (externally and internally) must be prescribed.

If the disorder is encountered in scrofulous subjects, one or more of the following must be had recourse to: *Aurum* or

Asafœtida; or *Sulphur*, followed by *Calcarea;* or *Belladonna*, followed by *Mercurius* and *Hepar s.* When the disease has been excited by the abuse of *mercury: Hepar s., Acidum nitricum, Aurum, Belladonna*, or *Sulphur*, will be found the most efficacious. When attributable to the habitual use of *spirituous liquors: Calcarea, Arsenicum, Nux v., Pulsatilla, Sulphur;* or *Lachesis, Bellad., Merc., Hepar s.* Finally, *Bellad., Merc.*, and *Hepar* have been found most serviceable in cases where the tumefaction was red and very painful; in similar cases of an obstinate character: *Bryonia, Sulphur, Calcarea* and *Rhus* have proved efficacious. When black spots in the nose are met with at the same time, *Sulphur* and *Graphites* have chiefly been recommended; and where there are *scabs, Silicea, Sepia, Carbo v.* and *Natrum m.*, for the most part. Red spots, *Acidum phosphoricum.* Redness of the *point* of the nose, *Calc., Carbo animalis*, or *Rhus toxicodendron.* Coppery redness, *Arsenicum* and *Cannabis.* WARTS on the nose, *Causticum* chiefly; but in some cases, also *Thuja* and *Acidum nitr.*

Against swelling of the *interior* of the nose (Schneiderian membrane), *Teucrium marum verum* especially.

In CARIES of the bones of the nose, whether of a scrofulous or mercurial origin, *Aurum* is the most important remedy. When of syphilitic origin, *Mercurius* is to be preferred, provided the patient has not already been placed under an injurious course of that powerful medicine, in which case the affection is as likely to have arisen from the *remedy* as from the disease, and will consequently require to be combated by *anti-mercurial* medicines, amongst which *Aurum* will in this instance form the most valuable remedial agent; the other general antidotes to the injurious effects of mercury on the constitution, such as *Hepar s., Acidum nitr., Sulphur*, and *Calcarea;* or, *Lachesis, Carb. v., Staphysagria, Lycopodium, Asafœtida, Acid. phosph.*, and *Silicea*, etc., may in some cases become necessary, particularly when the system generally has become impaired by the cause in question.

OZÆNA. This disorder consists of an ulcer having its site in the nose, from which a fetid purulent matter is discharged.

It usually commences with slight inflammation and tumefaction about the alæ nasi, accompanied with sneezing, increased flow of mucus, with which the nostril becomes obstructed, and sometimes slight hemorrhage. The ulceration soon spreads from the schneiderian membrane to the nasal cartilages, the mucus gradually assumes the nature of pus, and if the disease be not checked, the bones become implicated, and caries results; a thin, acrid, offensive matter or sanies is then constantly discharged, and often excoriates the lips and throat, and the sense of smelling becomes abolished; eventually the ossa spongiosa inferior, and also the vomer, and in the worst cases, particularly when there is complication with scrofulous and venereal or mercurial disease, even the palate and superior maxillary bones exfoliate, the bridge of the nose falls in, and leaves a frightful deformity of countenance.

Therapeutics. The remedies which have chiefly been employed in this malignant disease are: *Teucrium marum verum, Pulsatilla, Sulphur;* or *Magnes. m., Bryonia, Belladonna, Lachesis, Lycopodium, Natrum m., Causticum,* in the first stage, with mucous obstruction; *Mercurius* and *Aurum* in the second, with discharge of pus, and also affection of the bones; followed, if required, in Ozæna scrofulosa, by *Sulphur, Silicea, Acidum nitricum, Phosphorus, Conium,* or *Potassæ bich.* In SYPHILITIC OZÆNA, *Mercurius* forms the principal remedy; but if the patient has already been subjected to an injurious course of that medicine, *Aurum* is to be preferred, and succeeded, if requisite, by *Acidum nitricum, Hepar s., Asafœtida, Lachesis, Conium,* or *Thuja.*

In disease in the *Antrum Highmorianum,* the following have been recommended: *Teucrium marum verum, Arsenicum, Lycopodium, Sulphur, Silex, Aurum, Mercurius, Hepar s., Mezereum, Staphysagria, Carb. v., Antimonium c., Kali hydr., Phosphorus;* and *Spigelia, Nux, China, Phosphorus,* as palliatives when the pains are very severe.*

* Goullon considers *Arsenicum* and *Lycopodium* as almost specific in this disease. He recommends Arsenicum to be given when the pains are excessively severe, of a throbbing and splitting, or bursting description, when at their height. Lycopodium when there is a thick and yellow discharge. A. H. Z. 2, 24.

POLYPUS: *Teucrium*, *Staphysagria*, *Phosphorus*, *Sulphur*, *Sepia*, and *Silicea*, have chiefly been recommended.

CANCER NASI: *Arsenicum*, *Carbo v.*, *Aurum*, *Sepia*, *Silicea*, *Sulphur*, and *Calcarea*, are the remedies which have principally been pointed out as the most appropriate to combat this serious and frightful malady.

CANKER OF THE MOUTH. SCURVY IN THE MOUTH.

Cancrum Oris. Gangrena Oris. Stomacace.

This affection consists of a fetor in the mouth, with a viscid, bloody discharge from the gums, which are at the same time hot, red, tumid, spongy, very sensitive, retracted from the teeth, and subsequently ulcerated along their margins. Sometimes there is also glandular swellings, salivation, or ptyalism; and usually looseness of the teeth, impeded mastication and deglutition, great debility, and slow fever.

THERAPEUTICS. *Mercurius* is the most useful remedy here, and may generally form the first prescription in almost every case of the kind, as it will rarely fail to prove serviceable, if not sufficient to effect a perfect cure. When, however, we have reason to conclude that the symptoms above described have in reality been created by the injurious employment of that remedy, under allopathic treatment, it will be necessary to have recourse to the appropriate antidotes to these effects of the said powerful mineral, amongst which *Carbo v.* will be found of primary importance; should the improvement effected by *Carb. v.* be only of a partial character, the treatment must be followed up by *Hepar s.* and *Acid. nitricum* alternately; or by *Staphysagria*, if fungous excrescences form on the gums. *Carbo v.* is, moreover, of great service when the disorder has arisen from unwholesome food, the daily use of kitchen-salt in *excess*, or the prolonged use of salt meat;* when the gums smell most offensively, and bleed

* Constantine Hering recommends a drop of *Spiritus ætheris nitrosi* once or twice a day, in the event of *Carbo v.* or *Arsenicum* failing to bring about a favourable action in such cases.

during mastication; the teeth loose, mouth hot, tongue much excoriated, and with difficulty to be moved.

After the employment of *Carbo v.* we may have recourse to *Arsenicum*, if the ulceration continues extensive, and the patient complains of *burning* pains in the gums, with great prostration of strength; or *Arsenicum* and *China* in alternation; if, in addition to the foregoing, the gums present a black, spongy, and somewhat gangrenous appearance.

Nux v. is an admirable remedy in this disorder, particularly when it occurs in meagre, dark-complexioned subjects, of bilious temperament and choleric disposition, who lead a sedentary life; the gums presenting a putrid aspect, and so much swollen as completely to cover the teeth; countenance pale and sunken.

Capsicum has been found useful, under nearly similar circumstances, but the affected party of a plethoric habit and phlegmatic temperament.

Dulcamara may be used with advantage after *Mercurius*, when the glands of the throat are implicated in the derangement; or it may be selected in preference to *Mercurius* when the disease is prone to be excited by the least exposure to cold, during damp, or cold, raw, wet weather.

Natrum m. is frequently a valuable remedy in completing the cure after the administration of *Carbo v.*, *Acid. nitr.*, *Hepar*, etc. It is more especially indicated when the ulcers are indolent, and do not put on a healing aspect; the gums being at the same time much swollen, very sensitive to heat or cold, and disposed to bleed at the slightest touch; moreover, when painful vesicles or blisters are observed on the tongue, inner surface of the lips, and cheeks; which impede speech, and, together with the irritable gums, render the act of mastication a work of labour and excessive torture. When, notwithstanding the employment of the last mentioned remedy, the complaint seems disposed to linger, *Sulphur* may be prescribed, and followed or alternated with *Acidum sulphuricum*, *Sepia*, or any of the other medicines already treated of, if required by the bent of the succeeding changes in the features of the case, etc. *Silicea*, *Sub-boras Sodæ*, *Helleb.* and *Iodium* may also prove useful in some cases.

Lemon-juice, which is well known as a most valuable remedy in *scurvy*, is equally useful as a domestic remedy in stomacace.

Sage is equally useful in some varieties of the disorder. Rinsing the mouth with brandy has also been found of service.

The use of wholesome, easily digested food, with a due proportion of *vegetables*, must be enjoined in order to expedite the cure.

SCURVY. (*Scorbutus.*)

This disorder is characterized by excessive debility, pale and bloated countenance; œdematous swelling of the inferior extremities; hemorrhages; livid spots on the skin, or foul ulcers; offensive urine and extremely fetid stools. The gums spongy, or otherwise diseased, as described in the preceding article.

It chiefly affects sailors, or others who from circumstances are deprived of fresh provisions and an adequate quantity of ascescent food, and are exposed to cold and moisture together with fatigue. Intemperance, want of exercise, impure air, uncleanliness, with depressing emotions, further tend to predispose to the disease, when combined with unwholesome food, or the before-said alimentary deficiency.

In the cure, as also the prevention of this malady, it is requisite, in the first place, to remove the probable cause of its invasion where that is practicable ; and to furnish the patient, if possible, with wholesome diet, fresh vegetables, and those fruits which furnish citric acid, such as lemon, the juice of which made into a drink forms an invaluable remedy. Sour-kraut, and other substances which have undergone the acetous fermentation; cider, spruce beer, and the like, as also vinegar, have, moreover, been recommended.

The homœopathic medicines which may be prescribed with the most advantage against the ulcers and diseased gums are: *Carbo v.*, *Nux v.*. *Arsenicum*, *Mercurius*, *Staphysagria*, and *Sulphur ;* or also, ***Acid nitr.***, ***Cistus***, ***Nat. m.***, ***Ammonium c. et*** *m.*, *Causticum*, *Dulcamara*, *Kreasotum*, *Acid. mur.*, *Sepia*, etc. (See the preceding article, and also that on ULCERS.)

The use of lemon or wine-juice and other acids must be discontinued during the employment of the homœopathic remedies.

GUMBOIL. *Silicea*, *Staphysagria* and *Calcarea*, but particularly the former, are the principal remedies against this affection. When there is much inflammation, and considerable swelling, *Belladonna* may be prescribed, followed by *Mercurius* and *Hepar sulph.*, if little relief is obtained from the former. *Nux v.*, *Pulsatilla*, and *Sulphur*, are sometimes very useful. In swelling of the jaw, with suppuration, whether in consequence of carious teeth, or from the unskilful abstraction of a tooth, *Silicea* is the most important remedy. Irritation, arising from the cutting of the wisdom-teeth : *Aconite* and *Calcarea ;* also *Belladonna*, *Arnica*, and *Chamomilla*, when there is inflammation with swelling of the face.

INFLAMMATION OF THE TONGUE.

Glossitis.

DIAGNOSIS. Tumefaction, with heat and redness of the tongue; the swelling is sometimes so great as to fill the whole cavity of the mouth, rendering swallowing impossible, and threatening suffocation; unless re-solution take place, it may terminate in induration, suppuration, or gangrene.

CAUSES. Besides a general strumous habit, local injuries, acrid substances, rheumatism, catarrh, and metastasis.

THERAPEUTICS. The following medicines will be found most appropriate in the treatment of this affection, according to the exciting cause : *Arnica*, *Urtica urens*, *Mercurius*, *Aconitum*, *Belladonna*, *Pulsatilla*, *Lachesis*, and *Arsenicum*.

ARNICA, in cases of lesion of the tongue from the points of decayed teeth, etc., or of burns or scalds. (*Acid phosph.* is occasionally required after, or may, in severe cases, be given in preference, to *Arnica ;* in other instances, *Silicea* and *Sulphur* will be required to complete the cure.

Administration. A few drops of the matrix tincture to a cupful of water, rinsing the mouth with the mixture two or three times a day.

Urtica urens has been recommended in preference to *Arnica* in burns and scalds of the mouth.

Administration. The part affected slightly touched with a soft brush dipped in the tincture.

Mercurius is almost specific when it presents itself in the form of a disease of the tongue, attended with excessive inflammatory swelling or induration.

Administration. Half a grain of the third trituration to an ounce of water; a dessert-spoonful of the mixture every two, three, or twelve hours, according to the violence of the disease.

Aconitum may, with advantage, precede the above remedy should the inflammation be very intense.

Administration. $\frac{0\,0}{6}$; if needful, repeated in two hours, followed by *Mercurius* in from three to six hours.

Belladonna. When the affection does not speedily yield to *Mercurius*, or when the inflammation is of an erysipelatous or active phlegmonous nature.

Administration. A few globules of the sixth potency to an ounce of water; a dessert-spoonful every six to eight hours, until the inflammation abates; after which we may, in many cases, return to *Mercurius*.

Pulsatilla has been found useful in cases arising from suppressed hemorrhoidal and arthritic affections.

Against indications of threatening gangrene, *Arsenicum* and *Lachesis* are the principal remedies. They may both be given at the sixth potency, and repeated according to results.

In some cases when, from great tumefaction of the tongue, suffocation threatens, we must have recourse to longitudinal incisions; and after having thus warded off the more pressing danger, exhibit *Cinchona*, and then fall back upon the more specific remedies.

In some *extreme cases* of this nature, where the disease having made head before the arrival, it may be found necessary to resort to tracheotomy. This is, however, a dangerous mode of relief from the risk of consequent tracheal inflammation; but, when it has been found absolutely necessary, we may, by the exhibition of *Arnica*, $\frac{00}{6}$, internally; and in the form of lotion, in the proportion of four minims of the mother-tincture to a hundred of water, materially diminish the risk of this taking place. In cases of soreness or ulceration of the tongue: see ULCERS.

Such cases will, however, rarely, if ever, occur to the homœopathic practitioner, if the disease be taken in time, and his remedies judiciously selected.

OFFENSIVE BREATH.

The most frequent causes of this unpleasant affection are: uncleanliness, leaving particles of food in the teeth; and accumulation of tartar; or carious teeth; a diseased state of the gums; aphthæ in the mouth; derangement of the stomach; or an abuse of mercury.

THERAPEUTICS. When there is reason to suppose that the first named circumstance is the chief cause of the complaint, its removal will be readily effected by proper attention, rinsing the mouth with tepid water, and brushing the teeth with a moderately hard brush night and morning, as also after every meal.

When attributable to the second cause, a dentist of known skill and respectability ought to be consulted. Lastly, when the annoyance can be traced to any of the remaining sources enumerated, the remedies given under those different headings ought to be had recourse to.

When, on the other hand, no apparent cause of derangement can be assigned or detected, benefit will often be derived from one or more of the following medicines: *Nux v.*, *Silicea*, *Pulsatilla*, *Sulphur*, and *Chamomilla*; or *Arnica*, *Bellad.*, *Hyos.*, etc.

If the heaviness or fetor of the breath is chiefly perceptible in the morning: *Nux v.* and *Silicea* will frequently be found successful in affording relief. *Arnica*, *Bellad.*, and *Sulph.*, have also proved effectual in similar cases. If after a meal, *Nux v.*, succeeded by *Chamomilla* and *Sulphur*. If in the evening, or during the night, *Pulsatilla* or *Sulphur*.

Mercurius, *Bryonia*, *Arsenicum*, *Hyoscyamus*, *Agaricus*, *Ambra*, *Carbo v. et a.*, *Sepia*, *Lycopodium*, etc., may also prove useful in particular cases. In young girls at the age of puberty, *Aurum* is often the most appropriate; but occasionally *Pulsatilla*, *Sepia*, *Belladonna*, or *Hyoscyamus*, will be found preferable here. When the abuse of mercury has evidently been the cause of the evil: *Aurum*, *Carbo v.*, *Lachesis*, *Sulphur*, *Hepar*, *Belladonna*, or *Acidum nitricum*, etc., will be found the most suitable.

FACE-ACHE. FACE-AGUE.

Neuralgia Facialis. Tic Douloureux. Prosopalgia.

This distressing malady consists in an excruciating pain, which has its seat in the branches of the fifth pair of nerves, and is accordingly experienced with great acuteness under the eye, and sometimes before the ear, from whence it shoots over the entire half of the face, and frequently into the orbit and cranium. The paroxysms occasionally continue, with shorter or longer intervals, for several days or weeks in succession, and when at their height, are frequently accompanied with spasmodic twitchings in the facial muscles.

The disease is unfortunately generally of great obstinacy, and, in some melancholy instances, utterly incurable. In its idiopathic form, the remedies which have hitherto been employed in homœopathic practice with the most success are: *Belladonna*, *Platina*, *Lycopodium*, *Colocynth*, *Arsenicum*, *China*, *Mezereum*, *Veratrum*, etc.

Belladonna. When the pain chiefly pursues the course of the infra orbitary nerve, but sometimes also the other branches of the fifth; and is prone to be excited by rubbing the usual seat of the sufferings; darting pains in the cheekbones, nose, jaws, or zygomatic process; or cutting and tensive pains, with stiffness at the nape of the neck, and clenching of the jaws; twitches in the eyelid, or violent shooting and tearing and dragging pains in the ball of the eye; convulsive jerking in the facial muscles, and distortion of the mouth; heat and redness in the face. The pain is generally preceded by itching and creeping in the affected side of the face, and at times becomes so severe as to be almost insupportable.

PLATINA. Feeling of *coldness* and *torpor* in the affected side of the face, with severe spasmodic pain, or tensive pressure in the zygomatic process, with a sensation of creeping or crawling, and aggravation or renewal of the sufferings in the evening, and when in a state of rest; lachrymation; redness of the face, etc.

LYCOPODIUM is often useful, when the symptoms are much the same as described under the preceding remedy with the exception of the torpor and creeping, but particularly when the right side of the face is the part affected.

COLOCYNTH. Violent rending and darting pains, which chiefly occupy the left side of the face, are aggravated by the *slightest touch*, and extend to the head, temples, nose, ears, teeth, etc.

ARSENICUM. When there is a tendency to periodicity in the attacks or paroxysms, and the pains partake more especially of a *burning*, *pricking*, and rending character, and are experienced chiefly around the eye, and occasionally in the temples, the sufferings being occasionally of so severe a description as almost to drive the patient distracted; great anguish; excessive prostration, with desire for the recumbent posture; sensation of coldness in the affected parts; exacerbation during repose, after fatigue, in the evening, when in bed, or after a meal; temporary melioration from external heat.

CHINA. Also, as in the instance of the foregoing remedy, when there is a tendency to periodicity in the attacks, and when the pains are excessive, attended with extreme sensibility of the skin, and consequent *aggravation from the slightest touch;* sensation of torpor and paralytic weakness in the affected part; great loquacity, with ill-humour, paleness of the face, frequently followed or alternated with redness and transient heat of the face.

MEZEREUM. Pains which occupy the *left zygomatic process*, consisting chiefly of a spasmodic stupifying description, and extending to the eye, temple, ear, teeth, neck, and shoulder, with exacerbation from partaking of warm food or drink, or on coming into a warm room after being in the open air.

VERATRUM. Insupportable pains which almost drive the patient to distraction; excessive weakness even to fainting; general chilliness; exacerbation of suffering on getting warm in bed, or towards morning; temporary relief on moving about.

SPIGELIA is frequently a useful palliative remedy in all cases when the pain is excessive.

In other cases: *Lachesis, Phosphorus, Hyoscyamus, Mags. arc., Manganum, Merc., Rhus, Ignatia, Arnica, Capsicum, Causticum, Staphysagria, Coffea*, etc , may be found useful.

When the malady is symptomatic of derangement of the digestive functions,—*Nux v., Pulsatilla, Bryonia, Chamomilla*, or *Lycopodium*, will usually be found the most serviceable.

In RHEUMATIC FACE-ACHE, or prosopalgia,—*Aconitum, Bryonia, Rhus, Causticum, Mercurius, Phosphorus, Pulsatilla, Mezereum, Phosphorus, Sulphur, Nux v., Lachesis*, etc., are those that have generally proved the most effectual.

In ARTHRITIC,—*Nux v., Rhus, Colocynth, Mercurius, Causticum*, etc.

FACE-ACHE from the effects of *mercury* will chiefly require the employment of *Aurum, Hepar, Carbo v., Sulphur, China*, etc. Finally, in prosopalgia generally, the following have proved more or less useful: *Aconitum, Arnica, Verbascum, Sulphur, Calcarea, Capsicum, Pulsatilla, Stannum, Conium, Thuja, Baryta c., Coffea, Kali, Camphora*, etc.

PALPITATION OF THE HEART.

Palpitatio Cordis.

When this disorder occurs in plethoric individuals, *Aconitum, Belladonna*, and *Nux v.* will be found the most appropriate remedies, followed by *Sulphur*. Should the affection prove obstinate, *Arsenicum* and *Veratrum* alternately are sometimes useful after *Sulphur*, when the palpitation has resulted especially in consequence of the suppression of an eruption, or the sudden healing up of an old sore. ***Causticum*** and ***Lachesis*** are also occasionally useful in the latter case.

When it results after debilitating losses, such as hemorrhage, etc., *China* is the principal remedy, but may require to be followed by *Acid. phosph.*, *Sulphur*, *Calcarea*, or *Nux v.*

Palpitation of the heart from a *fright*, usually yields readily to *Opium;* from *fear* or anguish, to *Veratrum;* after sudden joy, to *Coffea;* and if from contradiction, or a fit of passion, *Acon.*, *Cham.*, or *Nux v.*, and *Ignatia.* When the derangement occurs in nervous individuals, and particularly hysterical females, *Pulsatilla, Coffea, Cocculus, Veratrum, Lachesis, Chamomilla,* and *Asafœtida* will generally be found the best adapted to afford relief. In other cases, *Aurum, Cocculus, Phosphorus, Spigelia, Ferrum,* or *Acid. nitr.*, etc., will be required.

CRAMP IN THE LEGS.

Veratrum, Nux vomica, Sulphur, Calcarea, Lycopodium, Acidum nitricum, Sepia, Camphora, Argilla, Colocynth, and *Rhus*, are amongst the best remedies for cramps in the calves of the legs. *Veratrum* has been recommended as one of the most useful remedies in eradicating the tendency to frequent returns of this painful and troublesome disorder, succeeded by *Sulphur* and *Colocynth*, should it not suffice to effect a cure. *Rhus* when the attacks occur during the day when sitting, as well as at night. *Sepia, Lycopodium,* and *Acid. nitr.* when it occurs chiefly in walking. *Sulphur*, after *Nux v.* or *Rhus*, when the attacks occur chiefly during the night. *Calcarea* when stretching out the limb brings on the cramp. *Argilla* in cramps on crossing the legs, or even on descending stairs. *Colocynth* is frequently beneficial when stiffness and pain are always experienced in the limb for some time after the attack.

GOITRE. BRONCHOCELE.

This disfigurement arises from a tumefied state of the glandula thyroides, a large glandular body situated on the front of the throat (upon the cricoid cartilage, trachea, and horns of the thyroid cartilage). As the enlargement increases, it is productive of a considerable degree of obstruction to free inspiration, from the pressure which it exerts against the windpipe. The disorder is most frequently encountered amongst the inhabitants of mountainous districts. Women are more prone to be afflicted with it than men, and particularly those who have suffered from severe labours. An inherent constitutional taint seems, however, to be the chief predisposing cause.

In the treatment of this affection, *Spongia marina* has been found the more generally useful remedy, administered in repeated doses, from the sixth potency downwards. In cases of long standing, one or more of the following remedies may prove of service in materially diminishing the size of the tumour, if not sufficient to disperse it entirely: *Calcarea, Staphysagria, Lycopodium, Iodium, Ammonium c., Causticum,* and *Natrum c. et m.;* or *Ferrum, Sepia, Thuja.*

SWEATING FEET.

Some individuals are much troubled with a disagreeable, clammy, sweating of the feet, to such an extent as to render it necessary to change the stockings several times daily. This evil is, moreover, a source of extreme annoyance to others, from the offensive odour which is usually exhaled at the same time. The utmost attention to cleanliness is insufficient to remedy the state of matters; and to attempt to suppress the secretion by cold water, or powerful astringents, is highly culpable, from the dangerous consequences which are liable to ensue from a sudden suppression thereby effected.

Amongst the homœopathic remedies, through the instrumentality of which, a safe and permanent cure has most frequently been brought about, *Rhus toxicodendron* and *Silicea* merit priority of notice. A few globules of the first named, may be taken every four days for a fortnight or three weeks; at the expiration of which period, a few days may be allowed to elapse, and if improvement then set in, the medicine may be continued at intervals of increasing length until the cure is effected. But should no melioration result, *Silicea* may be had recourse to in the same manner. After *Silicea*, *Rhus* may again be resorted to, if required. These two remedies are also the most appropriate to be administered against the deleterious consequences of a suddenly checked foot-sweat.

Other remedies may be required in obstinate cases of this complaint, or in those where derangement of the system generally coexists. The following may therefore be pointed out as worthy of being referred to in such cases: *Mercurius*, *Baryta c.*, *Graphites*, *Kali c.*, *Cyclamen;* or *Sulphur*, *Calcarea*, *Lachesis*, *Carbo v.*, *Lycopodium*, *Sepia*, *Acid. nitr.*, etc.

SLEEPLESSNESS. *Agrypnia.*

Sleep is essential to renew the vital energy which has been exhausted during the day, as also to assist the function of nutrition. When, therefore, anything occurs to deprive us of this indispensable necessary for a protracted period, or, at all events, so materially to disturb it as to render it inadequate to fulfil its requisite purpose, the health will, as an all but invariable rule, eventually give way under the deprivation.

The average duration of sleep is from six to eight hours; but it is liable to variation from several causes. Some, from peculiarity of constitution, require less, others a little more. Habits of idleness, etc., tend to prolong it; and it may here be remarked, that when not restrained within proper limits, instead of repairing, it exhausts the strength; and is, as well as the derangement of which it is our object at present to treat, consequently productive of serious diseases, such as madness and idiocy,—these distressing maladies having unquestionably been traced, in some instances, to indolent habits of prolonging sleep beyond the period required for healthy recreation.

In almost all cases, sleeplessness is but symptomatic of some other disease, and can only be remedied by the removal of the abnormal source. It frequently, however, forms so prominent a feature as to render it necessary that we should treat it as an idiopathic disease, and direct our attention to the selection of medicines comformably.

Intense mental application, continued up to the period of going to rest; sedentary habits; the habitual use of coffee, (often for the express purpose of warding off inclination to sleep,) also weakness of the digestive functions, are frequent causes of sleeplessness. Under such circumstances, *Nux v.* will generally be found the most appropriate remedy; but, unless the acquired habits above detailed are given up, or materially altered, no permanent benefit can be expected from the employment of the remedy referred to.

Overloading the stomach, particularly towards night; the habitual employment of stimulating, or rich, indigestible food; thereby producing constipation, excessive flatulence, and other signs of derangement in the digestive functions, are additional fertile sources of disturbed sleep, which can only be obviated by the observance of a more simple mode of living. The attainment of the desired relief may, however, be considerably forwarded by means of a dose or two of *Pulsatilla.*

Mental emotions often originate sleeplessness.

When excessive joy is the assignable cause, *Coffea* is a useful remedy. When from dejection, caused by grief, unpleasant ideas, vexation, etc., *Ignatia.* If attributable to fear, or fright, or when the sleep is disturbed by fantastic or frightful visions, *Opium;* followed, if required, by *Belladonna* in the latter instance; and when anxious, annoying, or agitating events disturb or retard sleep, *Aconitum.*

Sleeplessness arising from nervous excitement in sensitive or irritable subjects will often yield to *Hyoscyamus,* or to *Belladonna* where there exists a strong but ineffectual desire to obtain sleep. The latter medicine is further indicated when agitation or anguish, with frightful visions, timidity or terror, apprehension of real objects, etc., are complained of; or when the sleep is disturbed by frequent starting, and is attended with extreme sleeplessness early in the evening, or towards morning.

Moschus is a useful remedy in sleeplessness occurring in hysterical or hypochondriacal individuals, arising from nervous excitement. *Acid. phosph.* and *Sepia* are also occasionally useful in such cases.

STANNUM has been recommended as a *general* remedy (?) in sleeplessness.*

Sleeplessness in old people can scarcely be considered a disease. But when it occurs in children, it almost invariably arises from some bodily ailment, which ought to be attended to and removed as early as possible, if practicable, as deprivation of sleep is more detrimental during infancy and childhood than at any other period of life. (See SLEEPLESSNESS IN CHILDREN, Part. III.)

Coldness of the feet is a frequent cause of retarded or disturbed sleep. Daily exercise in the open air is here, as in most other cases, to be recommended; also gentle and general friction, when there is at the same time, chilliness or stiffness of the limbs. The application of a vessel containing hot water to the feet is the only mode of obtaining any refreshing sleep in some cases, when coldness of the feet is the disturbing cause:—

This languid state of the circulation is often capable of being permanently removed by means of homœopathic remedies, combined with appropriate exercise. *Ammonium m.* and *Carbo v. et a.*; as also *Graphites*, *Kali c.*, *Nux v.*, or *Sulphur*, etc. will generally be found the best adapted to the attainment of this.

When, on the other hand, sleep is prevented or retarded by burning heat in the feet,— *Lachesis*, and, in other cases, *Pulsatilla*, *Acid. phosphoricum*, *Stannum*, *Lycopodium*, *Kali c.*, *Sepia*, or *Secale c.*, etc., must be selected.

Sleeplessness from a harsh, dry, and imperspirable state of the skin, may be remedied after the removal of the said cause, when not impracticable from too long continuance, etc., by means of *Graphites*, *Natrum c.*, *Silicea*, *Sepia*, *Acid. nitr.*, or *Calcarea*, etc. (The warm bath forms a useful palliative, occasionally.)

Sleeplessness and other derangements resulting from tea, require the employment of the antidotes to that drug for their removal. Of these, *Cinchona* will usually prove the best;

* A. H. Z. No. 12. Band 28.

should it not be adequate to effect the purpose required, *Ferrum* will often succeed. (*Coffea* is to be preferred in recent cases of indisposition from green tea; but it must be followed by the exhibition of *Cinchona*, if relief is not soon obtained.)

When from coffee, *Nux v.*, as has been already remarked, is the principal remedy; on other occasions, *Chamomilla* will be required, particularly when sleeplessness and other sufferings, such as headache, colic, etc., occur in nervous, highly excitable, and irritable subjects, who are extremely impatient under sufferings even of a description that would be deemed trivial by ordinary people. *Ignatia*, particularly in the case of mild, sensitive, or changeable dispositions. *Cocculus*, in nearly similar circumstances as described under *Chamomilla*, with the distinction of a sensation of emptiness or lightness in the head.

NIGHT-MARE. *Incubus. Ephialtes.*

When this well-known and distressing disturbance occurs very frequently in an aggravated form, it becomes necessary to prescribe for it. The homœopathic remedies which have chiefly been employed against it to the best advantage are *Aconitum*, *Nux vomica*, and *Opium*.

Aconitum. When there is considerable febrile excitement, with quickness of pulse, thirst, palpitation of the heart, oppression at the chest, anxiety, and agitation.

Nux v. When night-mare is occasioned by sedentary habits, the habitual indulgence in spirituous, or malt liquors, etc.

Pulsatilla. When there is derangement in the digestive functions, arising from gross living, heavy suppers, etc.

Opium is a remedy of importance in all cases of a severe character; but particularly when, during the attack, the respiration is nearly suspended, or stertorous, the eyes only half closed, the mouth open, the countenance expressive of extreme anguish, and bedewed with cold perspiration; subsultus tendinum. When any of the foregoing remedies, but especially *Nux v.* and *Pulsatilla*, are insufficient to effect a cure,—*Sulphur* or *Silicea* may be resorted to in repeated doses. In other cases, one or more of the following may prove useful: ***Phosphorus*, *Ruta*, *Valerian*, *Ammonium c.***, and ***Hepar***. Any apparent exciting causes of the attacks must at the same time be avoided; the diet should be light and wholesome; suppers altogether abstained from, and a glass of cold water partaken of instead, on retiring to rest.

Daily exercise in the open air, the shower-bath, or sponging with cold water every evening, are useful preventives, or auxiliaries during treatment.

ACUTE INFLAMMATION OF THE SPINAL CORD AND ITS MEMBRANES.

Myelitis. Meningitis spinalis.

This affection is indicated by pain, more or less severe, in some cases of an intermittent character, either confined to the lumbar, dorsal, or cervical region, or embracing the entire length of the spine. The pain is aggravated by the slightest movement, and an exalted sensibility of various parts of the cutaneous surface is often perceptible in the dread and shrinking which the patient exhibits at the slightest touch. Sharp pain at the epigastrium, sometimes spreading over the whole of the abdominal region, and increased on pressure; palpitation of the heart; sensation of constriction and weight in the fore part of the chest, with oppressed respiration; small, quick, hard pulse,—are symptoms which are generally encountered in the course of the disorder.

When the inflammation occupies only a *part* of the cord, the symptoms vary according to its locality. Thus, when the commencement, or the cervical portion is principally affected: spasm of the pharynx, trismus with loss of voice; spasm or other abnormal conditions in the muscles of the neck, chest, and superior extremities, with general clonic convulsions, declare themselves. When the dorsal portion of the cord is the seat of the inflammation, opisthotonos usually results. And when that of the lumbar region is seized: retention of urine, or paralytic or spasmodic affections of the pelvic viscera generally, are met with. In each of the latter cases, the inferior extremities are commonly either convulsed or paralyzed.

When the membranes of the cord are principally or solely affected, the sensibility of the surface is said to be always increased, and the spasms more frequently general, and of a tonic character. While, in inflammation, confined to the substance of the cord, the sensibility is usually lessened, the muscles of the extremities affected with clonic spasm or paralysis, and only those of the back in a state of tonic contraction. In the former, moreover, the bowels are for the most part constipated,—while in the latter, diarrhœa has almost uniformly been found to predominate. Finally, according as the interior or posterior columns of the spinal cord happen to be the seat of the inflammation, so, it may be concluded, will the power of *motion* or the *sensibility* be abnormally altered.

CAUSES. Exposure to cold and damp, and external injuries, appear to form the leading causes of this inflammation.

CHRONIC INFLAMMATION of the spinal cord and its coverings is generally accompanied with a trivial degree of local pain, and its prominent features chiefly consist in derangement of the functions of the viscera, deprivation or diminution of the sense of feeling, paralysis, cramp, and emaciation. The chronic variety is even more dangerous than the acute.

The disease, when confined to the substance of the cord, may terminate in *softening* (ramollissement); *induration; suppuration; gangrene*. And in effusions of serum, pus, or blood; or in thickening of their structure, when the membranes have been the seat of the inflammation.

THERAPEUTICS. *Aconitum* must be prescribed in repeated doses, in all cases where the accompanying fever is intense; and on the completion of its beneficial action, recourse must be had to *Belladonna, Dulcamara, Arsenicum, Digitalis, Pulsatilla, Bryonia, Nux v., Cocculus, Rhus, Ignatia, Opium, Veratrum*,—according to the portion of the cord which is evidently attacked.

BELLADONNA is the most important remedy when the upper part is the seat of the disorder. If, from the invasion of delirium, etc., there is some reason to apprehend an extension of the inflammation to the brain, this remedy will still be the most appropriate, and that on which we must rest our chief hope in so serious a complication of a malady already sufficiently dangerous. *Hyoscyamus*, *Stramonium*, *Bryonia*, and in some instances *Sulphur*, may be found necessary, however, and prove useful in warding off a fatal result. (Vide PHRENITIS.) *Dulcamara** may follow *Aconitum* and *Belladonna*, when the more acute symptoms of spinitis have been removed, and particularly when the disease has been excited by exposure to cold and wet. *Arsenicum*, *Pulsatilla* and *Digitalis*, have been recommended as useful auxiliary remedies when the thoracic viscera are prominently affected, evidenced by laborious and anxious respiration, palpitation of the heart, etc.; and *Veratrum*, *Nux v.*, *Cocculus*, and *Ignatia*, when the abdominal viscera are seized with coldness and spasms.

Should opisthotonos result from inflammation of the dorsal division of the cord: *Belladonna*, *Rhus*, *Ignatia* and *Opium* are chiefly to be recommended. Again, when the inflammation is restricted to the lumbar portion of the cord: *Nux v.*, *Cocculus*, *Digitalis*, and *Bryonia*; or *Pulsatilla*, *Rhus*, *Veratrum*, and *Sulphur*. In general tonic spasms resulting from inflammation of the entire cord, or rather its enveloping membranes,—*Belladonna*, *Lachesis*, *Hyoscyamus*, *Opium*, *Natrum m.*, and *Ignatia*, are the remedies from which, in general cases, we may expect to derive the greatest benefit. *Arnica*, *Hyoscyamus* and *Opium* may claim a preference in myelitis arising from external injury; but we must be guided in our selection by the nature of the symptoms, and not hesitate to have recourse to one or more of the above-mentioned medicines if called for. (Vide HYDROPHOBIA and TETANUS.) In the chronic form of the malady, the medicines from which the most benefit may be looked for when the disease has not reached an irremediable stage are, in addition to most of those required in the acute variety,—*Sulphur*, *Silicea*, *Lachesis*, *Baryta c.*, *Stannum*, *Causticum*, etc.

* *Rhus* is perhaps more appropriate than *Dulc.* in such cases.

PALSY. *Paralysis.*

This affection consists in the abolition or diminution of the power of voluntary motion. It usually comes on suddenly, but in some instances it is preceded by numbness, coldness, paleness, and slight convulsive jerking or twitching in the parts. The treatment must be regulated according to the originating cause. When it results from apoplexy, see that article. When occurring as a sequel of rheumatism: *Arnica*, *Ferrum*, *Ruta*, as also *Bryonia*, *Rhus*, *Lycopodium*, *Sulphur*, and *Causticum*. When in consequence of debility from loss of fluids: *China*, *Ferrum*, *Baryta c.* and *Sulphur*. From the sudden suppression of an eruption, or of a wonted discharge: *Sulphur* and *Causticum*. And when it is attributable to exposure to the fumes of lead, or the constant handling of white-lead: *Opium* and *Belladonna*; or, *Platina*, *Alumina*, *Pulsatilla*, and *Nux v.* (These remedies are equally useful in LEAD COLIC, *colica pictonum.*)

With reference to the parts which are affected with the disorder: *Belladonna*, *Graphites*, and *Causticum* are chiefly recommended in paralysis of the facial muscles. *Belladonna*, *Opium*, *Hyoscyamus*, *Stramonium*, *Lachesis*, *Graphites*, and *Causticum*, in that of the tongue. *Belladonna*, *Nux v.*, *Cocculus*, *Lycopodium*, *Calcarea*, *Silicea*, *Opium*, *Zincum*, *Ruta*, etc., in paralysis of the upper extremities. And in that of the inferior extremities: *Cocculus*, *Nux v.*, *Opium*, *Sulphur*, *Silicea*, *Stannum*, and *Oleander* principally.

Electricity or galvanism, in moderation, is frequently of considerable service in facilitating the cure, or at all events, in promoting improvement in obstinate cases.

RUPTURE. *Hernia.*

By this term is understood a swelling occasioned by the protrusion of some of the viscera from the cavity of the abdomen. In most cases, the displaced intestines are included or contained in a bag, derived from the peritoneum, which they push before them in their descent. The situations in which the swelling most commonly makes its appearance are the groin, the navel, the scrotum, the labia pudendi, and the upper and interior part of the thigh. It also occurs in the vagina, perinæum, foramen ovale, and sciatic notch, and occasionally at every point of the fore part of the abdomen. The viscera which are most frequently protruded are the omentum, and the small and large intestines, or a portion both of omentum and intestine. But the stomach, liver, spleen, bladder, uterus, and ovaria, etc., have been known to enter into the formation of hernial tumours. In consequence of the tumour escaping at the above-mentioned different situations, it has received the appellations of *inguinal,** *umbilical,*† *scrotal,*‡ *prudendal,*‖ *crural* or *femoral, vaginal, perinæal, thyroideal,*§ *ischiatic and ventral,* etc. Further, from containing different kinds of viscera, it has been designated *epiplocele,* when its contents consist of a piece of the omentum only; *enterocele,* when of a fold or portion of intestine; and *entero-epiplocele* if both intestine and omentum contribute to form the swelling. A hernia or rupture, for the most part, appears suddenly after some violent corporal exertion, and presents an indolent, usually soft and elastic tumour, at some of the points or situations already referred to, but most frequently at the lower and lateral part of the abdomen (the groin); or towards the inner part of the bend of the thigh, or at the navel (descending from the abdominal ring in the first mentioned instance; from below Poupart's ligament in the second; and out of the umbilicus or navel in the third.) The swelling is subject to a change of size, being smaller, or quite imperceptible, when in the recumbent position; larger or only apparent on assuming the erect posture, and particularly when taking a full breath, coughing or sneezing, also on walking or standing long after a hearty meal. It is frequently diminished, or caused to recede completely, when pressed, but returns as soon

* Or a bubonocele.

† Or an oscheocele.

‡ Or hernia foraminis ovalis.

‖ Or an exomphalos. Omphalocele.

§ Or a bubonocele.

as the pressure is removed. Vomiting, constipation, colic, and other signs of a deranged state of the stomach and intestines, are frequent concomitants of rupture, arising from the abnormal situation of the viscera.

The nature of the contents of the hernial tumour are generally known by the following distinctions: if the case be an *enterocele*, the swelling is smooth, elastic, rendered tense by coughing, or by holding the breath; is in general very easily returnable, and is usually attended with a gurgling noise when ascending. An *epiplocele*, or omental hernia, is, on the other hand, of a more uneven and doughy or flabby feel; it is neither made tense, nor receives any impulse from coughing; is more compressible, and, if large, or in the scrotum, is more oblong and heavier than enterocele; it recedes very gradually, and its reduction is unaccompanied by any gurgling noise.

An *entero-epiplocele*, or a hernia composed both of intestine and omentum, has the characteristic marks less clear than either of the preceding cases; when reducible, in pressing back the contents, it is known by the gurgling noise which attends the ascent of the intestinal portion, while that of the omentum is reduced without noise, and with greater difficulty; otherwise, the feeling communicated to the touch is sufficient to render this variety distinguishable from the others.

CAUSES. The predisposing causes of hernia are: general relaxation, or unusual largeness of the natural openings of the abdomen. When any such proclivity exists, particularly in children and the aged, the viscera are occasionally protruded by trivial circumstances, such as crying, coughing, sneezing, or even by the act of a somewhat full inspiration; but in other cases, or where there is no marked predisposition, the protrusion only takes place under great bodily exertion. When rupture ensues in consequence of predisposition, or seems to take place spontaneously, its formation is very gradual; but when it results from extreme corporal exertion, it appears very suddenly; and if the opening through which the bowel protrudes be small, as is generally the case in such instances, there is much danger of strangulation.

Hernia is termed *reducible* when it can at any time be readily returned into the abdomen, and when, in an unreduced state, it is productive of no pain, or hinderance to the performance of the intestinal functions; *irreducible*, when it cannot be replaced in consequence of its bulk, or from the contraction of adhesions; and *strangulated*, when the protruded parts are not only incapable of being returned, but are moreover affected with constriction, pain, and inflammation, attended with nausea, frequent retching, or vomiting, tension of the abdomen, obstruction of the bowels, quick, hard pulse, and more or less fever. If the return of the intestine be not effected under such a state of matters, an aggravation of all the said symptoms at first ensues, and subsequently the vomiting is exchanged for a convulsive hiccough, with frequent bilious eructations; after the abdominal tension, fever and extreme restlessness have continued for a few hours in an increased degree, the patient suddenly becomes relieved from pain, the pulse low, feeble, and intermittent, the eyes dim and glassy, the belly ceases to be tumid and tense, and the skin, particularly that of the extremities, cold and moist; the hernial swelling disappears, and the skin over the part often changes to a livid hue, but invariably conveys an emphysematous feel or crepitus to the touch, indicative of the establishment of gangrene; finally, spasmodic rigours and convulsive twitching in the tendons supervene, and death soon terminates the scene.

THERAPEUTICS. When the disease has not been neglected, or is not of long standing, it may be cured by the action of internal homœopathic remedies. No truss should be applied until the hernia is completely reduced, and care should be taken that the truss fits properly, as it is intended only to keep the hernia from protruding, and not for effecting the cure.

In effecting the reduction of a hernia by the taxis, the patient should be laid upon his back, and a pillow placed under the chest and pelvis, so as to curve the trunk of the body, and thereby relax the abdominal muscles. If the case be one of inguinal or femoral hernia, the muscles, etc., of the thigh must also be relaxed, by putting the limb in a state of flexion, and rotated inwards, then gently compressing the tumour, and pushing upwards and outwards in the case of *inguinal* hernia; and first backwards and then upwards in the case of *femoral*, if the tumour be small; but first downwards, and then backwards and upwards, when it is large and reflected over Poupart's ligament.* In most cases, the following simple method may be pursued by the uninitiated: place the left hand on the swelling as if for the purpose of grasping it, then introduce the fore and middle fingers of the right hand between the thumb and fingers of the left, on the top of the tumour, and rub and press it gently; persevere softly and patiently for half an hour and upwards when the hernia is considerable.† The palm of the hand should also be occasionally employed, by giving it a rotatory motion combined with gradually increasing pressure, especially when the tumour begins to diminish in bulk, or when it has been small from the first. Even strangulated hernia is capable of being reduced by the taxis with facility, after the employment of the proper remedies, particularly *Aconite* and *Nux vom.*, and the operation, which is always more or less dangerous, thereby avoided.—When the rupture is painful, and very tender to the touch, medicine must first be prescribed to remove the irritability; after which the protrusion has often been found to recede of itself. In some cases, the application of warm fomentations to the part reduces the hernia, and the general relaxing effects of a warm bath are well known as being useful in facilitating reduction. The following treatment has been strongly recommended when the symptoms encountered are as described.

ACONITUM $\frac{000}{3}$. When there is considerable fever, with quick, hard, full pulse, *inflammation* of the affected parts, with excessive sensibility to the touch; violent burning pain in the abdomen; *bitter, bilious vomiting;* agonizing restlessness and cold perspiration. A second dose to be given, if required, an hour after the first. In the majority of cases, marked benefit has resulted after the administration of the first dose of *Aco-*

* In *Umbilical* hernia the pressure is to be made directly backwards.

† Hering's Hausarzt.

nitum, under the circumstances mentioned; but when no change for the better resulted after the third exhibition, or when the bilious eructations and vomiting become converted into an acid character, SULPHUR must be prescribed, and if the patient fall asleep thereafter, he should be allowed to repose quietly.

When the tumour is not so painful or tender to the touch as above mentioned, and the vomiting less severe, but the respiration oppressed and laborious, and the strangulation has arisen from errors in diet, the effects of exposure to cold, from being overheated, or from a violent fit of passion, etc., *Nux v.* is to be preferred, and may be repeated every two hours or so.* If no change results in about two hours after the socond dose of *Nux v.*,—*Opium* should be prescribed, or this remedy may be had recourse to from the first, and repeated every quarter of an hour, until improvement takes place, should there be hardness and distention of the abdomen, putrid eructations, or even vomiting of fecal matter. (PLUMBUM may be given after the third or fourth dose of *Opium*, if no decided change for the better become perceptible.)

When there is retching and vomiting, with cold moist skin and *coldness of the extremities*,—VERATRUM should be administered, and repeated in from half an hour to an hour or so; and in the event of no favourable turn taking place after the second dose,—BELLADONNA should be prescribed.

When the case has been neglected, or the progress of the malady already advanced so far on reaching the patient, that the integuments over the rupture have assumed a livid hue, and there is reason to apprehend the invasion of gangrene, the patient may yet be saved by the administration of LACHESIS in repeated doses; if no relief follow in the space of about two hours, ARSENICUM may be tried. RHUS has also been spoken of as being serviceable in extreme cases. The operation should not be delayed when symptoms of a serious character do not speedily yield to be remedies indicated; but the latter should always be tried first, as no bad consequences

* Vide note, page 21.

will result from the delay under the precautions stated; on the contrary, the subsequent manual treatment has been found to be thereby facilitated.

FAINTING. SWOONING. *Syncope.*

Individuals of weak nerves and delicate constitutions, particularly of the female sex, are frequently subject to fainting fits, which, although rarely dangerous, yet when utterly neglected, or inappropriately treated by violent or very debilitating means, are prone to become serious, and even fatal.

The usual causes are: sudden transitions from cold to heat; breathing vitiated atmospheres; great fatigue; loss of blood; long fasting; grief, fear, and other mental emotions.

When fainting occurs, let the patient be immediately removed to where a stream of pure fresh air can be obtained, and let all tight clothing about the neck, chest, and abdomen be loosened; the patient should at the same time be placed in a comfortable position, with the head low. If the foregoing prove insufficient to effect restoration, sprinkle cold fresh water on the face and neck, and, if necessary, on the pit of the stomach. Should there still be no marked benefit produced, or if the patient becomes cold, a little spirits of camphor may be applied to the nose. When the fainting has arisen from fright, the best medicines for the consequences are *Aconite* or *Opium*, and sometimes *Colocynth*. (See MENTAL EMOTIONS.) After great depletion, or other debilitating causes,—*Cinchona*, and, in some instances, *Nux v.*, *Carb. v.*, and *Veratrum;* also a little wine in very small quantities at a time, or a little bread or biscuit, soaked in wine, and sometimes a little strong soup may be administered. Should the fainting arise from mental emotions, *Ignatia* and *Chamomilla* are the remedies in general cases. (See MENTAL EMOTIONS.) When slight pain causes fainting, *Hepar sulph.* Fainting from violent pain, *Aconite*, *Chamomilla*, or *Cocculus*. If liable to result from even the most trivial degree of fatigue, *Veratrum*. From excessive mental application, or in those who have been addicted to the use of ardent spirits, *Nux vomica*.

In other cases, the following remedies have been recommended where the symptoms met with are as described.

Aconitum $\frac{0\,0\,0}{3}$. When there is *palpitation* of the heart, with determination of the head, humming in the ears; or when the paroxysms come on usually *on assuming the erect posture*, and are accompanied with shivering and flushing of the face, succeeded *by deadly paleness.*

Coffea $\frac{0\,0\,0}{3}$ may be prescribed after *Aconitum* in highly excitable or nervous subjects, when the fainting fit has arisen from fright, and the last-named medicine has not relieved much.

Hepar Suplhuris, when the fits generally come on towards evening, and are preceded by vertigo.

Lachesis $\frac{0\,0}{6}$. When the fainting fits are either preceded, accompanied, or followed by *asthmatic symptoms, vertigo, paleness of the face,* nausea, vomiting, convulsions, spasms of the jaw, rigidity of the body; bloated appearance of the face; epistaxis; *aching pain or stitches in the fore part of the chest; cold perspirations.* (See Veratrum.)

Moschus $0\frac{0\,0}{3}0$. Fainting fits, attended with spasms in the chest, or succeeded by headache, and occurring towards evening, during the night, or in the open air.

Veratrum $0\frac{0}{3}0$, when the attacks are excited by the slightest fatigue; or when they are often preceded by a feeling of *extreme anguish* and excessive dejection, or despair, and accompanied by spasmodic clenching of the teeth, and convulsive movements of the eyes and their lids.

Nux v. is a beneficial remedy when the fits take place particularly in the morning, *after a meal,* or after taking exercise; and there is *nausea,* with paleness of the face; also, when the patient complains, on recovery, of pain in the stomach, sparks before the eyes, or dimness of sight, together with a feeling of anxiety; and is, further, affected with anxiety, trembling, and congestion in the head, or oppression at the chest.

Acidum phosphoricum $\frac{0\,0}{6}$ has been found useful after *Nux v.*, when that remedy has not removed or diminished the tendency to suffer from fainting fits *after a meal.*

When, as is frequently the case, the fits of swooning or

fainting take place in hysterical females, the remedies which will commonly be found the most appropriate are: *Ignatia, Nux moschata, Cocculus, Chamomilla, Nux v., Natrum m.*, or *Arsenicum*, etc.

In conclusion, it may be added, that *Caladium*, in addition to *Acon.*, is useful in cases that are liable to come on after assuming the erect posture. *Kreasotum* and *Spigelia*, when occurring from the heat of the room. *Lycopodium* and *Silicea*, when in the recumbent posture. *Caladium*, when engaged in meditation. *Carbo v., Natrum m., Kreasotum*, in addition to *Nux v.*, when in the morning. When writing, *Caladium.*

If the attacks are attended with asthmatic symptoms, *Kreasotum* and *Berberis*, in addition to *Nux v.* When accompanied with headache, *Lycopodium, Moschus, Graphites, Natrum m., Stram.;* loss of consciousness, *Lycopodium, Oleander, Arnica*, etc. Creeping or crawling in the limbs, *Nux v., Borax.* Humming, buzzing or tingling in the ears, *Aconitum, Nux v., Petroleum*, etc. Paleness of the face, *Berberis, Natrum m., Pulsatilla*, etc., in addition to *Nux v.* Copious perspiration or sweating, *Calcarea.* Pain in the heart, *Lachesis*, etc. Benumbed limbs, *Natr. m.* Coldness or shivering, *Aconitum, Calcarea, Colocynth*, etc. Vertigo, *Sulphur, Arsenicum, Berberis, Lachesis*, etc. Vomiting, *Lachesis, Nux v., Pulsatilla, Kali c.*, etc.

Those who are subject to fits of fainting or swooning should, if possible, strictly avoid those frequent causes of fainting fits, which have been alluded to at the commencement of this chapter; as also, where practicable, any other cause known by experience to be productive of the attacks; otherwise the cure will be rendered difficult, or even hopeless.

ADMINISTRATION of the remedies. The dose may generally be repeated in from five to ten minutes, or if after the second or third dose no effect is produced, another remedy must be selected.* $\frac{000}{3}$ or $\frac{000}{6}$.

* Vide note, p. 21.

HEADACHE.

Cephalalgia. Cephalæa. Cephalalgia Arthritica. Cephalalgia Nervosa. Hemicrania (megrim). Clavus Hystericus.

Headache is often but symptomatic of disease, and in such cases is only to be cured by the removal of the primary affection. When, therefore, it arises from derangement of the stomach, or dyspepsia, constipation, cold in the head, mental emotions, congestion of blood in the vessels of the head, etc., the remedies most appropriate to the treatment of these different disorders must be had recourse to.

In the treatment of nervous headaches, hemicrania or megrim, the following remedies have generally been found the most useful: *Nux v., Veratrum, Colocynth, Pulsatilla, Sepia, Ignatia, Bryonia, Rhus, Ipecacuanha, Chamomilla, Coffea, Hepar, China, Sicuta, Belladonna, Arsenicum, Arnica, Acid. nitr., Petroleum, Sulphur, Silicea, Platina, Causticum, Graphites, Natrum m., Phosphorus, Zincum*, etc. Rheumatic headaches: *Aconitum, Chamomilla, Mercurius, Nux v., Pulsatilla, Lycopodium, Spigelia, Sulphur, Bryonia, Belladonna, China, Ignatia, Phosphorus*, etc. Arthritic: *Bryonia, Nux v., Belladonna, Colocynthis, Sepia, Ignatia, Veratrum*, etc. Hysterical: *Ignatia, Moschus, Platina, Veratrum, Valerian, Sepia, Aurum, Acid. nitricum, Magnesia c. et m., Cocculus, Phosphorus*, etc. Against headaches occurring in extremely sensitive individuals: *Aconitum, Ignatia, Chamomilla, Coffea, Spigelia, Veratrum, Cina*, or *Ipecacuanha*, have usually proved the most appropriate. Headaches arising from the habitual use of *Coffee* are generally curable by means of *Nux v., Chamomilla*, or *Ignatia*. Those from long-continued, *excessive mental application: Nux v., Opium*, and *Sulphur*, chiefly; but also, *Lachesis, Pulsatilla, Calcarea, Aurum, Natrum m., Silicea, Lycopod.*, etc.

If from sitting up late, or prolonged watching at the bedside of a sick person: *Cocculus, Nux v.*, or *Pulsatilla*. When headache is always excited by exposure to a current of air: *Aconitum, Belladonna, Colocynth, Nux v.*, or *Cinchona*, have often been found successful either in removing the said susceptibility, or in shortening the attacks, and rendering them of a much more bearable character. And when cold, damp, or boisterous weather is generally productive of headache: *Bryonia, Nux v.*, and *Carbo v.:* these last named medicines, together with *Silicea*, are frequently equally useful, if headache is always experienced during hot, sultry weather,—the air being overcharged with electricity. Against headaches arising from the effects of mercury in large doses: *Carbo v., Pulsatilla, Cinchona;* or *Hepar sulphuris, Acidum nitricum, Aurum*, or *Sulphur*. Headache after drinking cold or iced water, etc.: *Aconitum, Arsenicum, Opium, Belladonna, Pulsatilla, Sulphur*, and *Natrum*.

In general cases, the subjoined remedies will prove useful, and may be selected according to the indications given:

BELLADONNA $^0\frac{0}{3}{}^0$. When headache is periodic, or nearly constant, and the pain is increased by the slightest movement either of the head or body, and particularly on stooping, or by moving the eyes; or when a bright light or the most trivial noise tends to aggravate the pain, which consists of a dull pressure at the vertex, or is of a lancinating description, and occupies either the entire head (cephalæa), or merely one side (hemicrania), extending from the occiput into the orbit and root of the nose, and is then described as a violent, screwing, piercing, bursting or tearing pain, sometimes attended with great heat at the vertex; or the seat of the pain is in the forehead, and is of a dull, aching, or cutting description, attended with a sense of fulness, or a feeling as if the brain would be forced through the forehead in stooping. At times these pains become so violently increased as almost to deprive the patient of consciousness whilst they last; or the headache attended with extreme restlessness, sleeplessness and delirium; falling off of the hair in consequence of the headaches. *Platina* answers well, in some cases, after *Belladonna*, when the pain is chiefly lateral, and of the same description; or when there is, at the same time, coldness of the one half of the face, etc., with humming or buzzing in the head. *Mercurius* and *Hepar s.*, and in very obstinate cases, *Sepia* and *Silicea*, are frequently very useful after *Belladonna*.

Bryonia $\frac{000}{3}$. Aching, piercing, or digging, tearing pain, at a small fixed spot (clavus hystericus); or piercing, aching pain in the forehead daily after a meal, or coming on in the morning, and afterwards becoming lancinating; or pain coming on in the morning, disappearing in the afternoon, and returning again in the evening with great violence, when it is attended with a sensation as if the head were pressed together; burning, tearing pain over the entire head; shootings in one side of the head. The pains are increased by movement, and are attended with irascibility, and disposition to chilliness or shivering; they are sometimes relieved or terminated by a fit of vomiting. *Nux v.* and *Rhus* often serve to complete the cure of the foregoing symptoms, or, at all events, to curtail or remove each attack after the previous administration of *Bryonia.*

Rhus $\frac{000}{3}$. Shooting and rending pains, extending to the ears and root of the nose; burning or pulsative pains; headache after a meal, with desire to assume the recumbent posture, and remain quiet; fulness and weight in the head; renewal of the headache at the slightest contradiction, or on going into the open air; *undulation of the brain at every step;* or sensation as if water were in the head, or as if the contents of the cranium were in a relaxed or loosened state, and shifted about with every movement of the head; feeling of creeping or crawling in the head.

Sepia $\frac{00}{6}$. Periodic cephalalgia, aggravated by mental emotion, particularly in hysterical subjects; the pain is either of a lancinating description, and affects the whole head, or is merely seated under the eye, or occupies the one half of the head or forehead; in the latter case, the pain is experienced chiefly in the morning, and is frequently attended with extreme sensibility of the eyes to the light. *Sepia* is also very efficacious in cases of chronic hemicrania, with violent piercing or rending pain, intermingled with lancinations, so excruciating that the patient is afraid to move, and can only obtain a trivial degree of relief by remaining perfectly quiet with the eyes closed; at other times, the pain is so violent as to cause the patient to scream out, and is attended with heat in the head, or faintness and giddiness, followed by nausea and vomiting.

SILICEA $\frac{00}{6}$, is especially useful where a sensation is experienced as if the brain were about to protrude through the forehead or orbits; or pain so severe as if the head would split; or semilateral, shooting, rending pains, commencing at the temple, and extending to the nose, the upper and lower jaw-bones, and teeth of the same side. When there is a tendency to frequent sweating of the head, or when there is frequently great tenderness of the scalp, *Silicea* is further indicated; as also in cases where the parties affected are subject to the formation of small tubercles on the head.

HEPAR SULPHURIS $\frac{000}{6}$ is also a good remedy to follow *Belladonna* in the treatment of headaches, when only partial relief has been obtained from the said medicine, or it may be administered alternately with *Silicea* in cases where there are painful tubercles on the head. The pains chiefly piercing, generally aggravated at night, and frequently limited to a small fixed spot, with a sensation as if a nail were being driven into the head. Against this latter species of headache, (clavus hystericus,) *Nux vomica, Ignatia, Coffea, Mosch., Magn.*, and *Staph.*, are also most important remedies; the former may be selected when the following symptoms are complained of: Pain commencing with a slight pressure, or a sensation of coldness at the part which is subsequently affected; succeeded by throbbing, and then an intense shooting, piercing, rending, or stunning pain confined to a small space, which can frequently be covered with the point of the finger, and is extremely sensitive to the touch; or the pain causes a sensation as if a nail were driven into the head; at other times, the pain extends over the nose down to the lip, and also to the gums; or, on the other hand, it commences at the eyelid or the orbit, causing constant lachrymation, and extends over the forehead and temples to the ears, back of the head, and nape of the neck; or it is seated in the crown of the head, and produces a sensation as if the head would split, or were being opened at the coronal suture; intense, piercing pain, confined to a small place, which can frequently be covered with the point of the finger; or rending, aching pain, affecting only one side of the head, sometimes combined or alternating with shootings; the pain becomes heightened to such a degree occasionally, and more particularly in the morning, as well nigh to drive the patient to despair, or deprive him of consciousness;* great heaviness of the head, and sensation as if the brain were bruised or lacerated; tenderness of the scalp. The pains are aggravated by movement, such as walking or stooping, or by reflection; also after eating, or on going into the open air, and are frequently attended with considerable giddiness or confusion in the head; the headache is generally attended with extreme irascibility, and is renewed or aggravated after partaking of coffee, the constant habit of drinking which is not an unfrequent cause of the complaint; sudden attacks of it are frequently excited by a fit of passion, a fright, the effects of a chill, or an overloaded stomach.

IGNATIA $\frac{000}{3}$ is, as already stated, also an excellent remedy in cases in which the pain is confined to a small space, and causes a sensation *as if a nail were driven into the brain;* nausea; dimness of the sight, and sensibility of the eyes to light; paleness of the face, and temporary alleviation from change of posture; aggravation from noise or strong odours, or after partaking of coffee. *Ignatia* is sometimes serviceable in completing the cure after the previous administration of *Nux v.*, or *Pulsatilla.* It is especially applicable to nervous, hysterical females of a mild and sensitive disposition.

COFFEA $\frac{000}{3}$. In cases of megrim, brought on by meditation, vexation, or exposure to cold, attended with irritability, sensibility to noise, great anxiety; and chilliness, and a sensation as if *a nail were driven into the brain,* or a feeling as if the brain were bruised, occurring in individuals who are extremely impatient under suffering, and who are not habituated to the use of coffee, this remedy is frequently a very efficacious one.

PULSATILLA $\frac{000}{3}$. Megrim, characterized by rending or shooting pains, with heaviness of the head, dimness of the sight, sensibility to light; or buzzing or singing in the ears, and ear-

* Compare with *Belladonna* and *Arsenicum.*

ache; nausea; paleness of face, lowness of spirits; headache with pain in the nape of the neck; aggravation of the headache, with chilliness towards evening, during repose, or particularly when sitting; melioration in the open air. Disposition mild; temperament phlegmatic.

CHINA $\frac{0000}{3}$. Headache worse at night, accompanied with a sensation as if the head would split; or dull, aching, pressive, or boring pains, particularly at the crown of the head, increased by movement, or by the open air; tenderness of the scalp; great sensibility to pain; taciturnity and obstinacy.

VERATRUM $\frac{000}{3}$. Headache preceded by coldness and shivering; pain in the head as if the brain were bruised or lacerated; or lateral aching, constrictive, and throbbing pains, sometimes attended with a sensation of constriction or tightness in the throat; feeling of coldness at the crown of the head, as if ice were placed upon it; or sensation both of coldness and heat on the exterior of the head, with deep-seated or internal burning heat; headache with paleness of the face, nausea and vomiting, and preceded by a copious discharge of colourless urine; headache, with pain at the pit of the stomach, or painful stiffness of the neck; headache with extreme weakness and melancholy; painful sensibility of the hair to the touch; chilliness, with general cold perspiration. *Arsenicum* and *Acidum phos.* are sometimes useful after *Veratrum*.

LACHESIS $\frac{00}{6}$. Deep-seated pains in the head, or severe aching pain in the occiput, in the sockets of the eye or above the orbits, with stiffness of the neck, particularly at the nape; heaviness and feeling of expansive pressure, sometimes to such an extent as if the head would burst; tension in the head as if caused by strings or threads drawn through the occiput towards the eyes; lancinations in different parts of the head; headache every morning on waking, or after dinner, or at every change of weather.

MERCURIUS $\frac{000}{6}$. Rending and burning or lancinating and piercing pains, generally lateral, sometimes extending to the teeth and neck, with shootings in the ears; tightness round the head; excessive nocturnal aggravation of the headaches, often accompanied by profuse sweating.

COLOCYNTH $^{0}\frac{0}{3}{}^{0\,0}$. Nervous headaches attended with smarting in the eyes; excruciating lateral action; rending, dragging pains; nausea and vomiting; feeling of compression in the forehead, increased by stooping or lying on the back; headache every afternoon or evening, with great anguish and excessive restlessness, rendering it impossible to remain in the recumbent posture; offensive perspiration; profuse discharge of colourless urine during the headache.

CHAMOMILLA $\frac{0\,0\,0}{3}$. Headaches occurring in individuals who are extremely impatient under suffering, and whom the slightest pain exasperates or calls forth symptoms and expressions of suffering apparently uncalled for by the nature of the complaints; the headaches are often confined to one side of the head (hemicrania), and the pains are of a rending, aching, or shooting character, and sometimes extend into the upper and lower jaw; sweating at the head is a frequent concomitant symptom.

Chamomilla $^{0}\frac{0}{3}{}^{0}$, is further occasionally very useful after the previous administration of *Coffea* when not called for from the commencement. Or in hemicrania attended with extreme excitability arising from the daily use of black coffee, but which is generally relieved for the time by partaking of a cup of coffee, will generally be materially relieved, if not cured, by *Chamomilla*; sometimes a subsequent dose or two of *Nux* is required to complete the cure.

SULPHUR $\frac{0\,0\,0}{6}$. Chronic headache; headaches occurring daily, or every eight days; worse in the morning, or during the night, and attended with heaviness of the head, aching or pressive pains in the forehead above the eyes, (causing the patient to knit the brows, or keep the eyes closed,) or over the entire head; incapability of mental exertion from the pains in the head; pains as if the head would split; or rending, shooting, dragging, jerking, pains on one side of the head; aggravation of the headaches from meditation, the open air, or from movement; extreme tenderness of the scalp to the touch; falling off of the hair.

CALCAREA $\frac{0\,0}{6}$. Chronic headaches frequently attended with a sensation of extreme coldness, either interiorly or on the scalp; the pains either affect the entire head, or merely the forehead, the side, or the crown of the head, and are chiefly of a stunning, aching, throbbing, or hammering description, compelling the patient to retain the recumbent posture; at times the head feels as if compressed in a vice; or the forehead feels as if it would burst open, particularly when in the open air; headache, with humming noise in the head, confusion of ideas, with aggravation from intellectual employment, or from movement; falling off of the hair; *Calcarea* is generally very useful after *Sulphur;* and *Silicea*, *Lycopod.*, *Ac. nitr.* after *Calc.*

Arsenicum $\frac{0\,0}{6}$. Headaches so intolerable as almost to drive the patient to despair, occurring periodically and aggravated by partaking of food; the pain sometimes extends to the gums, where it is so excruciating as to render it impossible to fall asleep; tenderness of the scalp to the touch; temporary amelioration of the headaches from the application of cold water.

Aurum $\frac{0\,0\,0}{6}$. Headaches in hysterical persons attended with buzzing or other noises in the head; and pain as if the head had been bruised, especially on rising in the morning, or during mental occupation.

Eugenia $\frac{0\,0\,0}{3}$. Severe one-sided headache (megrim) *coming on in the evening*, attended with a sensation of pressure or forcing outwards behind the eyes, lachrymation, and sometimes nausea and vomiting which produce exacerbation; aching pains in the entire head at night (cephalæa) with burning in the eyes, thirst, and copious discharge of urine.

One remedy is seldom sufficient to effect a cure of cephalalgia of long standing, particularly when of a nervous character: in some cases of this description, it is only possible to effect a degree of melioration. In comparatively recent cases, the medicines may be repeated at intervals from an hour to six or twelve hours,* when the headache is excessively severe; but in those of a more chronic and obstinate nature, in which it is necessary to have recourse to such remedies as *Sulphur*, *Calcarea*, *Silex*, &c., considerably longer intervals must be

* Vide note, page 21.

observed between the doses, when our object is to attempt to eradicate the disorder, or destroy the susceptibility to headache from trivial causes.

HEADACHE.—ADDENDA.*

Headache is one of the most frequent and annoying ailments with which the human organism is afflicted. It requires distinct consideration. Although it is generally associated with or dependent on other maladies, it so often predominates that its phenomena should no doubt occasionally control the selection of the appropriate remedy, which should, however, include as far as possible the totality of the suffering. It may also depend on accidental causes; still the remedy, while antidotal to them, must carefully embrace all the existing symptoms. Again, it may occur perfectly independent of any assignable cause, and thus render the following arrangement of the remedies essential to the successful selection of the therapeutical agent.

CONGESTIVE HEADACHES, or those attended with pressure of blood to the head. Examine carefully the symptoms of *Congestive Headache* under the following remedies: *Aconite, Arnica, Belladonna, Bryonia, Coffea, Ignatia, Mercurius, Nux vomica*, and *Pulsatilla.*

CATARRHAL HEADACHE. Examine *Aconite, Belladonna, Mercurius, Nux vomica*, and *Pulsatilla.*

RHEUMATIC HEADACHE. *Aconite, Belladonna, Bryonia, Chamomilla, Mercurius, Nux vomica*, and *Pulsatilla.*

NERVOUS HEADACHE. *Aconite, Arnica, Belladonna, Bryonia, Chamomilla, Coffea, Ignatia, Nux vomica,* and *Pulsatilla.*

DIGESTIVE OR GASTRIC HEADACHE. *Antimonium crudum, Bryonia, Nux vomica,* and *Pulsatilla.*

* In the British edition of Laurie, from which the third American was reprinted, no article on Headache was inserted. We supplied the omission at the time, and, although Dr. Laurie has furnished a chapter for his last edition, we do not find it sufficiently complete to obviate, in all respects, the repetition of our own paper. We consulted Hahnemann, Hering, Jahr, and other best authorities of our school in its composition. —ED.

HEADACHE FROM HEAT. *Aconite*, and *Bryonia*.

HEADACHES FROM CHANGEABLE WEATHER, CURRENTS OF AIR, COLD, COLD DRINKS, AND BATHING. *Aconite*, *Antimonium crudum*, *Belladonna*, *Bryonia*, *Chamomilla*, *Nux vomica*, and *Pulsatilla*.

HEADACHE FROM TOBACCO. *Aconite*, *Antimonium crudum*, and *Ignatia*.

HEADACHE FROM SUPPRESSED ERUPTIONS. *Antimonium crudum*, and *Sulphur*.

HEADACHES FROM MECHANICAL INJURIES. *Arnica* and *Belladonna*.

HEADACHES FROM DEBAUCH AND SPIRITUOUS DRINKS. *Belladonna*, *Coffea*, *Nux vomica*, and *Pulsatilla*.

HEADACHE FROM COFFEE. *Chamomilla*, and *Nux vomica*.

HEADACHE FROM ANGER. *Chamomilla*, *Ignatia*, and *Nux vomica*.

ACONITE.

ACONITE deserves attention in headaches connected with *Congestion to the head*, *Catarrh*, *Rheumatism*, *Neuralgia*, and those caused by *Heat*, *Currents of Air*, *Cold*, *Bathing*, *or Tobacco*; and for *females*, *children*, and *nervous* invalids.

Aconite is indicated in *Congestive* headaches, when a *violent throbbing pain* seizes the forehead and temples, with a sensation of ardent *heat* through the entire brain, *red* and *bloated* face; *redness* of the eyes, visible pulsation of the neck, excessive sensibility to the least noise or movement, and, sometimes, great irritability or delirium.

When congestive headaches are habitual, the patient should sponge the forehead and temples every morning with cold water, or take a shower-bath and drink one or two tumblerfuls of cold water on retiring and rising, night and morning.

In *Catarrhal* headaches the indications are: dull, *pressive*, and constrictive pains and *heat* in the forehead, especially above the root of the nose, with flowing from the eyes, running at the nose, but more frequently obstruction of the same, dry heat in the nose, buzzing in the ears, colic, frequent chilliness, alternating with feverishness, occasional cough; *amelioration* of the symptoms in the *morning*, and in the *open air; aggravation* in the *evening*, and from speaking and exercise.

The *Rheumatic* headache is characterized by *darting* or *rending* pains, sensitive to the touch, which fly from one part of the head to another, as from the nape of the neck to the ears, temples, vertex or forehead, are sometimes connected with rheumatism of the neck and shoulders, are attended with *active fever, dry and hot skin, thirst, redness* or varying pallor and redness of the cheeks, are insupportable at *night* with mental disquietude and vexation, are palliated by *sitting*, and aggravated or renewed by *wine*, stimulants, or great mental excitement.

The *Nervous* headache generally occurs above the root of the nose or on one side of the head. The pains, which are intolerable, especially at night, are *throbbing, darting*, and *stinging*, producing by their intensity, lamentations, inconsolable anguish, fear of death, and, at times, temporary insensibility, and are attended by thirst, *flushed cheeks*, small, quick, weak, and occasionally, intermittent pulse, *and intolerance of touch, light, and sound.* Headache from exposure to *Heat* usually assumes the characteristics of the *Congestive*, which are recorded above. The headaches which arise from *Currents of Air, Cold, or Bathing*, are in every respect analogous to the sufferings we have described as *Catarrhal.*

The *Tobacco* headache, whether from chewing or smoking, is very similar to the *Congestive* headache of Aconite, marked, particularly by sensation of great weight on the vertex and over the eyes, *nausea* and amelioration in the open air. All the preceding forms of headache to which Aconite is applicable, have the distinctive peculiarities of an *increase* of suffering from *motion, rising* from *a recumbent position, speaking* and *drinking ;* and a *diminution* in the *open air.*

Administration $\frac{000}{3}$. The *Aconite* may be repeated in *severe* forms of headache every two or three hours; in milder forms, from six to twelve hours, increasing the intervals in proportion to the improvement effected. We have acquired great service from *Aconite* in acute paroxysms of headache, by using it as a precursor to, or in alternation with, *Arnica*, *Belladonna*, *Bryonia*, *Chamomilla*, *Nux vomica*, *Pulsatilla* and *Veratrum*. Thus a single dose of *Aconite* may precede the administration of these remedies some two or three hours, or may be alternated with them every three or four hours.

ANTIMONIUM CRUDUM.

ANTIMONIUM CRUDUM $^{0}\frac{0}{6}{}^{0}$ has been used for headaches dependent on *Chills*, *Suppressed eruptions*, *Tobacco*, or *Indigestion*. They are characterized by a *pain in the forehead as if it would burst*, or dull, boring, rending, piercing, spasmodic pains in the forehead, temples and vertex, with a sensation as if in the *bones* of the head, especially of the *vertex*. The pains are *increased* by ascending stairs, and *mitigated* in the open air. If the headache arise from *Tobacco*, it is attended with *dizziness*. If it depend on *Indigestion*, it is frequently preceded by *nausea*, want of appetite, *aversion to food*, *eructation*, and efforts to vomit. It is sometimes followed by *loss of hair*.

The *Antimonium* may be taken every *twelve* or *twenty-four* hours, and is often more efficient after the use of *Pulsatilla*, especially for the headache of *Indigestion*.

ARNICA.

ARNICA is indicated in headaches connected with *Congestion to the head*, *Neuralgia*, and in those caused by *Mechanical injuries*.

The *Congestive* headache is characterized by a spasmodic *pressing* in the forehead, as if the brain were contracted into a hard mass, principally when near the fire, whirling dizziness with nausea, *heat and burning in the head* with coldness of the remainder of the body, and occasional prickling or numb sensations in one or more of the extremities.

The *Nervous* headache manifests itself by *crawling*, *pricking*, and *stinging* pains in one or both temples, or on one side of the head, which feel as if they had been bruised, or by an intense pain, as if a nail had pierced the brain.

The headache which follows ***Mechanical injuries***, such as blows, falls, or strains, in the same as the *Congestive*, attended, at times, by pressive sore pain in the part injured or over one or other eye, and *green vomiting*.

This remedy is the more appropriate when the sufferings are *aggravated* at *evening* or *night*, *after eating*, or by *mental* or *physical exercise*.

ADMINISTRATION. $\frac{0\,0\,0\,0}{3}$ *Arnica* follows and alternates admirably with *Aconite* when the *febrile action* is prominent, and may precede the use of *Belladonna*, *Calcarea* and *Rhus*. The rule of repetition is the same as that given for Aconite.

BELLADONNA.

BELLADONNA obtains in headaches, complicated with *Congestion to the head*, *Catarrh*, *Rheumatism*, *Neuralgia;* and those from *Heat*, *Spirituous drinks*, *Mechanical injuries*, *Cold*, and *Currents of Air*. It is especially suitable for *females* and *children*.

It is appropriate in *Congestive* headache when the indications given for this form of suffering under *Aconite*, are not promptly or permanently relieved by that remedy; also if the pains are more *deeply seated*, are *violent*, *pressive*, *heavy* and *full*, as if the brain would protrude through the forehead or side of the head, with pale, haggard face, drowsiness, loss of consciousness, murmurs and delirium; or if this form of headache develop itself *after eating*, with great lassitude, drowsiness, painful stiffness of the nape of the neck, imperfect speech, distortion of the face, especially of the *mouth*, and other symptoms of *Apoplexy*.

The *Catarrhal* headache is marked by *pressive aching in the forehead* and congestive feeling of the entire head, as if it would split open, with sneezing, *swelling*, *redness and excoriation* of the nose, profuse flow of acrid water from the nose, or flowing from one nostril, or alternating with stoppage of the nose, *smell too acute*, especially for tobacco smoke, or *too obtuse*, shivering or feverish heat, thirst and pains in the limbs. (*Hepar sulphuris* or *Mercury* may precede or follow *Belladonna* for this variety of *Catarrhal* headache.)

Rheumatic headache is attended by *violent shooting and*

burning pains, especially of one side of the head, congestion to the head, swelling of its veins and *visible pulsation of its arteries*, *redness of the eyes and face*, and fever.

The *Nervous* headache is characterized by *burning*, *shooting* pains, generally of one side of the head in the mildest form of attack, attended by sensitiveness of the scalp, distention of the veins of the head and hands, roaring and buzzing in the ears, and clouded sight. In a severe form, the pains become pressing, *burning*, *shooting*, *rending*, and distracting, appearing on one side of the head or above the eyes and nose, with a sensation as if water fluctuated or undulated in the head. The neuralgic pain may also commence very *gently*, increase in intensity through one side of the head, producing irritability, lamentations, and delirium.

The headache which arises from *Heat* is similar to the *Congestive*, and indicates *Belladonna*, especially, when the head seems as if it would split open and the suffering is *increased* by walking and *mental excitement*, and is attended by hot fever, thirst, vomiting, sleepiness, anxiety, tears, lamentation, despair or rage, and delirium.

Spirituous drinks produce pressing aching in the forehead with congestive fulness of the entire head, red and bloated face, loss of appetite, especially for meat, thirst and feverishness.

The headache from *Mechanical injuries* is similar to the *Congestive*, and requires the *Belladonna*, most frequently, after the previous use of *Arnica*.

The effects of *Cold* and *Currents of Air* accord with the *Catarrhal* headache, attended at times by imperfect vision, *sore throat* and indigestion.

All these symptoms of *Belladonna* are *aggravated* chiefly at *night*, also about three or four o'clock in the afternoon, and after *sleeping*, also by the *warmth of the bed*, recumbent position, *motion*, especially that of the eyes, the slightest touch, shock or noise, open air or currents of air, *contradiction*, even the slightest, and *mental excitement*; they are *mitigated* by flexing the head *backward* and *supporting* it.

ADMINISTRATION $\frac{0000}{3}$. *Belladonna* is frequently preceded by, and alternated with *Aconite*, and *Mercury*. Its rule of repetition and alternation is the same as that directed for *Aconite*.

Bryonia.

Bryonia is available in headaches associated with *Congestion to the head*, *Derangement of the stomach*, *Neuralgia and Rheumatism*, and those caused by *Heat* and *Changeable weather*. *Congestive* headache is manifested by severe pain in both sides of the head, *pressing* from without inwardly, with a sensation as if the contents of the skull would protrude through the forehead, especially on stooping; bleeding at the nose, affording no relief; burning of the eyes, effusion of tears, and *constipation*. The Bryonia is of the greatest value if this form of headache occur with *Constipation of the bowels*. It is generally worse in the *morning*.

For headaches of the *Stomach*, see Indigestion.

Nervous headache has pressing, burning, rending and shooting pains, as if a tumour were forming under the skin, and as if the brain would press through the forehead, which seize the forehead, *dart to one or other side of the head*, or extend to the cheek-bone, shooting and pulsating at times violently; rheumatic and passionate patients suffer most from this form of headache.

Rheumatic headache is complicated with local or general rheumatism, manifested by *rending* and *shooting* pains which fluctuate from the nape of the neck, sides of the head, and forehead, attended by *coldness* or *shivering*, or fever and perspiration of the head or entire body, and aggravated by the *least movement* and at *night*. *Changeable* weather frequently excites the *Rheumatic* headache.

Headache from *Heat* is marked by *pressing pain* and *fulness* of the entire head, attended by want of appetite, especially in the morning, *nausea*, *vomiting* and *diarrhœa*, thirst, fever, agitation, trembling and apprehension of the future. The *Bryonia* may be used in alternation with *Belladonna*, when that remedy is not promptly efficient for headache from *heat*, as described under *Belladonna*.

The headaches of *Bryonia* appear most frequently in the morning and *after meals*, and are *aggravated by motion*, walking, stooping, &c., and *touch*.

ADMINISTRATION. $\frac{0\,0\,0\,0}{3}$. *Nux vomica* may be used after and alternated with *Bryonia*. The repetition and alternation of the dose the same as directed for *Aconite*.

CHAMOMILLA.

CHAMOMILLA is useful for *Digestive*, *Nervous*, and *Rheumatic* headaches, and those caused by *Coffee*, *Anger*, and *Cold;* and for females, children, and persons excited by the slightest pain.

For *Digestive* headache, see "Indigestion."

Nervous headache is characterized by *drawing*, *rending* and pulsative pains of *one side of the head* which extend to the jaw, sometimes attended by a benumbed sensation, or *sensibility which renders the touch intolerable;* acute shooting pain in the temples, heaviness and throbbing above the nose; bloated face, *redness of one cheek and paleness of the other; hot perspiration of the head and scalp*, and painful and congested eyes.

Rheumatic headache is similar to the above, occurring in persons of a rheumatic habit or labouring under rheumatism.

Headaches dependent on *Coffee* and *Anger* are recognised by the same peculiarities.

The headache from *Cold* is marked, in addition, by weeping eyes, *sore throat*, *hoarseness*, and catarrhal irritation of the chest.

ADMINISTRATION. $\frac{0\,0\,0\,0}{3}$. *Chamomilla* may be used after *Aconite* and *Coffea*, and may precede *Belladonna* and *Pulsatilla*.

COFFEA.

COFFEA is applicable to *Congestive* and *Nervous* headaches, to those caused by *Debauch* or *Spirituous drinks*, and to nervous persons and children.

Congestive headache may arise from *excess of joy*, is attended by lively exaltation of the mind, heaviness of the head, with occasional *violent pain of one side*, redness of the eyes and sleeplessness, and is exasperated by *speaking*.

Nervous headache is marked by a sensation as if the brain were bruised and rent, or by severe rending pains of *one side of the head, as if pierced by a nail,* which seems *insufferable;* frequently *caused* by *Debauch or Spirituous drink,* meditation, vexation, and influenza; *attended* by extreme sensitiveness to noise and music, by agitation, great anguish, tears, cries, distraction, throwing about, chilliness, aversion to fresh air, and distaste for coffee.

ADMINISTRATION. $\frac{000}{3}$. The *Coffea* may be repeated frequently, from *half an hour* to two and three hours, according to the relief afforded. *Ignatia, Nux vomica* and *Pulsatilla,* may *precede,* and *Aconite* and *Chamomilla* succeed the use of Coffea.

IGNATIA.

IGNATIA $\frac{000}{3}$ relieves *Congestive, Hysterical,* and *Nervous* headaches, those dependent on *Grief, Anger,* and *Tobacco,* and those of nervous persons and children.

Congestive headache is characterized by a *painful sensation of fulness* and *expansion* of the head, as if it would burst, especially when conversing, reading, or listening to another; also by a pulsative and deep-seated pain, especially in the *forehead,* and above the root of the nose, attended by trembling of the body, palpitation of heart and great despondence.

Hysterical headache is generally owing to a high degree of mental excitement, and particularly *Grief* or *excessive Anger,* and is marked by *piercing, darting pains,* which penetrate the brain deeply, either in the *forehead* or *on one side of the head,* by alternations of extravagant gayety, and laughter, and extreme despondence and tears, imperfect sight, very red or pale face, nervous agitation and physical restlessness.

Nervous headache is attended by *rending,* boring, throbbing, and *lancinating* pains, which seize the *forehead as if a nail were driven through it* deep into the brain; or pressing pain in the *forehead* and *above the nose,* which progresses from without inwardly and is mitigated by stooping; paleness of face, nausea, darkness before the eyes, intolerance of light, profuse colourless urine, fickleness of disposition, sensitiveness, strong fears, taciturnity, sadness, mildness, &c.

Ignatia may be used as an antidote to a headache caused by *Tobacco*, when the symptoms are *similar* to those we have given as characteristics of Ignatia.

The headaches of Ignatia are *aggravated* by coffee, tobacco smoke, brandy, noise, and strong smells; *aggravated* or *mitigated* by stooping; mitigated by *lying down* and *change of position;* and are *renewed* after a meal, lying down in the evening and rising in the morning.

Rule of administration the same as for *Aconite*. It may be used to advantage after *Chamomilla*, *Pulsatilla* and *Nux vom.*

MERCURIUS SOLUBILIS OR VIVUS.

MERCURIUS SOLUBILIS OR VIVUS, is most efficient in headaches connected with *Catarrh*, *Congestion of the head*, and *Rheumatism*.

The *Catarrhal* headache frequently prevails *epidemically*, and is distinguished by *pressing, aching pain* in the *forehead*, frequent sneezing, profuse discharge of serous mucus, which is offensive at times, *redness* and *excoriation* of the nose with itching and aching pains on pressing the nose, chills or fever, nocturnal perspiration, violent thirst, *pains in the limbs*, and increased suffering from either heat or cold. (It may precede or alternate with *Belladonna* in this form of headache.)

Congestive headache has a *full and crowded feeling* of the head as if the forehead would fly apart, or as if the head were firmly bound by a band, especially with *aggravations at night*, when the pains become boring, burning, rending and darting, and are attended by easy, frequent and profuse *perspiration*, which affords *no relief*. (Here it is useful after *Belladonna and Opium*.)

Rheumatic headache is attended by *burning*, *shooting*, *throbbing* and *rending* pains, which *affect one side of the head*, extending to the teeth and neck, with pulsatory dartings in the ears. The pains seem to be imbedded in the *bones*, and the external flesh is frequently *tumefied*. It may be used before or after *Belladonna* or *Bryonia*.

It is a distinct peculiarity of the *Mercurial* headaches, that they are *aggravated at night*, towards morning, by the *warmth of the bed*, damp and cold air, heat and touch; and are *attended* by *profuse perspiration*, which affords no relief.

ADMINISTRATION $^{0}\frac{0}{6}{}^{0}$. The *Mercury* may be given in extreme cases every four hours, and in alternation with *Belladonna* every three or four hours. In ordinary cases it is preferable to administer a single dose in the *evening*.

NUX VOMICA.

NUX VOMICA is a very prominent agent of cure in *Catarrhal, Congestive, Gastric, Nervous* and *Rheumatic* headaches, and those dependent on *Coffee, Spirituous drinks, Intellectual labour, Anger, Chills or Currents of air, Prolonged watching, and Constipation.**

Catarrhal headache is marked either by *heaviness in the forehead* or shooting and rending pains; *obstruction* in the nose, or else fluent coryza of a mucus which is sometimes brown and corrosive in the *morning* and *dry* in the *evening or at night*, with parched mouth and absence of thirst; bruised sensation throughout the body; burning heat and redness of the cheeks; heat of the head and entire body, and alternations of chills and fever, especially in the *evening;* and hard fæces or *constipation.*

Gastric headache: vide Indigestion.

Congestive headache is attended by excessive *heaviness of the head*, especially on moving the eyes, and *during mental exercise, with a feeling as if the skull would fly apart;* painful sensitiveness of the brain, either from motion or external pressure; pressure on the temples; imperfect sight, with desire to shut the eyes, and inability to sleep; and aggravated in the morning and open air.

Nervous headache appears in the form of *rending, shooting and jerking* pains principally *on one side of the head, as if pierced*

* The *Nux* is most indicated in persons of a lively temperament, red face and full habit, who make a free use of *Coffee* and *Liquors*, and especially in those who lead a sedentary life and suffer from *Constipated* habit.

by a nail, with nausea and vomiting of sour water; also, pricking, stinging, or oppressive sensation of one side of the head, which commencing in the morning, gradually increases in intensity, until the patient becomes distracted and insensible; also, as if the brain were rent asunder, with pale, haggard face, dizziness when walking, buzzing noise, excitation, &c.

Rheumatic headache is marked by *tensive drawing* pains affecting the forehead on one side of the head, attended by a *bruised sensation* of the head and similar pains in the back, loins and *joints, a sensation of torpor or paralysis in the parts affected, with cramps and palpitation in the muscles;* shivering and constipation. (It is mainly indicated for *Rheumatic* headache after *Aconite, Chamomilla, Ignatia,* or *Arnica.*)

The headaches dependent on *Coffee, Spirituous drinks, Intellectual labour, Anger, Prolonged watching,* or *Constipation,* are *Congestive* or *Neuralgic,* and require a careful study of their respective indications.

The headache from *Chill or Currents of air,* is *Catarrhal,* which see.

The *Nux* headache is *aggravated* in the *morning, after meals,* by coffee, wine, tobacco smoke, noise, bright light, meditation, watching, and windy and chilly weather; it is mitigated by sitting or lying down without change of position.

ADMINISTRATION. $\frac{000}{3}$. The *Nux* may *succeed Aconite,* or alternate with it every three or four hours in acute febrile conditions. It may *precede* or alternate with *Bryonia* or *Pulsatilla* by the same rule.

Administered singly, the interval of repetition should vary from 4 to 24 hours, according to the severity of the case.

PULSATILLA.

PULSATILLA applies to *Catarrhal, Gastric, Congestive, Nervous,* and *Rheumatic* headaches, and to those caused by *Debauch, Spirituous drinks, Intellectual labour, Chill, Bathing, or Cold drinks.* It is especially suited to *females,* and persons of phlegmatic temperament, mild character and lymphatic constitution, with *pale complexion,* light hair, blue eyes, &c.

Catarrhal headache is marked by *dull heavy aching* in the root of the nose, *forehead*, or *over one eye*, or confusion of the head, and is attended by loss of appetite, taste and smell; swelling and obstruction of the nose; discharge of blood or of a thick and offensive mucus, sometimes yellow, and sometimes green; and absence of thirst, with chilliness.

For *Gastric* headache, see Indigestion.

Congestive headache manifests itself by wearying, debilitating, and oppressive pains, which seize *one side of the head;* or progress from the *occiput* to the *forehead* or *root of the nose*, or conversely proceed from the root of the nose to the occiput; attended by heaviness of the head, dizziness, paleness of the face, agitation, and inclination to weep.

Nervous headache offers *rending* pains, in single spots or in every part of the head, which are augmented toward evening; or *throbbing, darting* and *pricking* pains, after rising in the morning or lying down in the evening; or jerking, rending, *darting* and pricking pains in *one side of the head only;* attended by *heaviness of the head*, frequent dizziness, obscure vision, intolerance to light, sickness at the stomach, *buzzing, darting, rending, and pricking in the ears*, paleness and varied expression of the face, loss of appetite and thirst, agitation and chills, bleeding at the nose, and *palpitation of heart.*

Rheumatic headache is characterized by *similar* pains to those of the *Nervous;* and are connected with rheumatic pains of the body, *which pass rapidly from one joint to another*, with sensation of torpor in the parts affected, dartings and *coldness* on change of weather, and shiverings increasing in proportion to the intensity of the suffering.

For headaches arising from *Debauch, Spirituous drinks, and Intellectual labour*, carefully consult the indications of *Nervous* and *Congestive* headaches; and from *Chill, Bathing, or Cold drinks*, look to *Catarrhal* headache.

The *Pulsatilla* headache is *aggravated* or *renewed* in *the evening after lying down*, or *at night*, or in bed in the morning; at rest, especially *when seated;* and *mitigated in the open air*, by movement, walking, external heat, and *firm pressure.*

ADMINISTRATION. $\frac{000}{3}$ *Pulsatilla* follows, and is of great service in alternation with *Aconite;* may *precede Bryonia* and

Nux, and *succeed Chamomilla* and *Ignatia*, with which it may occasionally alternate.

The repetition and alternation the same as advised for the *Aconite*.—ED.

PAINS IN THE LOINS. *Notalgia.*

As these pains are frequently purely symptomatic, the treatment must be directed against the disease from whence they originate. Thus as *Hæmorrhoids*, *Leucorrhœa*, *Metritis*, *Myelitis*, etc., are frequent sources of the complaint, the reader is referred to the treatment of these affections in their respective chapters.

When they arise from the habitual indulgence in wine or spirituous liquors, coupled with confirmed sedentary habits, as late hours, an occasional dose of *Nux v.* (three to four globules of the 6th potency in a teaspoonful of water) will generally afford relief; and when a strain from lifting a heavy weight or from any sudden twist on turning the body, or throwing up a window, etc., has given rise to the pain, *Rhus tox.* must be had recourse to; followed, if required, by *Sulphur* and *Calcarea*. (Vide also LUMBAGO, RHEUMATISM, p. 314, etc., and for *pains in the back, or lumbo-sacral pains, occurring in females during pregnancy*, see that Article, Part IV., p. 518.)

DELIRIUM TREMENS POTATORUM.

This malady consists of an affection of the brain, and is nearly peculiar to drunkards, hence its name. There are a few instances on record, in which it has arisen from exhaustion caused by excessive depletion; from the effects of lead, and also from the prolonged use of opium. The intemperate use of ardent spirits, vinous or strong malt liquors, is, however, beyond comparison, the exciting cause in by far the major number of instances. The disease generally comes on in drunkards in the state of prostration which ensues when they have in a great measure given up, or been suddenly deprived of their accustomed stimulus.

The first symptoms of the malady are generally indicated

by extreme irritability of temper, weakness of memory, but constant activity of mind, anxiety, and incontrollable restlessness with increased muscular mobility.

The appetite is often pretty good, but more frequently impaired in consequence of the previous habits, and the tongue sometimes foul and moist. Soon after these premonitory signs, vigilance sets in, and little or no sleep can be obtained; or it is unrefreshing and disturbed by frightful dreams, imaginary visions and sounds. Fixed ideas then take firm possession of the patient's mind, such as the supposition that some one is bent upon poisoning him or doing him some other grievous injury, etc., yet he generally dreads being alone. The speech is frequently stuttering and inarticulate; the countenance quick, wild, and exceedingly variable, according to the prevailing impression on the mind; the face in most cases pale or sallow; the eye rolling, expressive, and restless, and the conjunctiva blanched; the skin damp, or covered with sweat, chilly and relaxed, very rarely above the natural temperature; the hands are commonly tremulous, and muscular twitchings are often observable. As the disease advances, sleep is completely banished; loquacity with perpetual bustling occupation, becomes incessant; and when it is fully developed, delirium supervenes. The pulse is soft and compressible, and rarely quick when not agitated by the struggles or exertions of the patient, for his corporal activity keeps pace with that of the mind, and it is difficult to confine him to his bed or apartment; at the same time, exhaustion is liable to come on very rapidly after great exertion, and the patient is prone to drop down from fatigue. Occasionally convulsions take place, but though sometimes serious, they are usually not of a fatal character. The history of the case, together with the distinctive nature of most of the above described symptoms, enable us to discern this disorder from that of inflammation of the brain or its membranes.

THERAPEUTICS. *Nux v.*, *Opium* (provided, of course, the attack has not been excited by the effects of Opium or its alkaloid, in large doses), *Aconitum*, *Belladonna*, *Lachesis*, *Hyoscyamus*, *Sulphur*, and *Calc.*, form our main remedial agents.

Nux v. is particularly useful in the first stage of the disorder, and may frequently be the means of arresting its further progress when administered at that period. The $\frac{000}{3}$, or $\frac{000}{6}$, or $\frac{000}{12}$th potency may be used, and the dose repeated in from six, twelve, to twenty-four hours, according to the effects produced.*

But when the disease has become fairly established, and the patient is affected with *delirium* or *convulsions*, and an aggravated degree of all the symptoms remarked at the commencement of the attack, we must have recourse to *Opium*, (potency $\frac{000}{3}$ or $\frac{000}{6}$,) in frequently repeated doses. The curative properties of this drug, in this malady, do not, as is erroneously supposed by the majority of allopathic practitioners, arise from its property of producing sleep, but from its *homœopathicity*, or *specificity*, if I may use the expressions; the pathogenetic properties which it possesses being exactly similar to those which are developed in the course of the disease as it occurs in drunkards.

In some cases, particularly where the patient exhibits extreme irritability of temper, with more or less derangement of the digestive functions, considerable advantage will be attained from the alternate employment of *Nux v.* and *Opium.*

In some rarer varieties of the affection, which are more liable to occur in young, robust, or plethoric subjects, we meet with symptoms indicative of active cerebral congestion, which call for the administration of a dose or two of *Aconite*, followed in a few hours by *Belladonna*, or by *Belladonna* and *Lachesis* alternately, if only partial benefit is obtained from the action of *Belladonna* alone, and the trembling of the hands and arms forms a very prominent symptom. *Hyoscyamus* may be prescribed in preference to *Belladonna*, when the patient's insanity is more particularly apparent in the exhibition of excessive and uncalled-for jealousy.

In extremely obstinate attacks, *Sulphur*, *Opium* and *Nux v.* may be given in alternation, at longer or shorter intervals according to the greater or less severity of the symptoms. *Calcarea* is also a remedy of considerable importance in such

* Vide note, p. 21.

cases, but more especially in plethoric habits. Finally, *Stramonium* may be mentioned as likely to be useful when *Belladonna, Hyosciamus*, and even *Opium*, fail to do much good, and the spasms or convulsions are very severe. *Coffea* and *Camphora* have likewise been named as likely to prove serviceable against the vigilance, or the mental and bodily activity, when the remedies already enumerated fail to answer expectation. But it may safely be averred, that there are few instances in which *Nux v.* and *Opium*, when timely administered, will not succeed in subduing the more violent features of the disease; and *Sulphur, Opium, Nux v.* and *Calcarea*, in removing any inveterate sequelæ. These medicines, together with *Arsenicum* and *Acid. sulphuricum*, administered at intervals of from four to eight days, have also been recommended as useful in correcting the vice which gives rise to this disease as ordinarily met with. Delirium tremens arising from exposure to the vapour of lead, chiefly requires: *Opium, Belladonna*, and *Nux v.;* and that from poisonous doses of *Opium: Nux v.* and *Belladonna* chiefly. (See Poisons.)

EPILEPSY. *Epilepsia. Morbus sacer.*

This well known and truly distressing complaint would require a treatise of itself were we to enter minutely into the treatment of the different forms in which it shows itself; it must therefore be sufficient for our purpose, at present, merely to enumerate the various remedies which have been employed against it with the most success.

In cases of recent origin the following are generally the most appropriate: *Belladonna, Ignatia, Chamomilla, Nux v., Opium, Ipecacuanha, Camphor*, &c. In chronic: *Sulph., Calcarea*, and *Silicea;* or, *Causticum, Cuprum, Stannum, Belladonna, Hyoscyamus, Stramonium, Veratrum, Cicuta, Zincum, Lachesis, Hepar, Arsenicum, Agaricus*, &c. When the repercussion of an eruption, or the suppression of an accustomed discharge has given rise to the malady: *Sulphur, Calcarea, Causticum, Lachesis, Stramonium, Ipecacuanha*, have chiefly been recommended. When the disorder is symptomatic of other diseases, such as derangement of the digestive functions, worms, teething, etc., our attention must necessarily be directed to the treatment of the primary malady.

During the epileptic seizure, all that is usually requisite is to take true measures to guard against any injury accruing to the patient in his struggles; further, to remove anything which is calculated to obstruct the circulation, from the neck. A dose of ACONITE $^{0}\frac{0}{3}{}^{0}$ followed by *Belladonna* if relief be not speedily obtained, is necessary in some recent cases, when the fit occurs in plethoric subjects, and is attended with strongly marked signs of congestion of the vessels of the head and neck.

ASTHMA.

This affection is characterized by the following phenomena: difficulty of breathing, recurring in paroxysms, attended with a sensation of suffocating constriction in the chest, cough, and wheezing. The paroxysm is frequently preceded by a sense of coldness, languor, headache, heaviness over the eyes, sickness or flatulence, and a sense of oppression in the chest. During the attack, the patient feels much worse in the recumbent posture, and consequently sits up, requests the door or window to be thrown open, to admit more air into his apartment, and uses every effort to dilate and empty the lungs. There is great restlessness, and frequent attempts to force something out of the air-passages which he thinks impedes the breathing, by coughing. The face is pale or livid, and wears an anxious expression. The extremities, and even the nose and ears, are frequently cold, and the face and chest covered with cold perspiration; the heart palpitates; the pulse is in various states, sometimes quick and full, small and quick, or weak and irregular; often intermitting. These symptoms continue with a greater or less degree of violence for some hours or even days, until expectoration takes place, which affords relief as it increases in quantity. A remission also sometimes takes place soon after the occurrence of an accession of copious perspiration, or a profuse discharge of urine.

The disease is more frequently met with at an advanced than an early period of life, and oftener in men than women. The attacks occasionally come on in the afternoon, or on retiring to rest, but much more frequently during the night, and in the midst of a sound sleep, from which the patient is suddenly awoke by a sense of suffocation.

The recurrence as well as the duration of the attacks is very various. One attack generally leads to another, and the paroxysms commonly become more and more frequent and distressing; still, if no organic disease result, patients who are subject to returns in considerable frequency, sometimes survive to an advanced age. But this is unfortunately not often the case: for unless the disease be arrested, the repeated obstruction and disturbance which is offered to the respiration and circulation, seldom fails, in the majority of cases, to induce organic lesions of the heart and large vessels of the lungs, with the usual concomitants of water in the chest or abdomen. The quantity of expectoration is small, and even entirely absent in some cases of asthma, whilst in others it is exceedingly copious; and hence, the disease has been divided into dry and humid asthma. In the former (*Asthma siccum*), the attack is usually sudden, violent, and of short duration; the cough slight; the expectoration scanty, appearing only towards the termination of the fit, and in some instances entirely wanting. In the latter, (*Asthma humidum*), the paroxysm is gradual and protracted; the cough severe; the expectoration supervenes early, is at first scanty and glutinous, and afterwards copious, and productive of great relief.

Therapeutics. In nervous or convulsive asthma (*Asthma sicca*) the remedies which have been employed with the most satisfactory results are: *Arsenicum, Cuprum, Ipecacuanha, Nux v., Bryonia, Pulsatilla.—Opium, Tartarus, Sambucus.—Aconitum, Belladonna, Phosphorus.—Sulphur, Lachesis, Sambucus.—Ferrum, Veratrum, Moschus, Stannum, Hyoscyamus, Stramonium, Chamomilla, Carbo v., Aurum, Lycopodium, Acidum nitr., Ignatia, Kali, Ambra, Mercurius, Silicea, Calcarea, Dulcamara, Coffea, Lobelia inflata*, etc. In moist, humid, pituitous asthma (*asthma humida*) : *Pulsatilla, Dulcamara, Stannum.—Sulphur, Sepia, Tartarus, Cuprum, Sambucus.—Ipecacuanha, Belladonna, Bryonia.—Ferrum, Calcarea, Lachesis, Graphites, China, Silicea, Hepar, Baryta c., Conium, Camphora, Zincum, Mercurius.* In flatulent asthma : *Nux v., Cinchona, Carbo v., Lycopodium, Chamomilla, Phosphorus, Sulphur, Opium, Zincum,* &c. In asthma spasmodica, Pulmonary spasm (*cramps in the chest*): *Cuprum, Nux, Bryonia, Belladonna, Hyoscyamus, Arsenicum, Lachesis, Stramonium, Cocculus, Nux m., Sambucus, Tartarus, Zincum, Sulphur, Kali, Causticum, Sepia, Stannum, Lycopodium,* &c. Asthma arising from exposure of irritating vapours (*asthma vaporosum*), such as copper or arsenic: *Ipecacuanha, Mercurius, Hepar s.—Camphora, Cuprum,* or *Arsenicum.* From the vapour of sulphur: *Pulsatilla* chiefly; and when caused by the continued inhalation of stone-dust, and other irritating particles: *Sulphur, Calcarea, Silicea, Hepar,* have principally been recommended; and in some cases, also the following: *Arsenicum, Belladonna, Nux v., Phosphorus, Ipecacuanha,* and *Cinchona.* Where the repercussion or retropulsion of an eruption, or the suppression of a habitual discharge has been the occasional cause (*asthma metastasicum*): *Sulphur, Carbo v., Arsenicum, Bryonia,* and *Phosphorus,* are the most appropriate in the majority of cases. If from suppressed catarrh : *Arsenicum, Ipecacuanha, Nux v.,* &c. Where a chill has given rise to an attack of asthmatical breathing, *Ipecacuanha* and *Arsenicum;* or, *Dulcamara, Aconitum, Belladonna, Bryonia, Chamomilla.* And when mental disturbance has brought on a paroxysm of dyspnœa: *Aconitum, Chamomilla, Ignatia, Coffea, Nux v., Pulsatilla, Veratrum.* When *Congestion of blood* in the chest forms the occasional cause of dyspnœa, see that article. When the disorder occurs as a sequela of bronchitis, see BRONCHITIS.

The remedies which are best calculated to afford relief during a paroxysm of asthma are: *Ipecacuanha,* followed by *Arsenicum* if the former produces but little benefit. In other cases: *Cuprum, Moschus, Opium, Tartarus,* and *Sambucus;* or, *Nux v., Bryonia, Chamomilla, Belladonna, Cinchona, Nux moschata*, or *Pulsatilla*, will prove more useful. And those which have principally been recommended to eradicate the tendency to suffer from repeated recurrences of the disorder, where that is practicable from the absence of serious organic disease, &c., are as follows: *Sulphur, Calcarea, Arsenicum, Nux v., Antimonium.—Stannum, Sepia, Silicea, Cuprum, Lachesis, Carbo v.—Lycopodium, Causticum, Graphites, Acidum nitricum, Phosphorus, Ammonium c., Ferrum, Zincum, Tussilago.* In ordinary cases the subjacent remedies will be found serviceable, when the leading symptoms are in accordance with those which are described.

IPECACUANHA $\frac{000}{3}$. During the paroxysm of acute asthma, this remedy is one of the most frequently useful, whether the attack occurs in children or adults. It is more especially indicated when the patient is awoke from a sound sleep, with a suffocating sensation of *constriction* in the windpipe, with quick, laborious breathing and gasping for breath; wheezing and mucous rattling in the chest; short dry cough; *paleness* and *coldness* of the face, sometimes alternately with heat and redness; coldness of the feet; anxiety and dread of suffocation; feeling as if dust were inspired during the act of respiration, and caused the suffocating feeling in the chest; spasmodic rigidity of the body, and livid hue of the face. After a dose or two of *Ipecac.*, it is occasionally requisite to have recourse to *Arsenicum* to afford further relief. In other instances, *Nux v.* or *Bryonia* will be found better adapted to remove the remaining symptoms.

ARSENICUM $\frac{000}{6}$. Is chiefly called for (either in acute or chronic asthma) when, during the attack, the respiration appears to become more and more laborious, and is attended with extreme agitation, moaning, and jactitation; *great exhaustion, and anguish, as if at the point of dea'h, with cold perspiration*. In confirmed asthmatics, it forms a most important remedy, when the breathing is liable to become much oppressed when walking rather quickly, or when going up a hill, or ascending stairs; and when, particularly in the case of old people, even the effort of laughing, or the exertion of getting into bed, brings on a fit of dyspnœa. *Arsenicum*, as well as *Ipecacuanha*, is further indicated when the paroxysms of asthma are most liable to occur on retiring to rest, or before midnight, the patient being disturbed from sleep by a sense of *spasmodic constriction in the chest and larynx*, which is soon followed by *laborious*, *panting*, and *whistling* respiration, with gasping for breath. These symptoms are occasionally relieved by remissions, but the attack is prone to recur on using the slightest exertion; for the most part, however, the paroxysm continues with more or less intensity until relieved by the accession of a fit of coughing, with expectoration of viscid mucus filled with vesicles. *Arsenicum*, though principally called for in cases in which the attacks come on at night, is also useful when they are prone to be excited during the day, on exposure to a cold bracing air, or on going out during the prevalence of disagreeable, damp, or stormy weather; likewise when changes of temperature, or tight and very warm clothing, are likewise liable to cause a fit of dyspnœa. Sensation of *burning heat* in the chest duriug the fit of asthma, is an additional indication for *Arsenicum*.

BRYONIA $\frac{000}{3}$. As already mentioned, this medicine is frequently useful after the previous employment of *Ipecacuanha*. The indications are chiefly: Obstructed respiration at *night or towards morning*, with frequent cough, pains in the hypochondria, and inability to recline on the right side, and not without inconvenience on the left, so that the patient is constrained to lie on the back; frequent coughing, with expectoration at first frothy, and subsequently thick and glutinous, and frequently attended with retching or vomiting; aggravation of the dyspnœa from *talking* or from the slightest *movement*; frequent efforts to obtain sufficient air by deep inspirations, accompanied with moaning, palpitation of the heart, and great anxiety. The attacks are often attended by shootings in the chest, on taking a full inspiration, also on coughing, or after any movement of the arms or trunk. At other times there are eructations of the taste of the food partaken of, colic, irritability of temper, and disposition to find fault with everything. (*Bryonia* and *Nux v.* are often administered with great advantage in alternation.)

Nux vomica $^{0}\frac{0}{3}{}^{0}$. Nocturnal attacks of *suffocating tightness, especially at the lower part of the chest*, preceded by disagreeable or anxious dreams; also when the paroxysms are prone to occur in the morning, or after a meal, and are attended with anxiety, aching and pressive pains in the precordial region, as also in the hypochondria; feeling of distention in the abdomen and epigastrium; flatulence; tension, pressure, and aching in the chest; palpitation of the heart; short hacking cough, with difficult expectoration; inability to bear the slightest pressure from the clothing, particularly around the chest and waist; the clothes seem to fit tightly and increase the difficulty of breathing, when in reality they are quite the reverse; dyspnœa when walking and conversing in the open air, especially if the temperature be somewhat cold; dyspnœa after trivial corporal exertion of any kind. Melioration of the asthmatic sufferings when reclining on the *back*, or on changing from one posture to another, such as sitting up, and then lying down again, or turning from one side to the other. Disposition irritable and passionate.

Pulsatilla $^{0}\frac{0}{3}{}^{0}$. Oppressed, rapid, and laborious breathing from a feeling of spasmodic *constriction* in the chest, especially at the inferior portions; or suffocating feeling in the wind-pipe, as if caused by the *vapour of Sulphur;* tension, and sensation of fulness, pressure and aching, attended with mucous rattling in the chest; short fits of coughing in rapid succession, and appearing to threaten suffocation; or cough with *copious expectoration of mucus.* The attacks usually coming on at *night*, or in the evening when in a *horizontal posture; extreme anguish, palpitation of the heart*, and sometimes lancinating pains in the chest during the paroxysms.

Pulsatilla $\frac{0\,0\,0}{3}$, is generally more suitable for hysterical females or individuals of a mild, timid, sensitive, or fretful disposition. In dyspnœa, with mucous rattling, and cough, occurring in children from taking cold, it is likewise a most useful remedy.

Tartarus emeticus $\frac{0\,0\,0}{6}$. Dyspnœa with suffocating cough and anxious oppression at the præcordia, arising from an *excessive secretion of mucus in the bronchi;* this remedy is frequently of great service, either in aged persons or in children.

Opium $\frac{0\,0\,0}{3}$. *Obstructed breathing*, either from congestion or from pulmonary spasms, with suffocating cough and livid hue of the face; loud mucous rattling in the chest, with extreme anguish from dread of suffocation; dyspnœa during sleep resembling nightmare (incubus).

CHINA $\frac{000}{3}$. Paroxysms of asthma at night, as if caused by an accumulation of mucus in the wind-pipe; *wheezing in the chest during inspiration;* difficult expectoration of thick transparent mucus; oppression at the chest, palpitation of the heart, and inability to breathe, unless the head and shoulders are propped up with pillows; great weakness, and tendency to copious sweating at the slightest exertion, or when too warmly clothed.

SAMBUCUS $\frac{000}{3}$. Rapid and laborious respiration, with *loud wheezing;* oppression at the chest as if from a weight, attended with *anguish and dread of suffocation*, and sometimes swelling and livid hue of the face and hands, general heat, tremour, inability to talk much above a whisper; suffocating cough; aggravation of the symptoms in the recumbent posture. In the case of children this remedy is often of great service, when, in consequence of a chill, they are seized with spasm in the chest, and awake from sleep with a start, and exhibit many of the symptoms detailed. (See SPASMS IN THE CHEST.)

MOSCHUS $\frac{000}{3}$. Acute asthma occurring in *hysterical females*, or in children from exposure to cold; sense of *spasmodic constriction in the larynx and bronchi;* or oppression at the chest with *paroxysms of suffocating feelings*, as if caused by the inhalation of the vapour of sulphur, commencing with a fit of coughing, and succeeded by distressing oppressive constriction, sometimes to such a degree, as almost to drive the patient to exasperation and distraction.

BELLADONNA $\frac{000}{3}$. Difficulty of breathing, particularly when occurring in females of an irritable habit, and subject to spasms, with tension in the chest, and lancinating pain behind the sternum; *dry cough at night*, with *moaning respiration which is sometimes deep and full, at others, short and rapid*, with gasping for breath and great efforts to dilate the chest to the utmost to obtain a sufficient supply of air; sensation of constriction in the larynx, and feeling as if suffocation would ensue on putting the hand to the larynx, or on turning the neck; paroxysms of asthma, with loss of consciousness, etc.

Lachesis $\frac{000}{6}$, is often useful when only partial relief has been effected by the action of *Belladonna.*

VERATRUM $\frac{000}{3}$, in violent attacks of acute spasmodic asthma, with symptoms of threatening suffocation, cold perspiration, coldness of the nose, ears, and lower extremities, this remedy will often afford relief when *Cinchona*, *Ipecacuanha*, and *Arsenicum* have failed to do so.

DULCAMARA $\frac{000}{3}$. In moist asthma (*asthma humida*) this medicine is one of the most useful remedies, and particularly when the attacks are liable to be excited by a cold and damp state of the atmosphere. In severe dyspnœa, with loose-sounding cough, rattling of phlegm in the chest, and copious expectoration, arising from exposure to wet, it is likewise a valuable remedy.

STANNUM $\frac{00}{6}$. *Humid asthma with obstructed respiration and fits of shaking*, particularly at night, or on preparing for bed, but also when the paroxysms come on during the day, and render it necessary to loosen the clothing. The attacks are attended with oppression at the chest, and mucous rattling; cough, with *copious expectoration* of viscid or grumous, or transparent and watery, or yellowish mucus of a *sweetish* or saline taste. *Phosphorus*, *Sulphur*, *Calcarea*, *Sepia*, and *Lycopodium*, are also of much value in humid asthma, and of great service in some of the most obstinate cases. In chronic asthma, a dose of the medicine required may be taken at intervals of from four to eight days or so; but in acute cases, or when the remedy is prescribed during the paroxysm, the dose may be repeated at intervals of from half an hour to two hours, and upwards, according to the severity of the case. When the medicine first prescribed affords no relief after from two to three repetitions, another must be selected, preference being given to that remedy which corresponds the nearest to the existing symptoms.*

* Vide note, p. 21.

CASUALTIES.

CONCUSSION, BRUISES, SPRAINS OR STRAINS, WOUNDS, DISLOCATIONS, AND FRACTURES.

In Concussion of the brain, (which may arise from a violent shaking of the brain or of the whole body, without any *direct* violence having been offered, such as a severe blow or fall on the head,) the symptoms vary according to the degree of injury which the brain has sustained. When the concussion is very severe, there is immediate deprivation of sense and power of motion, and death is the general result; but when slight, a temporary stunning or confusion, with some headache, is produced, followed by increased action of the pulse, vertigo and sickness. When, on the other hand, the violence done is greater than in the latter instance, though not so severe as to cause the fatal termination alluded to in the first, the patient is rendered insensible and incapable of movement; his limbs become cold; the pulse weak, slow, and intermittent; the respiration laborious, but usually without stertor. (This has been denominated the *first stage* of concussion.) As the patient begins to recover from this condition, the pulse and respiration improve, and warmth begins to be felt in the extremities; the sensibility to touch then returns, and the contents of the stomach are in most cases rejected; still he continues to remain in a dull, confused state, and inattentive to, or almost unconscious of slight external impressions (*second stage*). On the gradual subsidence of the first effects of the concussion, the patient becomes enabled to respond to questions spoken in a loud tone. When, however, the stupor has considerably or entirely abated, inflammation of the brain, of an active character, will, in many cases, then begin to develop itself (*third stage*), with all its wonted symptoms, (see PHRENITIS,) and if not checked, suppuration or effusion within the head, preceded by rigours, will result.

THERAPEUTICS. In all cases of injury arising from external violence, *Arnica* is the *specific* remedy, and its *timely administration* in cases of concussion of the brain, will in most instances, if the injury be not very severe, suffice to remove all traces and evil consequences of such misfortunes. We may administer internally two globules of the sixth potency, in a teaspoonful of water; and, if there be an external wound, we may bathe the injured part with a lotion, in the proportion of a few drops of the *Tincture of Arnica* to an ounce or about two tablespoonfuls of water, twice or thrice a day; should the swelling, pains, and other symptoms, increase, after one or two applications, we must *discontinue* the lotion, but will almost always find a marked improvement follow such aggravation.

When, however, the contusion has been serious, and extreme restlessness or jactitation, and irritability of temper with sensibility of the eyes to light, small quick pulse, delirium, or subsequently rigours, etc., supervene, the same treatment must be pursued as that which has been described under INFLAMMATION OF THE BRAIN, and also HYDROCEPHALUS, which see.* After an injury to the head, particularly if it has been of a somewhat severe character, the patient ought not to be allowed to partake of any stimulating liquids, such as wine, spirits, &c., until at least three or four weeks have elapsed, even although he appears to have entirely recovered from the effects of the accident; he ought likewise to be kept quiet, and not be permitted to expose himself to excitement of any kind, otherwise the most serious consequences may be the result. When the chest has been injured by a contusion or violent concussion, etc., and soreness or a sensation as if from incipient suppuration, with heat and throbbing, is experienced in some particular spot; fever or alternate chilliness and heat followed by fever which becomes aggravated in the evening; sleeplessness or

* In fracture of the cranium the same treatment must be pursued; but when compression of the brain takes place attended with its usual concomitants, such as stupor, stertorous breathing, etc., from the effects of a depressed portion of bone, the trephine must be employed, if the symptoms continue unabated notwithstanding the use of the medicines indicated.

disturbed sleep, with general heat, and sometimes perspiration towards morning; short dry cough which increases the pain, or cough with spitting of blood; further, when the pain in the chest is rendered more acute by taking a full inspiration, laughing or sneezing, or when pricking pains or a sensation of fulness or pressure, as if caused by extravasated blood, is experienced, together with a feeling of constriction that obstructs the freedom of respiration,—it will be necessary to have immediate recourse to *Arnica* and *Aconitum* alternately, at intervals of from three to six hours, until an improvement in the symptoms becomes manifest; but should a degree of fever continue after the exhibition of several doses of the foregoing remedies, attended with a sensation as if there were an internal excoriation or wound, *Pulsatilla* should be administered. In the event of a continuance or even an increase of cough, with expectoration of thick, yellow mucus occasionally streaked with blood, *Mercurius* must be prescribed; if on the other hand, the expectoration has a sweetish taste, and is accompanied by difficulty of breathing, *Nux v.* is to be preferred. When a degree of delicacy of chest remains behind, after the employment of any of the preceding medicines, with tendency to suffer from shortness of breath, and a short dry cough, combined with paleness of the face, impaired appetite, and restless unrefreshing sleep, *Cinchona* has been strongly recommended. In other cases, especially those which have been neglected, where we have reason to apprehend the development of *Phthisis pulmonalis*, the employment of *Stannum*, *Acidum nitricum*, *Silicea* and *Kali c.*, or *Phosphorus*, *Sulphur*, *Calcarea*, and *Lycopodium*, may yet enable us to arrest the progress of that ruthless malady.

The effects of a shock to the nervous system, with pains in the limbs, &c., from stumbling or making a false step, are generally relieved by *Bryonia* or *Pulsatilla*. When the accident has been accompanied with fright, *Opium* $\frac{0\,0\,0}{3}$ may be prescribed in the first instance; ACONITUM $\frac{0\,0\,0}{3}$ when there is syncope, and CHAMOMILLA $\frac{0\,0\,0}{3}$ when from extreme pain convulsions ensue.*

* *Ignatia* has also been recommended in the event of convulsions; and *Coffea* when uncontrollable agitation and agonizing jactitation result.

But in almost all such cases, *Arnica* may be employed with advantage, either subsequently or at the commencement; in the event of headache resulting from a contusion or from stumbling, and *Arnica* does not afford much relief, *Belladonna* $^{0}\frac{0}{3}{}^{0}$ may be given;* the patient should at the same time remain quiet, and avoid any exertion, whether of the body or mind, until the pain is removed.

SPRAINS. In the treatment of these troublesome casualties, at the commencement, prescribe a lotion of *Arnica*, when there is much tumefaction and redness, with great pain on the slightest movement. After the employment of the *Arnica*, we may have recourse to RHUS TOXICODENDRON, which is, properly speaking, more specific to this description of external injury, in the same manner, and two or three globules of the third or sixth potency may also be taken internally. If severe pain continue notwithstanding the employment of *Arnica* and *Rhus*, the following remedies have been recommended: *Bryonia*, *Ammonium c.* and *Ruta*, and in some instances, *Belladonna*, *Pulsatilla*, *Nux v.*, *Agnus*, or *Silicea* $^{0}\frac{0}{3}{}^{0}$, or $^{0}\frac{0}{6}{}^{0}$.

STRAINS. When pricking or other pains are experienced in the back, &c., after a strain caused by any powerful or sudden exertion, such as lifting a heavy weight, or throwing up a window, with aggravation from the slightest movement of the arms or trunk, *Bryonia* should be exhibited, and succeeded by *Sulphur*, if only partial relief is obtained. When headache results from a similar source, or when the pains are confined to the extremities, or if at all in the back or loins, are equally, if not more severe, during rest as well as on movement, *Rhus* may be prescribed, followed in turn by *Calcarea* $\frac{0}{6}{}^{0}$, if the sufferings remain almost unmitigated. When sickness and great pain in the abdomen are produced by the effects of a strain, *Veratrum* $\frac{000}{3}$ has been recommended as being speedily serviceable.

* *Cocculus*, *Cicuta*, or *Acid. phosphoricum*, may be required to remove prolonged headache arising from the above-named causes. (See also CEPHALALGIA.)

WOUNDS are divided into incised, lacerated, contused, punctured, poisoned, and gunshot wounds.

By an INCISIVE WOUND, is meant one which has been produced by a sharp instrument, as a sword, knife, &c., and is not accompanied with any contusion or laceration. Incised wounds, although more liable to be attended with a greater degree of hemorrhage, are, generally speaking, the least dangerous and the most easily healed.

LACERATED WOUNDS are those in which the muscular fibres, instead of being divided by a sharp cutting instrument, have been torn asunder with some violence; the edges, instead of being even and regular, are jagged and unequal. They are commonly attended with little or no bleeding, rarely heal without suppurating, and are frequently succeeded by violent inflammation.

The terms CONTUSED WOUNDS, or BRUISES, are applied to those wounds which are occasioned by some blunt instrument, or hard blunt surface, being brought in violent collision with a part of the body. When severe, they are dangerous, from being prone to terminate in mortification and sloughing.

PUNCTURED WOUNDS are those which have been caused by pointed instruments; they partake more of the nature of lacerated than incised wounds, and are dangerous from the great depth to which they frequently penetrate, and the serious consequences they often entail by occasioning violent inflammation of the fascia, and tetanus.

THERAPEUTICS. In the treatment of wounds of all kinds, our first object is to arrest the hemorrhage. This is to be done by means of the tourniquet, by compression, by the ligature, by cold water or ice, and astringents, &c., according to the degree and source of the discharge.

Wounds of the arteries are for the most part the most serious: they are to be distinguished by the bright colour of the blood, which moreover issues very rapidly and in jets; while that from a vein flows in a smooth, uninterrupted stream, and has a dark or deep purple hue.

When the injured vessels are of a small size, they spontaneously cease to bleed, or do so, at all events, as soon as the wound is dressed; but when the hemorrhage is considerable, one or more of the arresting measures above alluded to must immediately be put in requisition. When, therefore, there is reason to conclude that an artery has been punctured, a tourniquet should be applied around the limb to check the flow of blood; the external wound must then be closed, covered with a graduated compress, and firmly secured with a bandage. When a proper tourniquet is not at hand, its place may be tolerably well supplied by a handkerchief bound round the limb, and tightened by two or three turns of a stick passed under the handkerchief; or the substitute may consist of a cork cut longitudinally, and securely fixed over the artery, the site of which is readily to be found at the inner surface of the limb, in spare or emaciated subjects, by its pulsation; but as the finding of the artery is not so easily accomplished in the robust and muscular, it will be advisable first to tie a handkerchief, or non-elastic garter, tightly round the limb, above the wound; this will have the effect of rendering the artery more prominent. In order to make the compression of the cork the more effectual, several plies of lint or linen, or a piece sufficiently large to form a few inches square and one in thickness, should be placed over the cork, (which should be held firmly in the required position during the preparation of the compress,) and the whole then tightened, and retained as long as may be requisite. The application of ice to the wound, or of cold water frequently renewed, is also of unequivocal service. Compression may in some cases be effectually applied by pressing a piece of sponge (which has been dipped in bees' wax and stiffened) down upon the bleeding vessels, then adding compresses of lint and a roller. When the hemorrhage comes from a large artery, it must sooner or later be stopped by ligature. In wounds of veins, or when the bleeding is from any small arteries, also when it is from a vessel which lies over a bone, or when it proceeds from vessels situated too deeply for the convenient application of the ligature, compression, with the aid of ice or cold water, is the method to be adopted for the suppression of the hemorrhage.

Bleeding from wounds, &c., in the mouth, sometimes requires the application of styptics, such as alcohol, and kreosote water, &c. The same may be said of slight superficial wounds, as also of fungous tumours, and other diseased surfaces, when cold water fails to answer the purpose. *Arnica*, *Diadema*, or *Phosphorus*, internally and externally, have likewise been strongly recommended in such cases.

Copious hemorrhage after the extraction of a tooth is usually readily suppressed, by pushing a compress of lint into the hollow space left; or by the aid of styptics, and the medicines above mentioned, when requisite. A simple, and sometimes extremely efficacious mode of checking this current of blood, is by replacing the extracted tooth, and keeping it there until the risk of further hemorrhage is obviated.

When severe syncope, with deadly paleness of the face, or when the face assumes a livid appearance, and subsultus tendinum and other signs of extreme exhaustion set in from excessive loss of blood, *Cinchona* ought to be prescribed; and if the patient should not exhibit any indications of rallying thereafter, a little wine may be given, and subsequently *Arnica;* but if the stimulating effects of the wine prove only of temporary service, another dose of *Cinchona* must previously be had recourse to.

The next step to be taken in wounds of every description, after the hemorrhage is stopped, is to remove all extraneous matter, as sand, fragments of glass, splinters, shot, rags, &c.; then relax the muscles so that the wound may not gape; finally, to place the lips of the wound in accurate contact, and keep them so by bandages, plasters, sutures, &c. Bandages are usually indispensable in deep, and even in small, superficial, incised wounds, but care must be taken not to apply them too tight, nor when there is excessive inflammation.

Sutures are commonly requisite in wounds of the face, abdomen, and sometimes of the hands, and in old people generally. In the young and vigorous they are seldom necessary, and even improper, when the patient is of an irritable habit of body. Strips of adhesive plaster, cut narrow in the centre or portion which is to cross the wound, and sufficiently long that they may retain their hold the more firmly, and act with the required compressive power, form, in the majority of incised wounds, the most frequently useful means of bringing the sides into close approximation and effecting adhesion. It sometimes happens, however, that even incised wounds, particularly when deep and of considerable magnitude, terminate in suppuration, it is consequently necessary to leave intervening spaces between the strips of plaster, to admit of the exit of the matter in such an event. Again, when it is found impracticable to cleanse the wound of all foreign substances, it ought to be only lightly, and so to speak, incompletely dressed, as it will be necessary to renew the dressings repeatedly. In some cases it is necessary to dilate the wound, to obtain the abstraction of a splinter, &c.

With regard to the constitutional treatment of wounds of all kinds, we should commence with the administration of *Arnica*, of which a few globules at the sixth potency should be given, as soon as the patient shall be made as comfortable as circumstances will admit. The patient should at the same time be kept cool, free from anxiety or exertion, and as quiet as possible. He should live abstemiously, avoid every thing of a heating nature, and drink cold water. If he be robust and strong, and sympathetic fever run high, a dose of *Aconite*, at the third or sixth potency, should be prescribed; followed, in the course of from three to six hours, by *Arnica*, and so on alternately as long as may be found requisite; in favourable cases one dose of each is often found sufficient. The local application in the first instance, if required by excess of pain, heat, and swelling, should consist simply of lint dipped in cold water, and frequently remoistened.

In the treatment of LACERATED WOUNDS we must, after having carefully cleansed them, closely approximate all the parts that will admit of the process, and retain them in their place by means of plasters and an appropriate position of the body or limb, for the purpose of endeavouring to unite them by the first intention. Should the wound become inflamed, attended with much pain and swelling, dress it with lint dipped in cold water, which must be frequently renewed. If, on the other hand, copious suppuration ensue, and the pain be very severe, the cold water must be discontinued, and *Chamomilla* exhibited, followed by *Hepar s.*; and should these remedies fail to bring on an early healing action, *Silicea* will generally answer; or *Silicea* and *Sulphur* in alternation to promote granulation. (See ULCERS.)

In CONTUSED WOUNDS (or BRUISES) *Arnica* must be given internally, and cold water applied externally, in the first instance. When there is considerable extravasation of blood, the tincture of *Arnica** must be applied as a lotion, of the strength of a teaspoonful of this tincture to a teacupful of water, to stimulate absorption and otherwise forward the cure.† In the event of an ABSCESS resulting from the effects of a contusion, *see that article.*

When joints,‡ or the synovial membranes, are injured by a Contusion, *Rhus* has been particularly recommended; in some cases *Silicea* will be found of great utility, as we can testify from experience. If the periosteum be affected, *Ruta* is said to be useful; we would however recommend an incision to be

* We have already remarked that this useful medicament, when employed as a lotion to wounds, should always be discontinued whenever any aggravation of the pains, &c., is experienced; and I take the opportunity to repeat here, that individuals of what is ordinarily designated an inflammatory habit, or who have very irritable skins, and are liable to be affected with erysipelas, must be very guarded how they use it, and invariably dilute the tincture with a larger proportion of water than is indicated in various parts of this work, when they have occasion to employ it.

† ARNICA OIL.—Arnica flowers digested in sweet oil by heat—is the best form in which this medicament can be used for injuries attended by *abrasion of the skin*, or *laceration of the flesh.* The flowers of HYPERICUM PERFORATUM, or *St. John's wort*, heated with sweet oil, also, exerts an equally salutary influence when applied to *incised wounds.*—ED.

‡ In cases of swelling, with considerable pain, stiffness or inflexibility of the knee, from the effects of kneeling, to which housemaids (hence the name of *Housemaid's Knee*,) and others, from the nature of their occupations, are liable,—and which affection, it may be added, consists of a degree of inflammation and consequent thickening of the *bursa mucosa*, situated between the patella and the skin, attended with increased secretion of the slippery lubricating fluid contained in the sac,—*Silicea*, 3 glo-

made in the membrane, if ecchymosed blood or matter is evidently pent up beneath it, and the patient's sufferings are great; after which, the treatment to be pursued must be the same as described for open abscesses. When a bruise or contusion is so violent as to squeeze the limb nearly flat, or otherwise disfigure it, cold water ought to be constantly applied, and *Arnica* prescribed internally. But if gangrene threatens, *Cinchona* must be given; and when the skin has assumed a livid and black appearance, amputation may still be avoided, and life and limb saved, by having recourse to *Lachesis* and *Arsenicum* alternately, in frequently repeated doses. In the greater number of such unfortunate cases, however, amputation becomes imperative, and ought to be performed without hesitation, when it becomes evident that the patient will fall a sacrifice to further delay. When amputation has been found necessary, the stump ought to be dressed with lint dipped in cold water, and *Arnica* given internally; subsequently the said medicine may be employed in alternation with *Aconitum*, if required by the accession of traumatic fever. *Hepar*, *Silicea*, and *Sulphur* $\frac{0\,0}{6}$ may also be required at the ensuing stages in the healing of the stump. (See ULCERS, for indications for the employment of these and other remedies.)

bules of the potency 6, or 30, either administered daily, or at intervals of four to eight days in susceptible habits, is an important and successful remedy.

The same remedy is equally efficacious in similar swellings in other parts, such as the ball of the great toe, (where it is usually known under the denomination of a *bunion*,) or the joints of the fingers; and indeed in most of the situations where tendons play; the use of these little sacs, or *bursæ mucosæ*, being to facilitate the action of the muscles.

By means of the specific effects of *Silicea* in this disease, we are spared the necessity, even in obstinate cases in which the fluid of the bursa becomes altered in character and contains small granular bodies, of opening the sac for the purpose of obtaining the discharge of these substances; a procedure by no means free from danger, and but too often the source of considerable suffering and annoyance to the patient, for a length of time afterwards. During the treatment of these swellings, it is very necessary that the patient should at the same time be careful to avoid pressure on the affected part, and that he should walk about as little as possible. In the case of a *bunion*, when there is active inflammation, his own suffering will sufficiently remind him of the necessity of these precautions.

In the case of PUNCTURED WOUNDS, the treatment to be followed is the same as that described for wounds in general; but unless compression, by means of adhesive plaster or a bandage, can be brought to bear against their entire extent, the cure by the first intention must not be attempted.

When suppuration ensues, *Mercurius* $\frac{0}{6}{}^{0}$ may be prescribed; after which *Hepar s.*, and then *Silicea* if required. *Chamomilla*, *Belladonna*, and *Rhus*, may be found serviceable in the event of excessive local inflammation; the latter two particularly if it partake of an erysipelatous character (see ERYSIPELAS.) When spasmodic twitchings make their appearance, *Cicuta* is frequently serviceable; but *Arnica* will generally be found sufficient to subdue the symptoms when timely administered; when the constitutional disturbance is severe, *Aconitum* may be alternated with *Arnica;* and when they arise from violent inflammation of the fascia, incision may *in some instances* be necessary to be made in it transversely; in which event a dose of *Arnica* must be prescribed almost immediately afterwards.

If tetanus supervene, *Arnica* must be administered in repeated doses, and followed, if required, by *Angustura* or *Cocculus*, etc. (Vide TETANUS.)

GUNSHOT WOUNDS must be treated by the exhibition of *Arnica* internally, and cold water constantly applied by means of lint, externally. In some cases it may be found advantageous to apply a *very weak* lotion of *Arnica*, in preference to water simply, at the commencement. When splinters of bone, a ball, etc., are lodged in the wound, they ought to be extracted with as little irritation as possible, if they press on some important viscera, etc.; but if not, they may be allowed to remain, particularly when deeply seated or difficult to be found, until loosened by suppuration, which process will be materially forwarded by the administration of *Silicea*. In other cases, *Hepar s.* and *Sulph.* may afford valuable aid. In the event of fever, gangrene, etc., see CONTUSED WOUNDS.

When a joint is greatly injured, or much of the soft parts with the blood-vessels and nerves of importance are carried away by a gunshot wound, the bone remaining entire; when there is fracture of a bone with destruction of the soft parts; when the bone is shattered, and the principal vessels lacerated or ruptured; or when a limb is completely shot or torn off, or other serious injury done, which renders the prospect of saving the limb hopeless, amputation should be performed.*

It may be added, that *Staphysagria* has been recommended as a useful remedy in severe incised wounds; and *Aconitum*, *Cicuta*, or *Acid. nitr.* in addition to *Silicea* and *Hepar s.*, in wounds from splinters, $\frac{000}{3}$ or $\frac{000}{6}$, etc. (For *poisoned wounds*, see HYDROPHOBIA, p. 426.)

DISLOCATIONS. LUXATIONS. Violent pain, swelling, distortion of the joint, loss of motion, with an alteration in the shape, length, and direction of the limb, characterize the existence of this injury.

THERAPEUTICS. The reduction of a luxation ought to be effected as soon as possible by the surgeon. When such assistance is not immediately to be had, and there is excessive pain and inflammation, a dose of *Arnica* ought to be given, followed by *Aconitum* in an hour or two if the pain continues violent, and the inflammatory symptoms active. Cold water, or very weak arnicated water, (a few drops of the tincture to a teacupful of water,) should be applied locally. When the luxation is reduced, the same treatment may be pursued if called for; and the usual beneficial mechanical measures employed, such as the application of an appropriate bandage to support the joint, and prevent a recurrence of the displacement, together with frequent but careful flexion and extension of the joint. In compound luxations, the same treatment must be pursued in the first instance as above described; and

* $\frac{000}{3}$ Aconitum after amputations, extirpations, and other surgical operations.—Dr. Thorer employed, in preference to an *Arnica* lotion, the tincture *Calendula officinalis* as a lotion, especially in incised, punctured or lacerated wounds, and those with considerable loss of substance. Even after amputations, the cure was effected by the first intention, and in almost every instance where it was impossible to avoid suppuration.

the wound treated so that it may be healed if possible by the first intention. (See WOUNDS.)

FRACTURES. The symptoms of fracture are: pain, swelling, deformity, and sometimes shortening of the limb; loss of power, with preternatural mobility when we attempt to bend the limb, and crepitation on rubbing the broken surfaces of bone together. Fractures are divided into transverse, oblique, and longitudinal; and also into simple, compound, complicated, and comminuted. By a *simple* fracture is understood one in which the bone is broken, without there being at the same time a wound of the soft parts. A *compound* fracture consists, not only of a solution in the continuity of the bone, but also in the coexistence of an external wound, caused by the protrusion of the extremity of one or both fragments of the bone through the integuments. Again, a fracture is termed *complicated*, when it is attended with a wound of a large artery, extensive laceration of the soft parts, or with dislocation of a joint. Lastly, it is designated *comminuted*, when the bone is broken into several pieces.

THERAPEUTICS. As soon as a limb is discovered to be fractured, the patient ought to be placed on a litter of any kind which happens to be at hand, such as a board or shutter, and removed to some neighbouring place of shelter, or to his own abode if it be not far distant, and a surgeon sent for. Great care and gentleness ought to be exercised in lifting and transporting the patient from one place to another; otherwise a fracture, originally of the simple kind, is liable to be converted into a compound, or at all events into a complicated one, from laceration of the soft parts, etc., caused by the serrated extremities of the fractured bone, whereby the probabilities of recovery will be rendered much more unfavourable, particularly if the accident has happened to a debilitated or aged individual. In the case of a simple fracture, the reduction should be immediately effected by placing the limb in the position best calculated to relax the principal muscles attached to the broken bone; it should be then gradually extended, until the upper and lower fragments are brought into their proper position; after the accomplishment of which, splints and bandages must be applied to retain the fragments in their situation. When all this is accomplished, a dose of *Arnica* should be administered, for the double purpose of preventing the invasion of undue inflammation, and of promoting the reunion of the fracture. *Symphitum officinale* has also been most favourably spoken of, as being extremely valuable in facilitating the last-named most desirable end.* Those who have had ample opportunities of testing the virtues of these two remedies, and of the homœopathic treatment generally, in cases of fracture, unhesitatingly declare that the patients are thereby enabled to regain the use of their limbs, and to be discharged with safety from the hands of the surgeon, at an earlier period than when treated according to the old rules; and further, that the formation of false joints is, under the said mode of treatment, of less frequent occurrence.

In fracture complicated with a wounded artery, or with a dislocated joint, the artery should be ligatured, and the luxation reduced before the bone is set.

In compound fracture, the protruded extremities of the bone should be restored to their natural position as soon as possible, the limb supplied with splints, etc., and the external wound attempted to be healed by the first intention. Consecutive inflammation and constitutional disturbance must be suppressed by the measures alluded to in the treatment of wounds.

When the protruded part of the bone cannot be reduced by the ordinary method, the wound may be enlarged, and in those cases where it is evident that that will not prove of material assistance, it is recommended to remove a portion of the exposed bone. When a false joint is formed, in spite of every care and attention, (as is prone to occur when the limb has been kept in constant motion by patients in a state of delirium, or under other circumstances—also when the fracture has taken place in an aged person, or in one of an extremely bad habit of body,) most surgeons advise the ends of the osseous fragments to be cut off, or a seton passed between them.

* *Ruta* has likewise been mentioned as useful in some cases.

It is foreign to our intention to occupy further space by entering into a description of the means to be adopted in the reduction of the various specific fractures which are liable to be encountered in different parts of the body: such a proceeding would come more within the province of a purely surgical work. Let it suffice therefore to remark, in closing these observations, that in all cases, the same *medical* treatment is to be pursued, as has been previously noted for that of contusions, wounds, and fractures in general:—Finally, it may be stated, that from the great success which has attended the homœopathic practice, as employed by continental surgeons in the treatment of those numerous and serious diseases which are usually considered of a surgical character, it is earnestly to be hoped that their colleagues in this country may be induced to emulate their example, and thereby become enabled to raise their important branch of the profession to a still higher standing than it already, in many respects, has attained.

BURNS AND SCALDS.

Ambustiones.

We shall here content ourselves with merely treating of these lesions in their simple form. In slight burns or scalds, the injured part should be held for a couple of minutes to the fire; a temporary increase of pain will be amply repaid by the prevention of future suffering and annoyance. If, however, the injury be more severe, we may bathe the affected part with heated alcohol, or oil of turpentine, taking care to keep the surface continually moist, and well protected from the external air.

The application of *raw cotton* to the part, is frequently found very efficacious, particularly when the injury presents a large surface; having previously punctured any blisters that may have arisen, and bathed the sore with tepid water, cover it with carded cotton or wadding, in three layers; when suppuration sets in, remove the *upper layer only*, and substitute fresh. Exhibit at the same time Hepar sulphuris, a grain of the third trituration to an ounce of water, a dessert-spoonful every twelve hours, desisting after the fourth administration.

Soap, a remedy generally at hand, is extremely serviceable in burns where not only the cuticle but the true skin has been destroyed: pure white or curd soap is the best for this purpose. The following directions for its application may be found useful: make a thick lather or paste, by means of tepid water, and spread it upon linen, in the form of a plaster; apply it to the injured part, and secure by a bandage. Any blisters which may have formed should, as before prescribed, be carefully punctured, and any loose skin removed.

This application will, as in the instance of dry heat, &c. at first increase the pain; but this temporary inconvenience will be superseded by a marked amelioration; after a lapse of about twenty-four hours, the plaster may be gently removed, and a fresh one substituted; generally speaking, however, we must be guided by the feelings of the patient, and renew it as often as a return of pain is complained of; and so continue until the injury is completely healed. Sapo communis, $\frac{00}{3}$, may also be given internally from time to time.

Aconitum, $\frac{00}{6}$, may be exhibited when we find considerable *fever* present; and repeated in a few hours, if required.

Opium, $\frac{0000}{30}$ on the tongue, when the system has received a severe shock from fright at the time of the injury.

Urtica urens has recently come into repute as a specific remedy in burns of *every description;* but not having yet had an opportunity of proving its efficacy, I cannot offer any testimony of its virtues in this respect. The mode of application recommended is, applying linen cloths, saturated with the mother tincture, to the injured part; and in severe cases, a drop of the tincture may be taken internally also, either in a little water, or on a piece of lump sugar.

Kreasote water has likewise been recommended as a lotion in burns of all kinds, either at the commencement or subsequently, to induce healthy granulation and cicatrization. *Crocus saticus* (applied externally) has also been favourably spoken of as most serviceable for the latter purpose in burns or wounds with considerable loss of substance, and disposition to mortification and sloughing. (See ULCERS.)

FATIGUE.

When a feeling of *contusion* is experienced in all the limbs, *Arnica* will generally be found the most appropriate remedy to afford relief.

ADMINISTRATION $\frac{00}{6}$, repeated in twenty-four hours, should any of the symptoms remain. When the feet have become swollen and painful, they ought to be bathed in arnicated water.

Pain in the joints, &c., arising from lifting heavy weights, or from violent physical exertion of any kind, are usually speedily removed by *Rhus toxicodendron*.

ADMINISTRATION. Same as *Arnica*.

CINCHONA $\frac{000}{3}$, will frequently assist in renovating the strength when there has been profuse perspiration.

VERATRUM $\frac{000}{30}$, when tendency to fainting ensues from the effects of extreme fatigue; and

COFFEA $\frac{000}{30}$, when abstinence from food, combined with violent exercise, has produced a state of exhaustion.

COCCULUS $\frac{000}{12}$, when fatigue occurs after the most trivial exertion of either body or mind. (*Veratrum* and *Calcarea* are necessary when *Cocculus* does not give much relief.)

In fatigue from long watching, *Cocculus* is the most generally useful medicament; but *Nux v.*, *Ipecac.*, *Puls.*, and *Carbo v.*, are also of utility occasionally. *Aconitum* is a valuable remedy when dyspnœa, with palpitation of the heart, pain in the side, or aching in the extremities, arises from running a short distance, or even from walking quickly. (*Bryonia* is sometimes necessary when these symptoms continue notwithstanding the employment of *Aconitum*. At other times *Arnica* will be found more efficacious, particularly when the pain resembles what is termed a *stitch* in the side. *Ranunculus bulbosus* is also very useful in the latter case.)

ADMINISTRATION. Same as *Cinchona*.

STINGS OF INSECTS.

The severe pain and febrile irritation which sometimes ensues from the stings of insects, such as bees, wasps, &c., is frequently speedily alleviated by the olfaction of spirits of *Camphor*. Should, however, considerable inflammation with swelling supervene, *Aconitum* $\frac{2}{6}$, should be administered, and subsequently *Arnica*, internally and externally, as described under Wounds. Should the tongue or any part of the mouth be the part where the sting has been inflicted—as occasionally happens to children when biting a piece out of an apple or pear, &c., into which a wasp may have greedily inserted itself —the mouth ought to be rinsed with diluted *Arnica* tincture; and should that not suffice, *Belladonna* should be administered, as follows: $\frac{000}{6}$, in a wine-glassful of water, a dessert-spoonful every hour, until relief is experienced. In some instances it will be found necessary to have recourse to *Mercurius* after *Belladonna*.

Administration. $\frac{000}{6}$, in the same manner.

The bites or stings of gnats require an *Arnica* lotion; lemon-juice will likewise be found useful in relieving the pain and itching caused thereby.

Immediate relief when a person has been severely stung by nettles, will often be found by the application of a lotion of *Arnica*, prepared according to the formula given under Bruises.

SEA-SICKNESS.

Therapeutics. The medicaments found most useful in the treatment of this distressing and painful malady are, *Nux v.*, *Cocculus*, *Tabacum*, *Arsenicum*, *Ipecacuanha*, *Petroleum*.

Nux vomica $\frac{000000}{6}$, should be taken fasting, from six to twelve hours before embarkation; this precaution will in some cases prove sufficient to ward off the attack. (*Nux v.* and *Arsenicum* alternately every hour or so, at the commencement of the voyage, or oftener should a degree of nausea have already come on, frequently ward off the sickness, or at all events, afford great relief. As soon as decided improvement is experienced, the remedies must be discontinued, or taken at much longer intervals.)

Should, however, a feeling of giddiness, or a sensation of *emptiness* in the head, be experienced, shortly after going on board, attended with headache, nausea, and inclination to vomit, as the motion of the vessel increases, which is aggravated by standing erect, Cocculus $\frac{\circ\,\circ\,\circ}{6}$ may be had recourse to, and repeated every one, two, or three hours, as those symptoms recur. (This remedy has also been found useful in sickness arising from travelling in a carriage.)

Tabacum $\frac{\circ\,\circ\,\circ\,\circ\,\circ\,\circ}{6}$. Excessive giddiness attended with *distressing nausea*, headache, and *deadly paleness of the face;* or nausea, with *sickness*, or a sensation of burning in the stomach, *renewed by the slightest movement* of the head or body. This remedy is further indicated, when the symptoms are somewhat relieved by exposure to the fresh air.

Arsenicum $\frac{\circ\,\circ\,\circ\,\circ\,\circ\,\circ}{6}$, is extremely valuable when the sickness becomes excessive, and is attended with a feeling of *utter prostration and helplessness, violent retching,* burning sensation in the throat, and the other severe concomitants of this malady. It should be administered between the paroxysms, and will rarely fail of relief. This medicine may be followed by *Tabacum* or *Cocculus*, to dissipate the symptoms of nausea and swimming in the head that may supervene.

Ipecacuanha $\frac{\circ\,\circ\,\circ\,\circ\,\circ\,\circ}{3}$, is useful in attacks of vomiting *unattended* with the great prostration of strength given under *Arsenicum.* Of course, in order to avoid interfering with the action of the medicines, the homœopathic regimen should be carefully observed during the period of their administration.

Petroleum,* Silicea, and Therideon, from the close analogy of their symptoms to those of the ordinary forms of this distressing malady, deserve a trial. $\frac{\circ\,\circ\,\circ\,\circ}{6}$.

Administration of the above remedies: six globules of the medicament, at the potency mentioned, in an ounce of water, a teaspoonful every hour, and then until relief is experienced.

* Dr. *Chase* found that *Petroleum* is the best specific for sea-sickness.

APPARENT DEATH. *Asphyxia.*

APPARENT DEATH. ASPHYXIA. In every instance that an individual has to all appearances suddenly expired from external causes, animation may only be suspended; there are many cases of course where sudden death is no mere suspension of animation, but there are others where apparent death is far from uncommon; in all cases where there is the least uncertainty, care should be taken to do nothing that may cause death, and interment should be avoided until certain signs of putrefaction set in.*

Apparent death from hunger. Give small injections of warm milk repeatedly; great care must be taken to give the food, when the patient begins to rally, in the smallest possible quantity at a time. Milk may be given drop by drop, and gradually increasing it to a teaspoonful, and after some interval a small quantity of beef-tea and a few drops of wine. After a sound sleep has succeeded, but not till then, a small meal may be given, but it is best that the patient should eat little at a time, but often, so that he may gradually return to his natural mode of living. It must be borne in mind, that in all persons suffering from starvation, eating too much and too quickly, is in the highest degree dangerous.

Apparent death from a fall. Place the patient cautiously on a bed, with his head high in a place where he can remain quiet; put a few globules of *Arnica* on his tongue, and wait till a medical man visits him to see if there is any fracture, or whether there are still signs of life; a bleeding here may be sometimes of benefit, but it requires great caution. *Arnica* may be repeated, and also *Arnica* in injections. If the patient has been bled, give *China;* but it is obvious that if much blood has been lost by the fall or wound, venesection would be injurious.

* The subjoined directions have chiefly been taken from Hering's Hausarzt.

Apparent death from suffocation, (hanging, pressure, choking.) Remove all tight clothing. Put the patient in a proper position, the head and neck rather high, the neck quite easy, not bent forward. Begin by rubbing gently but constantly with cloths, give an injection of a dozen or two globules, or a drop of *Opium*, dissolved in half a pint of water, and injected slowly. This may be repeated every quarter of an hour, whilst the ribs are being rubbed gently. Hold from time to time a mirror before the mouth, to see if the breath dims it; open the eyelids, and see if the eyes contract; put warm clothes on; hot stones wrapped in blankets to the feet, between the thighs, to the sides, neck and shoulders. If in an hour no change is produced, take a bitter almond, pound it fine, mix it in a pint of water, put a few drops into the mouth, or into the nose, and give the rest in injections.

Apparent death from lightning. The body should be immediately removed into a current of cool fresh air; cold water dashed frequently on the neck, face, and breast. If the body be cold, warmth with friction must be employed in the same manner as recommended for the drowned; as well as the means therein adopted for inflating the lungs. A few globules of *Nux vomica* may be put upon the tongue, and repeated in half an hour; if no effect is produced, a little *Nux vomica* in water rubbed on the neck, and some injected, may be of service. It has also been recommended to place the patient in a half-sitting, half-recumbent posture, and to cover him over with newly-excavated earth, (leaving the face alone exposed, which should be turned towards the sun,) until the first signs of returning animation become apparent, after which *Nux v.* is to be had recourse to as above directed.

Apparent death from drowning. Observe the following cautions: 1, lose no time; 2, avoid all rough usage; 3, never hold up the body by the feet; 4, do not roll the body on casks; 5, do not rub the body with salts or spirits; 6, do not inject smoke or infusion of tobacco, though clysters of warm water and salt, or spirits and water, may be injected, and the following means should not be delayed:—

1. Convey the body carefully with the head and shoulders in a raised position to the nearest house.

2. Strip the body and rub it; then wrap it in hot blankets, and place it in a warm bed in a warm room, or in warm sand or ashes.

3. Wipe and cleanse the throat, mouth and nostrils.

4. If the foregoing measures produce no reaction, place a few globules of *Lachesis* on the tongue, and in injections, and resume the rubbing. *Solanum mamosum* has also been recommended, and may be tried after Lachesis, when that remedy fails to do any good.

5. Again, should our efforts still fail, or should the medicines quoted not be at hand, we may, in order to restore the natural heat of the body, move a heated covered warming-pan over the back and spine. Place bottles, or bladders filled with hot water, or hot bricks, to the pit of the stomach, the armpits, between the thighs, and soles of the feet. Place the body in a warm bath, in the sun or at a proper distance from the fire; use friction with hot flannels, flour of mustard, or other stimulants; rub the body briskly with the hand; at the same time do not suspend the use of other means.

To restore breathing, introduce the pipe of a common bellows into one nostril, carefully closing the other and the mouth, at the same time drawing downwards, and gently pushing backwards, the upper part of the windpipe, to allow a more free admission of air; blow the bellows gently in order to inflate the lungs till the breath be a little raised, the mouth and nostrils should then be set free, and a moderate pressure made with the hand upon the chest; continue this process until signs of life appear.

6. Electricity, or a stream of galvanism passed through the chest, promise to be of great service.

7. Apply pungent salts, as sal volatile or spirits of hartshorn, to the nostrils.

These means should be persisted in for several hours, and till there are evident signs of death.

When the patient shows signs of life, and can swallow, small quantities of warm wine or spirits and water may be taken; but till then, nothing should even be poured down the throat, either by a flexible tube or otherwise. At this period the patient should never be left alone, as some have been lost for want of care who might otherwise have been saved.

Apparent death from being frozen. When an individual is found in a state of frost-bitten asphyxy, arising from exposure to intense cold, he should be removed with great gentleness and caution to guard against any injury, as fracture, etc., to a place of shelter, such as a barn or unheated apartment, since even a moderate degree of heat might annihilate all hope of restoring animation; at the same time the patient ought to be protected against the slightest draught.

He should then, especially if the limbs have become stiffened by the frost, be covered over with snow to the height of several inches, the mouth and nostrils alone being left free.

The patient ought to be put in such a position that the melted snow may run off readily, and its place supplied by fresh. When there is no snow, a cold bath, the temperature of which has been reduced by ice, (or a bath of cold sea or salted water,) may be substituted, and the body immersed therein for a few minutes.

The process of thawing is by these means to be effected, and when every part has lost its rigidity, the patient should be undressed by degrees, and the clothes cut from the body if requisite. As the muscular or soft parts become pliable, they may be rubbed with snow until they become red; or the body wiped perfectly dry if snow is not to be had, placed in flannel in a moderately warm room, and rubbed with the warm hands of several parties simultaneously.

In the event of no signs of returning animation declaring themselves soon after the foregoing treatment, small injections containing Camphor may be administered every quarter of an hour. As soon as any symptoms of approaching restoration become perceptible, small injections of lukewarm black coffee (coffee without milk) may be thrown up; and as soon as the patient is able to swallow, a little coffee may be given, in the quantity of a teaspoonful at a time.

The measures above detailed ought to be persevered in for several hours. Against the excessive pain which is generally experienced when life is restored, *Carbo v.* should be prescribed in repeated doses,* and if it fails to relieve the sufferings, *Arsenicum* may be given. The party rescued must avoid subjecting himself to the heat of the fire or stove for a considerable length of time after his recovery, as serious consecutive ailment, and particularly disease of the bones, is liable to result therefrom.

Apparent death from noxious vapours. The treatment consists in removing the body into a cool, fresh current of air; dashing frequently cold water on the neck, face and breast; if the body be cold, apply warmth, etc., recommended to the drowned; inflation of the lungs; early and judicious application of electricity or galvanism,—after life has been restored, give Op. or Acon.

HYDROPHOBIA.

It is acknowledged that no *allopathic* cure has hitherto been found for this disease when fully established. The plans of treatment which have been reported to have been successful in some few instances having generally failed in all others; thus rendering it probable, that in these supposititious cases of success, the persons bitten might have escaped without any treatment whatever. But it is not to my purpose to enter into the multitude of ineffectual remedies which have been recommended by the Allopathists.

Hydrophobia is a disease which arises in consequence of the bite of a rabid animal, and sometimes spontaneously, particularly in the course of some other disease; in which form it is known under the term of symptomatic hydrophobia.

Ere proceeding to the homœopathic treatment, a few remarks, descriptive of the disease as it appears in the human subject, may not be misplaced. The first symptoms that

* Vide note, page 21.

show themselves in a person who has been bitten, are usually, general uneasiness, anxiety and disturbed sleep; the eyes are glassy, inflamed and sensitive to light; there are also ringing in the ears, giddiness, and paleness of countenance; frequent paroxysms of chilliness; oppressed respiration, and quickness of pulse, which latter is usually at the same time small, contracted and irregular, and loss of appetite. These symptoms generally come on at some indefinite period, occasionally after the bitten part seems quite well. In the second or convulsive stage, the wound, which may have already become completely cicatrized or healed, begins to assume a somewhat inflamed appearance, and a slight pain and heat, now and then attended with itching, are experienced in it. It now breaks out afresh, and an ulcer, with elevated margins of proud flesh, which secretes a dark-coloured and offensive discharge, is subsequently formed; and wandering, drawing, and shooting pains from the lacerated part upwards towards the throat, present themselves. These symptoms, with the state of testiness and anxiety, increase daily; and the patient complains of a state of confusion in the head, or giddiness, with sparks before the eyes; is afflicted with sudden startings, spasms, sighing, and is fond of solitude; the pulse is small, irregular, and intermittent; the breathing laborious and uneasy; the skin cold and dry, and general chilliness, especially in the extremities, is complained of; then hiccough, colic and palpitation come on; the patient looks wild, and the eyes have a fixed, glassy, and *shining* appearance; the act of deglutition is impeded by a sense of pressure in the gullet, which occasionally renders every attempt to swallow liquids impracticable; convulsions also take place in the muscles of the face or neck. In this stage, however, the deglutition of any solid substance is performed with tolerable ease. In ordinary cases the sufferer remains affected in the above manner for a few days, after which, the disease passes into the *hydrophobic* stage, in which it is utterly impossible for him to swallow the smallest drop of liquid; and the moment that any fluid, especially water, is brought in contact with the lips, it occasions the individual to start back with dread and horror, although he may, at the same time, suffer the most excessive thirst; even the sight of water, or the very noise produced by pouring it from one vessel into another, in fact, anything that tends to remind him of that fluid, produces indescribable anxiety, uneasiness, convulsions, and even furious paroxysms of madness; he dreads even to swallow his own saliva, and is constantly spitting; vomiting of bilious matter soon comes on, succeeded by intense fever, great thirst, dryness and roughness of the tongue, hoarseness, and fits of delirium or madness, with disposition to bite and tear everything within reach, followed at intervals by convulsive spasms. These attacks commonly last for a quarter or half an hour, and at their expiration, the patient is restored to reason, but remains in a state of great despondency; finally, the paroxysms come on more violently and frequently, and in some instances a fit of furious delirium closes the frightful scene; in others, nature sinks exhausted after a severe attack of convulsions. The disease may be communicated to the human subject, from the bites of cats and other animals not of the canine race, which have been previously inoculated with the virus.

It may be remarked in this place, that the best and most experienced of our writers upon this subject, consider the human species as the least susceptible of contagion from the hydrophobic virus; scarcely one out of twenty, or even thirty, of those actually bitten by an animal in a state of rabies, suffering from its effects. I consider it my duty, while making this statement, which I hope may prove a means of relieving the minds of many from painful apprehensions, to enforce at the same time, the necessity of taking those precautions which are about to be pointed out against the danger.

It may also be added, before proceeding to the treatment of the malady, that the possibility of the poison being communicated through the medium of the epithelium is exceedingly questionable; but scarcely a doubt exists of the incapacity of the cuticle to absorb it. As many have been made wretched from having allowed a dog who has afterwards shown symptoms of rabies to lick their hands, it may be stated with confidence, that if no abrasion of surface exists, ***there is not the slightest danger.***

In the homœopathic treatment of this disease, and its prevention, the following are the principal remedies employed: *Belladonna*, *Lachesis*, *Hyoscyamus*, *Stramonium*, and *Cantharides*.*

* The use of *dry or radiating heat* in this disease, and in envenomed wounds by snakes, etc., is recommended by Dr. Hering of America, whose directions for the treatment of envenomed wounds in general, are as follows:

Envenomed wounds. The best remedies against the bites of *venomous serpents, mad dogs*, &c., is the application of *dry heat* AT A DISTANCE. Whatever is at hand at the moment, a red-hot iron or live coal, or even a lighted cigar, must be placed as near the wound as possible, without, however, burning the skin, or causing too sharp pain; but care must be taken to have another instrument ready in the fire, so as never to allow the heat to lose its intensity. It is essential also that the heat should not exercise its influence over too large a surface, but only on the wound and the parts adjacent. If oil or grease can be readily procured, it may be applied round the wound, and this operation should be repeated as often as the skin becomes dry; *soap*, or even *saliva* may be employed, where oil or grease cannot be obtained. Whatever is discharged in any way from the wound ought to be carefully removed. The application of burning heat should be continued in this manner till the patient begins to shiver and to stretch himself; if this takes place at the end of a few minutes, it will be better to keep up the action of the heat upon the wound for an hour, or until the affections produced by the venom are observed to diminish.

Internal medicines must be judiciously administered at the same time. In the case of a BITE FROM A SERPENT, it will be advisable to take from time to time a gulp of *salt and water*, or a pinch of *kitchen salt*, or of *gunpowder*, or else some pieces of *garlic*.

If, notwithstanding this, bad effects manifest themselves, a spoonful of *wine* or *brandy*, administered every two or three minutes, will be the most suitable remedy; and this should be continued till the sufferings are relieved, and repeated as often as they are renewed.

If the shooting pains are aggravated, and proceed from the wound towards the heart, and if the wound becomes bluish, marbled, or swollen, with vomiting, vertigo, and fainting, the best medicine is *Arsenicum* It should be administered in a dose of 3 globules (30th) in a tablespoonful of water; and if after this has been taken, the sufferings are still aggravated, the dose should be repeated at the end of half an hour; but if, on the contrary, the state remains the same, it should not be repeated till the end of two or three hours; if there is an amelioration, a new aggravation must be waited for, and the dose ought not to be repeated before its appearance.

BELLADONNA. HAHNEMANN, the noble founder of our science, states, in the introductory article to *Belladonna*, in his *Materia Medica Pura*, that he considers the smallest dose of that medicine, repeated every three or four days, to be *the*

In cases in which *Ars.* exercises no influence, though repeated several times, recourse must be had to *Bell.; Sen.* also frequently proves efficacious.

Against chronic affections arising from the bite of a serpent, *Phos.-ac.* and *Merc.* will generally be most beneficial.

For the treatment of persons bitten by a *mad dog*, after the application of dry heat, as directed and described above. (See *Hydrophobia*, on the other side.)

If morbid affections or ulcerations exhibit themselves in consequence of a bite from a rabid *man* or *animal*, *hydrophobine*, a dministered in homœopathic doses, will often render essential service.

For wounds that are envenomed by the introduction of animal substances in a state of putrefaction, or of pus from the ulcer of a diseased man or animal, *Ars.* is generally the best medicine.

Lastly, as a PREVENTIVE against bad effects, when obliged to touch morbid animal substances, envenomed wounds, or ulcers of men and animals under the influence of contagious diseases, the best method that can be pursued is the application of *dry burning heat at a distance.* To effect this purpose, it will be sufficient to expose the hands for five or ten minutes to the greatest heat that can be borne ; and after this, it will be proper to wash them with soap.

The use of *Chlorine* and muriatic acid, in similar cases, is well known.

HYDROPHOBIA. Apply *distant heat* to the recent wound, as described under "envenomed wounds," or until shudderings appear ; and continue this practice three or four times a day, until the wound is healed, without leaving a coloured cicatrix.

At the same time the patient should take, every five or seven days, or as often as the aggravation of the wound requires it, one dose of *Bell.* or *Lach.*, or also of hydrophobine, till the cure is completed.

If, at the end of seven or eight days, a small *vesicle* shows itself *under the tongue*, with feverish symptoms, it will be necessary to open it with a lancet or sharp-pointed scissors, and to rinse the mouth with salt and water.

If the raging state has commenced before assistance can be procured for the patient, the medicines that ought to be administered, will be according to circumstances, especially, *Bell.* or *Lach.;* or else again, *Canth.*, *Hyos.*, *Merc.*, or also *Stram.* or *Verat.* (See the indications above given for *Belladonna*, *Lachesis*, *Hyoscyamus*, *Stramonium*, and *Cantharides.*

most certain preventive against hydrophobia; and when we refer to the pathogenetic powers of that medicine, described in the aforesaid work, it is impossible not to be struck with the great resemblance which many of them bear to the symptoms of that malady; and it is from this circumstance, according to Hahnemann's doctrine of *similia similibus*,* that *Belladonna* is found to be both a prophylactic and curative remedy.

Administration. A drop of the third tincture in an ounce of water, a teaspoonful morning and evening, for two days. These precautions taken, the patient may be allowed to pursue his usual occupations, care being taken by those around him to avoid making any allusion which may tend to remind him of his misfortune. *Belladonna,* in the same dose, should be given on the third or fourth day, and subsequently at longer intervals. The effect of each exhibition should be attentively watched, and care taken that a fresh one be not given, as long as any symptoms of the action of the previous dose are perceptible. Generally speaking, from two to three administrations may be deemed sufficient to prevent the outbreak of the disease; or, at all events, to modify it in such a manner, as to render it less dangerous, and more easy of removal, by one or more of the other remedies, which must then be selected according to the symptoms that present themselves.

Lachesis, however, may generally be administered at the commencement of the convulsions.

Administration. $\frac{000}{6}$, repeated every two or three hours, or at every return of the convulsions, until benefit result or decided symptoms of medicinal action make their appearance;† but should this remedy appear to exert no perceptible influence in checking the progress of the malady, we must again have recourse to

Belladonna, particularly when the following characteris-

* The curing of a disease by the administration of a remedy which has been found to possess the property of producing a train of symptoms in a healthy person, similar to those observed in the disease.

† Vide note, p. 21.

tics are present: drowsiness, with constant but useless efforts to sleep, chiefly in consequence of excessive anguish and great agitation; sense of burning; great burning in the throat, *with accumulation of frothy mucus in the mouth or throat*, frequent desire for drinks, which are immediately pushed aside when presented, or a *suffocating or constricting sensation in the throat, on attempting to perform the act of deglutition*, or complete incapability of swallowing, with glowing redness and bloated appearance of the face; pupils immovable, and generally dilated; great dread; occasionally desire to strike, spit at, bite, or tear everything; inclination to run away; continual tossing about, and great physical activity, with twitching in various muscles, especially *those of the face;* ungovernable fury, with foaming at the mouth, and tetanic convulsions.

ADMINISTRATION. $^{0}\frac{0}{3}{}^{0}$ or $^{0}\frac{0}{6}{}^{0}$ to be placed on the tongue at every threatening of a return of the convulsions, the same precaution as enjoined under *Lachesis*. See also remarks upon this subject in the INTRODUCTION, *Article*—ADMINISTRATION and REPETITION OF THE MEDICINES.

HYOSCYAMUS is more particularly indicated either before or after *Belladonna*, when the *convulsions are severe and of long duration;* where there is not so much inclination to bite or spit, but a desire to *injure* those that stand around, in some manner or other. The spasms in the throat are not so violent, but great dryness and burning are complained of, attended with a sense of shooting or pricking, which causes a difficulty in swallowing, resembling a sensation of constriction in the throat, and threatening to produce suffocation on attempting to satisfy the thirst; *dread of liquids* in consequence of the pain and difficulty that is experienced in deglutition, with ejection of the saliva from the same reason; *excessive convulsions, with loss of consciousness*, come on soon after the *distressing act of swallowing has been performed.* There is, moreover, foaming at the mouth, with constant raving; sometimes the patient seems wrapped up in his own thoughts, or is full of fear, and inclined to run away from the house, being afflicted with a sort of *Anthropophobia;* there are also attacks of excessive fury, attended with apparently supernatural physical power; or excessive anguish and fear, alternating with fits of trembling and convulsions; the individual exhibits a peculiar dread of being bitten by animals; the pupils are dilated; sleep much disturbed by great *nervous excitement;* starts, and agonizing dreams.

ADMINISTRATION. Same as *Belladonna.*

STRAMONIUM is chiefly indicated in this disease, when we observe *severe convulsions taking place whenever the eye becomes fixed on brilliant objects,* or on whatever tends to remind the patient of water; great thirst; *dryness of the mouth and throat, with horror of water and all liquids;* spasmodic constriction in the gullet, with foaming at the mouth and frequent spitting; mania, with great loquacity and gesticulations; *fits of laughter and singing,* sometimes alternately with acute fits of passion and moaning; the convulsions, when severe, are generally attended with *ungovernable fury,* restless, agitated sleep, sudden shrieks, and starting up with wild gestures; insensible and dilated pupils; and great disposition to bite, or tear everything with the teeth.

ADMINISTRATION. Same as *Belladonna.*

CANTHARIDES. This medicine also possesses various pathogenetic properties, that bear a close resemblance to the symptoms that are met with in many cases of this disorder,* and should be selected in preference to any of the foregoing remedies, when we meet with the following symptoms: great *dryness* and *burning* in the mouth and throat, *much aggravated on attempting* to swallow; paroxysms of fury, alternating with convulsions, which are renewed by any pressure on the throat or abdomen, and also by the sight of water; fiery redness and sparkling of the eyes, which become prominent and

* Drs. Hartlaub and Trinks consider *Cantharides* to be the most certain prophylactic against hydrophobia, when administered early; they recommend a drop of the 30th potency, to be given every three or four days, and are of opinion that the virus is not eradicated as long as the cicatrized wound presents a *livid hue*, and is attended with induration, but affirm the danger to be over as soon as the part assumes a healthy and natural appearance. (Vide Hartlaub and Trinks, R. A. M. L., vol. i., p. 173.)

frightfully convulsed; spasms in the throat, excited by the pain produced by the act of swallowing, especially fluids; continual burning, titillation and other irritating sensations in the lower part of the abdomen, etc.

ADMINISTRATION. Same as *Belladonna.*

We have thus enumerated and described the characteristic indications for the principal Homœopathic remedies which have been successfully employed against *Hydrophobia*;* others have also been strongly recommended, but those mentioned have generally proved sufficient, *when administered early,* and exclusively adhered to throughout the course of the disease. *Belladonna* has frequently been tried by the Allopathists, but the cases in which it seemed to fail were *evidently attributable to the improper manner in which it was administered.* We shall not treat of the several remedies which have from time to time appeared, and have by their inventors been highly eulogized, as time and experience alone will prove whether they possess any virtue or not; it is to be feared, however, that like many other once celebrated "*specifics,*" (?) they will soon fall into oblivion. In fact, no medicine can be confidently relied upon for the cure of this or any other disease that has not been carefully tested by, and found in accordance with, THE GREAT LAW OF SIMILARITIES.

POISONS.

When any poisonous substance has been taken into the stomach, our first care must be its immediate evacuation by producing vomiting, or its neutralization by its antidote; our next, the removal of any injurious consequences that may remain after warding the more imminent danger.

To promote a speedy evacuation of the contents of the stomach, the stomach-pump should be immediately put in requisition, particularly when any vegetable or narcotic substance has been swallowed; but when the poison is of a corrosive nature, an antidote which will prevent its action upon

* Vide Hartmann's Acute Diseases, by Dr. C. Hempel, vol 2, p. 178.

the coats of the stomach, or neutralize it by chemical affinity, should be forthwith resorted to.

Vomiting should be promoted by the following means:

Swallowing large quantities of tepid water, tickling the throat or fauces with a feather, and, if these fail, placing snuff or mustard mixed with salt upon the tongue; or still better—particularly with those who are habituated to the use of tobacco—a tumbler of warm water, to which a teaspoonful of the flour of mustard has been added, should be taken at one draught, and then again warm water, as before. Finally, in extreme cases, the desired object must be effected by means of a clyster of tobacco-smoke.

It is not my intention to enter at any length into this subject, but merely to point the means which have been recommended to be adopted against the most common poisons, in order to give time for proper assistance to be sent for.

MINERAL POISONS. The mineral poisons and acids are, almost without exception, of a corrosive nature. When such have been swallowed by accident or design, soap-water in large quantities, the carbonate of magnesia—two or three drachms to half a pint of water, or the same quantity of chalk in water, or common potash or soda, should be swallowed; enemas of the same may be also exhibited, particularly when the poison seems to have affected the lower intestines. When the pain and vomiting have ceased, mucilaginous drinks, such as barley-water or milk, must be given in large quantities, to lubricate the surface of the stomach.

After mineral poisons, when vomiting ensues, in consequence of the substance swallowed, we must promote and sustain it by copious drinks, of the same nature.

ARSENIC. If vomiting sets in, sustain it by the means above mentioned; if not, provoke it, and give soap and water—white of egg in water—sugar and water, or milk in large quantities; the specific action of *Arsenic* being upon the stomach and rectum, inject also soap and water. The various preparations of iron, so much lauded some time back, although, no doubt, possessing a chemical affinity for this acid, and forming with it an arseniate of iron, are pronounced by the best Toxicologists to be extremely uncertain in their action.

OXALIC ACID. The best antidote to this powerful poison is new milk in large quantities; if taken *immediately*, it rarely fails to neutralize its effect.

LEAD. Its antidotes are Epsom or Glauber salts, two drachms dissolved in half a pint of water, and the same remedies given under *Arsenic*, both by the mouth and in the form of enema. Against the sequelæ which are sometimes encountered after the use of these remedies: *Opium*, *Platina*, *Alumina*, *Belladonna*, and *Nux v.*, are generally the most suitable, particularly when paralysis, colic, or delirium tremens result. $\frac{0000}{3}$ or $\frac{0000}{6}$.

VERDIGRIS and CORROSIVE SUBLIMATE. The remedies given under Arsenic may be resorted to; moreover, for *Verdigris*, iron-filings in vinegar, mixed with gum water, have been recommended; for *Corrosive sublimate*, in addition to the above remedies, starch, either in a large quantity of water, or in the form in which it is generally used for domestic purposes; and white of egg alternately with *eau sucré*.

In the After-Treatment, the following medicaments will be found useful: After ARSENIC, *Ipecacuanha*, *Cinchona*, *Nux vomica*, and *Veratrum*.

ADMINISTRATION. $\frac{0000}{3}$ or one drop of the tincture.

Ipecacuanha may first be exhibited to allay the irritation of the stomach, and the tendency to nausea and vomiting. $\frac{0000}{3}$.

Cinchona, if great irritability, with disturbed sleep and febrile motions during the night, remain behind. $\frac{0000}{3}$.

Nux vomica. Worse during the day, and especially after sleeping, with constipation or loose slimy evacuations. $\frac{0000}{3}$.

Veratrum, if after Ipecacuanha there still remain nausea, vomiting, heat, and coldness in the body, and prostration of strength. $\frac{0000}{3}$.

VEGETABLE AND NARCOTIC POISONS. The substance must be dislodged from the stomach as soon as possible; or if this be impracticable, among the best means to counteract its effects, are camphor by olfaction, sometimes spirits of ammonia, and *strong* black coffee taken internally; the patient must be kept continually in motion, and his attention roused by every means in our power; electricity has also proved useful in many instances.*

MUSHROOMS, POISONOUS. Provoke vomiting; give copious draughts of *cold water*, and administer charcoal in sweet oil, at the same time applying sal volatile to the nose of the patient.

After narcotic poisons have been evacuated from the stomach, vegetable acids may be used with advantage.

ANIMAL POISONS.

SEBACIC ACID. This poison develops itself in the rancid fat of pork, or hog's lard; against it, vinegar diluted with an equal bulk of water, or the juice of a lemon in strong black coffee, or better still, *strong black tea*, are the antidotes.

If any dryness of the throat remain after the more immediate danger has passed off, we may have recourse to BRYONIA, a drop of the third potency in a little water, repeating it as often as the symptoms seem to require. In some instances also benefit has been derived from the employment of *Acidum phosphoricum*, *Arsenicum*, and *Kreasotum*, $^{0}\frac{00}{6}{}^{0}$.

MUSCLES. *Antidote:* charcoal mixed with sugar and water; afterwards, camphor by olfaction, and strong coffee without milk or sugar.

POISONOUS FISH. *Antidote:* charcoal in a small quantity of brandy; if this does not speedily relieve, strong coffee—and this failing, sugar and water in large quantities; or again, if it should not relieve, vinegar with twice its bulk of water.

AFTER-TREATMENT. *Belladonna*, should an eruption or redness of the skin declare itself, particularly if accompanied with swelling of the face and angina.

ACIDUM HYDROCYANICUM. *Prussic acid.* The inhalation of *Ammonia*, or one drop of *liquid ammonia* dissolved in 12 oz. of water, and a teaspoonful taken every five minutes.

* In the case of *Opium*, a few doses of *Ipecac* often do good after the previous use of strong black coffee or vinegar; and when any morbid sequelæ remain, after *Ipecac.*: *Bell.*, *Nux v.*, or *Mercurius*, may be had recourse to.

Afterwards, strong black *coffee* should be administered in large quantities, both as a potion and as an enema. The vapour of *Camphor* or *Vinegar* have likewise been found useful, as also the cold affusion.

When the first alarming symptoms have disappeared : *Coffea*, or *Ipecacuanha*, and *Nux v.*, have been mentioned as being useful against any remaining effects.

Recently, a compound of *per-* and *prot-oxide of Iron* has been recommended by the Messrs. Smith, chemists, Edinburgh.

MENTAL EMOTIONS.

I shall conclude this part of the work with the consideration of those particular Mental Emotions which exercise so great a control over the human organism, among the more prominent and continually recurring of which we find fright, passion, or anger, and concentrated grief.

THERAPEUTICS. The remedies found most serviceable for derangements of the system arising from the above-mentioned causes are : *Opium*, *Aconitum*, *Pulsatilla*, *Belladonna*, *Ignatia amara*, *Chamomilla*, *Nux vomica*, *Staphysagria*, *Arsenicum album*, and *Bryonia*, *etc.*

OPIUM, when the sufferer has been exposed to sudden fright, with terror, horror, or fear, is generally efficacious if administered immediately, in restoring the patient, and obviating any evil consequences, such as convulsive fits, swooning, lethargic sleep, involuntary evacuations, diarrhœa, etc. (When *Opium* is not sufficient to remedy the mischief, *Aconitum* may be administered, or *Aconitum* and *Opium* alternately. In other cases *Ignatia* will answer better than *Aconitum*, especially when the convulsions continue ; *Belladonna* or *Hyoscyamus*, and *Veratrum*, are also serviceable in some cases, when none of the other remedies are sufficient to remove all the effects. *Causticum* is a useful remedy when a constant dread haunts the child, after a previous fright, etc.) See also *Samb.*

ADMINISTRATION of Opium. $\frac{0\,0}{6}$ or $\frac{0\,0}{3}$, repeated in from half an hour to an hour or so.*

ACONITUM is the appropriate remedy when the system is labouring under the joint influence of fright and passion; and especially when there is headache, feverishness, *heat in the face and head*, (congestion,) fear.

ADMINISTRATION. $\frac{0\,0}{6}$, in the same manner as *Opium*.

PULSATILLA, in cases of fright, fear, or timidity, particularly where accompanied with an effect upon the stomach and bowels, as also heat of the body with coldness of the extremities; or passion in people of generally mild temper; it is also suitable for highly nervous but not easily irritable temperaments.

ADMINISTRATION. $\frac{0\,0}{12}$, repeated if required in from six to twenty-four hours.

BELLADONNA $\frac{0\,0}{30}$, where there is present particular liability to be startled by trifles, or extreme general nervous excitement, after a fright, &c.

ADMINISTRATION. Same as *Aconitum*.

IGNATIA where the cause is gnawing, inward grief. *Acid. phosphoricum* and *Staphysagria* are sometimes requisite after *Ignatia*.

ADMINISTRATION. $\frac{0\,0\,0}{12}$, every three or four days, watching the effect.

CHAMOMILLA, where suffering has arisen from vexation, or a disposition to irritability, or great anguish and mental depression are present.

ADMINISTRATION. Same as *Pulsatilla*.

NUX VOMICA, suffering arising from a sudden fit, or outbreak of passion or rage.

ADMINISTRATION. $\frac{0\,0\,0}{30}$, repeated from six, twelve to twenty-four hours if necessary.

STAPHYSAGRIA $\frac{0\,0\,0}{30}$. Anger and vexation, arising from just cause.

ADMINISTRATION. Same as *Nux vomica*.

ARSENICUM is useful where passion is followed by great weakness and dangerous prostration of the vital powers.

* Vide note, p. 21.

ADMINISTRATION. Same as *Ignatia*.

BRYONIA $\frac{0\,0}{3\,0}$, is indicated where a fit of passion is followed by coldness and shivering over the whole body, great irascibility, want of appetite, nausea, vomiting, and bilious sufferings.

ADMINISTRATION. In the same manner as *Pulsatilla*.

COLOCYNTH $\frac{0\,0\,0}{3}$. Where indignation accompanies the above described effects of a fit of anger.

Against the injurious effects which occasionally result after excessive joy, such as headache, trembling, and tendency to fainting, *Coffea* $\frac{0\,0\,0}{3}$ is the most useful remedy. But when the consequences are more serious, and violent headache, with congestion to the head, vomitings, diarrhœa, swooning, &c., result, *Opium* must be given.

HYOSCYAMUS $\frac{0\,0\,0}{3}$ is the most useful remedy against any injurious consequences arising from jealousy, or disappointed love. In the latter instance *Ignatia* and *Acid. phosphoricum* are also beneficial.

Against the effects of mortification, or wounded vanity or self-esteem: *Colocynth*, *Ignatia*, *Staphysagria*, *Pulsatilla*, *Platina*, or *Belladonna*, have proved useful, $\frac{0\,0\,0}{3}$ or $\frac{0\,0\,0}{6}$.

SAMBUCUS $\frac{0\,0\,0}{3}$. When oppression at the chest, with stertorous breath, has ensued in consequence of a fear or fright, and not yielded to the influence of *Opium*.

END OF PART II.

PART III.

TREATMENT OF INFANTS AND CHILDREN;

AND OF

THEIR PECULIAR AFFECTIONS.

INTRODUCTORY REMARKS.

The homœopathic system of medicine possesses many advantages in the treatment of the diseases of infancy and childhood. In the first place, when any constitutional taint exists, by the selection of suitable remedies, it meets disease upon the very threshold of life, and destroys it in the germ; it substitutes a rational mode of treatment for the nostrums of the nursery, since the application of the remedies requires, even in the most trifling cases, a certain degree of education, and a careful study of medicinal action. How many lives, sacrificed by the overweening self-confidence and prejudices of those intrusted with the life of man, at the most precarious period of his existence, might have been preserved, had this system been more extensively known and acted upon!

As before remarked in the Introduction, to which the reader is referred, the receptivity of the infant organism to the influence of homœopathic remedies, has been established by experience. Here again our system possesses the faculty of modifying the energy of the remedial agents used, and to administer them of sufficient power to overcome disease, without incurring the risk of danger.

The tasteless nature of the medicaments is another point of no small importance in affections of infants and children, and by means of which, nausea and annoyance are avoided. This has been touched upon in another part of this work.

In such complaints as occur at all periods of life, and which have been treated in the Second Part of this work, we should be guided in the selection of the dose by the age of the patient; with infants we may use the highest potencies, and rarely ever in acute diseases give more than a single globule; children from four to eight years of age may take about one-fourth to one-third of the dose prescribed for an adult, and above that age one-half to two-thirds. A great deal, however, depends, upon the constitution of the patient, whether delicate or robust, and upon their susceptibility to medicinal influence, a point only to be determined by experience: in very acute diseases we may sometimes be called upon to administer as low as the sixth potency, a single globule; from the great receptivity, however, of the system, above remarked, we should be particularly careful in repeating the medicines.

TREATMENT AFTER BIRTH.

As soon as the child is born, it should be wrapped in fine flannel, with a piece of soft linen rag inside, the flannel itself being too rough for its delicate skin; the wrapper should be heated to a temperature of 98 degrees, as it is only gradually that the infant becomes inured to the temperature of the surrounding atmosphere. The skin should be gently washed with a little lukewarm water and bran, applied with a sponge, taking care not to continue the first washing too long, for fear of irritation; soap must on no account be used; the room should be kept rather dark, and perfectly quiet, and all strongly scented substances removed. After washing, the body ought to be dried immediately, to avoid the risk of taking cold; the child should be bathed twice a day, to keep up the action of the skin, gradually lowering the temperature of the water, after weaning.

The best time for bathing the infant is in the morning, when taken out of bed, and again on returning to it for the night; immersing the whole body, with the exception of the head, is preferable to any other mode of washing, as the practice of placing it in a tub, with part of the frame alternately laved with tepid water, and exposed to the action of the atmosphere, is apt to bring on a chill.

Nothing can be more evidently opposed to nature, and the dictates of common sense—although like many of the absurdities bearing the impress of custom,—than the practice of swathing and bandaging the tender bodies of infants, and loading them with a superfluity of clothing, which, by its weight and length, presses upon their lower extremities, and is the frequent cause of deformity and weakness in after-life; in this opinion we are fully borne out by the corroborative testimony of the most eminent practitioners of the old school.

ASPHYXIA.

The first danger that the infant incurs on its entrance into life is *Asphyxia.*

Diagnosis. Suspension of the functions of vitality, of respiration, circulation, and motion.

Causes. Natural debility; difficult parturition; injury from the forceps; pressure of the umbilical cord round the neck; tying the navel-string too tightly; accumulation of mucus in the throat; too sudden an alteration of temperature, the respiratory action of the lungs not having commenced. The usual mechanical means, under the direction of a competent person, must, of course, be instantly had recourse to; I shall, therefore, simply content myself with pointing out the homœopathic remedies most useful in such cases.

They are *Tartarus emeticus*, *Opium*, *Cinch.*, and *Aconitum.*

Tartarus emeticus, Administration of. A grain of the first trituration in eight ounces of water, a few drops into the mouth of the child every quarter of an hour.

Opium. If after half an hour no change for the better take place, and the face is livid and bluish.

Administration. A few globules of the third, in a wine-glassful of water, a few drops into the mouth of the child every ten or fifteen minutes, until some effect is produced.

Cinchona $\frac{000}{6}$. If the face be *pale,* also when the infant is reviving and respiration commencing—if the same indication presents itself.

Administration. Same as *Opium.*

Aconitum. When the child is reviving and beginning to breathe, if the face has been previously flushed red or of a bluish tint.

Administration. $\frac{0}{6}$ on the tongue, repeated if necessary, after shorter or longer interval, according to the effects produced.

SWELLING OF THE HEAD.

Immediately after birth, the head of the infant appears more or less swollen; this is in most cases but a trifling affection, and generally goes off of itself. The administration of ARNICA $\frac{0}{12}$ or $\frac{0}{30}$, will materially hasten its disappearance; should, however, the swelling be at all excessive, bathe the part affected in a weak lotion consisting of three drops of the tincture of *Arnica* to a wine-glassful of water.

Occasionally a considerable swelling in the larger mould, (*fontanel*,) consisting of fluid, is observable; this is of greater import than the other, though seldom dangerous; if it does not disappear in a day or two, we may administer RHUS TOXICODENDRON $\frac{0}{30}$ in globule to the infant. *Calcarea carbonica* $\frac{0}{18}$ repeated in six days, in cases where the fontanel is long in closing. In some instances *Silicea* or *Sulphur* is also requisite in addition, if not in preference to *Calcarea.*

NAVEL RUPTURE IN INFANTS.

In cases where there is an evident tendency to navel rupture, we may take the half of a nutmeg, cover it with very soft linen, like a button, and sew it to a bandage, with the base of the cone in the centre; then press the apex into the umbilical opening, and secure it there by the bandage, which should be of sufficient length to pass two or three times round the body of the child. This mechanical process* will usually prove sufficient to effect a cure; if not, we must exhibit NUX VOMICA $\frac{0}{30}$, dissolving it in six teaspoonfuls of water, and administering one, which, if no alteration takes place, may be repeated in the same manner in five or six days, and if no effect declare itself,

* The following is a simple and commonly efficacious mode of applying a compress:—Take a piece of lint, just sufficiently large, that when folded five or six times, it will cover the rupture effectually; then press in the protrusion, and keep it reduced with the hand until the compress is rightly adjusted and secured in its position by means of two strips of adhesive plaster (which have been previously warmed by being held at the fire, so as to make them adhere) placed over the compress in the form of a cross. (It is still better, however, to get an efficient bandage made to measure by an intelligent and experienced maker.)

again repeat, bearing in mind the directions upon the Repetition of Medicines given in the Introduction; if, however, we discover no amelioration from the administration of *Nux v.*, we may have recourse to VERATRUM $\frac{0}{30}$ in the same manner. Obstinate cases are frequently found to yield to the application of the NORTH POLE of the MAGNET.* All these medicines are equally useful in those cases of inguinal hernia, or rupture in the groin, we occasionally meet with, generally effecting a cure with wonderful promptitude. (See HERNIA, Part II., p. 361.)

This disease being frequently brought on by the violent fits of crying that delicate children are subject to, the bandage may be worn, and retained for some time after the cure, as a precautionary measure against its return. In cases of soreness of the umbilicus or navel, remaining after the falling off of the ligature, or even before, we may give SULPHUR $\frac{0}{30}$, a single dose, and repeat in six days. If, however, during that time *no* amelioration has been observable, we should exhibit SILICEA $\frac{0}{30}$, which, if marked benefit resulted, may be at the same interval repeated with advantage.

MECONIUM, EXPULSION OF.

After having been permitted to sleep for five or six hours undisturbed. the infant should be applied to the breast as soon as the mother feels herself sufficiently recovered to permit it, which is generally from six to eight hours after delivery, and should never be deferred, as we elsewhere observed, longer than twelve; the milk of the mother exciting a mechanical action of the alimentary canal, and assisting in the expulsion of the meconium. Here again we cannot too strongly reprobate the too general practice of administering *laxative medicines* for this purpose, possessing, as they do, a most deleterious effect upon the tender organism of the infant, and, if not productive of jaundice—a too frequent consequence of their repeated administration—at least laying the foundation of bowel complaint, debility of the stomach, and a host of diseases in after-life.

* *Chamomilla, Aurum* and *Sulphur,* are occasionally found necessary, particularly the last-named, in order to effect a permanent cure.

Mothers need not be under apprehension should a temporary delay occur in the passing of the meconium; far greater evil results from the violent methods taken for its expulsion, than could possibly occur from its continuance in the alimentary canal for a few hours later than ordinary.

Should, however, an unusually long period elapse, and the child appear costive, which in many instances arises from the mother having indulged in the use of ptisans, such as chamomile tea, &c., or in coffee, the administration of a few teaspoonfuls of warm sugar and water will generally answer every purpose; if it fail of immediate relief, we may then make use of a lavement of equal parts of sweet oil (or pure honey) and water; if these simple means do not effect the desired object, and the infant appear to suffer from inconvenience, more particularly when the origin of the constipation seems to be from the mother or nurse, we may administer *Nux vomica, Bryonia, Tinctura sulph.* $\frac{0}{30}$ or *Opium* $\frac{0}{3}$ to the female herself—for the indication of which medicines see CONSTIPATION.

SUCKLING OF THE INFANT.

While upon this subject, we shall quote the expressions of a well known writer, in whose opinion, in this respect, we perfectly coincide.

"Unless very peculiar urgent reasons prohibit, a mother should support her infant upon the milk she herself secretes. It is the dictate of nature, of common sense, and of reason. Were it otherwise, it is not probable that so abundant a supply of suitable food would be provided to meet the wants of an infant, when it enters upon a new course of existence.

"It is difficult to estimate the mischief resulting from infants being deprived of their natural nourishment; for, however near the resemblance may be between food artificially prepared and breast-milk, still reason and observation demonstrate the superiority of the latter to the former." (*Conquest's Outlines of Midwifery,* p. 193.)

And again:—

"As a further inducement, it should be remembered that medical men concur in their opinion, that very rarely does a constitution suffer from secreting milk; whilst the health of many women is most materially improved by the performance of the duties of a nurse." (Ibid., p. 194.)

Upon the same subject, he says in another place:

"But few mothers, comparatively, are to be found who, if willing, would not be able to support their infants, at least for a few months, and parental affection and occasional self-denial would be abundantly recompensed by blooming and vigorous children.

"Presuming that the laudable determination is formed to indulge the child with that nutriment which is designed for its support, it becomes necessary to state, that unless very strong objections should exist, *twelve hours* should never elapse before the infant has been put to the breast. Instinct directs it what to do, and the advantages of allowing it to suck soon after birth are many and important, both to the mother and child.

"By this commendable practice, the patient is generally preserved from fever, from inflamed and broken breasts, and from the distressing and alarming consequences resulting from those complaints.

"If the breasts should not have secreted milk previous to delivery, the act of sucking will encourage and expedite the secretion. Thus the mother will be saved from much of the pain connected with distended breasts. Besides which, if the infant be not put to the nipple till the breasts become full and tense, the nipple itself will sometimes almost disappear, on account of its being stretched; and without much, and often ineffectual labour on the part of the child, it cannot be laid hold of, and even then the pain endured by the mother is exquisitely severe, and not unfrequently the cause of sore nipples." (Ibid., p. 195.)

Having premised thus much upon the advantages resulting to both mother and child from following the law of nature, which enjoins the female to nourish her own offspring, and having, moreover, elsewhere noted some of the causes which may prevent its being fully carried into effect, we shall now proceed to that important point—for those who do not intend nursing their own children—the choice of a nurse, and the regimen to be observed, which is equally applicable to both parties.

THE CHOICE OF A NURSE.

In the selection of a nurse, the medical attendant ought generally to be consulted; the following points merit particular attention:

She should be apparently of sound health, full and moderate plumpness, with a fresh complexion, and clear *eyelids free from any appearance of redness, scurfiness, or thickening.* She should be thoroughly exempt from glandular enlargements; possess deep red lips without cracks, sound white teeth; and well-formed, moderately firm breasts, with nipples free from excoriation or appearance of eruptions; the child of the nurse is one of the best criterions to judge by—its being plump and healthy is a great point in her favour. We should also endeavour to discover if she is free from any hereditary taint; she should, moreover, be of a mild, patient, and equable temper, not irritable, nor disposed to fits of passion, or nervous; of regular and temperate habits, neat in person, and fond of children. She ought also to be about the same age, and delivered about the same time, or, at least, within three months of the same period as the mother; with respect to the age, we must, of course avoid extremes. A women, having given birth to a child very late in life, should choose a nurse several years her junior, and fully qualified for her duties; the reverse of the rule applies to extremely young mothers.

DIET DURING NURSING.

As regards her diet, it should be simple and easily digested, and she ought to live upon a proper proportion of animal and vegetable food. Nature generally provides for the increased call upon her powers, by the suppression of the menstrual discharge, and moderate increase of appetite, which may be safely indulged; but all food of a highly concentrated, nourishing nature, is injurious, causing the milk to become too rich, and unsuited to the delicate digestion of the infant; the best guide is the regular homœopathic regimen, which may be consulted with advantage.

I cannot too strongly repudiate the too prevalent, but deeply erroneous idea, that women, during the period of suckling, require *stimulants* to keep up their strength; under this impression, both wine and malt liquors—and, among the latter, more particularly porter—are frequently resorted to. Porter is not only injurious from its stimulating properties, but the deleterious effect of the different ingredients which enter into its composition have upon the milk, forms one of the most prolific causes of the many evils that attack infancy. My opinions in this respect are corroborated by the physicians of the old school, though, I regret to say, not to the same extent. I shall here content myself with a single quotation from a well-known medical writer:

"There is an evil too generally prevalent, and most pernicious in its consequences on individuals and society, and by no means confined to mothers in the lowest classes of the community, which cannot be too severely reprobated; it is the wretched habit of taking wine or spirits to remove the languor present during pregnancy and suckling. It is a practice fraught with double mischief, being detrimental both to mother and child. The relief afforded is temporary, and is invariably followed by a greater degree of languor, which demands a more powerful stimulus, which at length weakens, and eventually destroys the tone of the stomach, deteriorates the milk, and renders it altogether unfit to supply that nutriment which is essential to the existence and welfare of the child."

SUPPLEMENTARY DIET OF INFANTS.

Unfortunately, some mothers do not possess sufficient milk for the proper nourishment of their offspring; if this arise merely from a deficiency in the secretion, and the female is in other respects healthy, we must have recourse to supplementary diet, to make up for the diminished quantity of the natural nutriment. Goats', asses', and cows' milk, are excellent substitutes, especially the latter, diluted with one third of water; goats' milk being apparently objectionable from its peculiar aroma. The milk, therefore, of the cow ought, when possible, to be obtained, and, if given undiluted, boiled; cows' milk being generally considered too heavy, which boiling in a great measure obviates; it ought also to be slightly sweetened, so as to resemble as closely as possible that of the nurse; it should, moreover, be about the same temperature, say ninety-six to ninety-eight degrees, a point less regarded than it should be, and easily determinable by the thermometer. If any constitutional taint exist in the mother, the sooner the child is transferred to another breast, the better for both parties; if a nurse be not procurable, the above will generally prove sufficient nourishment until the front-teeth appear, which is a clear indication that the digestive organs are prepared for more solid food; if, however, the milk diet appears to disagree with the infant, we may mix a little thin arrow-root, rusk, or well-toasted bread in water, to which the milk may be afterwards added; such alterations in diet are, however, but rarely required.

We may remark, that no portion of the milk ought to be retained for a subsequent meal, from the quickness with which it becomes sour; the same remark applies to any of the above preparations, in which milk forms the principal ingredient.

In the cows' milk, which was at first diluted, we may, after two or three weeks, gradually diminish the quantity of water, as the digestive organs become stronger; but we cannot too stringently press the point, that where it is at all practicable, the child ought to derive as great as possible a portion of its nutriment from the breast, as no food can efficiently supply the place of that which nature intended for it at its birth.

When it is necessary to give supplementary nourishment, a suckling-bottle ought to be used, as the best imitation of nature in giving the food slowly; particular care being taken to observe the utmost cleanliness. The child ought, in feeding, to be kept in a reclining, not supine, position, as the latter frequently causes it to incur the risk of suffocation; and when it evinces disinclination to its food, no more should be offered. When the front teeth appear, which is about the fifth or sixth month in healthy children, an alteration may take place in the diet; and a well-made panada, diluted milk sweetened, and thickened with a small quantity of arrow-root, sago, semolino, or rusk, may be given twice a day. When milk, even prepared with farinaceous substances, disagrees, barley-water, fine well-boiled gruel, or weak chicken-broth, and beef-tea, may be substituted, adhering to that which seems best to agree with the infant, and taking care to vary as circumstances require it, as too long an adherence to barley-water may occasion looseness in the bowels, while the animal diet is liable to lead, if too long continued, to a contrary result; the best precaution in these cases, when the predisposition becomes evident, is an immediate change of aliment.

The child should be accustomed to take its nourishment from each breast alternately; as, if this precaution be not adopted, inflammation is likely to arise in the one not used, and the child is apt to become crooked from being always retained in the same position.

The physician is frequently asked, how often the child ought to be applied to the breast? The best rule is to give it when the infant appears to desire it, and to withdraw it when it appears satisfied. As it increases in strength, it may easily be accustomed to regular hours, giving it the breast late at night, and again early in the morning; but during the first six weeks or two months, three times during the hours of rest, late in the evening, middle of the night, and early in the morning, will generally be found sufficient.

DURATION OF SUCKLING AND WEANING.

The period of suckling ought seldom to last longer than forty weeks; but in this we must be guided, in a great measure, by the constitution of the infant; weak, ill-conditioned children, in whom the teeth are long in making their appearance, it has been recommended to continue at the breast for eighteen months, or even a longer period. Weaning ought, in fact, to be regulated both by the constitution of mother and child; the full *development* of the front teeth, which in healthy children is from nine to ten months, but in delicate or scrofulous constitutions, is delayed for several months later, is the best indication for weaning. If, however, the strength of the mother appear unequal to the task, and the supply of milk begin to fall off, the child may be gradually weaned, even before the teeth appear;

but if the infant is healthy, a continuance of suckling beyond the tenth month is injurious to both parent and child. Weaning should not take place *suddenly*, but the infant should be gradually accustomed to other food, and a less frequent administration of the breast, till entirely weaned; the time to commence this gradual course, is from the first appearance of the front teeth, so that the weaning terminate with their full development; thereby the secretion lessens by degrees, preventing all evil consequences of swollen or inflamed breasts, and the child also becomes quietly reconciled to the deprivation. Weaning ought not, however, to take place, if the child suffers considerably from the irritation of teething, or any acute infantile disease. When, however, it is found absolutely necessary to wean, *Belladonna* $\frac{0}{30}$ should be given as a *precautionary* measure against the inconveniences and not unfrequent dangers which sudden weaning entails. Among these may be mentioned, restlessness, sleeplessness, fretfulness, and excitability, nay, even a degree of irritability sometimes amounting to inflammation of the brain. The value of this remedy in affections of that organ has already been commented upon in several parts of this work. Although, perhaps, slightly out of place, it may be remarked that *Phosphorus* is the remedy best calculated to prevent inflammation of the breasts consequent upon a sudden cessation of suckling.* See the articles relative to this subject in Part IV., TREATMENT of Females and their peculiar Affections, p. 496.

After the child has been weaned, his nourishment should generally consist of the same simple food before mentioned, with an occasional light pudding, without spice or eggs, made from semolino, tapioca, or other farinaceous substance. The transition to a more substantial diet ought to be extremely gradual and guarded, and no material alteration made, till after the appearance of the eye-teeth.

SLEEP. SLEEPLESSNESS.

The sleep of the child is the next consideration; from the inability of the infant itself to maintain a proper degree of

* Vide A. H. Z., p. 8, No. 23.

warmth, it should sleep by its mother's or nurse's side, for at least the first six weeks, particularly during winter or early spring. Care must be taken not to over-burthen it with bed-clothes, and to place it in such a position as to prevent it slipping under them, and thereby becoming exposed to the risk of breathing a vitiated atmosphere, or even of suffocation; after six or eight weeks, when the organism becomes stronger, and able to preserve a proper degree of natural warmth, placing it in a separate bed or cradle, will be more conducive to its thriving; this change of arrangement will be found beneficial to both parties—to the child, by its breathing a purer air, and by the continual appetite for the breast being diminished; and the mother being freed from the necessary watchfulness and restlessness consequent upon its sleeping with her, will enjoy better health, and be more likely to secrete good and nutritious milk. Moreover, it is generally known, that sleeping in the same bed with an adult, is detrimental to the health and proper development, not only of infants, but even of children: a child sleeping in the same bed with a very old person, will very soon begin to exhibit signs of a falling off in its general appearance.

With regard to the kind of bed best suited for the infant, the suspended cradle seems the most eligible; we must, however, be careful not to allow the nurse to abuse its use by continual rocking, which frequently causes irritation of the brain; it should not be closed up with curtains, but the room may be a little darkened; in cases where there is danger of draughts, a screen will answer every purpose.

As to the length of sleep allowed, the chief business of the first months of its existence being sleep and nourishment, we may safely leave the point to nature, and not attempt to coerce the inclinations of the child; if the infant is lively on waking, we may conclude it has not slept too much; as it increases in vigour, with longer intervals of wakefulness, we may proceed (recollecting that night is the proper period for sleep) so to regulate its habits of taking its food and rest, as to accustom it to a uniform system, and particular hours. Children, up to two years of age, require rest during the day, and the nurse ought to endeavour to get them into the habit of taking it in the forenoon, for if in the afternoon, it generally interferes with the night's sleep. Whether by night or day, we must carefully exclude both light and noise from the nursery, for although they may be insufficient to *arouse* the infant, still they cause its sleep to be disturbed and unrefreshing, and by acting upon the nervous sensibility, predispose it to convulsions or spasmodic attacks from slight accidental causes.

It is true, that during the first month, the infant sleeps immediately on leaving the breast, and no evil consequences ensue; but it must be borne in mind, that it takes but little at a time, and the tenuity of the milk is at that time wisely adapted to its delicate digestion; but as the secretion becomes richer, and suited to the increasing power of those organs, it is injurious to put the child asleep immediately after a full meal; his rest is then restless and disturbed, from the process of digestion being interfered with, more particularly when nurses foolishly endeavour to force nature, by resorting to the baneful practice of rocking.

Nothing causes greater annoyance, and even anxiety, to the mother, than a disposition to wakefulness on the part of her infant. A healthy child should always be prepared for its rest at the usual hours; if, instead thereof, it appear restless, fretful, and disinclined for its accustomed sleep, it is an evident indication of some derangement of its general health; frequently through ignorance, nurses, instead of attending to this warning voice of nature, which by the sleeplessness of the infant demands appropriate relief, endeavour to stifle it, and sometimes to free themselves from a little temporary annoyance, administer opiates, which induce an unrefreshing slumber, and not unfrequently a deep stupor, mistaken for sleep, while the original evil still continues to make head against the vital power. This baneful practice has not only been the ruin of many constitutions in after-life, but to it, conjoined with diet, drinks, carminatives, and other quack medicines, together with the highly erroneous practice—sanctioned though it be by names of medical repute—of a frequent administration of that active mineral preparation, *calomel*, in infant maladies, to say nothing of laxatives, an infinite number of diseases and deaths are annually attributable. Every mother should not only caution her nurse against the use of opiates, but use her utmost vigilance to detect any breach of her injunctions, which should be visited with the immediate discharge of the person so offending; for she must be truly unfitted for such an important trust who, after being warned of its injurious tendency, will persevere in a practice placing in jeopardy the life of her infant charge.

Amongst the homœopathic remedies which have been found the more generally useful in removing *restlessness* and *sleeplessness* in children, *Coffea, Opium, Chamomilla,* and *Belladonna,* deserve notice. COFFEA $\frac{0}{30}$, is very efficacious when the child seems unusually lively, restless, and wakeful; but will commonly fail to answer its purpose when the nurse is in the daily habit of taking coffee as a beverage. In such circumstances, OPIUM $\frac{0}{6}$ may be substituted, particularly if the face of the child looks red. CHAMOMILLA $\frac{0}{12}$ will do good when the child is tormented with flatulence, and distention of the bowels, and appears to suffer from colic, indicated by drawing up the legs, screaming, etc. Against the sleeplessness after weaning, BELLADONNA $\frac{0}{6}$ is the most efficacious remedy. When these remedies do not seem indicated, or fail to relieve, an experienced homœopathist ought to be consulted. (See also CRYING and WAKEFULNESS, p. 462.)

EXERCISE.

For the first six or seven months the great business of nature seems to be the proper development of the infant organism, and of the respiratory and digestive functions. During this period the cartilage is gradually forming into bone, and its delicate muscles acquiring power and strength. We find also that consciousness is yet indistinct, and the infant evinces no anxiety to indulge in voluntary motion, the muscles of the neck and back not possessing sufficient power to support the head, or to keep the body in an erect position; for this reason, children during this period should, when carried in the arms, be kept in a reclining position, so as to avoid an undue pressure upon the vertebral column; a neglect of this precaution, and a premature carrying of the infant in an upright position, are a too frequent cause of deformities of the spine, and derangement of the internal functions in after life.

As its powers gradually develop, the infant seems inclined to exercise them, and evinces a desire to sit upright, which we may safely indulge, taking care that they be not overtasked by keeping it sitting up during the greater part of the time it is awake. A careful attention to nature in this, as in all other cases, is the best guide.

The practice of dandling the child in an upright position, seems rather to proceed from the pleasure of indulging the feeling of parental affection, than from any benefit the child can, by any possibility, be expected to derive from it; in fact, it is highly injurious, even at a rather more advanced period, as exciting a premature involuntary exercise of the muscles, and consequent deformity. The act of respiration bringing into play a great variety of muscles, occasionally crying seems sufficient active exercise during this period.

In mild spring and summer weather the child may, after the first fortnight has elapsed, be carried out into the air for a quarter of an hour, and the period of exercise gradually increased; in fact, if the weather be fine, it can scarcely be too much in the open air. Should its birth occur in winter, advantage may be taken of a fine day, after it is a month or five weeks old, as the frame is gradually acquiring the power of generating heat; but at the same time *great care* must be taken to prevent its catching cold; and should it exhibit the slightest sign of being affected by the atmosphere, the practice should be immediately discontinued, and it should be carried up and down in a well-ventilated room, the nurse moving it quietly in her arms from side to side. Many children are lost through a foolish idea of *making them hardy*, by accustoming them to endure cold; this can occur only through ignorance, for nature, in very early infancy, does not possess sufficient energy of reaction to overcome the power of a sudden or long-protracted chill. We may recommend an occasional gentle friction of the hand over the body and limbs, which materially assists in the promotion of the circulation of the blood, and will, in unfavourable weather, serve in some measure as a substitute for exercising the infant out of doors.

In carrying the child, it should be from time to time transferred to different arms, as a continuance on one side is a frequent cause of deformity, and in some cases of squinting.

The child, as the organization develops itself, seems to evince a desire for independent movements, in which it may very properly be indulged, by removing every impediment in its dress, and allowing it to roll about, or crawl upon a soft carpet. The practice of assisting children to walk, or of exciting them to a premature exercise of their powers, is highly reprehensible, causing curvature of the limbs, the bones not being yet sufficiently formed to bear the burden imposed upon them. By allowing nature to act, the infant's powers will become more gradually, but at the same time, more fully developed, its carriage will be more firm and erect, and its limbs straight and well-formed; moreover, it will walk with greater confidence and independence by the expiration of the first year, than those who have been *taught to walk* by the assistance of the nurse, leading-strings, or mechanical inventions. When the period at which a child should make attempts to walk is retarded by evident debility of constitution, Homœopathy affords us the means of obviating this evil, by acting against the constitutional cause. Dr. Gross has found CALCAREA $\frac{0}{30}$, very useful in a case of this nature; and Dr. Hartmann has frequently administered CAUSTICUM $\frac{0}{30}$, with great effect. (*Silicea*, *Sulphur*, *Belladonna*, *Mercurius*, or *Staphysagria*, etc., may be required in particular cases.)

DISEASES OF INFANCY.

INFLAMMATION OF THE EYES IN NEW-BORN INFANTS.

A SUDDEN exposure to the strong light of day, or the glare of a fire, is the general cause of this affection; and no doubt many children who are, what is vulgarly denominated born blind, owe their misfortune to the neglect of those precautions which we have so strongly enforced under the head of TREATMENT OF INFANTS, in many cases the external indications of this affection being so very slight as to escape observation.

As soon, however, as, on a careful examination, we become aware of the existence of this evil, we should administer ACONITE $\frac{0}{24}$, which will generally be found promptly efficacious in its removal.

When, from the constitution of one or both of the parents, we have reason to suppose that the exposure to light has been merely the exciting cause, but that the real origin of the evil is more deeply seated; or if the *Aconite* seems to produce no effect, and the disease continues to aggravate, we may have recourse to TINCTURA SULPHURIS $\frac{0}{30}$, and in some cases CALCAREA $\frac{0}{30}$, alternating them every eight or ten days, if we find it necessary to resort to the *Calcarea*—the *Tincture of Sulphur* having been found in many cases to act as a specific.

CHAMOMILLA $\frac{0}{12}$, is useful some weeks after birth, when the perceptive faculties are more developed, and the child exhibits great intolerance of light; also when redness, swelling, and agglutinations of the eyelids, with other indications, given under ACUTE INFLAMMATION OF THE EYE (Part II., p. 324), are present. LYCOPODIUM may also be named as a useful remedy in some inveterate cases.

HICCOUGH.

This affection, though in itself of slight importance, frequently causes no small degree of uneasiness to young mothers; it generally arises from exposure of the body, even in a warm room, to the atmospheric air, even during the operations of dressing and undressing the new-born child; wrapping it warmly in the bed, or, better still, applying it to the breast, will frequently lead to its cessation; should it, however, continue, the administration of a small quantity of white sugar as much as will cover the end of a teaspoon, dissolved in a teaspoonful of water, will effectually abate the evil.

COLD IN THE HEAD. CORYZA.

This affection frequently becomes exceedingly distressing to the infant, when it appears in the form of *an obstruction of the nose*, impeding the action of the suckling, by not allowing the breath to pass through the nostril, obliging the infant to release the nipple frequently in order to breathe, causing it to become fretful and irritable, sometimes leading to irritation and excoriation of the nipple, and thus in its repeated efforts to suck causing suffering to both itself and the nurse.

Whilst this state continues, it operates considerably against the infant's thriving, both by hindering it from taking a sufficient quantity of nutriment, and by the impediment it causes to respiration, preventing the child sleeping at night. When the nose is dry, and the secretion of mucus suspended, we may, while administering a remedy calculated permanently to remove the evil, afford relief, by imitating the natural secretion by the application of a little almond oil or cream to the interior of the nostrils with a feather.

This malady is often excessively obstinate, and presents itself under many different phases, which of course demand remedies suited to the entire group of the symptoms. Among these, NUX VOMICA $\frac{0}{30}$, has been most frequently successful, particularly when the following symptoms are present:—

Obstruction of the nose, with dryness or nocturnal obstruction, slight discharge during the day; irritability and peevishness.

SAMBUCUS NIGER, $\frac{0}{6}$, is frequently efficacious when *Nux v.* fails to relieve; but is also of service in cases when there is an accumulation of thick and viscid mucus in the nostrils; or when, in addition to the cold in the head, there is a suffocating cough, with wheezing in the chest, and quick laborious breathing, *Tartarus* should be had recourse to if *Sambucus* does not soon relieve the latter symptoms; and if no amelioration quickly appear, we may without hesitation have recourse to a globule of the first dilution, and repeat the dose every four to six hours, or oftener, if apparently called for,* until improvement is effected, or another remedy required.

CHAMOMILLA, $\frac{0}{12}$, is very useful when there is cold in the head, *with a watery discharge from the nose*, more particularly when there are febrile symptoms, soreness of the nostrils, and redness of one cheek.

CARBO V. is chiefly useful in obstinate cases, and particularly when the cold in the head becomes aggravated towards evening. CALCAREA, when the nose is stuffed with mucus, and the affection occurs in stout, lymphatic children. PULSATILLA, thick discharge from the nose, attended with frequent sneezing.

ADMINISTRATION. The doses already given repeated in from one to two days. (See also CORYZA, Part II., p. 193.)

CRYING AND WAKEFULNESS OF NEW-BORN CHILDREN.

As we have already remarked, the occasional crying of new-born children is a wise provision to bring the respiratory organs into play, and to expand the chest. When, however, the crying becomes excessive, and threatens to prove injurious, we must, in the first place, endeavour to discover its origin, which frequently will be found to be some mechanical cause, such as derangement in the infant's dress, or a pin sticking into its flesh, etc.

THERAPEUTICS. When, however, no exciting cause or guiding symptoms of disease presents itself, and the infant is peevish and irritable, with incessant whimpering and wakeful-

* Vide INTRODUCTORY REMARKS.

ness, or prolonged fits of crying, BELLADONNA, $\frac{0}{30}$,* will frequently be found sufficient to remove the evil.

When a fit of crying comes from the child having been irritated or excited by any cause, such as suddenly rousing it from its rest, and when it seems willing to sleep, but finds a difficulty in composing itself to slumber, COFFEA CRUDA, $\frac{0}{3}$, will prove efficacious. (*Aconitum*, $\frac{1}{24}$, may follow *Coffea* when there is considerable heat of skin, and extreme restlessness.)

CHAMOMILLA, $\frac{0}{12}$, is often more efficacious than *Belladonna* when the infant is of a very spare and delicate habit; or when we can trace the fits of screaming and wakefulness to a derangement of the digestive functions, and the child appears to suffer from griping pains, indicated by contortions of the body, drawing up of the little limbs upon the abdomen; and when a whitish, yellowish, or greenish, or watery excoriating diarrhœa is present.

JALAPA, $\frac{0}{3}$, in similar cases, but without diarrhœa, or with motions tinged with blood.

In other cases, when the screaming and vigilance are attended with colic and flatulence, SENNA, $\frac{0}{6}$, will answer best.

RHEUM, $\frac{0}{9}$ is more appropriate when, in addition to screaming and wakefulness, combined with griping, there are also *ineffectual* efforts to relieve the bowels by frequent straining, or when, at the utmost, only scanty, sour-smelling motions are passed, of *grayish* appearance, and seem to afford no relief.

When flatulent colic, accompanied by constipation, appears to be the source of the disturbance, *Nux v.* $\frac{0}{30}$, will commonly succeed in restoring ease to the little sufferer.

PULSATILLA, $\frac{0}{30}$, is very efficacious when it arises from overloading the stomach, or improper food, and the crying or wakefulness is accompanied with flatulence and diarrhœa, or with constipation.

REMARKS. The milk of a nurse who has suckled for some months previously is much too heavy for a new-born infant;

* See the INTRODUCTORY REMARKS to this Part of the work, as also those in the INTRODUCTION, (Part I.,) for directions as to the repetition of the dose, etc.

here, the only alternative is a change of nutriment. When, however, the above-named or any other infantile derangement arises from congenital weakness of the stomach, the most useful remedies in addition to *Nux v.* and *Puls.* are *Sulphur*, *Calcarea carbonica*, and *Baryta c.*, $\frac{0}{6}$.

REGURGITATION OF MILK. ACIDITY, FLATULENCE, ETC.

Children, in sucking, sometimes overload their stomachs, and regurgitate a *portion* of their milk; so far, mothers have no cause for uneasiness, nor is medical assistance requisite; but when this changes into vomiting, and the whole of the nutriment is returned from the stomach, or when sickness and regurgitation of food occur in children who have been weaned, at times followed by mucus and watery fluid, and even bile, it must be looked upon as a disease, and treated accordingly

THERAPEUTICS. IPECACUANHA, $\frac{0}{6}$, will generally afford relief, and may be repeated, if not followed by some amendment, giving the medicine from twelve to twenty-four hours to allow time for its action.* In the case of spoon-fed infants, or in children at a more advanced age, this remedy is equally efficacious, when the derangement is evidently owing to their having been over-fed, (a most culpable error, which most nurses are prone to fall into by cramming the stomach of their little charges, and but too often with food of an indigestible nature, whenever they are seized with a fit of crying.) Should the vomiting or flatulence, and also the diarrhœa when present, not decrease after some doses of *Ipecacuanha*, *Pulsatilla* $\frac{0}{12}$ may be exhibited in a similar manner, and succeeded in turn by *Antimonium crudem*, $\frac{0}{12}$, or $\frac{0}{18}$ if the symptoms continue, though in a mitigated form.

NUX VOMICA, $\frac{0}{30}$, in the same manner as the above, and that failing, BRYONIA, $\frac{0}{30}$, in case the disease is attended with flatulence, constipation, uneasiness, or irritability of temper.

Gentle friction with the extended hand, which has previously been warmed, is a simple and frequently efficacious

* Vide note, page 21.

mode of affording temporary relief in cases of flatulent distention of the stomach and bowels. But permanent relief is only to be attained from *Pulsatilla*, *Nux v.*, *Chamomilla*; or *Carbo v.* and *Sulphur*, when the former are insufficient. The diet must at the same time be attended to, and altered if of an indigestible nature and the undoubted cause of the mischief. When there is diarrhœa and *excessive* flatulency, *China* is very useful.

CHAMOMILLA. Same dose as described for Ipecacuanha, when attended with *convulsions*, or *diarrhœa*, as described elsewhere under this medicine. (See those articles).

A single dose of *Sulphur*, $\frac{0}{30}$, followed by *Calcarea carbonica*, $\frac{0}{30}$, in from five to ten days, and then again one or more of the preceding remedies, according to indications, will often be the means of effecting a cure in inveterate cases.

SPASMODIC ASTHMA. SPASMS IN THE CHEST.

Children are sometimes seized during the night with sudden attacks of suffocating spasm in the chest. The little patient suddenly awakes from sleep, and utters a shrill cry, in consequence of the feeling of suffocation which is experienced. The countenance soon assumes a livid hue, and is expressive of extreme anxiety. A dull, hollow-sounding, dry cough, usually accompanies the attack, and the breathing is rapid, very laborious, and painfully distressing to witness. In such cases a globule or two of *Ipecacuanha* (potency 3 or 6) ought immediately to be dissolved in about a wine-glassful of water, and a few drops of the liquid put into the mouth of the patient. If relief follows, the medicine must be allowed to act, and only repeated when the symptoms threaten to become worse again. But in the event of no favourable signs resulting in from a quarter of an hour to half an hour or so, according to the severity of the symptoms, *Sambucus* may be given in the same manner.

In other cases, *Arsenicum* $\frac{0}{6}$ will be found more efficacious than either of these; or the employment of *Ipecacuanha* and *Arsenicum* alternately every ten or twenty minutes, until improvement takes place. Whenever a sudden aggravation ensues after the administration of any of these remedies, nothing further should be done, as on waiting patiently for a few minutes, if the change arise from the effects of the medicine, the symptoms will subside, and gradually give way to unequivocal signs of improvement. (See ASTHMA of MILLAR, p. 486.)

Some children are liable to be seized with obstructed respiration or asthma, although otherwise in good health, whenever they are exposed to sudden changes of temperature, or to a cold and high wind. This form of asthma is always attended with considerable, hard, distention of the pit of the stomach and region of the lower ribs; the child affected is at the same time thrown into a state of great anxiety and uncontrollable restlessness, attended with crying or screaming, tossing about, etc. Against this indisposition *Chamomilla* $\frac{6}{6}$ has repeatedly proved to be an effectual remedy. A dose ought therefore to be given as soon as the attack declares itself.

MILK-CRUST. MILK-SCAB.

Crusta lactea. Porrigo larvalis. Tinea faciei.

This affection, as it occurs in infants at the breast, usually consists of an eruption of numerous small whitish pustules, which appear in clusters upon a red ground. These generally show themselves in the first instance on the face, particularly the cheeks and forehead, but sometimes spread over the whole body. The lymph contained in them soon becomes yellow, dark, or even sanguineous, and, on their bursting, forms into thin yellowish crusts.

Frequently there is considerable surrounding redness and swelling, with distressing itching, which renders the little patient excessively restless and fretful, and causes it to keep continually rubbing the affected parts, by which the discharge and crusts are repeatedly renewed, often increased in thickness, and often to such extent, that the whole face becomes covered; the eyes and nose alone remaining free. The eyes and eyelids, as also the parotid and mesenteric glands, occasionally become inflamed, and sometimes marasmus supervenes.

THERAPEUTICS. The following medicines have been found serviceable in this affection: ***Aconitum, Rhus toxicodendron, Viola tricolor, Sulphur, Belladonna, Hepar sulphuris, Euphrasia, Staphysagria, Arsenicum,*** etc.

ACONITE $\frac{0}{24}$, should commence our treatment, when we find excessive restlessness and excitability produced by this affection, and when the skin around the parts is red, inflamed, and itching.

As soon as we have found beneficial effects result from the administration of the above remedy, we may follow it up with VIOLA TRICOLOR, which is often sufficient to effect a cure in the simple uncomplicated form of the disease.

ADMINISTRATION. $\frac{000}{3}$, in four teaspoonfuls of water, one night and morning. The prescription to be repeated in four days, or another remedy selected, if the affection threatens to extend, or otherwise become worse.

RHUS TOXICODENDRON may sometime succeed or supersede *Viola tricolor*, when the scalp is considerably affected and thickly studded with incrustations.

ADMINISTRATION. $\frac{0}{12}$, repeated in two to three days, if the same appearances remain.

If, after the employment of *Rhus*, the affection is found to have made but little favourable progress, as not unfrequently happens in debilitated or in strumous subjects, *Sulphur* $\frac{0}{30}$, may be given and repeated in four days.

The *alternate* use of *Rhus* and *Sulphur* every four or five days, has been found very efficacious in cases of the aforesaid description, and when the eyes are a good deal affected.

ADMINISTRATION. $\frac{0}{30}$, dry upon the tongue.

Sarsaparilla and *Mezereum* have also been strongly recommended in Crusta lactea; also *Arsenic.* $\frac{0}{30}$. The former in the earlier stage of the malady, when small, burning, itching pustules appear on the face. *Mezereum*, when from the bursting and discharge of the contents of the pustules, incrustations have formed from which an acrid exudation flows, and gives rise to a fresh eruption of vesicles wherever it comes in contact.

Graphites, as also *Sepia*, *Hepar*, *Baryta c.*, *Lycopodium*, etc., have been recommended as likely to prove of service in complicated cases. But the remedies above mentioned will rarely fail to cure the affection as ordinarily met with, if had recourse to in due time. (See also Scald Head.)

THRUSH, OR APTHÆ.

This disease commences by the formation of small isolated, round, white vesicles, which, if not checked, become confluent, and sometimes present an ulcerated appearance, filling the whole of the cavity of the mouth, and in severe cases extending to the throat. This affection, although of itself neither malignant nor dangerous, frequently causes not only considerable suffering to the child by preventing it from sucking, but great pain and inconvenience to the mother by its being communicated to the nipples, and causing excoriation, etc.

The complaint is most generally produced by the want of a proper attention to cleanliness, both as regards the constant personal laving of the infant, but especially from the suckling-glass, when employed, not having been carefully washed after use. Improper aliment is another of the principal causes; thus we find that children who are what is commonly called reared by the hand, either partially or wholly, are more liable to this affection than those whose sole nourishment has been from the breast.

One of the remedies in this affection, although perfectly homœopathic in its action, has long been in use, in its external application, by practitioners of the old school, namely, Borax; and a weak solution applied to the mouth with a brush has not unfrequently been found efficacious. Or we may prescribe this remedy, to be taken internally, as follows:

We may dissolve a few globules of the third or sixth potency in an ounce of water, and administer one teaspoonful morning and evening for two days, then allow an interval of three days to elapse; if at that period no amelioration has taken place, we must have recourse to Sulphur $\frac{0}{30}$, given dry.

In cases where there is much salivation, and the thrush indicates an inclination to ulceration, we may administer MERCURIUS SOLUBILIS $\frac{0}{12}$, twice in forty-eight hours, followed, in a few days, by SULPHUR, and then ACIDUM SULPHURICUM $\frac{0}{30}$, after a similar interval if necessary. In very bad cases, when the aphthæ assume a livid, blue, or violet appearance, attended with excessive weakness and diarrhœa, ARSENICUM $\frac{0}{30}$, is highly useful.

Great cleanliness ought to be observed in all cases.

When the disease frequently, notwithstanding every precaution, reappears in infants at the breast, we may safely infer that it arises from some virus in the constitution of the mother, or nurse, who ought to be changed, or immediately put through a proper course of treatment, under the direction of an experienced homœopathic practitioner.

CONSTIPATION. *Obstructio Alvi Neonatorum.*

This generally appears in children who are either wholly or partially reared by the hand, and also in those whose mothers or nurses are similarly disposed, which if it arises from a peculiar diet or want of exercise, such as too much animal food, &c., on the part of the last mentioned, may be removed by a proper attention to these points; but in many instances it is necessary for them also to have recourse to proper remedial agents at the same time with the infant.

THERAPEUTICS. *Nux vomica*, *Bryonia alba*, and *Opium*, are the principal remedies; and in more obstinate cases, *Sulphur*, *Veratrum album*, *Lycopodium* and *Alumina*.

Most of the medicaments have been already mentioned under *Constipation* (PART II., p. 123), which see.

ADMINISTRATION. $\frac{0}{30}$ of the three first-mentioned remedies, every three to four days, until relief is obtained, or another remedy called for;* and of the last, the same dose at intervals of a week.

An enema of tepid water may be occasionally had recourse to, if required, until the medicine has remedied the irregularity.

* Vide note, p. 21.

BOWEL COMPLAINTS OF INFANTS.

Diarrhœa Neonatorum.

Diarrhœa, like constipation, is to be regarded merely as a symptom, not as a *disease*; the real disease here consists in *irritation* or inflammation of the mucous membrane of the intestines, arising from the effects of aperients, indigestible food, cold, fright, &c.

I have already mentioned, (article MECONIUM,) that much mischief is too often occasioned by the deleterious practice of administering laxative medicines, and even drastic purgatives! to the tender new-born infant, for the purpose of hurriedly expelling the blackish green-looking matter, technically known by the name of *Meconium*, that collects in the large intestine of the fœtus during the last month or two of its uterine existence. This unwarrantable and extremely reprehensible conduct is frequently persevered in even for some time after the expulsion of the first discharge has taken place, and is in many cases the UNDOUBTED cause of *bowel complaints* and other sufferings in infants. I cannot, therefore, refrain from again expressing a warm disapprobation on the subject, and am convinced that in so doing, I but give utterance to the conjoint opinion of every experienced and enlightened practitioner, even of the allopathic school.

The introduction of unappropriate, indigestible food, such as thick gruel, &c., into the delicate stomach of a new-born infant, is another very frequent source of intestinal derangement; this unpardonable error is not unfrequently committed by ignorant nurses, in order, as they say, to keep it from *starving* during the few hours of necessary repose to which the mother is left after delivery.

This disturbance is, moreover, likely to be excited in those cases in which, either from a deficiency in the secretion of milk or other causes, it becomes incumbent to administer supplementary diet to make up for the diminished supply; and again at the period of *weaning*, when serious disturbances are occasionally produced in the stomach and bowels, from want of proper attention and caution in the selection and administration of the food. (See art. SUPPLEMENTARY DIET OF INFANTS, p. 451.)

Fright and exposure to cold are, as already noted, two other most frequent exciting causes of the disorder.

THERAPEUTICS. A healthy infant on the breast soils on an average, from four to six napkins in the twenty-four hours, but in some instances the evacuations are more frequent, yet, without in any degree affecting the health of the child, (as is likewise often the case when a constipated state of the bowels exists;) in such cases then, little or no interference ought to be made so long as the stools remain free from *fœtor*, possessing merely the slightly acid smell peculiar to the infantile state, and are evidently unattended with pain, or any other abnormal indication. When, however, the stools become green and watery, or yellow and watery, brown and frothy, or white and frothy, as if fermented, mixed with mucus, or consist entirely of mucus, and emit an offensive odour, and are generally preceded or accompanied by signs of suffering, it becomes imperative to have recourse to remedial aid. As already observed, the minuteness of the doses, and the absence of all nauseous taste in the homœopathic medicines, not to mention their other more important virtues, render them peculiarly well adapted to the treatment of children, and thereby spares many an affectionate and anxious parent the pain and difficulty which is so frequently encountered in inducing the little sufferer to swallow the nauseous allopathic drugs.

The following are the principal remedies employed in homœopathic practice against this derangement: *Aconitum*, *Belladonna*, *Chamomilla*, *Rheum*, *Pulsatilla*, *Ipecacuanha*, and also *Mercurius*, *Nux v.*, *Arsenicum alb.*, *Sulphur*, *Sepia*, *Opium*, and *Verat. alb.*

When there is *inflammation*, the constitutional symptoms are pretty clearly indicated by *heat of the surface of the body*, quickness of pulse, and by rigours; in this case, we must have immediate recourse to ACONIT. $\frac{0}{24}$, and follow it if necessary by

BELLADONNA; when the more acute symptoms have been removed, but the infant continues to suffer much and scream constantly. (*Lachesis* may be preferred to *Belladonna*, when constipation suddenly supervenes, attended with swelling and apparent tenderness to the touch over the entire abdomen, but especially at one particular spot. *Mercurius* may follow Lachesis if the symptoms do not yield to the latter remedy.

ADMINISTRATION. $\frac{0}{3}\frac{0}{0}$, in six teaspoonfuls of water, one every six to eight hours, until relief is obtained.*

CHAMOMILLA is one of the most invaluable remedies in the treatment of the diseases of children, and particularly in bowel-complaints, whether arising from irritation caused by indigestible food excited by a chill, or occurring during teething; when the following symptoms are apparent: redness of the face, or of one cheek, hardness and tension, and fulness of the abdomen, attended by severe colic, which is indicated by the state of peevishness, *restlessness, constant crying*, and *drawing up of the legs* towards the abdomen, *sickness*, frequent evacuations, of a *bilious, watery, slimy*, or frothy description, of a *whitish, yellowish*, or GREENISH colour, sometimes bearing a resemblance to beat-up eggs, of an offensive odour, similar to that of rotten eggs. *Chamomilla* may be preferred to Belladonna after Aconite in cases of inflammation, when any of the above symptoms present themselves. (See also INFANTILE REMITTENT, p. 488.)

ADMINISTRATION. $\frac{0}{6}$, in four teaspoonfuls of water; a teaspoonful every six hours, until benefit results.†

RHEUM is another remedy of great utility in the treatment of this affection, provided the disorder has not been actually *excited* by frequent use of this medicine itself in allopathic doses, in which case it will be necessary to have recourse to *Pulsatilla, Chamomilla*, or *Mercurius*, as antidotes, according to the nature of the symptoms. Rheum is particularly appropriate when *acidity* or bilious derangement has been generated by indigestion, or has arisen from the prolonged use of antacids, such as magnesia, &c., and when there is flatulent distention of the abdomen, colic, crying, restlessness, *tenesmus* before and after the evacuations, which are either of the consistence of

* Vide note, page 21. † Ibid.

pap, or watery and somewhat slimy, occasionally of a grayish, or of a brown colour, and when a sour smell is emitted from the body of the infant. It is sometimes necessary to give *Chamomilla* after *Rheum*, to complete the cure.

ADMINISTRATION. $\frac{0}{3}$, in the same manner as *Chamomilla*.

PULSATILLA. *Diarrhœa*, arising from "*indigestion*," or *from a chill*, with *watery*, *slimy*, *whitish*, or *bilious*, *greenish-*looking evacuations, occurring chiefly at night; want of appetite, fretfulness. *Pulsatilla*, as stated, is also very serviceable in obsinate cases, where the affection has been brought on by the abuse of *Rhubarb*, or by *Rhubarb* and *Magnesia*, when the symptoms are as *above described*; it is further often efficacious under similar conditions, when *fright* has been the exciting cause, and *Opium* has not sufficed, or has been administered too late. (See VERATRUM, p. 474.)

ADMINISTRATION. $\frac{0}{12}$, in six teaspoonfuls of water, one every twelve hours, until improvement ensue.

IPECACUANHA is particularly valuable when the diarrhœa is excited at the *period of weaning* (*weaning-brash*), from the *sudden change of food*, which the stomach is unable to digest; and when the following symptoms result in consequence: bilious derangement, with repeated attacks of *vomiting*, paleness of the face, frequent crying, diarrhœa with stools of a bilious, slimy, or greenish *yellow*, sometimes blackish, or streaked with blood, and of a putrid odour; on other occasions, evacuations resembling matter in a state of *fermentation*, or containing substances like white flocks or flakes, followed by straining. When this remedy is insufficient to effect a complete cure, we should have recourse to *Pulsatilla* or to *Antimonium crudum*, should the vomiting not speedily subside.

ADMINISTRATION. $\frac{0}{6}$, in four teaspoonfuls of water, a teaspoonful night and morning.

MERCURIUS. This medicine will be found very serviceable in some cases where the irritation owes its origin to the abuse of aperients, such as *Rheum*, etc., or when it has arisen from A CHILL. The following are the principal indications: watery, slimy, or bilious stools, (sometimes *streaked* or mixed *with blood*,) of a blackish, "*greenish*," or of a whitish yellow colour:

frothy, or having the appearance of beat-up eggs; attended with symptoms of severe colic, and frequently also with *severe tenesmus* and protrusion of the intestine.

ADMINISTRATION. $\frac{0}{12}$, in the same manner as *Chamomilla*. It is necessary to state, however, that the employment of mercury in the form of calomel or some other mercurial preparation in allopathic doses, is a fruitful source of bowel complaints in children; when, therefore, the complaint is attributable to the abuse of that powerful mineral, the homœopathic *Mercurius* must of course be avoided, and its place supplied by an antidote, which will generally be found in *Hepar sulphuris* or *Acidum nitricum*, should the former not suffice.

DULCAMARA. This is an admirable remedy in derangements of every description arising from exposure to wet; and is indicated in cases of diarrhœa from *this cause*, with the following symptoms: *Watery*, bilious, or *slimy* evacuations, of a greenish yellow colour, and occurring chiefly at night.

ADMINISTRATION. $\frac{0}{6}$ or $\frac{0}{12}$, in a teaspoonful of water, and repeated in twenty-four hours, if necessary, (*Merc.* or *Cham.* may be required to complete the cure in some instances.)

NUX VOMICA is very useful in cases arising from a chill, or from indigestible food at the period of weaning, or earlier; it is also useful in some cases in which the disorder has been created by the frequent employment of *laxative* medicines.

Its indications are: very frequent but scanty evacuations of watery, *slimy*, whitish, or greenish stools, attended with colic and tenesmus, sometimes followed by protrusion of the intestine; extreme fretfulness. This medicine is also of great service in many cases when the diarrhœa alternates with constipation.

ADMINISTRATION. $\frac{0}{30}$, in three teaspoonfuls of water, one each night at bedtime.

BRYONIA is a useful remedy in cases of diarrhœa which recur whenever the weather becomes very warm.

ADMINISTRATION. $\frac{0}{6}$, repeated in from twelve to twenty-four hours. (*Carbo-v.* has been found efficacious when only temporary benefit resulted from *Bryonia*, in diarrhœa during the heat of summer.)

ARSENICUM. This medicine becomes indispensable in neglected cases, or in those at an advanced stage of the disorder, when there is reason to fear that it will terminate in marasmus. The following are its characteristic indications: Watery or slimy stools, of a greenish, whitish, dark, or brownish colour, or of a putrid or gangrenous odour, taking place chiefly during the night, or after *drinking* or partaking of any kind of food, *great thirst*, sleeplessness, paleness of the face, sunken cheeks, and blue circles round the eyes, *enlargement* of the *abdomen*, with *extreme weakness* and *excessive emaciation*. $\frac{0}{30}$, in four teaspoonfuls of water, one night and morning.*

SULPHUR is an invaluable remedy in protracted cases, or in those occurring in children who are the offspring of delicate parents,—when there is great weakness, emaciation, distention of the abdomen, and excoriations between the thighs and neighbouring parts. (*Calcarea* is required to complete the cure after *Sulphur.*) In other cases, *Sepia, Hepar s., Acid. sulph., Magnesia* or *Veratrum* may be required. (See DIARRHŒA, Part II., p. 137.) $\frac{0}{30}$, in four teaspoonfuls of water, one night and morning.

OPIUM, as has been stated in another part of the work,† is a most valuable remedy, when immediately employed, for averting the bad results which sometimes arise in consequence of a sudden fright. When convulsions, with derangement in the stomach and bowels, are excited in children by such a cause, we ought to administer *Opium* $\frac{00}{3}$, followed by *Veratrum* $\frac{0}{3}$, should *Opium* prove insufficient, and the vomiting and diarrhœa become excessive; or we may select a remedy from amongst those above mentioned, in preference, such as *Pulsatilla*, &c., if the symptoms correspond.

SMELL OF THE ALVINE EVACUATIONS. Acid: *Rheum., Merc., Sulph., Calc., Graph., Natr.;* or *Cham., Arn., Hep., Sep., Phosph.*—Cadaverous: *Bismuth.*—Mouldy: *Coloc.*—Eggs, rotten, resembling: *Cham.*—Fetid, putrid: *Ars., Ass., Carb v., Puls., Sil., Sulph.;* or *Arn., Bry, Aur., Calc., Cam., China, Graph., Nux v., Phosph. a., Dulc., Sep.*—Involuntary

* Vide note, p. 21. † Vide MENTAL EMOTIONS.

discharge of fæces: *Phosph.*, *Phosph. a.*, *Verat.*, *Ars.*, *Bell.*, *Ac. mur.*, *Natr. m.*, *Sulph.*; or *Rhus.*, *Bry.*, *Nux v.*, *China.*, *Staph.*, *Dig.*, *Merc.*, *Puls.*, *Sep.*, *Zinc.*—When urinating: *Ac. mur.*—When expelling flatus: *Ferr. mag.*—When sleeping: *Rhus.*, *Puls.*, *Arn.*, *Moschus.*

DIET. When the derangement can be traced to any particular kind of food, an alteration in the diet becomes imperative; at the same time the quantity of food or drinks must be diminished until improvement sets in.

EXCORIATION. *Excoriationes Neonatorum.*

Against this affection cleanliness is the best preventive; however, we frequently find it proceed to such an extent as to require the aid of medicines for its removal.

CHAMOMILLA will be found, in most instances, speedily effective, when we are certain that the disease is not the medicinal result of chamomile-tea taken by the nurse or child, in which instance IGNATIA, PULSATILLA, BORAX, or CARBO VEG., at the same potency, have been recommended to be given.

ADMINISTRATION. $\frac{0}{6}$ or $\frac{0}{12}$, repeated in three days.

MERCURIUS. When a yellow colour of the skin is present, which *Chamomilla* has not removed, and when the excoriation is extensive and severe. In very obstinate cases we may have recourse to *Carbo v.* 30, followed in four to six days by *Tinctura sulph.*, at the same potency. *Acidum sulph.*, *Graphites*, *Silicea*, *Lycopodium*, and *Sepia*, are also useful in this malady.

ADMINISTRATION. $\frac{0}{12}$ in the same manner as *Chamomilla.*

JAUNDICE. *Icterus Neonatorum.*

This disease, as we have before observed, frequently takes its rise from the mischievous practice of administering aperients immediately after birth; exposure to cold is also one of its exciting causes.

When it has arisen from the last mentioned, and when there is, together with the distinguishing characteristic of the disease—a yellow hue of the skin—considerable distention of the stomach, the administration of CHAMOMILLA will be found prompt in affording relief. Mercurius may, in many cases, follow this remedy if it has only partially relieved; after which, if any symptoms still remain, we may exhibit CINCHONA.

NUX VOM., when the complaint is combined with costiveness, and the little patient appears *generally* of irritable temper.

ADMINISTRATION of the remedies:—A globule in four teaspoonfuls of water, one night and morning; again repeating, or selecting another remedy, after an interval of from three to five days, if the case seem to require it. (See remarks on this point in INTRODUCTION; *Article*, ADMINISTRATION AND REPETITION OF THE MEDICINES.)

For more particular indications for the medicines above given, and further information, see article JAUNDICE, in part. II., p. 161 of this work.

INDURATION OF THE CELLULAR TISSUE.

Erysipelas Neonatorum.

DIAGNOSIS. Fever with red spots, generally appearing first upon the nates, but sometimes on the extremities, afterwards upon the abdomen and genital organs, accompanied with induration of the skin and even of the maxillary muscles, which prevents the child from uttering other than a dull sound; the skin at last becomes as dry and hard as parchment. Sometimes, instead of fever, the induration is accompanied with cold.

This affection generally presents itself in the first two months of infancy; its duration is from four to fourteen days, and if not promptly treated, it is generally fatal.

THERAPEUTICS. The remedies principally required in this affection are: *Aconitum*, *Belladonna*, *Rhus toxicodendron*, *Arsenicum album*, *Lachesis*, and *Sulphur*.

ACONITUM. At the commencement, when fever is present.

ADMINISTRATION. $^{0}\frac{0}{6}{}^{0}$, in four teaspoonfuls of water, one every six hours, until diminution of the febrile symptoms ensues.

BELLADONNA may follow the exhibition of *Aconitum*, particularly when the spots present an erysipelatous appearance.

ADMINISTRATION. $\frac{0}{6}$, in a teaspoonful of water; to be repeated in twelve to twenty-four hours, and so on if the same indications continue, but at shorter or longer intervals, according to the effects produced.*

Rhus toxicodendron, if the appearance of the skin exhibits a vesicular character.

Administration. Same as *Belladonna.* (In some cases *Belladonna* and *Rhus* alternately may be found necessary.)

Arsenicum, should the dryness and hardness of the skin remain undiminished, or become increased; should we also find rejection of food from the stomach, evacuations green, watery, acrid, and very offensive; moreover, when there is a tendency to gangrene, with livid spots and vesication.

Administration. $\frac{0}{30}$, repeated as *Belladonna.*

Lachesis may in some cases be called for after *Belladonna*, when that remedy does not appear sufficient to combat the malady; or it may occasionally be advantageously exhibited in alternation with *Arsenicum.*

Administration. $\frac{0}{30}$, in the same manner as *Belladonna.*

Sulphur may be usefully employed against the sequelæ of this affection, such as torpidity of the intestines, and is also indicated where we have reason to suspect some constitutional taint. *Graphites. Hepar s.*, or *Clematis*, may also prove useful.

The body during this disease must be kept as dry as possible, and lint applied to the parts affected; when practicable, the infant's only nourishment should be from the breast, to which it should be frequently applied, but only allowed to suck little at a time.

LOCK-JAW OF INFANTS. *Trismus Nascentium.*

This serious, and so generally fatal disease, under the old mode of treatment, usually occurs in the first few days of infant life; at first the child vainly attempts to suck, and even if it succeed, the milk is returned. On examination, from stiffness of the masticator muscles, the lower jaw cannot be depressed—the jaws gradually close, the whole frame becomes rigid, and death ensues.

The duration of the malady is from two to four days.

* Vide note, p. 21.

Causes. Foul air; vitiated milk; taking cold; and local irritation; for example, the umbilical cord being too tightly tied.

Therapeutics. We must in the first place remove the causes where known. When local irritation has given rise to the attack, Arnica ought to be immediately given internally; at the same time the seat of the injury may be bathed once or twice with a weak lotion, a few drops of the tincture to a wine-glassful of water. When we can trace the occasional cause to a bad state of the milk, Lachesis, 30, may first be given, and followed by Belladonna, 30, (which, it may be observed, is to be held as a most important remedy in all cases where the affection cannot be assigned to any particular cause,) if no signs of improvement transpire after the first or second dose. Mercurius, 12, may also prove useful in similar cases. If cold or sudden chill has evidently given rise to the disorder, *Chamomilla*, $\frac{0}{6}$, may first be administered, and then *Belladonna*, if required; or *Nux v.*, $\frac{0}{30}$, may be given in preference to *Chamomilla* when catarrhal symptoms are present and indicate that remedy especially. (See Cold in the Head, Parts II., p. 193, and III., p. 461.) *Hyoscyamus*,—or *Belladonna*, *Lachesis* and *Hyoscyamus* in alternation, may be useful in some cases. (See also Trismus and Tetanus, Part II., p. 276.)

Administration. One globule of medicine chosen may be inserted, if possible, between the gums, or dissolved in a little water, of which a drop or two may be let fall upon the joining of the gums, if closely locked; repeat in from three to twelve hours, according to results.

HEAT SPOTS.

New-born infants and young children with an eruption consisting of small vesicles filled with a pellucid or slightly tinged fluid, surrounded by an inflamed base. When the vesicles break, they generally form into thin incrustations, but often the parts are inclined to ulcerate. The eruption is attended, especially at the outset, by more or less fever. Warm weather, or a warm room, and an excess of clothing, favour the development of the eruption. The daily use of the bath, with attention to ventilation and clothing, remove the disorder; if considerable fever, restlessness, $\frac{0}{3}$ of *Aconite* may be dissolved in three teaspoonfuls of water, and a teaspoonful given every twelve hours. *Rhus* $\frac{0}{3}$ may follow *Aconite* after 12 or 24 hours, when the eruption is extensive. *Sulph.* or *Ars.* $\frac{0}{6}$, if the eruption should still increase. *Cham.* $\frac{0}{3}$ after *Aconite* when the child is fretful and much excited; Bryon. $\frac{0}{3}$ when it is peevish, sleepless, and cannot bear to be moved.

DERANGEMENTS DURING TEETHING.

As already stated, about the fifth or sixth month the teeth generally begin to protrude. Under a proper system of treatment, if a due attention has been paid to the rules for exercise and diet which we have already laid down, and the child is free from any constitutional infirmity, we may calculate upon the period of dentition being exempt from much suffering.

Broths and jellies should, during the acute stages, be wholly prohibited, and its food, if it take other nourishment than the breast, be of the lightest and simplest description. The mother or nurse should pay particular regard to her regimen, and avoid all substances of a stimulating and indigestible nature. Here, we remark, that the indulgence in vinous or fermented liquors is, from their irritating properties, one of the most frequent causes of the suffering of children during this period.

During dentition there is always a tendency of blood to the head, which from simple irritation may, if not quickly checked, terminate in inflammation of the brain; the best remedy against this affection is keeping the head perfectly cool.

In order, as much as possible, to allay the anxiety of parents, who may be led to mistake the natural symptoms attendant upon dentition for those of disease, we shall in the first instance briefly enumerate those which frequently take place in healthy children, and may be safely left to nature; and afterwards proceed to point out in what cases, from any of the symptoms diverging from the usual track, it may be necessary to have recourse to medicines, or to call in a physician.

During the teething, the child is more restless than usual, especially at night; has flushes of heat, alternating with paleness; the gums gradually swell and become hot; it evinces a difficulty in sucking, sometimes forcibly bites, and frequently lets go the nipple; it drivels at the mouth, and its bowels become relaxed; the two latter symptoms may, in some measure, be looked upon as a wise precautionary measure of nature, to prevent a congestion to the head and lungs, to which all children are at this time more or less disposed; and the sudden cessation of either after having once set in, is a sign of derangement of functions, demanding prompt attention.

THERAPEUTICS. The medicines most generally required are *Coffea, Chamomilla, Nux v., Bellad., Cuprum acet., Calc. carb.*

When the child is in an excited state, and unable to sleep, irritable, liable to start, and difficult to soothe, a globule of *Coffea* may be administered; if the symptoms remain without alteration, we may have recourse to *Aconitum*. When benefit results from either one or the other remedy, the dose must only be repeated in the event of a threatening relapse.

CHAMOMILLA may be given after the foregoing remedies when they are merely productive of partial relief; or it may be given in preference thereto, if the following symptoms are encountered: extreme excitability; the infant starts at the slightest noise; evinces great thirst; spasmodic twitches or convulsions in the limbs during sleep; short, quick, and loud respirations, sometimes with a hacking cough; *excessive* diarrhœa, with *green*, whitish, or watery evacuations; and especially when the mother has been in the habit of taking *coffee*, which we have already so strongly reprobated as an article of diet to women nursing. *Mercurius* and *Sulphur* are sometimes requisite after *Chamomilla* against the diarrhœa. (See DIARRHŒA.)

ADMINISTRATION. $\frac{0}{6}$, in a teaspoonful of water, repeated at first in twenty-four, then in forty-eight hours, but oftener *if called for.*

When in the assemblage of these symptoms, *constipation* takes the place of diarrhœa, we may administer NUX VOMICA, $\frac{0}{30}$, repeated in from two to three days if necessary.

When strong symptoms of cerebral irritation exist, we should have instant recourse to BELLADONNA, or

Cuprum aceticum $\frac{0}{6}$. When marked *cerebral sensibility* declares itself, and the child almost spasmodically clenches the spoon or cup with its gums when drinking.

Administration, according to the formula given under *Scarlet Fever*, one fourth of the dose there specified.

When the irritation seems to arise *from difficulty of teething*, we may administer Calcarea, $\frac{0}{30}$, repeating it every eight days for about a month, which will materially assist the protrusion of the teeth.

When *obstinate constipation* is present, see that article in this part of the work. See also Convulsions in Children.

CONVULSIONS IN CHILDREN.

Early childhood is, from various causes, peculiarly predisposed to this distressing malady. They generally arise from the anatomical and physical peculiarities of infancy, in the preponderance of the nervous and cerebral systems over the other parts of the frame; hereditary predisposition called into activity by dentition—repelled eruptions, irritating substances in the stomach, intestinal worms, mechanical injuries, fright, and lastly, from some occult cause, frequently a derangement of the organic structure, in many instances bidding defiance to the powers of medicine. When no physician or medicines are at hand, and the danger is imminent, we may, in the first place, recommend immersing the lower extremities up to the knees in water, as hot as can be borne with safety to the infant, for the space of eight or ten minutes, until the paroxysms seem in a measure subdued; after which, the child should be wiped perfectly dry, and placed in a warm wrapper; if the first immersion be followed by no relief, it should be repeated; at the same time pour a small stream of cold water upon the crown of the head, until reanimation becomes apparent, when the child ought again to be warmly covered up; this course, *frequently repeated*, has been found to restore children, although the prior attempts have proved inefficient. When improper food or foreign substances in the stomach or intestines are the causes, lavements of equal parts of sweet oil and warm milk should precede the foot-bath;* if homœopathic medicines be not immediately at hand, the careful administration of *Camphor* by olfaction, or a drop or two of the tincture, considerably diluted, placed on the tongue, will frequently be found efficacious in giving relief, awaiting the arrival of a physician.

THERAPEUTICS. *Chamomilla, Belladonna, Ignatia amara, Cina, Mercurius, Cicuta virosa, Arsenicum, Bryonia, Sulphur, Nux vomica, Pulsatilla, Arnica, Opium, Stramonium, Secale, Cornutum*, and *Hyoscyamus*, are the most important remedies.†

Among these, *Chamomilla* stands in the first rank, particularly in very young children, when the convulsions have been excited by *dentition*, as well as for children who have passed that period, who are of a *nervo-sanguine* temperament, *extremely* sensitive, and *peevish*, or when the attacks have been excited by fever, colic, a chill, or a fit of passion, or vexation. The characteristic indications for its administration are: restlessness, fretfulness, and disposition to drowsiness when awake; one cheek red, the other pale, diarrhœa; (if this remedy be exhibited at this stage of the disorder, it will frequently prevent the fit from becoming fully developed;) eyes half-closed; great thirst; quick and loud breathing: rattling in the throat; moaning; cessation of consciousness; twitches of eyelids and muscles of the face; contortion of the eye-balls; *jerks and convulsions of the limbs, with clenched thumbs;* constant rolling of the head from side to side; loss of consciousness. (*Belladonna* may be substituted after *Chamomilla*, should this fail to do much good.)

ADMINISTRATION. We may, for very young children, dissolve one globule of the sixth potency in four teaspoonfuls of water, and administer one at the commencement of the attack; if fresh paroxysms come on some hours after, but *decreased in intensity*, we ought not to repeat the remedy, but allow it to exhaust its action; if the convulsions increase, on a second or

* Some useful remarks upon this subject may be found in the "HOMŒOPATHIC EXAMINER," (published in New York, vol. i, No. 2.)

† I may remark, that in plethoric, well-nourished children, great advantage will frequently be derived from administering a dose of *Aconite* prior to any of the other remedies.

third attack, we may give another spoonful; *unless other symp toms* declaring themselves, intimate that we ought to have recourse to any other of the undermentioned.

Belladonna, besides being useful in cases of suppressed eruptions, is more particularly indicated when the child starts suddenly, when asleep, or stares about wildly; the *pupils are much dilated;* the body or individual members become rigid; the forehead and hands dry and burning; occasionally followed by clenching of the hands; involuntary micturition after returning to consciousness; the *slightest touch* will sometimes provoke a renewal of the attack. This medicine is also indicated when the *paroxysms are preceded by smiles or laughter.*

Administration. $\frac{00}{30}$, in the same manner as *Chamomilla.*

It is frequently found that *Chamomilla* and *Belladonna* answer in alternation, and that when one has alleviated the evil, the other, sometimes followed by the one first administered, will dissipate the remaining symptoms.

In cases that withstand the exhibition of these two remedies, particularly during dentition, we frequently find Ignatia successful, more especially in children that appear of a *melancholy* temperament, or in pale, delicate infants, of peevish dispositions, with alternations of vivacity and sadness, and laughing and crying almost in the same breath.

Administration. Same as *Belladonna.*

The characteristic symptoms are:—The infant, while reposing in a moaning, light slumber, becomes suddenly *flushed with burning heat,* awakes, and springs with a convulsive start, and the utmost soothing scarcely quiets the excitement; *a tremor of the entire body,* attended by *violent crying* and agonizing shrieks; and the muscles of single limbs seem convulsed. Ignatia is further indicated when the fit returns *every day at a regular hour,* followed by fever and perspiration, or *every other day at variable hours.* (In other instances *Belladonna* will be found requisite after *Ignatia.*)

Ipecacuanha is useful when *great difficulty of breathing,* nausea, aversion to food, vomiting, either precede, accompany, or follow the attacks; and when the child has a constant inclination to remain in the recumbent posture.

Cina is useful, particularly during the second teething, for children of a melancholy temperament, scrofulous constitution, and who are troubled with worms, or habitually wet the bed; the characteristic symptoms are: spasms, commencing with constriction of the breast, followed by stiffness of limbs, pallor, and rigidity of the whole frame.

Administration. As *Chamomilla.* But in some cases it will be found useful to prescribe $\frac{0}{6}$ every four days for a week or a fortnight, in order to remove the susceptibility to the attack.

Mercurius in spasms which are caused by the presence of worms; *the stomach is swollen and hard before, during and after* the fit; the child is attacked with painful eructation, and a species of salivation; the limbs tossed and convulsed, attended by fever and moist skin; after the paroxysms the child lies for a long time exhausted and apparently dying.

Administration. Same as *Chamomilla.*

The foregoing are the more generally useful in ordinary cases; but the subjoined are sometimes called for in the particular instances specified.

Cicuta virosa is exceedingly serviceable when there is a clear indication of the presence of worms; when the child is first attacked with severe griping and colic, terminating in convulsions; the characteristic features of the fit are: *tremour of the limbs;* jerks like electric shocks, terminated by insensibility.

Administration. Same as *Cina.*

Arsenicum has proved very valuable in severe cases of convulsions, during dentition, when a *burning heat* diffuses itself over the whole body of the child; it stretches its feet out, and the hands convulsively backwards, then throws its hands about, and rolls over with violent shrieks; changes its position, and bends forward with *clenched fingers and extended thumbs;* it is irritable, restless, and perverse; evinces *insatiable thirst,* but drinks little at a time, with diarrhœa, sometimes of *undigested food;* frequently vomits immediately after taking food; the paroxysms recur frequently, and all attempts at soothing seem only to irritate the child.

Administration. Same as the foregoing.

BRYONIA is valuable in convulsions arising from suppressed measles. (See MEASLES, p. 59.)

ADMINISTRATION. Same as *Arsenicum*.

SULPHUR is particularly indicated in spasms arising from *repelled chronic eruptions ;* but such cases should be confined to experienced medical care, as until the disease is completely eradicated, the constant liability to such attacks still exists.

When the disease arises from indigestible substances being taken into the stomach, NUX VOMICA or PULSATILLA may be given according to the symptoms and disposition for which the indications have been already given in different parts of the work, to which the reader is referred. (See tabular Index.)

In cases of mechanical lesion, ARNICA, $\frac{0}{6}$, and externally in lotion, where any wound or contusion exists.

In cases of convulsions from FRIGHT, we may have recourse to OPIUM, $\frac{0}{3}$ or $\frac{0}{6}$, when the following appearances are present: general trembling; throwing about of limbs; vacant stare; cries seemingly unconscious; stertorous breathing, and final insensibility.

STRAMONIUM $\frac{0}{6}$, when the child becomes suddenly convulsed and senseless from fright.

SECALE CORNUTUM, $\frac{0}{12}$, in alternation with *Stramonium*, in cases where the latter does not afford relief.

HYOSCYAMUS, $\frac{0}{12}$, when *sudden fright* causes very violent convulsions. (See MENTAL EMOTIONS, Part II., p. 438.)

WATER IN THE HEAD. *Hydrocephalus.*

This fatal and frequent disease is liable to be excited by a variety of causes, and is particularly prone to take place in scrofulous children, who are born with unusually large heads, and in whom the fontanels remain long unclosed. The *symptoms* are sometimes so mild and insidious, that parents are thrown off their guard, and attribute the apparently slight indisposition of the little patient to some comparatively trivial circumstance; such as teething, or gastric derangement. In other instances, the symptoms are much more striking, and in many respects strongly resemble those described under Inflammation of the brain. In general, the skin is hot, pulse rather quick, chiefly at night, and the child becomes *peevish* whenever it is *raised from the horizontal position*; at other times it is affected with fits of screaming; grinding of the teeth; redness of the face and eyes; peculiar expression of countenance; convulsion and stupor.

THERAPEUTICS. The most appropriate remedies are: *Aconite, Belladonna, Bryonia, Helleborus, Mercurius,* and *Sulphur,* or *Sulphuris Tinctura.* The indications for the two former have already been given under INFLAMMATION OF THE BRAIN, Part II., p. 271.

ADMINISTRATION. Two globules at the potency mentioned, in four teaspoonfuls of water, one daily; in severe attacks every six or twelve hours, carefully studying the effects of each dose, and acting accordingly.*

BRYONIA, $\frac{0}{6}$, may be administered *after Aconite* or *Bellad.*, if necessary, or may be given at the commencement, when there is heat in the head, with dark redness of the face, and great thirst; eyes convulsed, or at one time closed, and at another wide open or fixed; delirium; sudden starts, with cries, or constant inclination to sleep; continual movement of the jaws as if engaged in chewing; tongue coated yellow; abdomen distended; urine suppressed, or the passing of urine appears to cause pain; great thirst, especially at night; skin hot and dry; respiration hurried, laborious, and anxious; constipation.

HELLEBORUS NIGER $\frac{0}{3}$. This remedy, as stated by Dr. Wahle,† will generally prevent a fatal termination, when BRYONIA merely produces only temporary benefit. The same authority quotes it as being the most important medicine in all serious cases, and that it should be given in these at the very commencement in preference to all other remedies; followed by *Sulphuris Tinct.* when danger is not removed within a few hours, and when spasms are present.

MERCURIUS, $\frac{0}{12}$, will sometimes be found useful after *Belladonna,* or previous to that remedy, when the bowels are much relaxed. *Hyoscyamus, Opium, Cina,* and *Stramonium,* may

* Vide note, p. 21.

* Brit. Journ. of Homœopathy, No. vii., p. 286.

likewise prove valuable in cases wherein the indications correspond with those described in PART II., and in some cases, *Lachesis*, particularly when the disease has reached an advanced stage. *Kali hydriod.*, *Digitalis*, *Arnica*, and *Conium*, have also been named as likely to prove serviceable in this malady. In chronic cases, Dr. Wahle recommends *Helleborus*, *Arsenicum*, and *Sulphur* in particular.

ASTHMA OF MILLAR. *Laryngismus Stridulus.*

This affection is by some denominated the Spasmodic Croup, or Acute Asthma of infants; it bears a considerable resemblance to croup, but differs from it in many respects, by the extreme suddenness of the attack, while that of croup is generally preceded one or two days by hoarseness and a slight cough, and by the cessation from suffering the patient enjoys between the attacks; while, when croup has once set in, the excitement is permanent; moreover, this disease generally attacks in the evening or at night, whereas croup in most cases makes its first appearance during the day.

Croup, as we mentioned in the article upon that subject, is an inflammation of the membrane of the windpipe, exciting the formation of a peculiar secretion, which if not checked, concretes into an abnormal membraneous tissue, constituting what is technically called the *false membrane* of croup; whereas, in the Asthma of Millar, the suffering appears to arise from a *spasmodic contraction of the top of the windpipe*, impeding the progress of respiration.

The attack commences with a sudden spasmodic inspiration, with a species of stridulous or crowing noise; if the fit continues, the face becomes purple, and the extremities partake of the same hue, frequently accompanied, as in convulsions, with a clenching of the thumbs inside the palm, and spasmodic constriction of the toes, giving an appearance of distortion to the foot; if proper means are not promptly taken, these attacks recur frequently, and at short intervals, and occasionally the little patient perishes during one of the paroxysms.

The disease rarely occurs except in infants of delicate constitution, which due means should be taken to endeavour to eradicate by a proper course of treatment; it is a frequent accompaniment of the period of dentition, and excited by similar causes to those bringing on convulsions.

THERAPEUTICS. *Aconite, Ipecacuanha, Arsenicum, Sambucus, Moschus* or *Pulsatilla*, are the medicines which have been employed by homœopathists with the most successful results.

ADMINISTRATION. A globule every one or two hours, according to symptoms.

ACONITE, $\frac{0}{12}$, when a suffocating cough comes on at night, with shrillness and hoarseness of voice; respiration short, anxious, and difficult, more particularly if any marked febrile symptoms be present, or we have reason to dread determination of blood to the head.

IPECACUANHA, $\frac{0}{3}$, when there is *rattling in the chest*, from an accumulation of mucus, with spasmodic constriction, and symptoms as from suffocation; anxious and short, or sighing respiration, with purple colour of the face, and cramps, or rigidity of the frame; it may be advantageously followed by

ARSENICUM, $\frac{0}{30}$, when many of the above symptoms are still present, or in a measure subdued; also if we find *great anguish, cold perspiration and considerable prostration of strength*, during and after the paroxysms; when these last indications are particularly prominent, *Arsenicum* may supersede *Ipecacuanha* at the commencement.

SAMBUCUS, $\frac{0}{3}$. Lethargy, or ineffectual inclination to sleep, with oppressed respiration and wheezing; livid hue of the face, agonizing jactitations, dry heat of the trunk; no thirst; pulse small, irregular, and intermittent.

MOSCHUS, $\frac{0}{3}$, is frequently of value in cases that occur at *a more advanced period of life*, when a *constriction in the larynx, as if caused by the vapour of sulphur*, is complained of; difficult respiration and short breathing; *severe spasms in the chest*, with inclination to cough, after which (especially in children) the paroxysms become *much exacerbated*.

PULSATILLA, $\frac{0}{12}$, will often be found successful in cases in which the foregoing remedy fails in producing the desired effect.

THE RICKETS. *Rachitis.*

This malady almost invariably begins to show itself at the tender age of from one to two years, and is distinguished by great development of head, abnormally prominent forehead, projecting sternum, flattened ribs, enlarged abdomen, with emaciation of the extremities, and extreme general debility. As the disease progresses, the muscles become more flaccid, the epiphyses of the limbs increase in size, the bones and dorsal spine become more or less distorted, the bowels relaxed and the motions frequent; and frequently, if the disease be not arrested, slow fever, with cough, oppressed breathing and atrophy supervene, and a fatal termination results.

Therapeutics. The remedies which have hitherto been employed with the greatest success in the treatment of this distressing affection by homœopathists are: *Belladonna, Mercurius, Arsenicum, Sulphur, Calcarea, Silicea ;* also *Asafœtida, Acidum phosphoricum, Phosphorus, Baryta-muriatica, Staphysagria, Lycopodium, Acidum nitricum, Mezereum, Petroleum,* and *Rhus.** (See Atrophy, p. 493.)

INFANTILE REMITTENT FEVER.

By infantile remittent is here chiefly meant that form of fever which occurs in infants and children, arising from morbid irritability, inflammation or even ulceration in the mucous membrane of the stomach and bowels.

The affection is usually preceded by languor, irritability of temper, want of appetite, nausea, thirst, slight heat of skin, and very restless nights. Ere long these symptoms present themselves in a more aggravated form, together with an acquisition of abnormal phenomena, such as hurried and oppressive breathing, quickness of pulse, with occasional flushes in the face, vomiting of food or bile, distention and tenderness of the abdomen; obstinate constipation; sometimes diarrhœa, or frequent desire to go to stool with but little effect; motions discoloured,

* The author begs to refer the reader to a somewhat interesting case of Rachitis, which he published in the *Brit. Journ. of Homœopathy,* No. 10, p. 105.

fetid, frequently mixed with mucus, and occasionally with blood. The hands and feet are often cold, while the rest of the body is parched; the head hot and heavy, or attended with other symptoms resembling hydrocephalus, such as coma, etc. The tongue, at first moist, loaded, and occasionally very red along the margins, often becomes dry over a triangular spot at the point. When the febrile exacerbation takes place at night, it is accompanied by vigilance and jactitation; when during the day, there is, on the other hand, drowsiness and stupor. An annoying cough with bronchitic indications, succeeded by wheezing and expectoration, sometimes appears. Although, as is characteristic of remittent fever, the febrile symptoms never entirely subside, still the patient will frequently appear to be steadily recovering for a time, and the unwary or inexperienced may consequently be led to pronounce an unduly favourable prognosis, which will too often be contradicted by the occurrence of a relapse, followed perhaps again by another encouraging but deceptive remission; and so on, unless the progress of the disease be checked, until either the mesenteric glands become affected, dropsical effusion into the cavity of the abdomen ensues, or unequivocal signs of cephalic disease become established, or the little sufferer is so emaciated and reduced by protracted disease, that the vital powers give way, and he sinks exhausted.

THERAPEUTICS. In mild attacks occurring in tolerably healthy children, the disease is generally readily subdued in a few days, by means of one or more of the following remedies: *Ipecacuanha*, *Pulsatilla*, *China*, *Nux v.*, *Aconitum*, *Belladonna*, *Mercurius*, *Bryonia*, *Lachesis*, *Chamomilla*, and *Sulphur*, combined with light farinaceous diet. Solid food must be strictly prohibited, even although the appetite should be good, which it occasionally is, and even ravenous at times.

With regard to the indications for the remedies quoted, *Ipecacuanha* may be given if, as is generally the case, the attack has been excited by over-feeding, or by indigestible food, and particularly when the patient has contracted a habit of *bolting* the food without having previously masticated it properly, and the symptoms encountered are as follows:—General dry heat, or harsh and parched skin, especially towards evening; thirst, extreme restlessness, burning heat in the palms of the hands; perspiration at night, quick oppressed breathing foul tongue, nausea, vomiting, or fastidious appetite with sickness after eating; great languor, apathy, and indifference. Should these symptoms remain unaltered after several doses of *Ipecac.*, or should the bowels become very relaxed, the motions fetid, whitish, bilious, or of variable colour at different times, and accompanied with griping and distention of the abdomen; fever during the night—*Pulsatilla* must be prescribed, followed, if required, by *Cinchona*, especially if the nausea or vomiting has subsided, but the bowels remain relaxed, and are considerably distended, or tense and tympanitic.

Nux vomica $\frac{0}{3}$ is also a most efficient remedy in mild cases, or in the early stage of the disorder of any variety, when the bowels are confined, or very costive, with frequent inclination to go to stool; or when there is tenesmus, followed by scanty watery motions, generally mixed with mucus, or occasionally with a little blood; abdomen tumid and rather painful; further, when the child is excessively peevish and ungovernable; the tongue foul; appetite impaired, or there is nausea with disgust at food; restlessness; fever towards morning, but also in some degree during the night.

Chamomilla $\frac{0}{3}$ is sometimes useful after *Nux v.* when burning heat of skin continues, or when bilious vomiting or diarrhœa supervenes; the tongue red and cracked, or coated yellow; sleep lethargic, or restless and agitated, attended with frequent starts and jerkings of the limbs; flushes of heat in various parts of the body. Also when the little patient is of a plethoric habit, or in all cases in which the head is hot and heavy, the skin dry or parched, the face flushed, the pulse quick; and when there is thirst, foul tongue, nausea, bilious vomiting; no motions, or frequent and scanty evacuations, with tenesmus.

Belladonna $\frac{0}{3}$ may succeed the former remedy if the head continue hot, the pulse excessively quiet and full, the tongue loaded, or coated white or yellow in the centre, and very red at the edges; thirst; nausea or vomiting; great heat of the abdomen with tenderness on the slightest pressure; oppressive breathing. If the more active inflammatory symptoms yield to the action of *Belladonna*,—Mercurius $\frac{0}{6}$ will often serve to complete the cure; but more particularly when the following symptoms remain: loaded tongue, nausea or vomiting, with continued tenderness of the abdomen; thirst, sometimes with aversion to drinks when offered; no motions, or diarrhœa with excessive tenesmus. If, on the other hand, the head continue hot and heavy, the pulse quick, the tongue foul, and other symptoms of gastric derangement prominent, together with a tumid and painful state of the abdomen, constipation, excessive restlessness, and quick, laborious respiration, particularly at night, with drowsiness during the day, *Bryonia* is to be preferred.

Lachesis $\frac{0}{6}$ may follow *Belladonna* $\frac{0}{3}$ or $\frac{0}{6}$ *Mercurius* when the signs of intestinal irritation or inflammation continue with but little abatement. Or it may precede these remedies, when the tenderness and distention is more marked at one particular spot (the most trivial pressure there being intolerable) than over the entire abdomen; and when the fever is highest at night.

Sulphur $\frac{0}{6}$ may be given with advantage to complete the cure in many cases, after the previous employment of any of the foregoing medicines. It is, however, when the attack is characterized by the following features that this remedy is more directly called for: feverish heat, especially towards evening, but also in the morning, or during the day; flushes alternately with paleness of the face; dryness of the skin; hurried and laborious breathing; palpitation of the heart; nocturnal perspiration; languor and great weakness, particularly in the inferior extremities; tense, tumid and painful abdomen; dry, hard, or loose and slimy motions.

These, then, are the more generally useful remedies in cases of the above description, and will materially tend to facilitate recovery, and prevent the disease from assuming an obstinate character. When, however, the malady occurs in children of relaxed and feeble habits, or of a decided strumous diathesis, it becomes, especially if neglected, and not checked at the commencement of its course, a most intractable and frequently fatal disease, from the proneness which it then has to become complicated, and terminate in one or other of the serious forms alluded to in the diagnosis.

The remedies from which the most benefit is to be anticipated under such unfavourable circumstances are, in addition to those previously mentioned: *Silicea, Sulphur, Calcarea, Baryta c., Arsenicum, Cocculus, Cina, Sabadilla,* etc.

Silicea $\frac{0}{6}$, when there is great emaciation, languor and debility, paleness of the face, want of appetite, or craving for dainties; shortness of breath on movement; feverish heat in the morning or towards evening. This remedy is also a most important one when the patient is afflicted with worms, and when the disease is in a great measure attributable to invermination. *Cina* and *Sabadilla* may likewise be found useful along with *Silicea* in the latter instance. (See Invermination.) The indications for sulphur have already been given.

Calcarea $\frac{0}{6}$. Great debility, with flabbiness of the muscles, dryness of the skin, and excessive emaciation; frequent flushes, or general heat, followed by shivering towards evening; exhaustion, or dejection after speaking; impaired, fastidious appetite, with weak and slow digestion, or, on the contrary, extreme voracity; perspiration towards morning, hard, tense, and tumid abdomen. (*Baryta c.* is sometimes useful after *Calcarea.*

Arsenicum $\frac{0}{6}$. Extreme prostration of strength and emaciation, with desire to remain constantly in the recumbent posture; dry, burning heat of the skin, with great thirst, but desire to drink little at a time, or merely to moisten the lips, which are frequently parched; impaired appetite, and sometimes excessive irritability of stomach, so that very little food can be retained; hard and tense abdomen; restless, unrefreshing sleep, and frequent starts, or subsultus tendinum; fretful and capricious disposition.

Cocculus $\frac{0}{3}$. Great weakness, with excessive fatigue, depression, and tremor, after the slightest exertion; heavy, expressionless eyes; flushes of heat in the face; nausea, or aversion to food, distention of the abdomen, constipation; oppressed respiration; perspiration on attempting any trivial exertion; lowness of spirits; mildness of temper.

Belladonna, Lachesis, or *Baryta c.,* will be required when the head becomes much affected. The former especially when there is heat, heaviness, flushing and delirium; or deep and protracted sleep with subsultus tendinum, coldness of the hands, pale cold face, small quick pulse, hot, tumid, and tense abdomen. LACHESIS:—Either, before or after *Belladonna*, when we encounter deep prolonged sleep; grinding of the teeth; or somnolency alternately with sleeplessness; tremulous, intermittent, or scarcely perceptible pulse.

BARYTA. $\frac{0}{6}$ Lethargy, jactitation, or agitation, moaning and muttering, feeble and accelerated pulse. (See HYDROCEPHALUS.)

Other remedies, such as *Antimonium*, *Acid. phosphoricum*, *Phosphorus*, *Hepar s.*, *Kali*, *Acidum nitr.*, *Lycopodium*, *Rhus*, etc., may be required according as the symptoms happen to vary; we have merely given some of those medicines which have been found of valuable service when the indications were as above given. It may be added, that when the skin is hot and parched, the sleeplessness and restlessness is often temporarily removed by sponging the body with tepid water: this is, however, only to be had recourse to when the remedies fail to afford this relief, and that in a more permanent degree. (See also ATROPHY.)

ATROPHY. *Atrophia.*

The medicines from which the most appreciable assistance has hitherto been obtained in this serious malady are:—*Sulph.*, followed by *Calcarea*; also *Ars.*, *Bar. c.*, *Bell.*, *Chin.*, *Nux vom.*, *Phosph.*, and *Rhus.*

SULPHUR $\frac{0}{6}$ in almost all cases at the commencement of treatment; craving appetite; enlargement of inguinal or axillary glands; slimy diarrhœa or obstinate constipation; pale complexion, sunken eyes, &c.

CALCAREA, $\frac{0}{6}$. Great emaciation, with craving appetite; enlargement and induration of the mesenteric glands; great weakness, clayey evacuation, a dry and flabby skin; too great a susceptibility of the nervous system.

ARSENICUM, $\frac{0}{6}$. Dryness of skin, which resembles parchment; hollow eyes; *desire to drink often, but little at a time; excessive agitation and tossing, especially at night*; short sleep interrupted by jerks; fæces of greenish or brownish colour, with evacuations of ingesta; extreme prostration.

Baryta, $\frac{0}{6}$. Enlargement of the glands of the nape of the neck; continual desire to sleep; great indolence, and aversion to exertion and amusement.

Bell., $\frac{0}{3}$. Capriciousness and obstinacy; nocturnal cough, with rattling of mucus; enlargement of the glands of the neck; unquiet sleep; precocity of intellect, blue eyes, and fair hair.

China, $\frac{0}{3}$. Excessive emaciation; voraciousness; diarrhœa at night, with frequent white evacuations, or of ingesta; frequent perspirations, especially at night; unrefreshing sleep.

Cina, $\frac{0}{3}$. Vermiculous suffering; wetting the bed. (See Worms.)

Rhus. Slimy or sanguineous diarrhœa; debility; voracity.

In children past the age of infancy, great attention should be paid to the diet; pure air and exercise are also of great importance.

VACCINATION.

This is an operation purely homœopathic, and one which, from its efficacy in the prevention of a disease exhibiting analogous symptoms, has been frequently quoted by our Great Founder and his disciples, as one of the best illustrations of the immutable law of SIMILIA SIMILIBUS CURANTUR.

Vaccination, when the child is strong and healthy, may be safely performed during the fourth and fifth month; but when the smallpox is rife as an epidemic, we may have recourse to this prophylax with infants of a still more tender age. If, however, we are allowed a choice of time, summer is the best period for performing the operation, as then the infant, after having taken the infection, incurs least risk of catching cold.

It is of the utmost importance to obtain the lymph from a perfectly sure source, as experience has too truly proved, that other diseases have, from a neglect of this precaution, been frequently transmitted to healthy children. For this reason, a child that has suffered from eruptions of the skin, affections of the glands, or soreness of the eyes, or one born of scrofulous parents, is an unfit subject for taking the vaccine matter from, although at the time apparently in health.

PART IV.

TREATMENT OF FEMALES,

AND

THEIR PECULIAR AFFECTIONS.

CHLOROSIS. Emansio Mensium.

This complaint generally declares itself in young females about their fourteenth year. Its proximate cause is an obstruction of the first menstruation; a disease very similar may be produced by great loss of blood.

Diagnosis. Pale blanched complexion and lips (sometimes with flushes of heat and redness), a depravity of appetite, a longing after innutritious substances, such as chalk, &c., and a general languor both mental and physical; the patient complains of weariness, lassitude and debility, and becomes emaciated; the lower extremities frequently assume an œdematous appearance, generally attended with cold in those parts, and headache, with flatulent distention of the abdomen, particularly after meals, and in the evening; bowels irregularly confined; sometimes at a later period very easily irritated and relaxed; a harsh harassing cough, occasionally with periodical expectoration of dark-coloured coagulated blood, and hurried respiration, frequently declares itself, if the affection has been allowed to proceed unchecked; and to an inexperienced eye, the sufferer appears to be on the verge, or even passing through the different stages, of a decline.

Therapeutics. The predisposing causes of this affection are very remote; we shall therefore be satisfied with confining ourselves to the treatment of the complaint in its more simple stage, as when we find an extremely obstinate case, we may feel confident that it requires a regular course of treatment, or originates in some organic derangement. The medicines hitherto found most useful in ordinary cases of this affection are, *Pulsatilla, Sepia, Bryonia, Sulphur*, and *Natrum m.*

Administration. Six globules of the potency mentioned after each medicine, in six tea-spoonfuls of water, one daily; and so on until benefit results, or it is found necessary to choose another remedy.*

Pulsatilla, $\frac{\circ\circ\circ}{12}$, or in light cases, 3 globules taken dry, when the complaint has been the effect of *dampness, or caused by damp or cold air*, or when it is accompanied by frequent attacks of semi-lateral headache, with shooting pains, extending to the head and teeth, *sometimes shifting suddenly to the other side*; also when we observe aching in the forehead, with pressure at the crown of the head, and *sallow complexion*, alternating with flushes of heat; difficulty of breathing, and sense of suffocation after the slightest movement; *palpitation of the heart; coldness of the hands and feet*, often changing to *sudden heat; disposition to diarrhœa and leucorrhœa;* pains in the loins; sensation of weight in the abdomen; spasms in the stomach, *with nausea, inclination to vomit, and vomiting;* periodical expectoration of dark coagulated blood; hunger, with repugnance to food, or want of appetite with dislike to food; great fatigue, especially in the legs. This medicine is peculiarly adapted to females of mild or phlegmatic disposition, disposed to sadness and tears.

Graphites, $\frac{\circ\circ\circ}{30}$, when there is retention of the period with congestion of the vessels of the head and chest; dark red flushing of the face, oppression at the chest; and a feeling of anxiety when in the recumbent posture. *Graphites*, together with *Causticum*, form two of the most important remedies in *scanty, insufficient* menstruation. *Belladonna* is often called for when the congestion of the head and chest is of an active character, with violent throbbing of the carotids.

Sepia, $\frac{\circ\circ\circ}{30}$, is also a very valuable remedy in this affection, when many of the above symptoms are present, with, at the same time, *hysterical megrims; complexion sallow, with dark-coloured spots;* frequent colic and pain as of a bruise in the

* Vide note, p. 21.

limbs. When the above symptoms declare themselves, advantageously follow *Pulsatilla*, if the latter have failed to relieve.

BRYONIA, $\frac{0\,0\,0}{6}$. Frequent congestion in the head or chest; *bleeding at the nose;* dry cough; coldness and frequent shivering, sometimes alternated with dry and burning heat; constipation or colic; bitter taste in the mouth, tongue coated yellow, sense of pressure *in the stomach, as if from a stone;* irascibility.

SULPHUR, $\frac{0\,0\,0}{6}$, is more particularly indicated when there *is pressive and tensive pain in the back of the head, extending to the nape of the neck;* or pulsative pain in the head, with determination of blood; *humming in the head; pimples on the forehead and round the mouth;* pale and sickly complexion, with red spots on the cheeks; voracious appetite; general emaciation; sour and burning eructations; *pressive fulness and heaviness in the stomach under the lower ribs and in the abdomen; bowels irregular;* difficulty of breathing; pain in the loins and fainting; *excessive fatigue, especially in the legs, with great depression after talking; great tendency to take cold;* irritability, and inclination to be angry; or, sadness and melancholy, with frequent weeping. In some cases, one or the other of the following medicines: *Conium, Kali carb., Phosph., Ferrum, Ignatia, Lycopod., Acid. nitr.*, etc.

CALC. CARB. $\frac{0\,0\,0}{12}$, has often completed a cure in the worst cases, with œdema of the extremities and extreme dyspnœa. It is necessary to follow up the treatment, on the disappearance of the more important symptoms under the employment of *Calc.*, with *Ferrum carb.* in repeated doses, to prevent a relapse. *Ferrum* is required when the pale and sickly hue of the face continues, notwithstanding the previous use of *Calc.* When *Ferrum* was given at the commencement, it did not aggravate the anxiety, cough, and other pectoral symptoms. Where there is a complication with tubercular diathesis, accompanied by cough, etc., coeval with the first appearance of chlorosis, *Sulph.* and *Calc.*, often prove beneficial in alternation. During the employment of *Calc.*, a dose of *Lycop.* is required, when there is constipation and extreme languor, or *Sepia*, when there is oppressive headache. Sometimes the menses do not appear for some time afterwards, although health may have been renovated.

Valeriana $\frac{000}{3}$, has been found of great service in daily-repeated doses, when a feeling of constriction was experienced in the gullet or chest, accompanied with signs of threatened suffocation, and followed by frequent yawning, as soon as the patient sat down to dinner.

Natrum muriaticum, potency $\frac{000}{6}$, $\frac{000}{12}$, or $\frac{000}{30}$, is a most valuable remedy in many obstinate cases, either exhibited as above described, or by giving a dose twice or thrice a week.

Plumbum aceticum has been found useful in cases with dyspnœa, œdema, and anasarca.

AMENORRHŒA. *Suppressio Mensium.*

Suppression of the menses occasionally takes place suddenly from some accidental cause, such as exposure to cold, powerful mental emotions, &c. In other instances the suppression is symptomatic of some other disease, either organic or functional, and can only be removed by the cure of the primary malady. It is of the former that we here propose to treat.

When a suppression takes place from the sudden effects of a chill, we may have recourse to *Pulsatilla*, when the symptoms generally correspond to those of that remedy, as detailed under Chlorosis. In other cases arising from this cause, *Nux moschata, Dulcamara, Sepia*, or *Sulphur* may be necessary. (See Chlorosis, for indications for *Sulph.* and *Sep.*, which are remedies of great service in a large number of cases, when the affection becomes chronic.)

When a sudden fright has given rise to the affection, *Aconitum* should be immediately administered, followed by *Lycopodium, Opium*, or *Veratrum*, if the bad consequences which frequently result do not yield, or if only partial relief is obtained from the employment of *Aconitum*. (See Mental Emotions, Parts II. and III.)

In chronic cases occurring in weak or debilitated individuals, in addition to *Sulphur* and *Sepia*, the following remedies are useful: *Natrum m., Conium, Arsenic., Cinch., Graph., Caust., Iodium*. Whilst in those which occur in plethoric subjects, whether of a chronic or recent description, *Aconit.*, *Bellad.*, *Sulphur*, *Bryon.*, *Nux v.*, *Sabina*, *Opium*, *Platina*, &c., will chiefly be found the most serviceable. When there is not a complete suppression, but the menstrual discharge is scanty and insufficient, *Graphit.*, *Causticum*, *Kali*, *Conium*, *Natrum m.*, *Phosph.*, *Pulsat.*, *Sulphur*, *Lycopod.*, *Magnesia*, *Silicea*, *Veratrum*, or *Zincum*, are the most important remedies. Dose: see ADMINISTRATION, under Chlorosis.

MENSTRUATIO NIMIA. MENOCHASIA. MENORRHAGIA.

The quantity of the menstrual discharge varies a good deal in different women. Considerable influence is for the most part exerted by climate, constitution, and the manner of living. The duration of the discharge and the period of return are also variable. In some, it continues from four to ten days, in others, it lasts only a few hours; from three to six days is, however, the most usual. The regularity is, in many, exact to a day, or even an hour, while in others a variation of several days is a usual occurrence, without the slightest disturbance to the general health resulting therefrom. When the discharge is excessive, and attended with pains in the back, loins, and abdomen, resembling those of labour, it becomes necessary to prescribe remedies calculated to arrest it, and to correct the tendency thereto. Amongst these the following are of great utility: *Ipecac.*, *Crocus*, *Sabina*, *Cinch.*, *Nux v.*, *Cham.*, *Platina*, *Sulph.*, *Calc.*, &c.

IPECACUANHA is generally useful in severe cases of this derangement, as well as in flooding after labour, and may in most instances be administered first, unless there are strong indications for a preference being given to any of the others.

ADMINISTRATION. $\frac{000}{3}$, repeated in from six to twenty-four hours.*

CROCUS is more especially called for when the discharge is of a dark colour, viscid, and very copious; and the menses have appeared before the usual time.

ADMINISTRATION. Same as the above.

* Vide note, page 21.

Sabina, when the discharge is excessive, of a bright colour, and occurs in plethoric females who are prone to miscarry, rheumatic pains in the head and limbs; great weakness; pains in the loins similar to those of labour.

Administration. $\frac{000}{6}$, repeated in from six to twenty-four hours.

Cinchona is of considerable utility after the previous employment of the foregoing, and in all cases where there is great debility in consequence of a more copious menstrual discharge than natural.

Administration. $\frac{00}{6}$, repeated in twenty-four hours.

Nux v., when the discharge is of too frequent occurrence, too profuse, and of too long duration; and when it commonly stops for a day or so and then returns, attended with spasms in the abdomen; sometimes nausea and fainting, especially in the morning; pains in the limbs; restlessness; irascibility. *Nux v.* is especially serviceable when the above symptoms occur in females who are addicted to the daily or frequent use of coffee, liqueurs and other stimuli.

Administration. $\frac{00}{3}$ or $\frac{00}{12}$ during the existence of the menstrual discharge, and a globule or two in a teaspoonful of water every fourth day during the interval before the next periodical return.

Chamomilla is frequently useful after *Nux v.*. but particularly when there is a discharge of dark, clotted blood, with severe colic, or pains like those of labour; great thirst; paleness of the face, and coldness of the limbs.

Administration. Same as *Nux.*

Ignatia is of considerable service when the derangement happens in hysterical females.

Administration. $\frac{00}{12}$ or $\frac{00}{30}$ during the period; the dose to be repeated once during the interval.

Platina. Preternaturally increased menstrual discharge, with painful bearing-down pains, and venereal orgasm; thick dark-coloured menstrual blood; great excitability.

Administration. $\frac{000}{6}$ during the discharge; to be repeated in twenty-four hours if the pains continue.

VERATRUM. Too early or too copious menstrual discharge, always attended with diarrhœa.

ADMINISTRATION. $\frac{000}{12}$ or $\frac{000}{30}$, repeated in twenty-four to forty-eight hours, if required.

SULPHUR administered thrice during the intervals, allowing ten or twelve days to elapse between the second dose, and followed by *Calcarea*, in the same manner, has frequently been found successful when any of the previous remedies afforded but temporary relief. In other cases *Belladonna*, *Bryon.*, *Natrum m.*, *Magnesia m.*, *Sepia*, *Silicea*, or *Phosphorus*, &c., may be useful. Dose: Same as *Nux v.*

DYSMENORRHŒA.

In painful and difficult menstruation, or menstrual colic, the most important remedies are the same as those enumerated under MENORRHAGIA and CHLOROSIS, but particularly *Chamom.*, *Pulsatilla*, *Belladonna*, *Nux*, *Coffea*, *Sulph.* and *Calc.*, &c.,* when the disorder occurs with great vehemence at the critical age (*tour d'âge*).

LACHESIS is of invaluable assistance, and particularly when diarrhœa, attended with almost insupportable tormina, usually sets in before and after the menstrual period; but the following are likewise of considerable utility: *Pulsatilla*, *Sepia*, *Sulphur*, *Cocculus*, *Ruta*, *Conium*. Against *uterine spasms*, *Cocculus*, *Pulsatilla*, *Ignatia*, *Platina*, *Cuprum*, form the most valuable remedial agents; but in some instances, *Nux v.*, *Cinchona*, *Sulphur*, *Graphites*, *Conium*, or *Natrum m.*, &c., may be more appropriate. Dose: see ADMINISTRATION under *Chlorosis*.

HYSTERICS. *Hysteria.* *Passio Hysterica.*

This disease appears in paroxysms, is preceded generally by depression of spirits, anxiety, effusion of tears, dyspnœa, nausea, and palpitatio cordis; also with pain is the left side, which seems to advance upwards till it gets to the throat, when it feels as if a ball were lodged there, (globus hystericus;) if it

* We have derived immediate relief from *Sabina* when all other expedients proved inefficacious.—ED.

advanced further, there is sense of suffocation, stupor and insensibility, with spasmodic clenching of the jaws; the trunk of the body is moved about, and the limbs agitated; alternate fits of laughing, crying, and screaming; incoherent expressions; the foaming mouth; relief ensues generally with eructation, and frequent sighing and sobbing, followed by a sense of soreness over the whole body. Hiccough is sometimes a concomitant, and a very distressing one, in hysteria. These are the usual symptoms accompanying this disease, but the complaint appears in a great variety of forms; and in many cases the patient is attacked with a violent spasmodic pain in the back, which extends from the spine to the sternum, and eventually becomes fixed at the epigastric region, and is often so intense as to cause clammy perspiration, a pale cadaverous countenance; coldness of the extremities; and a feeble thread-like, or scarcely perceptible pulse.

Hysteric affections are more frequent in single than in married life, and usually occur between the age of puberty and that of thirty-five, and generally about the period of menstruation.

The disorder is readily excited in those who are subject to it, by sudden mental emotions. They have been known to arise from sympathy and imitation.

Women of delicate habit, and of extreme nervous sensibility, are chiefly prone to be affected with hysteria, and are predisposed to the attack by an inactive or sedentary life, distress of mind, suppression or obstruction to the periodical illness, excessive depletion, or constant use of spare or unwholesome diet.

Those of a nervous, sanguine or plethoric temperament are chiefly liable to this disease.

The best medicines against hysterical affections are *Aurum, Bellad., Calc., Caust., Cocc., Con., Ignat., Lach., Mosch., N. mosch., Nux v., Phosph., Plat., Puls., Sepia, Sil., Stram., Sulp., Verat., Valeriana,* etc.

When the affection arises from CHLOROSIS or AMENORRHŒA, see the remedies mentioned under these headings.

When from MENORRHAGIA; see *that article.* MENTAL EMOTIONS; see the same.

When the attacks are attended with clenching of the jaws,

or general spasm, coldness of the extremities, and clammy sweat, particularly on the face and forehead, *Veratrum* is a valuable remedy. (See also the remedies mentioned under TETANUS, and likewise LOCKJAW IN INFANTS.)

When violent spasmodic *hiccough* predominates: *Nux v.*, *Bellad.*, and *Stramonium*:—*Hyoscyamus*, *Veratrum*, *Ignatia*, *Pulsat.*, *Cicuta*, *Bryonia*, and *Sulph.* will be found the most frequently useful. Dose: see *Administr.* under Chlorosis.

OBSERVATIONS ON PREGNANCY.

THIS period may be looked upon as one of the most interesting eras of a woman's life. She is now no longer acting for herself alone, but becomes invested with a new and serious responsibility, and upon some of the most apparently trifling of her actions may depend the future health and happiness of a being bound to her by the fondest ties.

From the mass of evidence, collected by careful observers of the operations of nature, we are warranted in drawing the conclusion, that the actions of the mother exercise a great influence over, not only the constitutional and physical, but also the mental organization of her offspring. Keeping this fact in view, we shall endeavour to point out the course that mothers, who prefer the welfare of their future offspring to their own indulgence, should pursue, from which they will derive a double benefit,—an improvement in their own health, with exemption from suffering, and the delight of seeing their children pass safely through the anxious period of infancy; while in after life beholding them flourishing around them, in the full enjoyment of health and vigour, they will reap the rich reward of a slight temporary self-denial, in the delightful consciousness of having performed their duty.

The leading causes of a weak and sickly offspring are, ill health, or constitutional taint of both or either of the parents; very early or late marriages; great inequality between the ages of the parties; errors in dress, diet, and general habits of life; and lastly, powerful mental emotions.

The first of these causes, medicine, under the present enlightened system, possesses powers considerably to obviate, not only by materially modifying or destroying the hereditary taint in the parents, but also by nipping it in the bud when transmitted to the infants. While upon this subject, we may remark, that in many families hereditary diseases are fostered and even exacerbated in virulence by intermarriages between their different members, sometimes disappearing in one generation, and again declaring themselves in the next; but when the habits or mode of life of communities become more adapted to the natural law, and Homœopathy, as it must do eventually, completely supersedes the present erroneous system of medicine, we may safely calculate upon the gradual extinction of all hereditary diseases; and so far, at least, children shall not have to suffer for the follies and faults of their progenitors.

Females should seldom, at least in this country, enter into the marriage bond before their twenty-first or twenty-second year; prior to that period, their organization is scarcely ever fully developed; those who marry at sixteen or eighteen years of age incur the risk of a severe after-suffering themselves, and of giving birth to weak and delicate children. How very often we see the first children of such marriages perish in infancy, or, after contending through a childhood of continued delicacy, sink into a premature grave! Women who marry late in life incur considerable personal risk and severe suffering in giving birth to children, and the offspring is seldom healthy.

The children of old men, although by a young wife, are very often extremely delicate and susceptible to illness; they not unfrequently precede their father to the grave, or linger on earth but to drag on a miserable and wearisome existence.

In concluding these observations, we may remark, that so far is the period of pregnancy from being destined for one of suffering or danger, that nature has taken every precaution for the protection of the female and her future offspring. While pregnancy runs its equable and uniform course, the expectant mother enjoys an almost complete exemption from the power of epidemic or infectious diseases, and chronic complaints are frequently suspended; in fact, with the exception of some slight morning sickness, and occasional trifling uneasiness, a well-constituted organism should enjoy as good health during pregnancy as at any other time; and many pass through this period, and give birth to vigorous children, without even the most trifling inconvenience.

Though, as we have said, nature seems, during this period, to adopt every possible precaution for the health and preservation of the parent and her future offspring, yet are her wise arrangements, in too many instances, rendered nugatory by a direct contravention of her laws. The expectant mother should therefore bear in mind, that the incumbency of a regular and systematic course of life, so essential to every individual, devolves upon her with double force, since every neglect or breach of these ordinances of nature upon her part, is frequently visited with fearful energy upon her yet unborn infant.

AIR AND EXERCISE.

Nothing tends more to the preservation of health than a proper attention to these two important points, and yet, unfortunately, there are perhaps few more completely lost sight of. Neither air nor exercise is *individually* sufficient, and those of the more opulent classes in this country, who merely take the air in their carriages, and shun the slightest physical exertion, from long-continued habits of acquired indolence, and who feel any attempt of the kind at this period attended with increased inconvenience, can scarcely expect to enjoy the benefit that nature has annexed to the observance of her laws in a course of pregnancy free from suffering, and the production of a fully-developed and healthy organized offspring.

During this epoch, passive or carriage exercise is not sufficient; walking brings not only the physical, but the whole of the organic muscles into play, and communicates the increasing vigour of the mother to her offspring; on the contrary, continual passive exercise in a carriage has been found particularly injurious during and towards the end of the second period of pregnancy; and is frequently the cause of premature and abnormal births; exercise on horseback, even not taking into consideration the risk of fright or accident to the rider, and the fearful consequences that may thence result, is still more objectionable for many reasons.

A second class, that of thrifty housewives, take a great deal of exercise, yet without a corresponding benefit, from their work occupying them wholly in-doors; this is a strong proof of the inutility of exercise of itself, unless combined with pure air. Moreover, these females, from too great activity of temperament, and others, coerced by hard necessity, frequently over-fatigue themselves, go to bed late, rise early, and sometimes unrefreshed, and thus in a manner deaden the energies of the organic powers, to their own injury, and that of the unborn child.

A third class of females injure their health, and frequently induce miscarriage, through their excessive levity and thoughtlessness, by unrestrained indulgence in active exercise, riding on horseback, but more particularly dancing. A female ought to recollect that, if through her own folly she has brought on miscarriage, the greatest possible care is necessary to prevent its recurrence; that a second attack increases her liability in future; and that she who has suffered twice or thrice from this misfortune, even when she escapes it, rarely attains her full time. Moreover, continued casualties of this nature not unfrequently terminate in premature death, from that serious and painful disease, uterine cancer.

The best exercise, therefore, for a female during this epoch is walking every day (when the weather permits it) in the open air. In order to prove beneficial, and not to interfere with the process of digestion, exercise ought to be taken two or three hours after a moderate meal, about mid-day, or in the afternoon, except during hot weather, when the evening may be preferred, care being taken to avoid the night damps, by not remaining out too late.

CLOTHING.

The dress of the female should of course be suited to the season, and if she pass from a warm into a cold atmosphere, she ought to have her neck and throat well protected, so as to avoid any risk of taking cold; but a point of far greater importance is the adaptation of her clothing to the form, so as, as much as possible, to preclude any pressure upon any part of the frame calculated to interfere with the functions of those important organs destined for the birth and nourishment of the infant; therefore lacing, at all times most objectionable, is particularly so during this period, inasmuch as it cramps the natural action of the body, and acting directly upon the abdominal muscles, the blood-vessels, lymphatics and the whole intestinal economy, produces narrowness of the chest, disturbed circulation, and induration or other derangements of the liver, and exercises a most baneful effect upon the breasts and uterus. We should bear in mind that a pressure upon these organs during development, is acting in direct contravention of the operations of nature. Females, in their efforts to preserve the elegance of their shape during pregnancy, are little aware that the constringing force exercised upon the abdominal muscles, destroys their elasticity, prevents a proper retraction after parturition, and thus proves one of the most common causes of permanent abdominal deformity; moreover, to the culpable vanity of their mothers, many, it is probable, owe their club-feet and other malformations; in addition to these evils, this practice not unfrequently deranges the position of the fœtus, which displacement, with the consequent want of energy in the muscles, and the parts concerned, generally brings on protracted and dangerous labours. Besides this, continual pressure on the uterus is liable to produce premature labours. To tight-lacing also may be attributed the difficulty many women of the present day experience in suckling their offspring, from the incipient process for the subsequent secretion of milk being deranged from the unnatural pressure on the beautifully constructed mechanism of the mammæ; from this also sometimes result those dangerous indurations, cancers, and other affections of the breast, and retraction and diminution of the nipple, from which the act of suckling is rendered difficult, and in some cases impracticable.

Young girls of seventeen or eighteen are frequently found

with pendulous breasts, from the artificial support having taken the office of the muscles, intended by nature for that purpose, and throwing them out of employment.

Garters too tightly bound are generally injurious, more particularly to pregnant females, for the pressure thereby exercised upon the blood-vessels encourages the development of varicose vessels in the inferior extremities (to which affection the system is already sufficiently predisposed), which in many instances become exceedingly painful and troublesome.

DIET.

The greatest simplicity should regulate the diet of the pregnant female; she should avoid taking too great a quantity of nourishment, because any excess in this respect, besides causing dyspepsia and general uneasiness, has a bad mechanical effect upon the future offspring; and, moreover, the fœtus shares in the derangements of the mother.

Much depends upon the *quality* of her food; nothing should be taken that is not of a simply nutritive nature, and every thing possessing a medicinal property avoided. Coffee and strong tea should be laid aside. Wine, liqueurs, malt, and other stimulating beverages, are also injurious. If the female has been long habituated to wine, it may be taken, if of good quality, in extreme moderation and diluted with water; *but better far if stimulants of every kind are altogether avoided;* indeed, the usual homœopathic diet (for which see the article Regimen, in Introduction) should be adopted as closely as possible during pregnancy.

EMPLOYMENT OF THE MIND AND HABITS DURING PREGNANCY.

It is not sufficient that the body may be in perfect health; the mind must also be kept in a state of serenity. An easy cheerfulness of temper is essentially useful in promoting the well-being of the unborn infant. Experience has presented us with many instances, in which the predominant feeling on the mind of the mother during pregnancy has influence on the future mental organization of the child. This shows how essential it is for females to keep their minds well employed during this period, to avoid both improper meditation, dissipation, and reading works not calculated to improve their understanding. Nothing can act more effectually against the future mental and corporeal health of the unborn infant than an oscillatory state of intellect, in combination with physical indolence; the late hours, turning day into night, and other practices of fashionable life, injurious as they are to the most robust constitutions, are *doubly* reprehensible on the part of the expectant mother.

INFLUENCE OF EXTERNAL OBJECTS UPON THE UNBORN INFANT.

The effect of any unpleasant or unsightly object upon the imagination of the mother, and its transmission of that effect to the offspring, evidenced in various mental or physical peculiarities after birth, is a theory as old as tradition; without entering upon the various arguments brought forward both for and against it, we would simply advise females to keep as much as possible out of the way of such objects, to preserve both body and mind in a state of health, which will lessen every fear of being affected by such occurrences; and endeavour, as constantly as possible, to direct their attention to pleasing subjects; as it must be perfectly evident that *brooding over such unpleasant impressions* can scarcely fail of being both physically and mentally injurious.

MENTAL EMOTIONS.

This subject has already been treated of in Part II., to which the reader is referred, as the remedies there mentioned are equally applicable to affections arising from these sources in either sex.

A not unfrequent symptom during pregnancy, is great DESPONDENCY OF MIND, and uneasiness about the future; some females, whose spirits are generally good at other times, suffer much from this affection during this period; and with others, we find the same feeling and excessive low spirits during the time of nursing; although not permanent, and when commencing early in gestation, usually disappearing before delivery, without material injury to the general health.

THERAPEUTICS. As this affection is apt to create some uneasiness, both to the sufferer herself and her friends, we have thought it advisable to mention it, and point out remedies which will frequently be found efficacious.

Such are *Aconitum*, *Bryonia alba*, *Nux vomica*, *Natrum muriaticum*, *Phosphorus*, *Calcarea carbonica*, and *Cinchona*.

ADMINISTRATION. Four globules of the potency mentioned after each medicine in four dessert-spoonfuls of water, one daily, after which the medicine may be allowed to exhaust its action; in the case of those who are known or found to be extremely susceptible to the impressions of the medicines, one or two globules may be given, and only repeated after an interval of from four to eight days or so, according to the effects produced.*

ACONITUM 6. If the state of despondency is preceded by one of excitement, marked by heat of skin, and frequency of pulse, attended *with apprehension and presentiment of approaching death.*

BRYONIA 30. *Great inquietude and fear of the future*, attended with irascibility and derangement of the digestive functions.

NUX VOMICA 30. Morning sickness and melancholy, with great uneasiness, impaired appetite, constipation, fretfulness.

NATRUM MURIATICUM 30. Melancholy, with weeping, uneasiness about the future, also obstinate cases of morning sickness, not yielding to *Nux vomica.*

When this affection comes on during lactation, arising from an over-secretion of milk, so that this fluid escapes involuntarily, and it is attended with great emaciation, melancholy, and apprehension of the future, we may give PHOSPHORUS 30.

CALCAREA 18, is also efficacious when the above symptoms present themselves, and more particularly so, when there is *excessive dejection with great lassitude.*

* In the treatment of pregnant women of exalted nervous sensibility, considerable caution is frequently requisite in the repetition of the doses. (See also the rules laid down for the repetition of the dose in ordinary cases, in the INTRODUCTION, Part I.)

This remedy is further very serviceable when there is suppression of the secretion, and also excessive obesity, or the individual is of *plethoric* habit. Both these remedies are also valuable when there is a disposition to consumption.

When there is lowness of spirits, attended with dyspepsia, which may arise from the energies of the mother being too severely tasked in the nourishment of her offspring, either from keeping the child too long unweaned, or from rearing twins, we may administer CINCHONA 6. The practitioner will further find occasion to select the following remedies in particular cases: *Belladonna*, *Pulsatilla*, *Veratrum*, *Stramonium*, *Platina*, *Aurum*, *Cuprum*, *Lachesis*, and *Sulphur*.

DERANGEMENTS DURING PREGNANCY.

MENSTRUATION.

VIRTUAL diseases during gestation are of rare occurrence, but when they do happen, they ought to be treated accordingly.

A continuance of menstruation is not an actual disease, but rather an exception to the general course of nature; nor must we here mistake their operation for an indication of the utility of the lancet, for neither in this nor in any other case, can the artificial supply the place of natural bleeding; however, when the female appears to suffer from the continuance of the menstrual flux, we must call in the assistance of medicaments, among which the principal are: *Cocculus*, *Phosphorus*, and *Platina*.

ADMINISTRATION. $\frac{000}{30}$, repeated every twenty-four hours until improvement takes place, or another remedy appears called for. (Vide note, p. 21.)

COCCULUS. A sanguineous mucous discharge, and very severe spasmodic pains in the lower part of the abdomen.

PHOSPHORUS. Discharge of blood, with incisive pains in the back, and occasionally vomiting.

PLATINA. Discharge very profuse, attended with a severe pain and bearing-down. (See also the remedies given under *Painful and difficult menstruation*. *Excessive menstruation*.)

MORNING SICKNESS.

Morning sickness, nausea, vomiting, and heartburn, are the most distressing symptoms attendant on the course of pregnancy; these troublesome complaints harass women most upon their first rising from a horizontal position in bed. They generally disappear soon after quickening, but sometimes continue during the whole period. The numerous palliative remedies recommended by Allopathists—leeches, cupping-glasses, blisters, aperients, sedatives, etc. etc., unfortunately too often fail in effecting their object; and in severe cases, when the stomach becomes enfeebled, the hazardous resource of artificially produced premature labour is resorted to.

THERAPEUTICS. The homœopathic treatment of this derangement, at once simple, prompt, and efficacious, has in almost all cases been stamped by the signet of success. In instances free from complication, with a tendency to relaxation of the bowels, IPECACUANHA is generally sufficient.

ADMINISTRATION. ${}^{0}\frac{0}{3}{}^{0}$, in four tea-spoonfuls of water, one morning and evening. (Vide note, p. 21.)

NUX VOMICA. When there is nausea or vomiting every morning on rising; heartburn, depraved appetite, or craving for chalk, earth, beer, etc., constipation, and irritability of temper.

ADMINISTRATION. $\frac{0\;0}{3\;0}{}^{0}$, repeated every fourth day, but if no improvement results after the second or third dose, another remedy must be substituted, such as *Pulsatilla*, or *Natrum m.*, etc., and then again *Nux v*, if required.

ARSENICUM. *Excessive* vomiting after eating or drinking, with attacks of fainting; great weakness and emaciation.

ADMINISTRATION. Same as *Ipecacuanha*, but at the twelfth or thirtieth potency.

PULSATILLA. Nausea after every meal; vomiting of ingesta, heartburn, depraved appetite, or *longing* for particular articles, such as acids, beer, wine, etc. Disposition peevish and sensitive, though naturally mild.

Conium, *Acidum nitricum*, *Magnesia*, *Phosphorus*, *Bryonia*, and *Lycopodium*, etc., will also be found useful in particular cases.

When this affection shows itself in a mild form, it may be

left to nature, adopting at the same time the homœopathic rules for regimen, and be careful not to overload the stomach. In severe cases depending upon plethoric tendency, *Aconitum* is an excellent substitute for the venesection recommended by the old school.

CONSTIPATION

Is a very common attendant upon pregnancy, and those usually suffer most who are naturally of a costive habit; when it does not arise from a mechanical cause, active exercise in the open air, and partaking frequently of cooked, or fully ripe sub-acid fruits, (at the same time avoiding coffee and other stimulating liquids,) are generally sufficient. When nature requires further auxiliary:—

Nux vomica $\frac{000}{30}$, taken at bed-time, will often answer; if after the completion of its action, there still remains some inconvenience, Ignatia, $\frac{000}{12}$, should be given as an intermediate, followed by a lower potency of Nux vomica ($\frac{000}{6}$); in other cases, when *Nux vomica* does not show a marked improvement, and the temper is extremely irritable, Bryonia $\frac{000}{6}$ will sometimes cure, or Opium $\frac{000}{3}$, which is especially indicated to follow *Nux vomica* when there appears to be a weight in the stomach, dryness of the mouth, and deep flushing of the face. In other cases, *Sepia*, *Lycopodium*, *Alumina*, etc., will be found useful. (See Constipation, Part II., p. 123.)

Dysuria. *Pulsatilla*, *Cocculus*, *Nux v.*, and *Acid. phosphoricum*, as also *Sulphur* and *Conium*, have chiefly been recommended.

DIARRHŒA DURING PREGNANCY.

See Diarrhœa, Part II., p. 137, and Diarrhœa in Lying-in Women, in this division of the work.

FAINTING AND HYSTERIC FITS.

Many delicate and nervous females are frequently attacked with fainting fits during pregnancy. The attack generally passes over easily and without deleterious consequences; exercise in the open air, and attention to the rules of regimen, are the best safeguards; but in cases where these are insufficient, and the attacks prove distressing, we must endeavour to ascertain their origin. If from tight-lacing, warm rooms, or any other obvious excitant, its simple removal is sufficient; should the sufferer remain long insensible, the speediest means of revival is sprinkling the face with cold water. When arising from plethoric habit, returns of the attack may be prevented by ACONITE, of which we have had occasion to speak several times, as a general regulator of the circulation.

CHAMOMILLA $\frac{000}{12}$, when the fainting is excited by sudden fits of anger.

NUX VOMICA $\frac{000}{30}$, when from general irritability of system, and consequent gastric derangement.

BELLADONNA $\frac{000}{30}$, when there is determination of blood to the head, with simultaneous flushing of face and perceptibly increased action of the arterial system. (Alternately with *Aconite* when required.)

CINCHONA $\frac{00}{12}$, when arising from general weakness, and especially from loss of blood.

PULSATILLA $\frac{00}{12}$. General excitability and disposition to hysteria, with hypochondriasis and great general susceptibility.

COFFEA. Abdominal spasms, with oppressed respiration, subsultus tendinum, cold perspiration, and uncontrollable agitation and jactitation. When the symptoms are generally preceded by a pain which proceeds upwards from the lower part of the bowels, left side, into the stomach, and from thence into the throat, where it creates a disagreeable and suffocative sensation, as if a ball were lodged there, *Lachesis*, *Belladonna*, *Sepia* and *Plumbum*, or *Ignatia*, *Sulphur*, *Nux v.*, *Conium*, etc., will prove useful, a preference being given to that remedy which corresponds the most closely to the whole features of the case.

IGNATIA $\frac{00}{12}$, when the patient suffers from severe headache, as if a nail were driven into the head; sadness; concealed sorrow, and sighing. (See SWOONING.)

ADMINISTRATION of the above remedies. The dose is given, repeated, if necessary, every two to four days, according to the urgency of the symptoms, until relief is obtained, or another remedy required. (Vide note, p. 21.)

TOOTHACHE

Is a frequent affection with pregnant women, and is sometimes too valuable an indication of some taint lurking in the constitution to be neglected; the female should, as soon as she is in a proper state, put herself under a course of treatment, as until this tendency is eradicated, no remedies can prove otherwise than palliative. We must particularly caution females in this situation against having teeth extracted, as the affection frequently occurs in sound ones.

THERAPEUTICS. To relieve the sufferings, the following medicines may often be given with advantage: *Sepia, Calcarea, Alumina*, and *Magnesia carbonica.*

For the ADMINISTRATION of the remedies, see TOOTHACHE, Part II., where, moreover, other useful remedies will be found.

SEPIA $\frac{000}{30}$, is particularly indicated when there is pulsative *shooting, drawing toothache*, with pain, extending to the ears, or to the arms and fingers, excited by compressing the teeth, or by cold air, and attended by impeded respiration, swelling of the cheek and enlargement of the submaxillary glands.

CALCAREA $\frac{000}{18}$, when it is *excited or aggravated by cold air, or anything hot or cold*, and attended with painful sensation of the gums, and pulsative gnawing or shooting pains, which are aggravated by noise.

ALUMINA $\frac{000}{30}$, when the *pains are excited by mastication*, or in the evening in bed, and when of a tearing nature, extending to the cheek-bone, temple, and forehead

MAGNESIA CARBONICA $\frac{000}{30}$. *Nocturnal pains in the teeth, insupportable when lying down*, and compelling the patient to get up and walk; pains generally boring, burning, drawing, tearing, and resembling those of ulceration, attended with swelling of the cheek of the side affected; throbbing and shooting in the teeth after a meal; pain aggravated by a cold. The above are the four leading medicines, though there are others which are demonstrable by peculiar symptoms. (See TOOTHACHE, Part II., p. 77.)

SWELLED FACE.

Tumefaction of the cheek arises from different causes; frequently it is the consequence of toothache, and will then be cured, or at all events much diminished, by the remedy given for the removal of that affection. Sometimes it happens, nevertheless, that from the employment of the proper remedy the toothache diminishes, but the swelling of the cheek remains unaltered. In this case *Arnica* is generally of great service, especially when the swelling is hard and stiff. If this treatment is of no avail, we may have recourse to *Pulsatilla* $\frac{000}{3}$, or to *Mercurius vivus* $\frac{00}{6}$, which is of especial service if the swelling of the cheek is accompanied by a drawing, tearing pain, and increased flow of saliva, and considerable erysipelatous redness; followed by *Belladonna* and *Hepar s.* $\frac{00}{6}$, if the inflammation threatens to extend. (See ERYSIPELAS.) *Cham.*, *Bryonia*, $\frac{00}{3}$, etc., are also occasionally of service.

Should we have neglected to employ the appropriate remedy at the proper time, or should the swelling have been maltreated by some external application, the swelling is frequently rendered of an obstinate character.

In most cases, however, the dispersion of the tumour, or, when matter is forming, the speedy completion of the suppurative process and consecutive bursting of the abscess, will be readily enough effected by means of *Hepar sulphuris*, one grain of the third trituration, repeated if necessary in from six to twelve hours.

In obstinate cases, *Lachesis* and *Hepar*, or *Mercurius* and *Hepar*, in alternation, are sometimes required; and occasionally *Silicea*, particularly in strumous habits. The application of a poultice to the cheek, or a fig boiled in milk and placed in the mouth between the affected cheek and gums, is sometimes useful. If the tumour has burst, and the opening is internal, no especial care need be taken of it; but if it has burst externally, a simple bandage, smeared with melted suet or fresh butter, must be applied. Dose $\frac{000}{6}$, twice a day.

VARICES, OR SWELLED VEINS.

Many females suffer much during pregnancy from distention of veins in the thigh and other parts, which becoming more exacerbated, eventually cause great pain and inconvenience. These varicose veins generally arise from obstructed circulation caused by the pressure of the gravid uterus upon the blood-vessels, but are also frequently a sure indication of the existence of constitutional debility, particularly when they occur in an aggravated form. They are much increased by partaking of stimulating liquids, which should consequently be avoided. Considerable alleviation is experienced by constant bathing with water, or with diluted alcohol; also by bandaging from the foot upwards with a gentle and equable pressure, and by preserving a recumbent posture, which is requisite in severe forms of the complaint accompanied with considerable swelling of the feet, ankles, &c. In order to afford a considerable relief, we may have recourse to the following remedies:—

PULSATILLA $\frac{0000}{12}$ is one of the most useful medicines, particularly when there is excessive pain and swelling, with a good deal of inflammation, or when the veins are of a livid colour, which is imparted to the whole limb. Should *Pulsatilla* give some relief, but the swelling and livid discolouration continue in much the same state, *Lachesis* may be substituted. *Arnica* is of material service when the occupations of the patient render it impossible for her to lay up, or avoid much standing and moving about in discharge of her domestic duties. *Arnica* and *Pulsatilla* in alternation, every six or eight days, have been found of great efficacy in such cases.

NUX VOM. $\frac{0000}{30}$, when attended with constipation, hemorrhoids, and irritability of temper. *Sulphur* is sometimes very beneficial after *Nux v.*

ARSENICUM $\frac{0000}{30}$, when the veins are of a livid colour, and are attended with severe *burning* pain.

CARBO VEGET. $\frac{0000}{30}$, where the former is not sufficient to subdue the constant scalding or burning.

BELLADONNA $\frac{0000}{30}$. Varices, with considerable erysipelatous inflammation.

LYCOPODIUM $\frac{0000}{30}$, has been employed with success in some inveterate cases.

Administration. Four globules of the potency named after each medicine in as many teaspoonfuls of water, one to be taken night and morning. (Vide note, p. 21.)

The simultaneous application of the remedy employed, is occasionally attended with benefit.

For a permanent eradication, a course of treatment is requisite, in which—*Sulphur*, *Graphi'es*, *Carbo veget.*, *Sepia*, &c., are useful. (See Ulcers, Part II.)

PAINS IN THE BACK DURING PREGNANCY.

Lumbo-sacral pains.

Some females suffer much from pains in the lower part of the back during pregnancy, which occasionally prove extremely distressing, particularly when they occur during the night, and tend to disturb sleep. They generally consist of an almost indescribable *aching*, or of an obtuse, heavy pressure, as if caused by a dead weight resting on the affected part. *Kali carb.* has repeatedly been employed against them with the most satisfactory results, especially when they partake of the character described. In other cases, *Bryonia*, *Rhus*, *Sulph.*, *Lycopodium*, *Pulsatilla*, *Nux v.*, *Sepia*, or *Causticum*, &c., may be given with advantage. If hemorrhoidal sufferings become added to these troublesome pains, and *Kali c.* prove insufficient to relieve the complaint in this complicated form, *Nux v.*, *Sulphur*, or *Sepia*, may be prescribed with advantage. (See Hemorrhoids; as also the indications given for the remedies under the heading of *False Pains.*) Dose: $^{0}\frac{0}{3}{}^{0}$ or $\frac{0\,0\,0}{6}$.

MISCARRIAGE. *Abortus.*

From the increasing number of homœopathic practitioners in this country, a point already alluded to in the Preface, we are justified in looking forward to a period, not far distant, when there will be no difficulty in obtaining professional assistance in misfortunes of this nature. I shall here endeavour as briefly, but at the same time as clearly, as possible, to point out the treatment best to be pursued both in preventing its occurrence, and in obviating the consequences it entails when medical aid has been called in too late, or when it has been found impracticable to avert the evil.

Women who have once suffered from this affection are exceedingly obnoxious to its recurrence, and this liability is still further increased if the event have taken place a second or third time. It may occur at any period between the first and seventh month, but in the majority of cases takes place about the third, or the beginning of the fourth. When *before* or *about* this period it is frequently attended with but little pain or danger, although repeated miscarriages, from the great discharge that is generally present, break down the constitution, and frequently develop severe chronic diseases. When miscarriage takes place at a more advanced period, it assumes a very serious complexion, and is often accompanied with a considerable degree of peril to the sufferer.

The premonitory and accompanying symptoms of miscarriage vary much in their nature; sometimes the discharge is exceedingly profuse, at others moderate or inconsiderable; the pains, in many instances, extremely severe and protracted, are in others very slight and of short continuance.

Sudden *mental emotions*, or great *physical exertion*, mechanical injuries, a *luxurious mode of life*, fashionable habits, powerful aperients, *neglecting to take air and exercise*, are a few of the exciting causes of this affection, which is particularly apt to occur in both highly plethoric or delicate and nervous habits. An abnormal condition of the constitution is undoubtedly the *predisposing cause*.

Miscarriage is, in most cases, preceded and attended by the majority of the following symptoms:—A sensation of chill, followed by fever, with more or less bearing-down, particularly when occurring late in pregnancy; also, *severe pains in the abdomen, drawing and cutting pains in the loins*, or pains frequently bearing a close resemblance to those of labour; discharge of viscid mucus, and blood, sometimes of a *bright red*, not unfrequently mixed with coagula, at others *dark* and clotted, followed by the emission of a serous fluid. The miscarriage generally takes place during this discharge, which occasionally continues, if not properly checked, to flow for hours after, placing the sufferer in considerable jeopardy. When the pains increase in intensity, and the muscular contractions become generally established, with their characteristic regular throes, and efforts to dilate the mouth of the womb, miscarriage is almost inevitable.

THERAPEUTICS. As *preventives* of this affection, the principal remedies are: *Sabina, Secale cornutum, Kali c., Lyc., Sep.,* and *Calc.*

When the premonitory symptoms *declare themselves, Chamomilla, Nux vomica, Ferrum metallicum, Ipecacuanha, Sabina,* and *Calcarea.* The same with the additions of *Hyoscyamus, Crocus,* and *Secale cornutum,* after the misfortune has taken place. *Cinchona* is also valuable when the indications which we shall give for that medicine are present.

In cases where there is an evident disposition to miscarriage, or where, from a variety of reasons, it is apprehended, the administration of SABINA, $\frac{000}{6}$, in the early stage of pregnancy, will frequently prevent its occurrence.

ADMINISTRATION. We may allow four or five days to elapse between the first and second dose, and gradually lengthen the interval for each successive administration, until the period of danger be past, being careful, however, on watching the effect of each dose, discontinuing the medicine whenever any indications of its action on the system become apparent, and not repeating until the symptoms attributable to the medicine have passed away, and then only with increased caution, and at longer intervals.

Hartmann* strongly recommends SECALE CORNUTUM $\frac{00}{12}$ as useful in similar cases, but particularly when this misfortune has already occurred more than once; it should be administered every fourteen days, commencing immediately after the cessation of the monthly period, and continuing until the period at which miscarriage usually occurs is past; one dose more, at the utmost, being allowed after this period.

Both these remedies are also extremely valuable after miscarriage has taken place, the latter particularly in *weak* or *exhausted* persons, or in those cases of hemorrhage in which the discharge consists of *dark liquid blood,* and is followed by *con-*

* Hartmann's Acute Diseases, by Chs. Hempel, M.D., vol. iii., p. 164.

siderable debility; this remedy is also efficacious in cases of *inevitable miscarriage,* attended with *feeble expulsive efforts;* the former (*Sabina*) when there are dragging and forcing pains, extending down the back and loins; profuse, bright-coloured hemorrhage; sensation of sinking or faintness in the abdomen; frequent desire to relieve the bowels; diarrhœa; nausea or vomiting; chilliness and heat, with fever.

Lycopodium and *Kali carbonicum* $\frac{000}{6}$ have also been recommended as useful preventive remedies against habitual tendency to abortion, the latter especially when the symptoms are always preceded or attended by severe pain in the loins.

We shall now treat of miscarriage when the premonitory symptoms have set in, giving under the same head the indications for the use of the medicaments, where the result is *unavoidable or has already taken place,* as even in these cases their administration is decidedly beneficial in obviating further injurious consequences, and in alleviating the sufferings of the patient. The remedies in these cases are, in addition to the two above mentioned, *Arnica, Chamomilla, Nux vomica, Ipecacuanha, Hyoscyamus, Belladonna, Crocus, Ferrum metallicum,* and *Calcarea.*

Arnica $\frac{000}{3}$. When the symptoms have been excited by an accident, such as a fall, blow, or concussion, etc., this remedy should be immediately administered.

Chamomilla $\frac{000}{3}$, when there are present: excessive restlessness, convulsions, twitching in the back and limbs; *severe pains in the loins and back,* worse at night, generally of a sharp cutting description, extending downwards, strongly resembling those of labour; sometimes also *abdominal spasms,* with a species of sanguineous discharge; or discharge of deep red or dark coagulated blood; frequent yawning; coldness and shivering.

Nux vomica $\frac{000}{6}$. Obstinate constipation, with a varicose condition of the internal organs of generation; also when the patient has been accustomed to a stimulating diet, and the use of coffee; severe burning, or wrenching pains in the loins; painful pressure downwards and mucous discharge. (*Bryonia* is sometimes of benefit, when *Nux v.* fails to do much good.) See also *Calcarea.*

IPECACUANHA $\frac{000}{3}$. Chill with heat; violent pressure downwards; *flooding;* cramp and rigidity of the frame; sometimes *convulsions;* vomiting, or desire to vomit; disposition to faint whenever the head is raised; cutting pains in the umbilical region. (*Platina* or *Cina* have been recommended when *Ipecac.* fails.)

HYOSCYAMUS $\frac{000}{30}$, when the convulsions are very severe, with cries, great anguish, oppression of the chest, and *loss of consciousness.*

BELLADONNA $\frac{000}{6}$, is perhaps more frequently required either at the commencement, or subsequently, than any other remedy. The following are its leading indications: great pains in the loins and entire abdomen; *severe bearing down,* as if the whole of the intestines would be pressed out; pain in the back, as if it were dislocated or broken; bruised pain in the sacral region; sensation either of spasmodic constriction, or of expansion in the abdomen. It is also particularly valuable in cases of profuse hemorrhage, the discharge of blood being neither very bright nor dark-coloured after miscarriage. *Platina* is sometimes to be preferred to *Belladonna,* when, along with bearing-down pains, there is a thick and dark-coloured discharge, attended with venereal orgasm.

FERRUM METALLICUM $\frac{000}{6}$, is a useful medicine in cases of miscarriage attended with fever, labour-like pains, and considerable sanguineous discharge.

CROCUS $\frac{000}{3}$, is especially indicated in cases which are attended or followed by discharge of *dark, coagulated* or viscid blood, with a sensation as of something moving or fluttering about in the umbilical region, and increased sanguineous discharge on the slightest movement. This remedy is frequently useful in obstinate cases, after the employment of one or more of the above-mentioned remedies.

CINCHONA $\frac{000}{6}$, is valuable in the *restoring the exhausted energies, after the hemorrhage,* or materially assists in checking the discharge should there be spasmodic pain in the womb, or bearing-down sensation, with considerable discharge of blood at intervals.

CALCAREA $\frac{000}{6}$, is a remedy of considerable importance in the treatment of cases where the affection has apparently been induced by a varicose state of the veins of the parts. It is also of value as a preventive, and especially where the patient is of a *plethoric habit*, with a tender or irritable skin, and other strumous appearances.

SEPIA, $\frac{00}{30}$. In threatening attacks of abortus from general plethora, or from local congestions and obstructed circulation, with sensation of weight in the abdomen, determination to the head and chest, and excessive nervous excitability, this remedy has been employed with success.

When MENTAL EMOTION has given rise to the symptoms of miscarriage, see the remedies given under that heading, Part II.

ADMINISTRATION. A few globules, or where necessary, one minim in an ounce of water, a teaspoonful every few minutes to half hour, hour, or only every three or four hours, according to the nature of the case, lengthening the intervals or discontinuing the medicine when decided benefit, or a stoppage of the hemorrhage is effected. When a favourable effect does not follow after the second or third dose in serious cases, another remedy must be had recourse to. Vide note, p. 21. When violent hemorrhage is present, and does not cease under the employment of any of the before-mentioned medicines, *Acidum nitricum* may be administered. Cold water is also useful.

I have thus enumerated some of the principal homœopathic remedies which are employed in the different stages of this misfortune, and have endeavoured to point out the peculiar indications for the selection of the proper medicament as succinctly, and at the same time as fully, as it is possible to do in a work like the present. In concluding the subject, I shall briefly notify a few precautionary measures that the patient ought to observe while threatened with, or after having suffered from the affliction.

When miscarriage is threatened, the individual must assume the recumbent posture, and in some cases, indeed, should be strictly confined to bed, sleeping with few bedclothes; the apartment should be kept cool, and every means must be employed to ensure perfect tranquillity of mind. The diet prescribed in cases under homœopathic treatment should be closely followed, and warm fluids generally avoided. When the misfortune has proved unavoidable, or has actually taken place, before assistance has been sought, the patient ought still to be confined to bed for a few days, lest a fresh discharge should be brought about by too early a change from a horizontal to an upright posture ; and on future occasions, when a *similar period* comes round, great care should be taken that the mishap may not again occur; in the attainment of this desirable object, we feel confident that nothing will tend so fully to ensure success, as a timely exhibition of one or other of the preventive remedies already commented on.

TREATMENT BEFORE PARTURITION.

PREPARATION OF THE BREASTS.

Young mothers frequently find great difficulty in suckling their children, in consequence of organic defect or incapacity of the nipple. In every case, a preparation of the breasts is necessary some weeks before delivery, in order to prepare them for their future offices. In many instances the structure of the breasts is disorganized from an ignorant nurse having compressed them in childhood, from the idea that such a process was needful for the expulsion of some matter in the breasts of the child—a vulgar error—a practice against which mothers ought to be particularly watchful. Inability of function is also likely to occur from the pressure of stays in after life, by which the cuticle is rendered so tender, as to preclude suckling.

The first two cases are beyond the power of art. If suckling be attempted, induration of the nipple and mamma ensue, attended with severe suffering ; when, however, a simple tenderness of the epidermis exists, this evil is much alleviated when the nipples are bathed with brandy twice a day, for several weeks anterior to delivery. Another difficulty, frequently accompanying this state, is a shortness or retraction of the nipple, so that the infant cannot take hold of it; this defect is frequently the cause of the first, from the ineffectual efforts of the child to suck injuring the part; in this case appropriate shields of soft wood may be applied to accustom the nipple to elongate and protrude, so as to present sufficient hold for the infant, when the period for suckling arrives, when the efforts of the child will still further contribute towards the effecting of this object. In this case also, bathing with brandy will naturally tend to correct any tenderness of the skin, and prevent subsequent excoriation. It may also be here remarked, that when any tenderness exists during the period of lactation, between the intervals of the infant being applied to the breast, the shield should be resumed, and the bathing continued, due care being always taken to lave the nipple carefully with tepid water, before it is again offered to the child.*

REMEDIES BEFORE LABOUR.

Many things are recommended by the old school previous to labour, such as frequent bloodlettings and aperients; but these, instead of promoting the object desired, have a contrary effect, by lowering the energies requisite at such an eventful period, and by placing the nervous system in an abnormal state of irritation and excitement; when this loss of humour is brought about in the first period of pregnancy, it defeats its own object, by what are commonly called *plethoric* symptoms, induced by the reaction in the organism, to supply this uncalled-for waste, and this always taking place with a correspondent expenditure of vital power. It is a species of infatuation to disturb the regular course of nature, by the ill-directed efforts of art, where an evident plethoric state exists; this object is much more safely and effectually attained, by the internal administration of a specific remedy, such as a dose or two of ACONITE $\frac{0\,0\,0}{6}$, which may be followed by *Belladonna*, should there be symptoms of

* When severe pains are experienced in the breast after each application of the infant, the employment of *Phellandrium aquaticum* has been found advantageous.

active congestion with fiery redness of the face, accelerated action of the carotids, etc.

An artificial evacuation, previous to delivery, may be obtained by a *lavement* of lukewarm water, repeated, with a small quantity of linseed oil, when necessary, from a failure in the first attempt to obtain the desired effect.

FALSE PAINS.

Before proceeding to notice parturition, a few words may be said upon the so-called false, spurious, or intestinal pains brought about by congestion of blood to the uterus, errors in regimen, emotions of the mind, effects of chill in the abdomen, and a variety of other causes :—they sometimes precede labour but a few hours, but in many cases come on some days, and even weeks, before delivery ; they chiefly differ from labour-pains *in the irregularity of their recurrence, in being unconnected with uterine contraction, and chiefly confined to the abdomen, with sensibility to touch and movement, and in not increasing in intensity as they return ;* sometimes, from their close resemblance, it is extremely difficult to discriminate between them and the real labour-pains, but in such cases we must be chiefly guided by the period of gestation ;* and our safest mode of procedure is, to endeavour to mitigate the patient's sufferings, if they be considerable, or come on a week or two before labour is expected, by the administration of a proper remedy, as, if we allow them to proceed unchecked, they not unfrequently continue till the moment of delivery, rendering the labour much more painful, exhausting, and difficult.

Therapeutics. The following medicaments may be had recourse to with effect: *Bryonia, Nux vomica, Pulsatilla, Dulcamara,* and *Aconitum,*—selecting the one most suitable for the affection, according to the causes and symptoms.

Bryonia, *when there are pains in the loins resembling a dragging weight,* attended with constipation and irritability, much *increased by motion, with abdominal pains preceding*

* If the os uteri be found unaltered, and consequently not enlarged or elongated, it may with certainty be concluded that the pains are spurious.

those in the back. (This remedy is more particularly indicated when the above symptoms have been excited by a fit of passion.)

ADMINISTRATION. $\frac{0\,0\,0\,0\,0\,0}{6}$, in four teaspoonfuls of water, one morning and evening, or oftener if necessary, until relief is obtained. (Vide note, p. 21.)

NUX VOMICA. Similar pains in the abdomen, and back; also when there is pain in the region of the pubis, as if from the effects of a bruise; the symptoms arise chiefly at night. When the exciting cause appears to be constipation, or mental irritation, or when a too luxurious mode of living, stimulants, coffee or spirituous liquors, there is additional reason for selecting *Nux v.*

ADMINISTRATION. $\frac{0\,0}{6}$, taken in a little water at bedtime, repeating it in six, twelve, or forty-eight hours, according to necessity, if required.

PULSATILLA $\frac{0\,0}{12}$. Similar abdominal pains; pains in the loins resembling those from continued stooping, or the pressure of a tight bandage, attended with a sensation of rigidity, and painful dragging and aching in the thighs; constipation or *relaxation;* mildness of temper or great sensibility. This remedy is particularly valuable when these pains appear to have arisen from indigestion brought on by rich, indigestible food.

ADMINISTRATION. Same as *Nux v.*

DULCAMARA $\frac{0\,0}{12}$, is chiefly useful when the origin may be traced to cold, and the pains are of a violent shooting and drawing nature, situated in the *small of the back,* generally coming on at night. When spurious pains arise from emotions of the mind, we may consult MENTAL EMOTIONS.

ACONITUM. When these pains occur in young plethoric subjects, attended with accelerated and strong pulse, flushing of the face, and increased temperature of the skin.

ADMINISTRATION. $\frac{0\,0\,0\,0\,0\,0}{6}$, in four dessert-spoonfuls of water, one every six, twelve, or twenty-four hours, according to the relief obtained or the violence of the symptoms.

The employment of this remedy completely obviates venesection.

PARTURITION.

Natural labour takes place at the end of the ninth month of pregnancy; the uterine contractions are regular and effective, and the whole process does not continue beyond twenty-four hours, rarely above twelve, and very frequently not longer than six. Were it not for the acquired habits of civilized life—improper diet—the proportions of the female frame being distorted by tight-lacing, &c.,* and their regular functions thereby disturbed—diseases generated by the want of proper air or exercise, or both—hereditary maladies, &c., parturition would be comparatively free from pain and remote from danger, as in fact it is, even at the present day, generally found amongst savages.

TEDIOUS OR COMPLICATED LABOURS.

When labour is protracted beyond the normal period stated, or is attended with an excessive degree of suffering, as is more prone to happen when the female is of a slender form and of a highly nervous and sensitive habit, it becomes incumbent on us to avail ourselves of all the means which art affords, in order to endeavour to alleviate those sufferings as much as possible.

Amongst the *medicines* best suited to attain this desirable result, we shall frequently find COFFEA CRUDA of considerable service in mitigating the pains when they are extremely violent and occur in rapid succession, scarcely allowing the female an interval of ease, and are attended with excessive agitation, bordering on despair. When *Coffea* $\frac{0\,0\,0}{3}$ affords but little relief, which is generally the case when the patient has constantly or frequently been in the habit of using coffee as a beverage, *Aconitum* should be resorted to, followed by *Chamom.* $\frac{0\,0\,0}{3}$, if required.

ADMINISTRATION. Four or five globules of the remedy se-

* It is to be regretted that the attention of mothers is not more particularly directed to the development of the female frame by means of calisthenic exercises, instead of distorting its symmetry by means of stays and tight-lacing; health being destroyed for the sake of that fashionable and unnatural absurdity—a thin waist!

lected, in two tablespoonfuls of water, of which a teaspoonful may be administered every five or ten minutes, until some relief is experienced. If little or no benefit ensue after several doses, another medicine may be prescribed. When we find that the throes are insufficient to accomplish their object, and the female becomes exhausted by the protracted nature of the labour,—

Belladonna, $\frac{000}{6}$, has been found of *the greatest value*, and will generally prove serviceable in almost every case of tedious labour which arises from the rigidity and unyielding state of the parts, (as is so frequently the case with elderly females giving birth to their first child;) but it is more particularly where labour is protracted by a spasmodic contraction of the inferior portion of the uterus, owing to which circumstance, notwithstanding the existence of powerful throes, *the os uteri does not become correspondingly dilated*, that the *Belladonna* is indicated. On the other hand, this valuable remedy is further of equal efficacy, when, on the escape of the waters, an almost complete cessation of the labour-pains ensues, or the uterine contractions are rendered so feeble as scarcely to be perceptible, and are only made known to the patient by a periodic sensation of pressure and aching at the sacral region—while the dilatation of the os uteri is found, as in the above instance, *to make no further progress*.

The following remedies will also occasionally claim attention: *Nux v.*, *Pulsatilla*, *Secale cornutum*, and *Opium*.

Nux v. $\frac{000}{6}$, when the labour is somewhat protracted, from the irregularity and insufficiency of the pains, and the female complains of a *continual urgency* to relieve nature.

Pulsatilla $\frac{000}{6}$, where the labour-throes are imperfect, and frequently extend upwards from the sacral to the epigastric region, attended with spasm of the stomach and vomiting; or when they are almost unfelt, and at long intervals, attended with acute pains in the loins, and *painful drawing sensations in the thighs*, which tend much to weaken the woman, without furthering the labour.

When *Pulsatilla* has not had the desired effect, and there is a continual deficiency of uterine contractile power; or when the labour-pains return every quarter of an hour, *not increasing in intensity*, Secale cornutum $\frac{0}{3}$ or $\frac{0}{6}$ ought to be administered. Again, when we find the pains, although powerful at first, suddenly cease, followed by a tremour of the whole body, occasionally interrupted by violent jerkings, and when the patient falls into a sort of *lethargic slumber, with open mouth, stertorous breathing, eyes half closed—and there is great difficulty in arousing the sufferer, even by violent means,* Opium $^{0}\frac{0}{3}{}^{0}$ is indicated.

Administration. A few globules of the remedy at the potency mentioned, may be dissolved in about an ounce of water, and a dessert-spoonful given between each pain, until benefit results, or a marked action of the remedy calls for a pause. When the pains suddenly disappear without other indications, one or two drops of the *Mother Tincture of Cinnamon* have proved of service, especially where the labour is far advanced.

We have now, in a great measure, treated of the course to be pursued when nature seems to call for our assistance to further her exertions; but we must at the same time reprobate a rash and ill-advised interference with her operations; and we cannot, in common with most men of eminence of the other school, too strongly reprehend the practice of administering spirituous beverages, or stimulants, such as chamomile tea, and other ptisans, coffee, and even opium, under the absurd impression of thereby facilitating delivery.

Spirituous liquors are objectionable, from their accelerating circulation, and consequently producing difficult labour, and too great a loss of blood; Coffee, from its causing high nervous excitability; Chamomile, from its pathogenetic property of producing or creating a tendency to metrorrhagia; ptisans, whose peculiar properties we need not enter upon here, are all more or less of a stimulative or irritative nature. Opium, given merely as a palliative of the severity of the throes, materially retards delivery.

As a general rule, every substance, possessing a medicinal property, administered upon the false premises above noticed, tends to injury, and must therefore be carefully avoided.

With regard to the after-birth, when common, gentle and

rational mechanical means* for its expulsion fail, we may have recourse to *Belladonna*, *Pulsat.*, *Secale corn.*, or *Opium*, $\frac{000}{3}$, selecting by the symptoms already mentioned, and will rarely be disappointed in our expectations of their beneficial effects.

When the parturition is complete, the ADMINISTRATION of ARNICA, $\frac{000}{8}$, in a little water, is always followed by the happiest results, frequently preventing much severe after-suffering; and we are convinced, that many critical cases of inflammation, &c., might thereby be warded off. In instances where the labour has been very protracted, the *Arnica* in lotion, one teaspoonful of the TINCTURE to two ounces of tepid water, applied externally, will be found to afford great relief.

SPASMODIC PAINS, CRAMPS, AND CONVULSIONS.

We sometimes, in *complicated* labours, find spasmodic pains set in, which occasion considerable suffering without advancing the birth.

THERAPEUTICS. The principal remedies against these affections are: *Chamomilla*, *Belladonna*, *Hyoscyamus*, *Stramonium*, *Cicuta virosa*, *Ignatia*, *Ipecacuanha*, and *Cocculus*; with regard to their Administration, two globules of the potency mentioned may be administered in a teaspoonful of water, and repeated after a shorter or longer interval if necessary, according to the effects produced, being guided in their selection by the following symptoms:

* We do not understand by the said term the exercise of *brute force*; it is truly melancholy, and almost impossible to conceive, that men who have undergone a medical education, and have had opportunities both of reading and hearing the *warnings* of enlightened and experienced obstetric practitioners, against the distressing and serious consequences which almost inevitably result from the employment of harsh and inconsiderate measures whenever the expulsion of the placenta happens to be somewhat tardy, could be guilty of the perpetration of such culpable and infamous conduct. Some of these reckless individuals do not appear to *wait* for any signs of tardiness, but as if in *anticipation* of an obstinate and prolonged retention, they set to work with their ruthless proceedings immediately, and are consequently, but too frequently, the authors of all the mischief, danger, and even the fatal termination, which sometimes result after *the natural process of labour.*

CHAMOMILLA, $\frac{00}{3}$, where there is extremely acute pain, chiefly of a cutting description, extending from the lumbar to the hypogastric region, attended by spasmodic convulsions; redness of the face, *especially of one cheek; excessive sensibility of the nervous system, and excitement.*

BELLADONNA, $\frac{00}{6}$, *when the bearing-down is excessive, as if the entire contents of the abdomen were about to be protruded;* convulsive movements in the limbs; great agitation with continual tossing; *occasional throbbing and distention of the vessels of the head;* bloated redness of the face, with profuse sweat. (See also the indications for this invaluable remedy at page 528.)

HYOSCYAMUS, $\frac{00}{6}$, when the convulsions are still more severe, accompanied with *great anguish and cries;* oppression of the chest and loss of consciousness.

STRAMONIUM, $\frac{00}{6}$, convulsions, *without loss of consciousness,* and trembling of the limbs.

IGNATIA, $\frac{00}{6}$, *spasmodic* and *compressive pains,* with sensation *of suffocation; confused feeling* in the head.

CICUTA VIROSA, $\frac{00}{6}$, general convulsions, or cramp-like contortions of the limbs; *pallor* or *sallow hue* of the face.

IPECACUANHA, $\frac{00}{3}$, spasmodic convulsions; paleness or bloatedness of the face, occasionally with desire to vomit.

COCCULUS, $\frac{00}{6}$, cramps or convulsions of the limbs and whole body, *more especially in the lower part of the abdomen, with heat, redness, and puffiness of the face. Acidum hydrocyanicum, Platina* and *Cina,* have also been recommended against convulsions during labour. Dose: $\frac{000}{3}$ or $\frac{000}{6}$.

TREATMENT AFTER DELIVERY.

AFTER the termination of delivery, both body and mind must be kept in a state of perfect repose; every thing which may tend to arouse the excitability of the patient, such as noise, strong light, and odour, must be carefully avoided, and the room kept at a moderate temperature. After the birth, the female should be allowed to enjoy that slumber, which in natural cases generally follows, without interruption; but it is commendable to feel the pulse from time to time, to ascertain if a healthy action is going on. Sometimes this desirable state of rest is kept off by great nervous excitement on the part of the female, with incessant tossing in bed and restlessness. A few globules of COFFEA CRUDA will often suffice to dissipate these symptoms, and to procure a refreshing slumber; should it fail, and any febrile symptoms be present, ACONITE will generally produce the desired effect. When these remedies, which answer in the majority of cases, fail of their accustomed success, we must endeavour to trace the cause, and will generally discover symptoms, pointing out a different remedy, which, if judiciously chosen, will, with almost absolute certainty, afford a satisfactory result. The practitioner will generally find but little difficulty in the selection of the fitting medicament; but there are so many circumstances to guide his choice, that it would be wholly foreign to our purpose, in a work of this kind, to enter upon the several contingencies applicable to individual or isolated cases. (See the article SLEEPLESSNESS, Part II.)

Here again, we must severely reprobate the practice of administering stimulating, and *even spirituous*, beverages, to females after delivery, which, far from possessing a strengthening property, tend only to excite and irritate the whole nervous system. For some time after parturition, nature calls for but little nourishment; it should be given only when the female *herself* expressly feels the want of it, and then be of the lightest and most digestible kind, and in very small quantities. It is highly reprehensible to endeavour to induce a female to partake of food, under the absurd idea of strengthening her. We must allow nature to pursue her own course, which prescribes but little nourishment for the first five or six days after delivery, and thereby avoids the necessity of calling the bowels into action, which state of *Constipation* (if it may so be called) is ordained for the wisest purposes, and attended with the most beneficial results; while the temporary inactivity of the alimentary canal is compensated by the vicarious action of the skin (demonstrating itself by increased perspiration), and the balance of the system thus kept up. We cannot, therefore, sufficiently condemn the use of aperients, which only tend to promote irritation, and bring on puerperal fever, and other evil consequences; in many cases, also, this artificial relaxation interferes with the proper secretion of milk. After the fourth or sixth day, nature generally acts spontaneously, and when it appears necessary to afford mechanical assistance, we may do so by the application of warm friction to the abdomen, or the employment of a simple lavement, consisting of tepid water, with a little linseed oil or thin gruel. When this state, which seldom happens, continues so long as to cause inconvenience, ***Bryonia***, or ***Nux vomica***, ***Pulsatilla***, and ***Opium***, may be resorted to. (See article CONSTIPATION.) Dose: $\frac{0\,0\,0}{3}$ or $\frac{0\,0\,0}{6}$.

AFTER-PAINS.

These pains are considered salutary, and perhaps justly so to some extent; at the same time, when they occur in an aggravated form, and are unduly protracted, as frequently occurs in females of exalted nervous sensibility, they tend to deprive the female of her rest, and ought, under such circumstances, to be subdued as speedily as possible; their early mitigation, in all cases, by means of homœopathic remedies, is, moreover, never attended but with the most satisfactory results.

In many instances the employment of *Arnica*, internally and likewise externally, as a lotion, (a few drops of the tincture to an ounce or so of tepid water,) when the labour has been somewhat severe, is sufficient to prevent their excessive development, as also in most cases to ward off fever and inflammation.* But when the pain still continues, and the patient is highly excitable and sensitive, we should give a few globules of CHAMOMILLA in a little water, followed in about an hour by *Nux v.* if no change is effected by the former. If the

* The soothing effects of *Arnica* are properly appreciated by those females who have had opportunity and occasion for its employment; and we believe there are few, who having once experienced the beneficial effects of the homœopathic treatment generally, during the entire period of confinement, would willingly return to the old method of treatment.

pain is of an insupportably intense description, or followed by convulsions, coldness and rigidity of body, COFFEA CRUDA ought to be selected. We may give PULSATILLA when the convulsions do not supervene, but the pains are protracted and the patient is of a mild and gentle disposition, but sensitive and easily alarmed about herself. Again, when the after-pains are very severe, and there is a continual inclination to relieve the bowels when in a recumbent posture, passing away when rising, followed by spasmodic pains in the lower parts of the abdomen, they are usually readily relieved by NUX VOMICA. Dose: $\frac{0\,0\,0}{3}$ or $\frac{0\,0\,0}{6}$.

SECALE CORNUTUM and CUPRUM METALLICUM have been strongly recommended in preference to any of the foregoing remedies, in severe and protracted after-pains occurring in females who have already borne many children.

ADMINISTRATION. With regard to the dose, we may dissolve a few globules at the potency named, in a wine-glassful of water, and give a teaspoonful every hour, or only every three or four hours, according to circumstances; carefully watching the effect produced, and discontinuing the medicine as soon as relief is afforded; in many cases a single dose will suffice. When, on the other hand, no improvement follows after a dose or two of the same remedy, another must be selected.

In the event of *flooding*, the following remedies must be had recourse to: *Ipecacuanha*—or *Crocus*, *Platina* or *Sabina*; also *Belladonna*, *Chamomilla*, *Cinchona*, in particular cases according to the symptoms. (For *indications*, see MISCARRIAGE.)

DURATION OF CONFINEMENT.

Even in strong and healthy females, during the first five days, the patient should remain in bed; in the four following, if she feels herself perfectly strong, and desirous to rise, she may gradually accustom herself to longer periods of sitting up; the great risk is from the extreme susceptibility of the system to cold. After this period, females who still find themselves weak and languid, should prefer the horizontal to the half-recumbent posture; and if this prove wearisome, she may sit up for an hour or two, but not so as to fatigue herself. The diet should be extremely light, and not of a very nutritious quality; she ought only gradually to partake of food of a more nourishing nature, never having recourse to any thing in the least degree stimulating; and all strong odours from flowers, or other aromatic substances, are to be carefully avoided, the mind kept in a state of perfect tranquillity, and the room dark.

DISEASES FOLLOWING PARTURITION.

SUPPRESSED SECRETION OF MILK.

It is of paramount importance that the normal operations of the organism peculiar to this state, proceed with due regularity. Among these, the secretion of milk takes a prominent position, and its sudden suppression is apt to be followed by internal and local inflammation, determination of blood to the head, and the usual array of symptoms which form the disease commonly denominated puerperal fever, which however also results from internal injuries, consequent upon difficult or protracted labour; but if the precaution of administering *Arnica*, already enjoined, has been taken, that source of danger will almost always have been effectually guarded against.

When, however, *puerperal fever* arises or threatens to set in, from a sudden *suppression* of the lacteal secretion, the immediate administration of PULSATILLA $\frac{000}{6}$ or $\frac{000}{12}$ in a teaspoonful of water, repeated in six, twelve, or twenty-four hours, according to necessity, will frequently be found sufficient to check it at the outset, restore the flow of milk, and re-establish the equilibrium of the organism; if any unpleasant symptoms still remain, they will, in most cases, yield to the administration of CALCAREA $\frac{000}{18}$ followed by ZINCUM $\frac{000}{30}$ if it appear called for. In other cases, particularly where serious metastases result, *Belladonna, Bryonia, Rhus,* or *Sulphur,* may be required.

If the suppression of the secretion arise from any sudden *mental emotion,* we must consult that article for the suitable remedy, giving perhaps a preference to *Bryonia*, *Chamomilla*, *Pulsatilla*, or *Coffea*.

Should active feverish symptoms, such as hot dry skin, &c., set in, ACONITE $\frac{6}{6}$, should be dissolved in six teaspoonfuls of water and a teaspoonful given at short intervals, according to the intensity of the symptoms;—when there is excessive restlessness along with the above, considerable advantage will accrue from the alternate use of *Aconitum* and *Coffea*.

We may here refer back to our remarks upon the evil effects of aperients, which, by their action upon the intestines, frequently cause a suppression of the lacteal fluid, and the consequent fever.

EXCESSIVE SECRETION OF MILK.

Sometimes, on the other hand, it happens that too *abundant* a secretion takes place, causing distention of the breasts, and involuntary emission of milk, productive of extreme emaciation, and sometimes development of phthisis. CALCAREA $\frac{}{18}$ will be found useful in this affection; or should it fail to relieve, PHOSPHORUS $\frac{}{30}$.

ADMINISTRATION. Six globules of the medicine at the potency mentioned, may be dissolved in an ounce of water, and a teaspoonful taken night and morning. Vide note, p. 21.

When febrile symptoms arise from distention of the breasts, induced by excessive secretion, and indications of what is generally denominated milk-fever, (which, however, frequently arises from other causes,) we may administer RHUS TOXICODENRON $\frac{6}{6}$, in six teaspoonfuls of water, a teaspoonful night and morning. (Vide note, p. 21.)

ACONITE $\frac{00}{6}$, as a precautionary measure when there is high febrile action of the whole system, and we are ignorant of the exciting cause. The dose to be repeated every six hours, or oftener, if necessary, until the rapidity of the circulation is diminished, and the skin rendered moist.

PERSPIRATION AFTER DELIVERY, SUPPRESSION OR EXCESS OF.

The increased perspiration which takes place after childbirth is, as we have before observed, a substitute for the suspended action of the alimentary canal; consequently its sudden *suppression* is unavoidably followed with an injurious result, and not unfrequently puerperal fever.

Exposure to cold, or a sudden chill, is the most frequent cause of this affection; we consequently find that the immediate administration of DULCAMARA $\frac{000}{12}$, will often suffice to restore the action of the skin, and prevent further injurious consequences. Should it fail, NUX VOMICA $\frac{000}{30}$, will frequently be found efficacious; or CHAMOMILLA $\frac{000}{6}$, in three teaspoonfuls of water, a teaspoonful every six hours; this latter remedy, particularly when there is excessive restlessness and excitability, with colic and relaxation of the bowels. When severe one-sided headache arises, combined or not with distressing pain in the neck, *Belladonna* may be prescribed. In other cases, *Bryonia* or *Sulphur* may be called for, $\frac{000}{6}$.

On the other hand, an *excessive* perspiration is almost equally prejudicial; it is generally brought about by keeping the room of the female at too high a temperature, too great a quantity of bedclothes, or stimulating beverages; it is chiefly injurious from the extreme debility and high susceptibility to taking cold it occasions. Our first care must be a removal of the exciting causes; and should the malady still continue, we may administer SAMBUCUS NIGER, which will generally be found effectual in its removal. In other cases, *China*, *Cocc.*, *Sulph.*, etc.

ADMINISTRATION. $\frac{6}{3}$. in six teaspoonfuls of water, a teaspoonful every twelve hours, until the desired relief is obtained.

MILK FEVER.

The secretion of milk must be looked upon rather as an operation of nature than one requiring medical aid for its regulation. Nevertheless, many females suffer some slight uneasiness for a few days following confinement, during the first period of that process; but when any of the under-mentioned group of symptoms present themselves, the affection is known by the name of milk fever:—

Thirst, shivering, and heat, terminating in perspiration; the pulse, at first weak, changing to various phases, sometimes quick and frequent, at others soft and regular; in some instances, these symptoms are attended with a drawing pain in the back extending to the breast, a disagreeable taste in the mouth, thirst, oppressed breathing, anxiety, headache, and diminution or suppression of the secretions of milk, etc.; the exacerbation declares itself regularly about evening, and towards morning perspiration comes on, with alleviation of suffering, or temporary termination of the attack, which not unfrequently recurs on the following day, but rarely rises to such a height as to threaten danger; nature herself, if not disturbed by improper treatment, will, in most cases, suffice to restore the equilibrium of the system. When the secretion is re-established, and the lochial discharge resumes its normal course, the derangement generally ceases: should, however, the affection become aggravated, we may dread the setting in of puerperal fever.

When the symptoms are as above described, and medical assistance is required for their alleviation, we must, if possible, in the first place, endeavour to discover the exciting cause;* when the affection is traceable to MENTAL EMOTIONS, we may consult that article for the remedy.

ACONITE, $\frac{000}{6}$, may be had recourse to in all instances where considerable fever is present, or administered alternately every six hours, with *Coffea*, when there is extreme restlessness, anxiety, and dread.

BRYONIA may with great advantage follow *Aconite*, when the active febrile symptoms are in a great measure subdued; and is further particularly indicated, when there is oppressed and laborious breathing, intense headache, and obstinate constipation.

ADMINISTRATION. $\frac{000}{12}$, in a teaspoonful of water, and repeated in six, twelve, or twenty four hours, according to circumstances. (Vide note, p. 21.)

PULSATILLA will be found particularly useful in severe cases, especially when caused by taking cold, and bearing a closer approximation to a rheumatic affection than to the general symptoms of milk fever; this medicament is very effica-

* Neglecting to put the infant sufficiently early to the breast, with consequent absorption into the circulation of the milk which has been secreted, is a frequent source of the derangement.

cious in restoring the lacteal secretion, and may be regarded as a prophylactic against puerperal fever, especially when the precautionary measure of the administration of *Arnica* has been neglected.

ADMINISTRATION. $\frac{000}{12}$, in a teaspoonful of water, repeated every twelve or twenty-four hours, according to the urgency of the symptoms, until benefit results.

BELLADONNA is very useful in particular cases; a reference to INFLAMMATION OF THE BREASTS, and other places where that medicament is mentioned, will serve to point out in what instances it is most likely to prove efficacious.

RHUS is also of considerable service in some cases of milk fever. (See the indications given for this remedy under the heading of EXCESSIVE SECRETION OF MILK.)

IRREGULARITIES OF THE LOCHIAL DISCHARGE.

This varies considerably in different females; with some it continues for several weeks, in others only a few days; sometimes it is thin and scanty, at others so profuse and long continued, as imperatively to call for medical assistance, which may be frequently traced to sitting up too soon after confinement, to errors in regimen, keeping the chamber of the female at too high a temperature, or mental emotions. If, after nine days, the discharge continues profuse, containing pure blood, whereby an abnormal state is indicated, *Crocus*, *Bryonia*, and *Calcarea*, are the principal remedies.

CROCUS. In most cases where the discharge is of too long duration, and particularly when the blood is of a black or dark colour, and viscid consistency.

ADMINISTRATION. $\frac{6}{6}$,* in an ounce of water, a dessertspoonful night and morning. (Vide note, p. 21.)

BRYONIA. When of a deep red, with internal burning pains in the region of the uterus.

ADMINISTRATION. $\frac{6}{6}$, in the same manner as the above.

CALCAREA is more particularly indicated when there is an itching kind of sensation in the uterus.

* In some cases the 3d, 2d, and even the 1st attenuation, or potency, of this medicine has been exhibited with marked benefit, when a higher number appeared to produce but little effect.

Administration. $\frac{6}{12}$, in six teaspoonfuls of water, one night and morning.

When the lochia are suddenly *suppressed*, which they sometimes are, from a variety of external causes, such as mental emotions, etc., and from this source puerperal fever threatens, the danger may frequently be warded off by the administration of Pulsatilla, $\frac{000}{12}$ repeated in six, twelve, or twenty-four hours, according to circumstances.

When the sudden suppression arises from fright, with febrile symptoms, Aconite $\frac{000}{24}$, will generally be found sufficient, or *Opium*, $\frac{000}{30}$, when the indications given under Mental Emotions are present. (See also the other remedies mentioned under that heading.)

When caused by exposure to cold or damp, Dulcamara $\frac{000}{12}$, will be found efficacious, and may be advantageously followed by Pulsatilla $\frac{000}{12}$.

On the other hand, when the discharge continues, but becomes sanious, fetid, and offensive, Belladonna $\frac{000}{12}$, in six teaspoonfuls of water, one daily, will generally suffice to restore it to its normal state; (vide note, p. 21); if it prove inefficient, we may administer Carbo animalis $\frac{6}{30}$, in the same manner; and if the occasion still seem to require it, Secale cornutum $\frac{00}{6}$, in a teaspoonful of water, repeated every twelve hours until benefit results.

Silicea, when *pure blood follows with the lochia each time that the infant is applied to the breast.*

Administration. $\frac{6}{30}$, in the same manner as directed for *Belladonna*. The following remedies may also prove useful: *Nux-v.*, *Hyoscyamus*, *Zincum*, *Colocynth*, *Veratrum* and *Secale cornutum*, chiefly in the event of a suppression. And *Platina*, *Secale cornutum*, *Hepar-s.*, *Rhus*, against too copious or protracted lochia.

DIARRHŒA IN LYING-IN WOMEN.

Diarrhœa, during this period, is a state to be looked upon as highly injurious, and immediate means should be taken for its suppression, by the administration of *Dulcamara*, *Hyoscyamus*, *Rheum*, *Antimonium crudum*, *Phosphorus*, and *Acidum phosphoricum*, etc.

The first remedy, $\frac{000}{6}$, is generally indicated by the cause, being the check of the natural increased perspiration in lying-in women, from a chill; and when timely administered, it will generally be found sufficient to answer the purpose required.

In painless and almost involuntary evacuations, HYOSCYAMUS $\frac{000}{6}$ is most effectual.

RHEUM $\frac{000}{6}$, and ANTIMONIUM CRUDUM $\frac{00}{8}$, in watery, or very offensive evacuations; the former when they emit a sour smell.

In very *obstinate* cases, when the discharge is watery, almost involuntary, and painless, PHOSPHORUS $\frac{00}{8}$, followed, if necessary, by ACIDUM PHOSPHORICUM, $\frac{00}{12}$ or $\frac{00}{30}$. (Vide also DIARRHŒA, in the second part of this work, and administer or repeat the remedies as there directed.)

ABDOMINAL DEFORMITY.

Although, in natural cases and healthy constitutions, no abnormal derangements should follow parturition, still we frequently find that a number of unpleasant symptoms, generally arising from maltreatment, supervene. Among these we may mention the thickening of the abdominal coats, occasionally ending in a permanent malformation and pendulous appearance. This affection is more commonly incident to females who have borne many children, or who present a predisposition to corpulency; and is found especially difficult of treatment, when tight stays, which we have already remarked upon as one of the principal exciting causes, have relaxed the abdominal muscles, and by so doing, increased the existing bias. When, however, it is caused by the natural strain upon these muscles during pregnancy, the inconvenience may be considerably alleviated by the internal and external use of RHUS TOXICODENDRON.

The internal administration of SEPIA $\frac{000}{30}$ is recommended by Dr. Gross as still more effectual, who at the same time advises the adoption of an elastic bandage, laced at the back, and exerting an equable pressure over the whole of the abdominal region. In some cases where there is a *tendency* to this affection, particularly in corpulent habits, we may, *soon after delivery*, have recourse to mechanical aid, by transferring the weight from the abdominal muscles to the shoulders, by the aid of a properly-constructed apparatus; but we must in the strongest manner object to this or any other pressure being exercised upon the abdominal region *during pregnancy* as calculated to entail malformation, such as club-feet, &c., upon the offspring.

FALLING OFF OF THE HAIR.

Another evil that some females, particularly those who nurse their infants themselves, suffer after confinement, is the falling off of the hair of the head.

This frequently arises from an innate delicacy of constitution, against which the following medicaments have proved efficacious, and may be repeated every eight days:

TINCTURA SULPHURIS $\frac{6}{30}$, NATRUM MURIATICUM $\frac{6}{30}$, and CARBO VEGETABILIS $\frac{6}{30}$, SEPIA $\frac{6}{30}$, LYCOPODIUM $\frac{6}{12}$, and CALCAREA $\frac{6}{18}$. The latter, particularly in those cases in which the lochial discharge has proved very profuse, or in which the catamenia are generally too abundant.

With regard to the other medicines, we would in most instances recommend a commencement with *Tinctura sulphuris*.

LEUCORRHŒA AFTER PARTURITION.

A third evil is Leucorrhœa, which, although at the commencement merely a consequence of the relaxation of the internal uterine economy, after the completion of the lochial discharge, and at first of an innocuous character, frequently proves exceedingly troublesome, and finally puts on a morbid appearance, becoming acrid, and productive of excoriation. We generally find a predisposition to the disease in scrofulous, torpid, and leuco-phlegmatic temperaments; in some families this malady is hereditary, and only to be removed by a careful course of anti-dyscratic treatment. It is frequently of a very obstinate character, requiring the exercise of considerable study and attention on the part of the medical attendant, on the one hand, with much patience and strict attention to dietetic rules on that of the patient, on the other, ere a successful result can be attained.

The remedies which have been found the most efficacious against the affection, either occurring after parturition or at other times, are: *Pulsatilla*, *Sulphur*, *Sepia*, *Bovista*, *Calcarea*, *Lycopodium*, and *Carbo v.*, *Causticum*, *Conium*, *Mezereon*, *Natrum*, *Magnesia c. and m.*, *Ammonium c.*, *Cannabis*, *Iodium*, *Petroleum*, *Stannum*, etc. Dose: $\frac{000}{3}$ or $\frac{000}{6}$.

INTERNAL UTERINE SWELLING AND PROLAPSUS.

A swelling of the interior economy is frequently the result of a difficult labour, and in some cases of mismanaged parturition; we sometimes find it complicated with uterine or vaginal prolapsus; if the precaution of exhibiting ARNICA $\frac{00}{6}$, which we have before noted, (page 411,) have been taken, this will frequently be prevented; if, however, symptoms of prolapsus set in, attended with a painful burning sensation, and bearing down, a dose or two of NUX VOMICA will generally remove the evil. *Sepia*, *Belladonna*, *Aurum*, *Mercurius*, *Lycopodium*, *Stannum*, *Cannabis*, *China*, *Platina*, and *Calcarea*, etc., have been employed with material benefit in cases of this description of longer standing, as also in other uterine affections, such as Metritis, Retroversio uteri, etc. Dose: $\frac{000}{3}$ or $\frac{000}{6}$.

WEAKNESS AFTER DELIVERY.

We frequently find a high degree of weakness or exhaustion remaining after delivery; when it has been caused by very considerable hemorrhage, during or after that period, CINCHONA is particularly indicated, and will generally be found efficient in restoring the vital energies.

ADMINISTRATION. $\frac{000}{3}$, in a teaspoonful of water, repeated in three or four days.

When however the derangement depends upon nervous weakness, and is attended with restlessness and want of sleep, we may administer ACONITE, followed, if necessary, by COFFEA, or substitute VERATRUM for the latter medicine, when the prostration of strength is excessive.

In some instances we must have recourse to KALI CARB., or to SULPHUR, CALCAREA, or ACID PHOSPH. Dose $\frac{00}{6}$.

INFLAMMATION OF THE WOMB.

(*Inflammatio uteri. Metritis.*)

Continuous burning, pricking, or shooting pain in the hypogastric region, with a sensation of weight. The utero-vaginal secretions are suppressed, sometimes also the evacuation of fæces and urine; and, in lying-in-women, the secretion of milk is likewise arrested. *Causes:* Severe, unnatural labours, harsh manual interference, and powerful stimulants, etc. *Aconit.* $\frac{0}{3}$, a few doses, when the accompanying fever partakes of a synochal type.—*Bellad.* $\frac{000}{3}$, when suppression of the lochia, sensation of weight, dragging or bearing down in the hypogastric region; burning, shooting pains in the lower part of the abdomen; shooting pains in the hip-joint; severe pain in the back, as if it would break; tenderness of the abdomen to the touch.—In consequence of severe labour, with laceration of the parts: *Arnica* in alternation with *Aconit.* $\frac{000}{3}$. *Nux v.* $\frac{000}{6}$, in uterine derangements of a shooting or cutting description, suppression of urine, constipation, tenesmus, etc.—*Merc.* $\frac{00}{6}$, when frequent fits of perspiration or shivering take place, with pains in the uterus.—*Cham.*, *Ignat.*, *Coff.*, or *Bryon.*, $\frac{000}{3}$, when mental emotions have preceded. In other cases: *China*, *Lach.*, *Plat.*, *Puls.*, *Rhus t.*, *Sec.*, *Thuja.*, etc. In *Irritable Uterus: Nux v.*, *Plat.*, *Bell.*, *Stann.*, *Cham*, *Ipec.*, *Sepia*, *Sulph.*, *Calc.*, *Cocc.*, *Con.*, *Graph.*, etc. Against *Uterine Spasms: Cocc.*, *Ignat.*, *Con.*, *Magn. c.*, *Magn. m.*, *Bell.*, *Cham.*, *Nux v.*, *Hyos.*, *China.* Against *Uterine Polypus: Staphys.*, *Thuja*, *Calc.*, *Ac. nitr.*, *Carb v.* Against *ulcerations* at the os uteri, etc: *Carbo v.*, *Graph.*, *Sulph.*, *Silic.*, *Sepia*, *Ars.*, *Merc.*, *Thuja.*—In *indurations* of the Uterus: *Aurum*, *Bellad.*, *Sep.*, *Staph.*, *Calendula.* In *Carcinoma: Bellad.*, *Ars.*, *Staph.*, *Thuja*, Carb. v., *Carb. a.*, Clem., *Con.*, *Silic.* Dose: $\frac{000}{3}$ or $\frac{000}{12}$ or $\frac{00}{30}$.

OBSTACLES TO SUCKLING.

DISINCLINATION OF THE INFANT.

WHERE there is a tendency to consumption in the mother, or she is of a strumous habit, the infant ought, for its own sake, to be reared with the spoon, or a nurse provided; but even some healthy mothers find a difficulty, before they become accustomed to it, in nursing their children, which a little perseverance will soon effectually overcome; but when (a rare instance, if applied soon after delivery) the child itself refuses to take the breast, the administration of CINA $\frac{0}{6}$, followed, if not speedily efficacious, by MERCURIUS SOLUBILIS $\frac{0}{12}$ is often found to remove this repugnance in the course of a few hours. SILICEA $\frac{0}{30}$, is also an excellent remedy in some cases, particularly when the child takes the breast readily enough, but returns the milk almost immediately after; the remedy selected ought to be given to the mother as well as the child.

EXCORIATION OF THE NIPPLES.

In the majority of those cases in which no malformation of the parts is present, the main difficulty arises from the nipples having become sore and cracked, which the efforts of the infant tear open afresh, and cause to bleed.

This excoriation of the nipples is frequently prevented by following up the treatment, of which we have already spoken, under the head of PREPARATION OF THE BREASTS, of course taking the precaution of laving them with a little warm milk and water before the child is applied to the breast; the shield before mentioned ought always to be worn during the intervals of suckling.

When there is a tendency, however slight, to rawness or excoriation, great care must be taken lest the shield adhere to the skin; it ought to be frequently removed, and together with the nipple, kept perfectly dry; attention to these particulars will generally remove this difficulty. The mother ought, however, gradually to accustom herself to nourish the infant, using a sucking-glass, which should be carefully washed every day. Should, however, the nipples have already become very sore and irritable, from the neglect of these precautionary measures, it is necessary to have recourse to specific remedies, without which, if suckling be persisted in, suppuration frequently ensues.

In the first stage of the affection, ARNICA $\frac{000}{6}$ should be administered internally, and the breasts laved with a *weak* lotion,* say one or two drops of the *Mother Tincture*, to one ounce of water. If this fail, we must have recourse to antidyscratic remedies, as this disease almost always arises from a constitutional cause, females of healthy temperament being generally exempt from it. Among these, TINCTURA SULPHURIS $\frac{00}{30}$ seems particularly indicated for most cases of this affection, and a dose of one or two globules may be administered every five or six days until improvement sets in, which will generally be the case in the space of a few days; and if this fail, CALCAREA $\frac{00}{18}$, administered in the same manner, will in most instances suffice. We may also mention GRAPHITES, SEPIA, LYCOPODIUM, MERC, and SILIC., as remedies of much value in some obstinate cases. In the choice of the fitting medicament in complicated cases, the physician can be guided by the aggregate of the symptoms. (*Nux v.* has been found of considerable service in soreness of the nipple, with painful excoriation of the adjacent surface.) Dose: $\frac{000}{3}$ or $\frac{000}{6}$.

* This lotion may also be applied with advantage in the PREPARATION OF THE BREASTS, when irritation or inflammation appears to arise from the pressure of the shield.

INFLAMMATION OF THE BREASTS.

Another, and one of the greatest obstacles to a mother nourishing her infant, is an erysipelatous inflammation and swelling of the breasts, of which any thing tending to disturb the lacteal secretion, such as fright, passion, cold, &c., serves for an exciting cause, although we frequently find it present, without being able to trace its origin ; it not unfrequently arises from a too tardy administration of the breast to the infant, or from a sudden cessation of suckling,—from the death of the child, or other reasons, —causing a distention of the lactiferous tubes. When a sudden suppression of the secretion occurs, the breasts become red, inflamed, and indurated, occasionally suppurating in some parts, which open and discharge, while others remain still hard and inflammatory, finally either ending in suppuration, or the formation of obstinate nodosities.

This disease, if not checked, and but too frequently under allopathic treatment, exhibits a variety of phases ; and the suppuration that takes place, leaves behind it disfiguring cicatrices; frequently the breasts are so far destroyed, as to be rendered ever after incapable of performing their functions; and in some instances, the foundation of cancer is laid.

The principal remedy in this affection before the inflammation becomes fully developed, is BRYONIA $\frac{0}{6}$, especially when the breasts are hard and tumefied, and the secretion of milk suppressed. BELLADONNA, when the inflammation is more intense, and the erysipelatous appearance of the skin clearly defined ; after which remedy, the disease is generally vanquished.

ADMINISTRATION. $\frac{000000}{6}$, in as many teaspoonfuls of water, a teaspoonful to be taken every six or eight hours, until improvement follows.

When, however, a degree of induration still remains, MERCURIUS SOLUBILIS, $\frac{000}{12}$, should be given, and repeated from two to three days; in more severe cases, ACIDUM PHOSPHORICUM should be resorted to, or HEPAR SULPHURIS, when *suppuration* has already commenced.

ADMINISTRATION, of the latter, one grain of the third trituration in an ounce of water, a dessert-spoonful to be given three or four times a day, in order to forward the suppurative process, when it becomes absolutely necessary to bring the matter to a head as speedily as possible.

In instances in which we find a fetid and serous discharge, which is frequently brought about by neglect or by improper treatment, such as the application of deleterious salves, etc., SILICEA $\frac{000}{30}$, repeated in five or six days, will generally be amply sufficient to restore the breast to its former condition; in some extreme cases, however, it will be found necessary to follow up the treatment with *Phosphorus*, *Calcarea*, or one or more of the remedies above mentioned, such as *Mercurius*, and *Hepar sulphuris*.

If this disease evidently arise from the effect of a sudden chill, DULCAMARA $\frac{000}{12}$ ought to be given immediately, and will frequently obviate all injurious consequences.

In cases where the disease has arisen from external injury, ARNICA $\frac{000}{6}$ should be administered, and a lotion, one part of the tincture to seven of pure water, locally applied.

In strumous habits, TINCTURA SULPHURIS, CALCAREA and GRAPHITES, will occasionally be found necessary to complete the cure, after *Belladonna* has removed the active inflammatory symptoms.

MENTAL EMOTIONS AFFECTING THE MILK.

It is a well known fact, confirmed by numerous examples, that Mental Emotions have a most powerful effect upon this secretion, in a moment changing it from a source of nutriment into a substance most injurious to the infant. Mothers ought to bear this in mind, and after having suffered from fright, passion, etc., should desist from suckling until they are perfectly composed; and ere the infant be again applied to the breast, a portion of the milk should be drawn off. Fortunately, for evils arising from these causes, Homœopathy presents prompt and efficacious remedies, (for which, see MENTAL EMOTIONS,) which, if at hand, should be administered immediately, according to the cause and symptoms.

DEFICIENCY IN THE SECRETION OF MILK.
SUPPRESSED SECRETION OF MILK.

Sometimes a deficiency of milk is found to arise from a want of energy, either functional or general. For disturbance of the secretion arising from an inflammatory action, Vide INFLAMMATION OF THE BREASTS.

When the deficiency or suppression arises from the first cause, the chief medicines useful in restoring a proper and healthy flow of milk, are PULSATILLA, CALCAREA, and CAUSTICUM. The physician is the best judge in the application of these remedies, as there are many minute symptoms by which his choice must be guided in the selection—in simple cases, Vitex agnus castus and Pulsatilla will frequently be found efficacious; but it is more generally requisite for the female to undergo a complete course of treatment, if she is anxious to persevere in nursing, in which the two latter, together with *Aconitum*, *Bryonia*, *Chamomilla*, *Belladonna*, *Sulphur*, *Sepia*, *Iodium*, will be found of great value. Dose: $\frac{000}{3}$ or $\frac{000}{6}$.

DETERIORATION AND DISCOLORATION OF MILK.

If the milk becomes too clear and watery, (or otherwise deteriorated in quality, or is repugnant to the child,) Cina $\frac{000}{6}$ and Mercurius solubilis $\frac{000}{12}$, ought to be administered alternately every twenty-four hours for three or four days; or Silicea $\frac{000}{30}$, in obstinate cases, (and particularly if the infant vomits immediately after suckling), will frequently bring about an amelioration.

Rheum will frequently be found of efficacy when the milk becomes thick and yellow, and disagrees with the child, rendering it restless and fretful; a globule of the third or the sixth potency ought to be given to the child while the mother is under the action of the same remedy.

MOTHERS NOT SUCKLING THEIR CHILDREN.

In the present state of society, there are many mothers who, from a variety of circumstances, find themselves necessitated to engage the services of a nurse for their offspring; in such cases, a female, who has the slightest regard for her health, should be particularly careful in her diet, and until the secreting process has entirely ceased, she should live as low as possible. The employment of dry cupping at the outer surface of the arm, a little below the shoulder, or to the inferior extremities, will materially hasten the suppression of the lacteal secretion. At the same time, material aid will be derived from the internal administration of Pulsatilla; indeed, the employment of that remedy alone will often be found sufficient to stop the secretion. A few globules of the third or sixth potency may be dissolved in a wine-glassful of water, and a teaspoonful taken night and morning. When suffering from inflammation ensues, we may have recourse to Phosphorus, Belladonna, and Bryonia, for which indications are given under Inflammation of the Breasts; Calcarea is serviceable when the breasts are considerably distended with milk. These same directions will serve as a guide during the period of weaning.

GLOSSARY OF MEDICAL TERMS

EMPLOYED IN THIS WORK.

ABDOMEN. The cavity situated between the lower part of the thorax and the region of the pelvis, containing the intestines; the belly.

ABNORMAL. A deviation from the course of nature; in medicine, unhealthy.

ABORTUS. Miscarriage; abortion.

ABRADE. To excoriate.

ABRASION. Excoriation.

ABSCESS. A collection of pus seated in any particular organ or tissue.

ABSORBENTS. In anatomy, this term is applied to small, delicate, transparent vessels which take up and convey any substances from the surface of the body, or from any cavity, into the blood.

ACETABULUM. A cavity of a cuplike form, receiving the head of the femur or thigh-bone.

ADHESION. In surgery, the reunion of parts that have been divided, by means of a special kind of inflammation denominated the *adhesive*. In pathology, the morbid union of parts which are naturally contiguous, though not adherent, through the instrumentality of adhesive inflammation.

ADHESIVE INFLAMMATION. The process by which wounds are united. It is often synonymous with *union by the first intention.*

ADYPSIA. The absence of natural thirst.

AGGLUTINATION. Adhesion.

AGRYPNIA. Sleeplessness.

AGUSTIA. Loss of taste.

ALÆ NASI. The lateral cartilages of the nose. Wings of the nose.

ALKALI. A substance which unites with acids in definite proportions, so as to neutralize their properties more or less perfectly, and to form salts. It changes vegetable blues to green.

ALKALOIDS. Substances having some of the properties of *alkalis.*

ALLOPATHY. A term used by homœopathic writers to designate the old practice of medicine in contradistinction to their own, now generally employed by both parties; literally implies curing one disease by another.

ALVINE. From the stomach or intestines.

AMENORRHŒA. Absence or stoppage of the menstrual flux.

AMNESIA. Loss of memory.

AMYGDALÆ. A popular term for the exterior glands of the neck, as also the *tonsils,* which are so called from their shape bearing some resemblance to that of an almond.

ANASARCA. Dropsy of the cellular tissue, or membrane, immediately under the skin.

ANCHYLOSIS. Stiffening of a joint, either from deposit of ossific or bone-forming matter, or contraction of the muscles or ligaments; adhesion of the articulating surfaces.

ANEURISM. Morbid enlargement of an artery.

ANGINA. Sore throat. The term is also applied to diseases with difficult respiration.

ANGINA MEMBRANACEA. Croup.

ANGINA PAROTIDEA. Mumps.

ANGINA PHARYNGIA. Inflammation of the membrane which forms the pharynx.

ANOREXIA. Want of appetite.

ANTACID. Substances possessing the property of neutralizing acidity.

ANTHRAX. Carbuncle.

ANTHROPOPHOBIA. A dread or horror of the human species.

ANTIPHLOGISTIC. Applied to remedies employed in the old system against inflammation; literally, against heat.

ANTRUM-HIGHMORIANUM. The maxillary sinus. A hollow or cavity above the teeth of the upper jaw, in the middle of the superior maxillary bone.

ANUS. The inferior opening of the rectum.

APEPSIA. Loss of appetite.

APHONIA. Loss of voice.

APONEUROSIS, plur. APONEUROSES. Tendons expanded upon a wide surface.

APOPLEXIA. Apoplexy; a loss of voluntary motion and consciousness. See *Diagnosis* under this head.

APYREXIA. The intervals between febrile paroxysms.

ARC. A segment of a circle.

ARTHRITIS. Gout.

ASCARIS, plur. ASCARIDES. Thread-worms.

ASPHYXIA. Apparent death.

ASTHENIC. Low; applied to disease; literally, want of strength.

ASTRINGENTS. Medicaments used in the old practice to contract the animal fibre.

ATONY. A want of tone or energy in the muscular power.

ATROPHY. A morbid state of the digestive system, in which the food taken into the stomach fails to afford sufficient nourishment. A wasting of the whole, or of individual parts of the body.

AUSCULTATION. The defection of symptoms by the ear in disease.

BILIARY. Connected with the secretion of bile.

BLEPHARITIS. Inflammation of the eyelids.

BORBORYGMUS. Rumbling in the intestines, caused by flatus or wind.

BRONCHIA; BRONCHI. The tubes into which the trachea or windpipe divides.

BRONCHIAL SOUNDS. Those which are heard in the bronchi.

BRONCHITIS. Inflammation of the ramifications of the windpipe.

BRONCHOPHONY. The resonance of the voice heard over the bronchial tubes.

BULIMY; BULIMIA. Canine, or excessive hunger.

CADAVEROUS. Resembling a corpse.

CÆCUM. The blind gut; so called from its being perforated at one end only.

CALAMINE. A preparation of zinc.

CALCULUS, plur. CALCULI. A concretion in the human body. *Calculosus.* Afflicted with the stone.

CANINE. Belonging to the dog species.

CANTHUS. The angle of the eye.

CARCINOMA. Cancer, adj. *Carcinomatous.*

CARDIALGIA. Spasm of the stomach.

CARDITIS. Inflammation of the heart.

CARIES. Ulceration of the bones.

CARMINATIVES. Medicaments used against flatulency.

CAROTIDS. The name of two large arteries of the neck.

CARPHOLOGIA. Picking at the bed clothes.

CARTILAGE. Gristle.

CATAMENIA. The menstrual flux.

CATARRH. Cold; used also to express inflammation of the mucous membrane.

CATARRHAL OPHTHALMIA. Simple inflammation of the conjunctiva.

CATHARTIC. Purgative.

CELLULAR TISSUE. The fine net-like membrane enveloping or connecting most of the structures of the human body.

CEPHALALGIA. Headache.

CEPHALIC. Pertaining to the head.

CEREBRAL. Appertaining to the brain.

CERVICAL. Belonging to the neck.

CESSATIO MENSIUM. Discontinuance of the menstrual flux.

CHLOROSIS. Green sickness.

CHOLERA. See article thereon.

CHOLERINE. A modified species of cholera.

CHRONIC. Long continued, in contradistinction to acute.

CICATRIX, plur. *Cicatrices*. A scar left after the healing of a wound, &c.

CLAVI PEDIS. Corns.

CLONIC SPASM. A spasm which is not of long duration. It is opposed to *tonic* spasm, which see.

COAGULA. Clots of blood.

COAGULABLE LYMPH. The term given to the fluid which is slowly effused into wounds, and afterwards forms the uniting medium or cicatrice.

COLIC. Griping in the intestines.

COLLAPSE. Failing of vitality.

COLLIQUATIVE. Excessive discharge of any secretion.

COMA. Drowsiness.

COMA SOMNOLENTIUM. Drowsiness, with relapse thereunto on being roused.

COMATOSE. Drowsy.

COMPRESS. Soft lint, linen, &c., folded together so as to form a pad, for the purpose of being placed, and secured by means of a bandage, on parts which require pressure.

CONGESTIO AD CAPUT. Determination of blood to the head.

CONGESTIO AD PECTUS. Determination of blood to the chest.

CONGESTION. Overfulness of the blood-vessels of some particular organ.

CONGLOBATE GLANDS. Glands of a globular form, composed of a texture of lymphatic vessels. They have no excretory duct.

CONJUNCTIVA. The membrane lining the eyelids, and extending over the forepart of the eye-balls.

CONTAGION. Propagation of a disease by contact.

CORNEA. The anterior transparent portion of the eye. It is of a horny consistence.

CORYZA. Cold in the head.

COXAGRA. Inflammation of the hip-joint. Literally, seizure or pain in the.

COXALGIA. Literally, pain in the hip; inflammation of the hip-joint.

CRANIUM. The skull.

CREPITATION. Grating sensation, or noise, such as is caused by pressing the finger upon a part affected with emphysema; by the ends of a fractured bone when moved; or by certain salts during calcination.

CREPITANT RHONCHUS, or RALE. The fine crackling noise heard in consequence of the passage of air through a viscid fluid. It is heard in the first stage of inflammation of the lungs.

CREPITUS. Crackling or grating.

CUTANEOUS. Appertaining to the skin.

CUTICLE. The outer or scarf skin.

CYSTICIS. Inflammation of the bladder.

DEBILE. Low.

DEFECATION. Alvine evacuation.

DEGLUTITION. The act of swallowing.

DELIRIUM. Derangement of the brain, raving.

DEPLETION. Abstraction of the fluids; generally applied to venesection.

DESICCATION. A drying up.

DESQUAMATION. Falling off of the epidermis in form of scales.

DIAPHRAGMITIS. Inflammation of the diaphragm (muscular partition between the thorax and abdomen).

DIAGNOSIS.—Distinction of maladies.

DIARRHŒA. Looseness of the bowels.

DIARRHŒA NEONATORUM. The same as the above, in infants.

DIATHESIS. Constitutional tendency.

DIETETIC. Relating to diet.

DIPLOPIA. Affection of the eyes, in which objects appear double or increased in number.

DIURETIC. Medicines which increase the secretion of urine.

DORSAL. Appertaining to the back.

DRASTIC. Powerful purgatives.

DUODENUM. The first intestine after the stomach, so called from its length; the twelve-inch gut.

DYSCRASIA. A morbid condition of the system; adj. *Dyscrastic.*

DYSECOIA. Deafness.

DYSMENORRHŒA. Painful menstruation.

DYSPEPSIA. Indigestion; literally, difficulty of appetite.

DYSPNŒA. Difficulty of respiration. Shortness of breath.

DYSURIA. Difficulty in passing urine.

EFFUSION. A pouring out or escape of lymph or other secretion.

EMACIATION. A falling off in the flesh.

EMETIC. Provoking vomiting.

EMPHYSEMA. Windy swelling. A swelling caused by the diffusion of air in the cellular tissue, rendering it tense, elastic, and crepitating. It is divided into the *traumatic* when the air has been introduced through a wound; *idiopathic*, or spontaneous, when the gas is developed within the cells, which is, however, of rare occurrence.

ENCEPHALITIS. Inflammation of the brain and membranes.

ENDEMIC. Peculiar to a particular locality.

ENDOCARDITIS. Inflammation of the internal parts of the heart.

ENEMA. A clyster.

ENGORGEMENT. Swelling up of.

ENTERALGIA. Colic

ENTERITIS. Inflammation of the intestines.

EPHEMERAL. Of a day's duration.

EPHIALTES. Night-mare.

EPIDEMIC. Diseases arising from general causes.

EPIGASTRIUM. The region of the stomach.

EPILEPSY. EPILEPSIA. Falling sickness.

EPISTAXIS. Bleeding from the nose.

EPITHELIUM. The cuticle.

ERYSIPELAS. St. Anthony's fire. Rose. A disease of the skin.

ERYSIPELAS PHLEGMONODES. Phlegmonous erysipelas.

ERYSIPELAS ŒDEMATODES. Œdematous erysipelas.

ERYSIPELAS ERRATICUM. Wandering erysipelas.

ERYSIPELAS GANGRENOSUM. Gangrenous erysipelas.

ERYSIPELAS NEONATORUM. Induration of the cellular tissue in infants.

EXACERBATION. Aggravation of fever, &c.

EXANTHEMA, plur. *Exanthemata.* Eruption terminating in exfoliation.

EXPECTORATION. Discharge of any matter; phlegm; pus from the chest.

EXUDATION. Discharge of fluid from the skin, &c.

FÆCES. Alvine excrement.

FALSE JOINT. When the two fragments of a broken bone do not become united by an osseus bond of union, the limb continues in a state of preternatural mobility, and, if not remedied, is converted into a *false joint*, admitting of flexion in various directions, without pain.

FASCIA. In anatomy, the tendinous expansion of muscles which bind parts together are called *fasciæ.*

FAUCES. The throat.

FAVUS CONVERTUS. Pustular ringworm, or ringworm of the scalp.

FEBRIS, plur. FEBRES. Fever.

FEBRIS NERVOSA. Nervous Fever, or typhus.

FEMUR. The bone of the thigh.

FETOR. Stench.

First Intention. See *Union by the.*

Fistula. An obstinate tube-like sore, with a narrow orifice; adj. *Fistulous.*

Fistula Lachrymalis. An ulcerated opening in the lachrymal sac.

Flatus. Wind in the intestines. Flatulency.

Fœtus. The infant in the womb.

Fomentation. The application of flannel wet with warm water.

Fontanel, plur. *Fontanella.* The mould.

Functional Diseases. Those in which there is supposed to be only derangement of action.

Furunculus. A boil.

Furunculus Malignans. Carbuncle.

Gangrene. Incipient mortification; adj. *Gangrenous.*

Gastralgia. Pain in the stomach.

Gastric. Belonging to the stomach.

Gastritis. Inflammation of the stomach.

Gastrodynia. Vide *Cardialgia.*

Gestation. Pregnancy.

Gland. A small body met with in many parts of the body, and consisting of various tissues, blood-vessels, nerves, &c.

Glossitis. Inflammation of the tongue.

Glottis. Opening of the wind-pipe. The superior opening of the larynx.

Granulation. See *Incarnation.*

Hæmatemesis, or *Hematemesis.*—Vomiting of blood.

Hæmoptysis, or *Hemoptysis.* Discharge of blood from the lungs. Spitting of blood.

Hæmorrhage, or *Hemorrhage.* Discharge of blood.

Hæmorrhoids, or *Hemorrhoids.* Piles.

Hectic Fever. Habitual or protracted fever.

Helminthiasis. Worm disease.

Hemiplegia. Paralysis of one side of the body longitudinally.

Hepatitis. Inflammation of the liver.

Hepatization. Structural derangement of the lungs, the result of inflammation; changing them into a substance resembling the liver, hence its name.

Hernia. Rupture.

Hernia Congenita. Congenital hernia. Literally, hernia from birth.

Herpes Circinnatus. Ringworm.

Hordeolum. Stye.

Hydrocephalus. Water in the head.

Hydrophobia Symptomatica. Symptoms resembling those arising from hydrophobic virus, appearing during the course of other diseases.

Hypertrophy. A morbid increase of any organ, arising from excessive nutrition.

Hypocratic. Sunken and corpse-like.

Hypochondrium. Region of the abdomen, contained under the cartilage of the false ribs.

Hypochondriasis. Spleen disease; great depression of spirits, with general functional derangement; adj. *Hypochondriacal.*

Hypogastrium. The lower anterior portion of the abdomen.

Hysteria. Nervous affection; almost peculiar to females.

Ichor. A thin watery discharge secreted from wounds, ulcers, &c.; adj. *Ichorous.*

Icterus. Jaundice.

Icterus Neonatorum. Jaundice of infants.

Idiopathic. Original or primary disease.

Idiosyncrasy. Individual peculiarity.

Ilium. The haunch-bone. It, together with the pubis, sacrum, and ischium, contributes to form the pelvis.

Ileus Miserere. A form of colic, a twisting pain in the region of the navel.

INCARCERATED. Strangulated or constricted; a term applied to rupture.

INCARNATION. The process by which abscesses or ulcers are healed; this takes place by means of little grain-like fleshy bodies, denominated granulations, which form on the surface of ulcers or suppurating wounds, &c., and serve the double purpose of filling up the cavities and bringing closely together and uniting their sides.

INCUBUS. The nightmare.

INFECTION. Propagation of disease by effluvia.

INFILTRATION. Diffusion of fluids into the cellular tissue.

INFRA ORBITARY NERVE. A twig of the second branch of the fifth pair of nerves. It passes out of a small hole immediately below the orbit, (the *foramen infra orbitarium*,) and is distributed upon the cheek, under eyelid, upper side of the nose, and joins with the portio dura of the seventh pair.

INGESTA. Food; aliment.

INSPISSATED. Thickened.

INTEGUMENTS. The coverings of any part of the body. The skin with the adherent fat and cellular membrane form the common integuments.

INTENTION. See *Union by the first.*

INTUMESCENCE. Swelling; puffiness.

INVERMINATION. The term given to the morbid states occasioned by the existence of worms in the intestines (intestinal canal).

ISCHIAS. Pain in the hip.

ISCHIUM. Hip-bone.

ISCHURIA. Suppression of urine.

LACHRYMAL SAC.

LACHRYMATION. Tear shedding.

LACTATION. Suckling; also the process of the secretion of milk.

LACTEAL. Appertaining to the process of the secretion of milk.

LACTIFEROUS. Conducting or conveying the milk.

LARYNGEAL. Belonging to the larynx.

LARYNGISMUS STRIDULUS. Asthma of Millar.

LARYNGITIS. Inflammation of the larynx.

LARYNX. Upper part of the windpipe.

LESIONS. Injuries inflicted by violence, etc.

LESION, ORGANIC. Structural derangement, or injury.

LEUCO-PHLEGMATIC. Torpid or sluggish; mostly applied to a temperament characterized by want of tension of fibre; with light hair, and general inertness of the physical and mental powers.

LEUCORRHŒA. Female sexual weakness; vulg. *Whites.*

LOCHIA. Discharge from the womb after delivery.

LUMBAGO. Rheumatism in the loins.

LUMBAR. Appertaining to the loins.

LUMBRICUS, plur. *Lumbrici.* The round or long worm.

LUXATION. Dislocation.

LYMPH. A colourless liquid, circulating in the lymphatics.

LYMPHATIC. As applied to temperament; same as Leucophlegmatic.

LYMPHATICS. Absorbent vessels with glands and valves distributed over the body.

LYMPHATIC GLANDS. CONGLOBATE GLANDS. These are composed of a texture of absorbents, or lymphatic vessels, connected together by a cellular membrane.

MAMMA. The breast in the female; adj. *Mammillary.*

MANIA. Insanity; madness.

MARASMUS. A wasting away of the body.

MATERIA MEDICA PURA. The title of that splendid work of the immortal HAHNEMANN, in which the true properties of medicaments are given, as determined by experiment upon the healthy body.

MAXILLARY Appertaining to the jaws. The superior and inferior *maxillary bones* form the upper and lower jaws.

Meatus Auditorius Externus.—The external passage of the ear.

Meconium. The excrementitious matter discharged from the intestines of a newly-born infant.

Megrim. A pain affecting only one side of the head.

Meibomian Glands. Small glands within the inner membrane of the eyelids.

Menochesia. Feeble menstruation.

Menorrhagia. Excessive discharge of blood from the uterus.

Menstrual Flux. The monthly period.

Meningitis Spinalis. Inflammation of the spinal membranes.

Metastasis. The passing of a disease from one part to another.

Meteorismus. Extreme inflation of the intestines.

Metrorrhagia. Discharge of blood from the womb.

Miasm, or *Miasma* (*Marsh*). Peculiar effluvia or emanations from swampy grounds.

Micturition. Urination.

Miliaria. Eruption of minute transparent vesicles of the size of millet seeds; miliary eruption.

Miliaria Purpura. Scarlet rash.

Minim. The sixtieth part of a fluid drachm.

Morbus Coxarius. Disease of the hip; hip-disease.

Mucous Membrane. The membrane which lines the sides of cavities which communicate with the external air, such as that which lines the mouth, stomach, etc.

Mucus. One of the primary animal fluids; secretion from the nostrils.

Myelitis. Inflammation of the spinal marrow.

Myopia. Short sight; near-sightedness.

Narcotic. Having the property of inducing sleep.

Nasal. Belonging to the nose.

Nasal Cartilages. The cartilages of the nose.

Nates. The buttocks.

Nephritis. Inflammation of the kidneys.

Neuralgia Facialis. Face-ache.

Nodosities. Swellings; nodes, a swelling of the bone or thickening of the periosteum.

Notalgia. Pains in the loins.

Obstructio Alvi. Constipation.

Obstructio Alvi Neonatorum. Constipation in infants.

Occiput. The posterior part of the head.

Octana. An intermittent fever which returns every eighth day.

Odontalgia. Tooth-ache.

Œdema. Swelling; dropsical swelling; adj. *Œdematous*.

Olfaction. The act of smelling.

Omentum. The caul. The viscus consists of folds of the peritoneum connected together by cellular tissue; it is attached to the stomach, lying on the anterior surface of the bowels.

Ophthalmia. By this term is now usually understood simple inflammation of the *conjunctiva*. (Catarrhal Ophthalmia.)

Ophthalmic Nerve. The first branch given off from the Gasserian ganglion of the fifth pair of nerves; it divides into the lachrymal, frontal, and nasal nerves.

Ophthalmitis. Inflammation of the entire ball of the eye.

Organic Disease. In pathology, diseases in which there is derangement or alteration of structure are termed organic.

Os Uteri. The mouth or opening of the womb.

Ossa Spongiosa. The spongy bones. They consist of a spongy lamella or plate in each nostril, which they contribute to form.

Ossicula Auditoria. The small bones of the ear. They are situated in the cavity of the tympanum, and are four in number:

termed—the malleus, incus, stapes, and os-orbiculare.

Otalgia. Ear-ache.

Otitis. Inflammation of the ear.

Otorrhœa. A discharge, or running from the ear.

Ozæna. An ulcer situated in the nose. See *Ozœna*.

Palate Bones. These are placed at the back part of the roof of the mouth, between the superior maxillary and sphenoid bones, and extend from thence to the floor of the orbit.

Palpebræ. The eyelids.

Palpitatis Cordis. Palpitation of the heart.

Panaris. Whitlow; panaritium; paronychia.

Pancreas. A gland situated transversely behind the stomach.

Paralysis. Palsy.

Paralysis Paraplegica. Paralysis affecting one half of the body transversely.

Parenchyma. The connecting medium of the substance of the lungs.

Paronychia. Vide *Panaris*.

Parotitis. Inflammation of the parotid gland; the *mumps*.

Paroxysm. A periodical fit of a disease.

Parturition. The act of bringing forth.

Pathogenetic. The producing or creating of abnormal phenomena.

Pathognomonic. Characteristic of and peculiar to any disease.

Pathology. The investigation of the nature of disease.

Pectoral. Appertaining to the chest.

Pectus. The chest.

Pediculi. Lice.

Pelvis. The basin-shaped cavity below the abdomen, containing the bladder and rectum; and womb in woman.

Percussion. The act of striking upon the chest, &c. in order to elicit sounds to ascertain the state of the subjacent parts.

Pericarditis. Inflammation of the Pericardium (sac containing the heart).

Perinæum. The space between the anus and the external sexual organs.

Periosteum. The membrane which envelopes the bones.

Peritonæum. The serous membrane which lines the cavity of the abdomen, and envelopes the viscera contained therein.

Peritonitis. Inflammation of the peritoneum.

Perniones. Chilblains.

Pertussis. Hooping-cough.

Petechiæ. Spots of a red or purple hue, resembling a flea-bite.

Phagedenic. A term applied to any sores which eat away the parts as it were.

Pharynx. The throat, or upper part of the gullet.

Phases. Appearances, or changes exhibited by any body, or by *disease*.

Phlebitis. Inflammation of the veins.

Phlegmatic. Vide *Leuco-phlegmatic*.

Phlegmon. An inflammation of that nature which is otherwise termed *healthy inflammation*.

Phrenitis. Inflammation of the brain.

Phthisis. (Pulmonalis) Consumption, abscess of the lungs.

Physiology. The branch of medicine which treats of the functions of the human body.

Plethora. An excessive fulness of the blood-vessels.

Pleura. The serous membrane which lines the cavity of the thorax or chest.

Pleuritis or Pleurisy. Inflammation of the pleura.

Pleurodynia. Pain or stitch in the side.

Pneumonia, Pneumonitis, Peripneumonia. Inflammation of the parenchyma of the lung.

Polypus. A tumour most frequently met with in the nose, uterus, or vagina.

Porrigo Scutulata. Ringworm of the scalp.

Porrigo Cervalis. Milk-crust; milk-scab.

Posterior Nares. The posterior nostrils which open into the fauces.

Poupart's Ligament. The tendinous portion of the *external* oblique muscle. It is stretched across from the anterior superior spinous process of the bone ilium to the pubis.

Præcordial Region. The fore-part of the chest.

Primæ Viæ. The stomach, and intestinal tube. (The first passages.)

Proctalgia. A severe pain in the anus.

Prognosis. The faculty of predicting what will take place in diseases.

Prolapsus Ani. Protrusion of the intestines.

Prophylaxis. plur. *Prophylaxes.* Means or remedies used as preservatives against disease.

Prosopalgia. Face-ache.

Prurigo. Itching of the skin.

Psoas Muscles. The names of two muscles situate in the loins.

Psoitis. Inflammation of the psoas muscle.

Ptisans. Domestic decoctions, such as of pearl barley, &c.

Pubis. The pubic or share bone.

Puerperal Fever. Appertaining to childbed.

Puriform. Pus-like, resembling pus.

Purulent. Of the character of pus.

Pus. Matter. A whitish, bland, cream-like fluid, found in abscesses, or on the surface of sores.

Pustule. An elevation of the scarf-skin, containing pus or lymph, and having an inflamed base.

Pyrosis. Heart-burn; water-brash.

Quinsy. Inflammatory sore throat.

Quotidian. Intermittent, about twenty-four hours intervening between the attacks.

Rabies. Madness arising from the bite of a rabid animal, generally applied to the disease showing itself in the brute creation.

Rachitis. The rickets.

Rale, Rattles. Sound in the chest, &c. on auscultation, &c.

Raucitas. Hoarseness.

Rectum. The last of the large intestines, terminating in the anus.

Remittent. A term applied to fevers with marked remissions, and generally subsequent exacerbation. The yellow fever of tropical countries.

Repercussed. Driven in.

Resolution. A termination of inflammatory affections without abscess, mortification, &c. The term is also applied to the dispersion of swellings, indurations, &c.

Rheumatic Ophthalmia. Inflammation of the tunica albuginea, and of the sclerotica.

Rhonchus. A wheezing or rattling sound. In auscultation, the term is applied to morbid sounds accompanying respiration, occasioned either by the passage of air through fluids in the bronchia or air-cells, or through partially contracted bronchial tubes.

Rigors. Coldness, attended more or less by shivering.

Risus Sardonicus. Involuntary spasmodic laughter.

Rose. A term applied to erysipelas, from its colour.

Rubeola. Measles.

Sacrum. The bone which forms the base of the vertebral column.

Saliva. The fluid secreted by the salivary glands into the cavity of the mouth.

Saturnine. Preparations containing lead.

Sanguineous. Consisting of blood.

Sanies. A thin greenish discharge of fetid matter, from sores, fistulæ, &c.

Scabies. **Psora.** Itch.

Scapula. The shoulder-blade.

Sciatica. A rheumatic affection of the hip-joint.

Sciatic Nerve. A branch of a nerve of the lower extremity.

Sciatic, or Ischiatic Notch. This

name is given to a notch in the *os innominatum*, which latter is formed of three bones termed the *ischium*, *ilium*, and *pubis*.

SCIRRHUS. Indolent, glandular tumour, generally preceding cancer in an ulcerated form.

SCLEROTICA. The hard membrane of the eye ; it is situated immediately under the conjunctiva.

SCROBICULUS. Pit of the stomach.

SCORBUTUS. Scurvy.

SCROFULOUS OPHTHALMIA. Inflammation of the conjunctiva, with slight redness, but great intolerance of light, and the formation of pimples, or small pustules.

SECRETORY VESSELS, or ORGANS. Parts of the animal economy, which separate or secrete the various fluids of the body.

SEMI-LATERAL Limited to one side.

SEQUELA, plur. *Sequelæ*.

SINUS. A cavity or depression.

SLOUGH. The part that separates from a foul ulcer.

SOLIDIFICATION. Vide *Hepatization*.

SOMNOLENCE. Disposition to sleep.

SORDES. The viscid, fetid, brownish, red-coloured matter discharged from ulcers. The matter which forms round the teeth in fever, &c. has likewise received this appellation.

SPECIFIC. A remedy possessing a peculiar curative action in certain diseases.

SPLEEN. A spongy viscous organ, of a livid colour, placed on the posterior part of the left hypochondrium.

SPLENITIS. Inflammation of the spleen.

SPLINTS. Long, thin pieces of wood, tin, or strong pasteboard, used for preventing the extremities of fractured bones from moving so as to interrupt the process by which they are united.

SPUTA. Expectoration of different kinds.

SPUTUM CRUENTUM. Spitting of blood.

ST. ANTHONY'S FIRE. Erysipelas.

STERNUTATION. Sneezing.

STERTOROUS. Snoring.

STOMACACE. Canker or scurvy of the mouth.

STRABISMUS. Squinting.

STRANGURY. Painful discharge of urine.

STERNUM. The breast-bone.

STETHOSCOPE. An instrument to assist the ear in examining the morbid sounds of the chest.

STRICTURE. A constriction of a tube or duct of some part of the body.

STRUMA. SCROFULA. The king's evil; adj. *Strumous*.

STYE. An inflammatory small tumour on the eyelid.

SUB-MAXILLARY. Under the jaw.

SUB-MAXILLARY GLANDS. Glands on the inner side of the lower jaw.

SUB-MUCOUS TISSUE. Placed under the mucous membrane.

SUDORIFICS. Medicines which produce sweating.

SUGILLATION. A bruise, or extravasated blood.

SUPPURATION. The morbid action by which pus is deposited, in inflammatory tumour, etc.

SUBSULTUS TENDINUM. Twitchings ; sudden starts of the tendons; weak convulsive movements which are often too feeble to elevate the limb itself, but sufficiently strong to be readily seen or felt in the muscles and their tendons. They are most frequently met with in states of extreme debility, particularly in low, nervous, or typhoid fevers, and are, in such cases, usually to be dreaded as prognostications of approaching dissolution.

SYNCOPE. Fainting or swooning.

SYNOCHA. Continued inflammatory fever.

SYNOVIA. A peculiar, unctuous fluid secreted within the joints, which it lubricates, and thereby serves to facilitate their motions.

SYNOVIAL MEMBRANE. The membrane which lines the cavities of

the joints, and secretes the synovia.

TÆNIA. Tape-worm.

TARTAR. A concretion encrusting the teeth.

TEMPORAL. Appertaining to the temples.

TENDON. The white and shining extremity of a muscle.

TENESMUS. Painful and constant urging to alvine evacuations, without a discharge.

TETANUS, adj. *Tetanic.* A spasmodic rigidity of the parts affected.

THERAPEUTICS. That branch of medicine which describes the action of the different means employed for the curing of diseases, and of the application of those means.

THORAX. The chest, or that part of the body situated between the neck and the abdomen.

THRUSH. Numerous small white vesicles in the mouth. See Thrush.

TIC DOULOUREUX. Face-ache.

TINEA ANNULARIS. TINEA CAPITIS. Ringworm of the scalp.

TINEA FACIEI. Milk-crust; milk-scab.

TINNITUS AURIUM. Ringing in the ears.

TITILLATION. Tickling.

TONIC. Medicines which are said to increase the tone of the muscular fibre when debilitated and relaxed.

TONSILS. The oblong, sub-oval glands placed between the arches of the palate.

TONSILLITIS. Inflammation of the tonsils.

TOPICAL. Remedies applied to a particular part.

TOURNIQUET. An instrument for stopping the flow of blood until some more permanent method of arresting the hemorrhage has been adopted, or until some operation has been performed.

TRACHEA. The windpipe.

TRACHEOTOMY. An operation by opening the windpipe.

TRAUMATIC. Appertaining to wounds; arising from wounds.

TREMOR. Trembling.

TREPHINE. A surgical instrument used for sawing a circular portion of bone out of the cranium.

TRISMUS. Lock-jaw.

TRITURATION. The reduction of a substance to minute division, by means of long-continued rubbing.

TROCHANTER MAJOR. One of the processes of the thigh-bone.

TUBERCLE. A small, round, eruptive swelling, anatomically speaking. In pathology, the name is applied to a peculiar morbid product occurring in various organs or textures, in the form of small, round, isolated masses of a dull whitish yellow, or yellowish gray colour, opaque, unorganized, and varying in shape and consistence according to their stage of development and the texture of part in which they are engendered.

TUMEFACTION. Swelling.

TUMEFIED. Swollen.

TUMID. Vide *Tumefied.*

TUNICA ALBUGINEA. The anterior part of the sclerotica, strengthened by the tendinous expansions of the muscles of the eye.

TUNICA ADNATA. That portion of the *tunica conjunctiva* which covers the sclerotic coat has been thus designated.

TUSSIO CONVULSIVA. Hooping-cough.

TYMPANITES. TYMPANY. DRUM-BELLY. An elastic distention of the abdomen, sounding like a drum when struck with the hand. It is attended with costiveness, but no fluctuation; and is distinguished into—*Tympanitis intestinalis,* flatulent obstruction, or lodgment of wind in the intestines, recognised by the emission of wind affording relief:—*Tympanitis abdominalis,* when the wind is in the cavity of the abdomen (*abdominal emphysema*).

Typhoid. Applied to diseases of a low character.

Umbilical Cord. The navel string.

Umbilicus. The navel.

Union by the first intention. The healing of wounds by adhesion; the growing together of the opposite surfaces of a wound when brought into close approximation, without suppuration or granulation. The latter process of healing is sometimes designated the *second intention*.

Urethra. The urinary canal.

Urticaria. Nettle-rash.

Uterus. The womb.

Varicella. Pimples, quickly forming pustules, seldom passing into suppuration, but bursting at the point and drying into scabs. Chicken-pock.

Variola. Smallpox.

Variola Spuria. (*Varicélla.*) Chicken-pock.

Varix, plur. *Varices.* Swelling or enlargement of the veins.

Venesection. The abstraction of blood by opening a vein.

Vesiccations. An eruptive elevation of the cuticle, containing a clear serous fluid.

Vertigo. Giddiness, with a sensation as if falling.

Vesicle. A small bladder-like eruption; an elevation of the cuticle containing a transparent watery fluid.

Vicarious. Acting as a substitute.

Virus. Contagion or poison.

Viscid. Glutinous and gelatinous.

Viscus, plur. *Viscera.* Any organ of the system. A bowl.

Vomer. A slender thin bone of the nose, forming the partition between the nostrils, and so called from its resemblance to a ploughshare.

Vomica. An abscess of the lungs.

Zygomatic Process. A thin narrow projection of bone, defining the squamous portion of the temporal bone at its base.

INDEX.

	PAGE
Abdominal Deformity . .	542
Abdomen, pendulous . .	ib.
Abortus	518
Abscess	288
Abscessus Nucleatus . .	283
Acidity, see Dyspepsia . .	95
Flatulence, &c. in infants	462
Administration of Medicines	9
Ægylops	330
After-pains	534
Agrypnia	354
Ague	39
Air and Exercise . . .	505
Ambustiones . . .	417
Amenorrhœa . . .	498
Angina, see Sore Throat .	81
Gangrenosa . .	89
Maligna . . .	ib.
Membranacea . .	210
Parotidea . . .	93
Perniciosa . .	210
Angylops	330
Anorexia	101
Anthrax	285
Anti-mercurial remedies .	341
Aphthous Sore Throat . .	81
Aphthæ	466
Apparent Death, Asphyxia 422,	443
from a Fall . .	422
Drowning .	423
Frost . .	425
Hanging .	423
Hunger . .	422
Lightning .	423
Noxious Vapours	426
Suffocation .	423
Apepsia	101
Appetite, Want of . .	101
Apoplexia	266
Apoplexy	266
Arthritis	307
Asiatic Cholera . . .	152
Asphyxia, Apparent Death .	422
in Infants . .	443
Asthma	395
Spasmodic in Children	463
Asthma of Millar . . .	486
Atrophia	493
Atrophy	493
Aversion of the Infant to the Breast	545
Bastard Pleurisy . . .	251

	PAGE
Bilious complaints . .	95
Birth, Treatment after .	442
Black Water . . .	119
Bladder Inflammation of .	180
Blearedness . . .	333
Blepharitis	333
Bleeding of the Nose . .	337
Blood, Spitting of . .	252
Blood-shot Eye . . .	330
Boil	283
Bowels, Looseness of . .	137
Inflammation of .	168
Bowel complaint of Children	468
Brain Fever . . .	271
Brain, Inflammation of the .	ib.
Concussion of the .	403
Breasts, Inflammation of .	547
Preparation of during Pregnancy . .	524
Breath, offensive . . .	348
Breathing, Difficulty of, see Asthma	395
Bronchial Tubes, Inflammation of	225
Bronchitis	ib.
Bronchocele, see Goitre .	352
Bruises	403
Bunions	412
Burns and Scalds . .	417
Bursæ, Injuries and Diseases of the	412
Cancer nasi . . .	341
Cancer in the face . .	331
Cancer in the lips . .	331
Cancer of the Mouth . .	343
Cancrum oris . . .	ib.
Carbuncle	285
Cardialgia	112
Carditis	313
Caries of the Bones . .	341
Carrying of Infants . .	456
Cataract	329
Catarrh	187
Catarrh bronchiorum, or Occulta . . .	239
Catarrhal Ophthalmia .	328
Cephalalgia . . .	370
Arthritica . .	ib.
Nervosa . .	ib.
Cephalæa . . .	ib.
Chest, Determination of blood to	221
Cold in . . .	225

	PAGE
Chicken-pox	71
Chilblains	285
Children, suckling of	549
Chin-cough, see Hooping-cough	204
Chlorosis	495
Cholera	149
Cholerine	155
Chronic Laryngitis	193
Clavi Pedis	287
Clavus Hystericus	370
Cleansings, see Lochia	540
Clothing	506
and Habits	4
Coffee, Derangements from the Use of	355
Cold, Common	187
in the head	193, 459
in the Chest	225
Colic	133
Concussion	403
Confinement, Duration of	535
Congestio ad Pectus	221
Caput	260
Congestive Pneumonia	240
Conglobate Glands, Diseases of	288
Constipation	123, 513
in Children	467
Consumption, pulmonary	259
Consumption, see Phthysis incipiens	241
Consumption of the Windpipe, see Phthysis Laryngea	193
Contagious Fever, (Typhus)	37
Contusions, see Bruises	403
Convulsions	531
in Children	480
Cornea, Ulceration of the	329
Opacity of, or Specks on the	ib.
Corns	287
Coryza, Cold in the Head	193, 459
Costiveness	123
Cough	196
after Measles	63
Cough after Smallpox	70
Hooping	204
Coup de Soleil	275
Coxalgia	318
Coxagra	ib.
Cramps and Convulsions	531
Cramp in the Legs	352
Critical Age, see Dysmenorrhœa	501
Croup	210
Crusta Lactea	464
Crying and Wakefulness of New-born Children	460
Cynanche, see Sore Throat	81
Laryngea	210
Maligna	89
Tonsillaris, see Quinsy	81
Tracheitis	210
Cynanche Parotidea	95
Cystitis	180
Death, Apparent	422, 443
Deafness	336
Decubitis	241
Deficiency in the Secretion of Milk	548
Delivery, Treatment after	532
Weakness after	544
Delirium Tremens	391
Derangement of the Stomach, Fever from	107
Derangement of Stomach	ib.
during Teething	478
Dentition	ib.
Determination of Blood to the Chest	221
Head	260
Abdomen	323
Deterioration and Discoloration of Milk	549
Diarrhœa	137
in Lying-in Women	541
during Pregnancy	513
in Children	468
Diet	508
Diet, Rules	14
in Fever	20
during Nursing	458
Difficulty in Breathing, see Asthma	395
Difficult Menstruation, see Dysmenorrhœa and Chlorosis	501
Discharge, Irregularities of the lochial	540
Disinclination of the Infant to Suck	545
Dislocations and Fractures	403, 414, 415
Dispepsia, see Dyspepsia.	
Dose, on the Repetition of the	9
Drowning, apparent Death from	423

PAGE

Duration of Suckling and Weaning . . . 451
 Confinement . . 535
Dyscrasia, Morbid Condition 336
Dysenteria . . . 141
Dysentery . . . ib.
Dysmenorrhœa . . . 501
Dyspnœa, see Asthma . 395
Dyspepsia 95
Ear-ache 333
Emansio Mensium . . 495
Emotions, Mental . 438, 509
Employment of the Mind during Pregnancy . . 508
Emprosthotonos . . . 276
Encephalitis . . . 271
Enteritis 168
Enteralgia . . . 133, 168
Ephialtes 357
Epilepsia 394
Epilepsy . . . . ib.
Epiphoria 330
Epistaxis 337
Eructations 107
Eruptive Fevers . . 48
Erysipelas . . . 280
 Neonatorum . 475
Excoriation of the Nipples 546
 in Children . 474
 see Decubitus . 241
Exercise 505
 in the case of Children 455
Expulsion of Meconium . 445
External injuries . . 403
Eyes, Bleareduess of . . 333
 Hemorrhage from . 330
 Inflammation of . 324
 Bloodshot . . 330
Eyelids, Inflammation of . 333
 Catarrhal Inflammation of the ib.
Face, Swelling of . . 516
Face-ache 349
Face Ague . . . ib.
 Scirrhus in the . . 331
 Warts on the . . 332
Fainting 367
Fainting and Hysteric Fits 513
False Pains . . . 526
Fall, Apparent Death from a 422
Falling down of the Womb, see Prolapsus . . . 543
Fatigue 419
Favus Confertus . . . 297
Feet, Sweating of the . 353
Fevers, or Febres . . 17

PAGE

Fever, Brain . . . 271
 Contagious (Typhus) 37
 Eruptive . . . 48
 Infantile Remittent 488
 Inflammatory . 22
 Intermittent . . 39
 Miliary . . . 72
 Milk . . . 538
 Nervous . . 24
 Putrid . . . 35
 Scarlet . . . 48
 Simple or Ephemeral 20
 Typhus . . . 24
 Contagiosus . 37
 Putridus . 35
Fistula in Ano . . . 306
 Lachrymalis . . 330
Fits, see Epilepsy and Convulsions . . . 394
Flatus 110
Flatulency . . . ib.
 in Infants . . 462
Fontanels, retarded closing of the 444
Fractures and Dislocations 414, 415
Frozen Persons . . . 425
Fungus Hæmatodes . . 306
 Oculi . 329
Furunculus . . . 283
 Malignans . 285
Galling, Excoriation . . 241
Gangrenous Sore-throat . 89
Gangrene 411
 Oris . . . 343
Gastralgia 112
Gastrodynia . . . ib.
Gastric or Bilious Fever, see Dyspepsia . . . 95
Gastritis 165
Glands, Conglobate, disease of the 288
Glossitis 346
Goitre 352
Gonorrhœal Ophthalmia . 329
Gout 307
Gravel or Stone . . . 181
Gripes, see Colic . . 131
Gumboil 346
Gun-shot Wounds . . 413
Habits during Pregnancy . 508
Hair, falling of . . . 543
Head, Determination of Blood to 260
 Swelling of, in Infants 444
 Cold in . . 193,459

	PAGE
Head, Water in the . .	484
Headache	370
Heart, Palpitation of the .	351
Inflammation of, see	
Carditis . .	313
Endocarditis . .	ib.
Heartburn	119
Helminthiasis	181
Hæmatemesis	119
Hemicrania (Megrim) . .	370
Hemorrhoids	128
Hemoptysis	252
Hemorrhagia Pulmonum .	252
Hemorrhage from the Lungs	ib.
after Delivery .	540
see Wounds .	407
Hepatitis	156
Chronica	160
Hernia	361
Herpes Circinnatus . .	296
Hiccough	502
in Infants . .	458
Hip-gout	318
Hip-disease . .	318, 320
Hoarseness	191
Hooping-cough	204
Hordeolum	332
Housemaid's Knee . .	411
Hunger, apparent death from	422
Hydrocephalus . . .	484
Hydrophobia	426
Hysteria	501
Hysterics . . .	501, 513
Icterus . . .	161, 474
Incubus	357
Indigestion	95
Induration of the Cellular Tissue	475
Infants, Treatment of .	442
Suckling of . .	446
Infants, Supplementary Diet of	449
Infantile, Remittent Fever .	488
Inflammation, Acute, of the Liver	156
Inflammation of the Bladder .	180
Brain . .	271
Bowels . .	168
Breast . .	547
Bronchial Tubes	225
Ears . .	333
Eyes . .	324
Eyes in new-born Infants .	458

	PAGE
Inflammation of the Heart .	313
Kidneys . .	177
Larynx . .	193
Liver . .	156
Lungs . .	234
Margins of the Eye-lids .	333
Peritoneum .	175
Psoas Muscle .	315
Pleura . .	242
Spinal Cord, etc.	358
Spleen . .	162
Stomach .	165
Tongue . .	346
Inflammatory Fever . .	22
Influence of External Objects upon the unborn Infant .	509
Influenza	219
Injuries external . . .	403
Insects, Stings of . . .	420
Intermittent Fevers . .	39
Intestine, Protrusion of the .	132
Introduction	1
Invermination . . .	181
Irregularities of the Lochial Discharge	540
Irritation of the Skin . .	294
Iritis	327, 328
Arthritica	329
Ischias	318
Itching of the Skin . .	291
Itch	291
Jaundice . . .	161, 474
Joints, Injuries of the . .	470
Kidneys, Inflammation of .	177
Knee joint, Diseases of the .	322
Labour	528
Labour, complicated . .	528
remedies before . .	525
tedious	528
Lacerations	407
Laryngismus Stridulus . .	486
Laryngitis Chronica . .	193
Larynx, chronic inflammation of the	193
Legs, cramp in the . .	352
Leucorrhœa	543
Lightning, apparent death from	423
Lips, Swelling of . . .	331
Scirrhus of the . .	ib.
Lippitudo, Blearedness . .	333
Liver Complaint .	155, 160
Acute Inflammation of	156
Chronic Inflammation of	160

	PAGE
Lochia	540
Lochial Discharge, etc.	540
Lock-jaw	276
of Infants	476
Loins, Pains in the	391
Looseness of the Bowels	137
Lumbago, Rheumatism in the Loins	314
Lumbo-sacral Pains	518
Lungs, Inflammation of the	234
Hemorrhage from the	252
Luxations	414
Lymphatic Tumours	288
Malignant Quinsy	89
Measles	59
Meconium, Expulsion of	445
Medical Terms, Glossary of	550
Medicines, Administration of	9
Megrim, Headache	370
Meningitis Spinalis	358
Mental Emotions	438, 509
affecting the Milk	548
Menochasia	499
Menorrhagia	ib.
Menstruation	499, 511
Scanty	498
Menstruatio Nimia	499
Miliaris Hahnemanni (Purpura)	55
Milliaris Purpurea	ib
Miliaria, Miliary Fever	72
Milk, excessive Secretion of	536
Deficiency in the Secretion of	548
Deterioration and Discoloration of	549
Fever	538
Mental Emotions affecting	548
Regurgitation of	462
Suppressed	536, 548
Miscarriage	518
Mind, employment of during Pregnancy	508
Milkcrust	464
Milkscab	ib.
Modified Smallpox	70
Morning Sickness	512
Morbus Coxarius	320
Mothers not suckling their Children	549
Mumps	93
Mouth, Canker of the	343
Scurvy in the	345
Moulds, Retarded closing of the	442
Myopia	331
Myelitis	358
Navel, Rupture of	444
Nearsightedness	331
Nephritis	177
Nervous Fever	24
Nettle Rash	74
Neuralgia Facialis	349
Nipples, Excoriation of	546
Nightmare	357
Notalgia	314, 391
Nose, Bleeding of the	337
Swelling of the	340
Cancer in	341
Coppery redness of	341
Nurse, the Choice of	448
Nursing, Diet during	ib
Obstipation	123
Obstructio alvi	123
Obstructio alvi Neonatorum	467
Occulta	239
Odontalgia	77
Offensive Breath	348
Ophthalmia	324
Opisthotonos	276
Otalgia	333
Otitis	ib.
Otorrhœa	335
Ozæna	341
Pains in the Back during Pregnancy	518
False	525
Pains in the Loins, Lumbago	314, 391
Spasmodic, during Labour	531
in the Hips, Sciatica	316-318
Palsy	361
Palpitation of the Heart	351
Panaris	293
Paralysis	361
Parotitis	93
Paronychia	293
Parulis, see Gumboil	346
Parturition	528
Passio Hysterica	501
Pentwind, see Asthma and Flatulency	110, 395
Peripneumonia	234
Peripneumonia Notha	239
(See also Bronchitis Chronica.)	
Peritonitis	175
Peritoneum, Inflammation of	ib.
Perniones	285

	PAGE
Pertussis	204
Perspiration after Delivery	537
Suppressed	ib.
Phthysis Laryngea	193
Incipiens	241
Pulmonalis	259
Phrenitis	271
Piles	128
Pleura, Inflammation of	242
Pleurisy	242
Pleuritis	ib.
Muscularus, see Pseudopleuritis	251
Pleurodynia	ib.
Pleurosthotonos	276
Pneumonitis	234
Pneumonia	ib.
Notha, Occulta	239
Typhoid or Congestive	240
Poison	434
Mineral	435
Vegetable	436
Animal	437
Polypus	343
Porrigo Scutulata	297
Lupinosa	300
Furfurans	ib.
Favosa	ib.
Decalvans	301
Larvalis	464
Potencies of Medicaments	5
Pregnancy, Observations on	503
During	511
Prolapsus Ani	132
Uteri	542
Prosopalgia	349
Protrusion of the Intestine	132, 349
Prurigo	294
Prunella, see Sore Throat	81
Pseudo-pleuritis	251
Psora	291
Psoitis	315
Purpura Rubra	55
Miliaris	ib.
Pustula Nigra	285
Putrid Fever	35
Sore Throat	89
Pyrosis	119
Quinsy	81
Malignant	89
Rachitis	488
Rickets	ib.
Raucitas	191
Rash, Nettle	74
from disordered Stomach	107

	PAGE
Regurgitation of Milk, Acidity, Flatulence, &c.	462
Regimen	1
Remedies before Labour	525
Rheumatism	310
in the Loins, Lumbago	314
Hip-joint, Sciatica	316, 318
Rheumatic Ophthalmia	329
Ringworm, Herpetic or Vesicular	296
Pustular	297
of the Scalp	ib
Rose	280
Rubeola	59
Rules of Diet	14
Rupture (Hernia)	361
Navel, in Infants	444
Scalds and Burns	417
Scabies	291
Scarlatina	48
Anginosa	49
Miliaris	53, 55
Maligna, see Ulcerated Sore Throat	49
	ib.
Sequelæ of	53
Dropsical Swellings after	53
Scarlet Fever	48
Rash	55
Scalled Head, see Porrigo Scutulata	297
Sciatica	316
Scirrhus, Cancer	331
Scrofula, see Glands	288
Scrofulous Ophthalmia	329
Scorbutus	345
Scurvy	ib.
in the Mouth	343
Sea Sickness	420
Shortsightedness	331
Sleeplessness	354
in Children	452
Smallpox	63
Sore Throat	81
Ulcerated	89
Sores, see Ulcers	301
Spasm of the Stomach	112
in the Chest in Children	463
Spasmodic Pains	531
Spleen, Inflammation of	162
Splenitis	ib.
Spitting of blood	252
Sprains or Strains	403
Sprains	406

PAGE

Spurious Pleurisy . . 251
Sputum Cruentum . . 252
Squinting, see Strabismus . 330
Strains 406
Strabismus 330
Stings of Insects . . . 420
St. Anthony's Fire . . 280
Stomach, Derangement of . 107
Inflammation of . 165
Stomacace 343
Stone or Gravel . . . 181
Struma, see Glands . . 288
Stye 332
Suckling . . 446, 451, 549
Suck, Disinclination of the Infant to 545
Sudor Miliaris . . . 72
Suffocation, apparent Death from 423
Supplementary Diet of Infants 449
Suppressio Mensium . . 498
Suppressed Dysentery . 148
Secretion of Milk 536, 548
Swelled Face . . . 516
Swelling of the head in Infants 444
Lips . . 331
Nose . . 340
Veins . . 517
Sweating at the Feet . . 353
Swooning . . . 367
Syncope . . . . ib.
Sycosic Ophthalmia . . 329
Synocha 22
Synovial Membranes, Injuries of 411
Syphilitic Ophthalmia . 329
Ulcers . . 306
Ozæna . . 342
Tea, Derangement from the Effects of 356
Teething 478
Tetanus 276
Thrush 466
Tic Douloureux . . . 349
Tinea Capitis . . . 297
Anularis . . . ib.
Faciei . . . 464
Tongue, Inflammation of . 346
Toothache 77
in Pregnant Females 515
Tonsillitis Maligna . . 89
Tonsillitis, see Sore Throat . 81

PAGE

Treatment of Infants . . 442
after Birth 442
Treatment after Delivery . 532
Trismus 276
Trismus Nascentium . . 476
Tumours . . . 288, 332
Tussis 196
Tussis Convulsiva . . 204
Tympanitis Intestinalis, see Flatulency . . 110
Typhoid or Congestive Pneumonia 240
Typhus Fever . . . 24
Contagiosus . . 37
Putridus . . 35
Ulcerated Sore Throat . . 89
Ulcers 301
Urine, Suppression of, see Cystitis, Nephritis 175, 180
Urine, Frequent, painful, or obstructed Emission of . . 180
See also Cystitis and Nephritis 175
Urticaria 74
Uterine Swelling and Prolapsus 543
Vaccination 494
Varices, or Swelled Veins . 517
Variola 63
Spuria, Varicella . 71
Veins, Swelled . . . 517
Vomiting in Infants . . 462
of Blood . . . 119
Walk, Teaching Children to 457
Slowness in learning to ib.
Warts on the Face . . 332
Nose . . 341
Water-brash . . . 119
Water in the Head . . 484
Watery Eye . . . 330
Weakness after Delivery . 544
Weaning 549
Weeping Eye . . . 330
Whitlow 293
Worms 181
Wounds 403
Contused . . 407
Incised . . . ib.
Lacerated . 407, 410
Punctured . . ib.
Gunshot . . . 413

www.ingramcontent.com/pod-product-compliance
Lightning Source LLC
LaVergne TN
LVHW021225110826
845150LV00002B/246

* 9 7 8 1 4 2 5 5 6 4 0 8 7 *